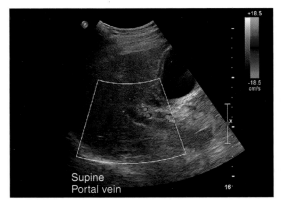

COLOR PLATE 1 Absence of flow within the portal vein. (See Fig. 3-3.)

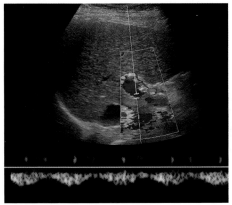

COLOR PLATE 2 Hepatofugal (reversed) flow in the main portal vein. (See Fig. 3-6, *B.*)

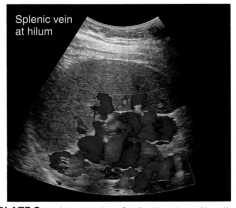

COLOR PLATE 3 Color Doppler of splenic varices. (See Fig. 3-15, *B.*)

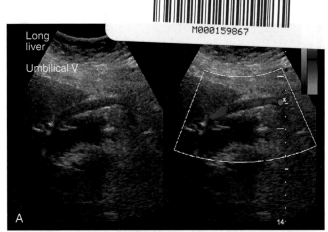

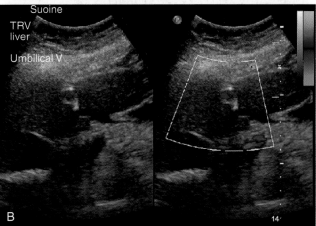

COLOR PLATE 4 A, Longitudinal image. Patent, recanalized umbilical vein. **B,** Transverse image. Patent umbilical vein in the ligament of teres. (See Fig. 3-17).

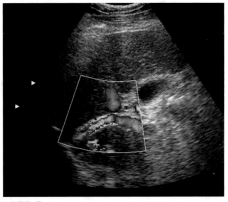

COLOR PLATE 5 Color Doppler of a TIPS demonstrating blood flow toward the IVC. (See Fig. 3-19, *B.*)

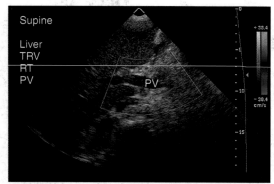

COLOR PLATE 6 Transverse midline image. (See Fig. 3-25.)

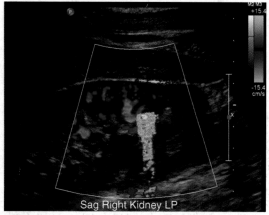

COLOR PLATE 7 Multiple colors are seen posterior to renal stone ("twinkle" sign). (See Fig. 5-6, *B*.) (*Courtesy Aubrey Rybyinski, BS, RDMS, RVT, Department of Radiology Ultrasound Section, Hospital of the University of Pennsylvania, Philadelphia, Pennsylvania.*)

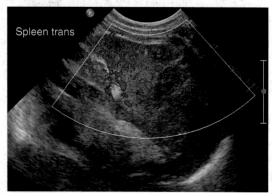

COLOR PLATE 8 Absence of color flow in the regions of hypoechogenicity. (See Fig. 8-1, *C*.)

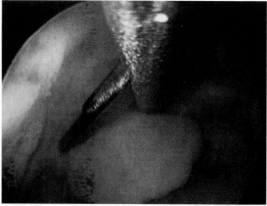

COLOR PLATE 9 Gynecologist removing endometrial polyp during hysterectomy. (See Fig. 13-23.)

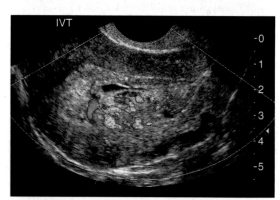

COLOR PLATE 10 Endometrial polyp demonstrating a vascular feeding stalk. (See Fig. 13-28.)

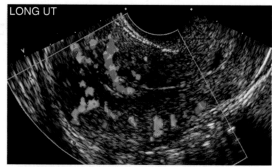

COLOR PLATE 11 Transvaginal sagittal image of a hypervascular uterus with a thick endometrium. (See Fig. 14-9, *A*.)

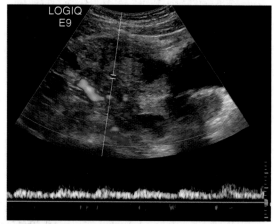

COLOR PLATE 12 Doppler imaging of right ovary. (See Fig. 17-1, *B*.)

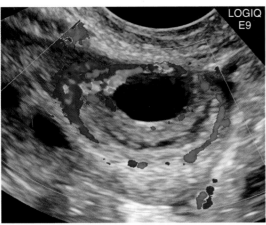

COLOR PLATE 13 Color Doppler image demonstrating flow around the highly vascular corpus luteum. (See Fig. 17-3, *C*.)

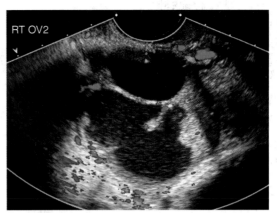

COLOR PLATE 16 Adnexal mass in a 60-year-old patient with increased CA 125. (See Fig. 17-24, *B*.)

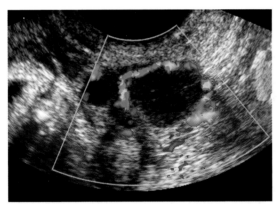

COLOR PLATE 14 Hemorrhagic cyst with peripheral flow shown on color Doppler imaging. (See Fig. 17-6.)

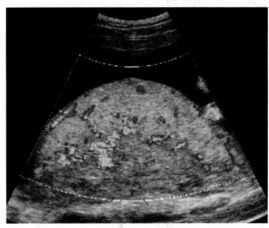

COLOR PLATE 17 Enlarged placenta. (See Fig. 19-1.)

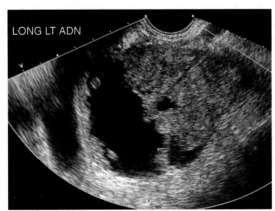

COLOR PLATE 15 Serous cystadenocarcinoma measuring 9.0 cm, demonstrating a solid component with internal vascularity evident on color Doppler imaging. (See Fig. 17-14.)

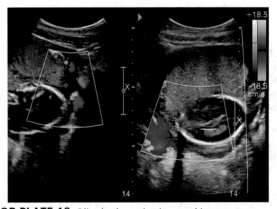

COLOR PLATE 18 Oligohydramnios is noted in a pregnancy at 19 weeks' gestational age. Only 1.9 cm of fluid is noted around the fetus. Color Doppler imaging helps identify the umbilical cord. (See Fig. 20-2.)

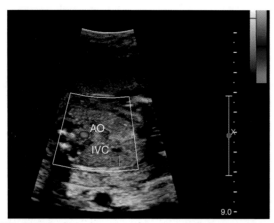

COLOR PLATE 19 Renal agenesis was confirmed in this breech fetus with severe oligohydramnios. Neither bladder nor renal arteries were identified. (See Fig. 20-3, *A*.)

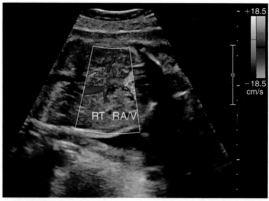

COLOR PLATE 20 Normal renal arteries are apparent. Color Doppler maps out renal arteries bilaterally in a growth-restricted fetus with oligohydramnios, confirming the presence of kidneys that are poorly visualized. (See Fig 20-3, *C*.)

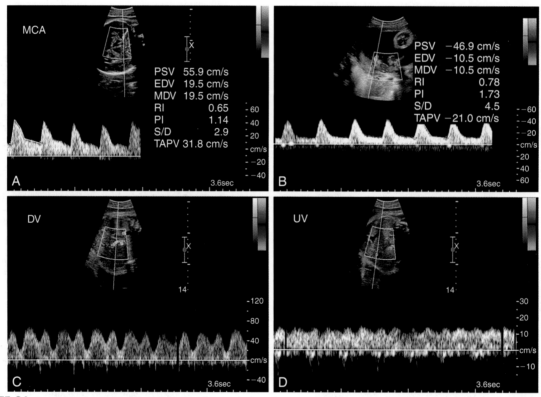

COLOR PLATE 21 **A,** Middle cerebral artery Doppler demonstrates decreased resistance. **B,** Umbilical artery demonstrates increased resistance. **C,** Ductus venosus is pulsatile. **D,** Umbilical vein is pulsatile. (See Fig. 20-10, *A-D*.)

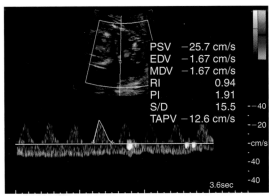

COLOR PLATE 22 Abnormal umbilical artery Doppler is demonstrated. (See Fig. 20-11, *B*.)

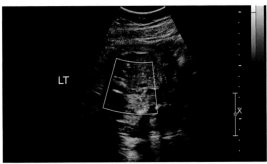

COLOR PLATE 23 Hyperechoic left kidney with no discernible blood flow. (See Fig. 20-12, *A-C*.)

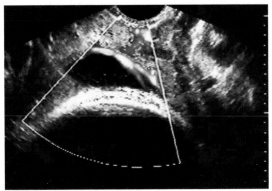

COLOR PLATE 24 Vessels are clearly shown covering the internal os and are enhanced with power Doppler imaging. (See Fig. 21-8.)

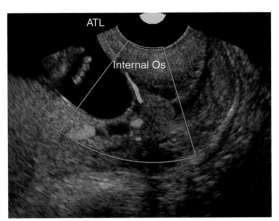

COLOR PLATE 25 Vasa previa in a twin gestation. Longitudinal image at the level of the cervix with vessels coursing over the internal cervical os. (See Fig. 22-5.)

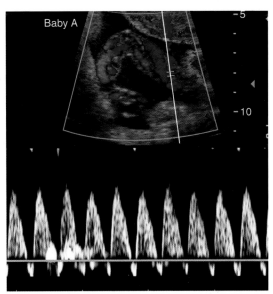

COLOR PLATE 26 Pulsed Doppler waveform of twin A's umbilical artery. (See Fig. 22-18.)

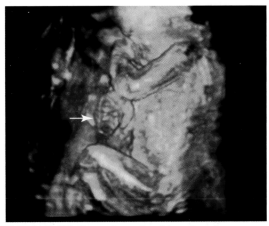

COLOR PLATE 27 Three-dimensional imaging demonstrates the gastroschisis. (See Fig. 23-6, *C*.)

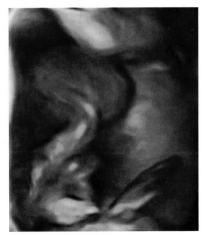

COLOR PLATE 28 Three-dimensional imaging shows the umbilical cord inserting into the defect. The karyotype was normal. (See Fig. 23-7, *B*.)

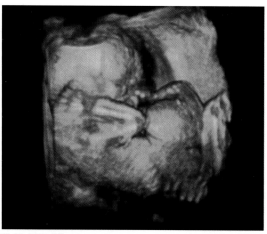

COLOR PLATE 29 Three-dimensional imaging further clarifies the anomaly. (See Fig.23-12, *B*.)

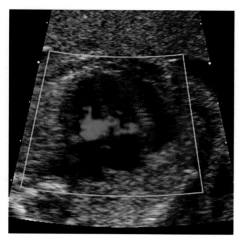

COLOR PLATE 30 Sonographic findings in a 25-week gestational age fetus. (See Fig. 24-1, *C*.)

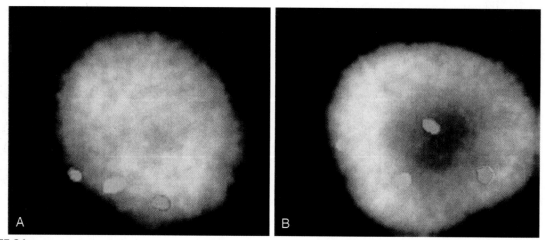

COLOR PLATE 31 A, Two copies of X chromosome coded in green and two copies of chromosome 18 coded in blue. **B,** Two copies of chromosome 21 are coded in red, and three copies of chromosome 13 are coded in green. (See Fig. 24-2, *B* and *C*.)

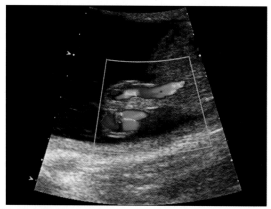

COLOR PLATE 32 Omphalocele with single umbilical artery. (See Fig. 24-13, *B*.)

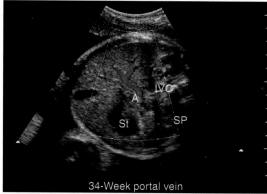

COLOR PLATE 33 The fetal situs is normal. Heart position is in the left chest, and the apex of the heart points to the left; stomach is to the left; aorta is anterior and to the left of the spine; and inferior vena cava is anterior and to the right of the spine. (See Fig. 26-1.)

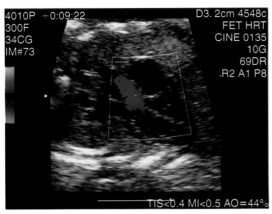

COLOR PLATE 34 Aortic outflow is shown in red in this four-chamber view. (See Fig. 26-7, *B*.)

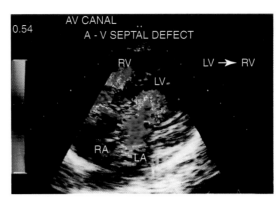

COLOR PLATE 36 Color flow imaging is helpful to map the flow across the defect and to track regurgitation into the atria. *LA,* Left atrium; *LV,* left ventricle; *RA,* right atrium; *RV,* right ventricle. (See Fig. 26-15, *C*.)

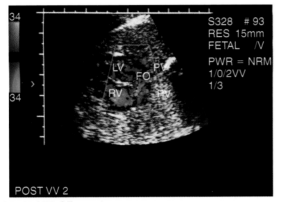

COLOR PLATE 35 In the fetus, normal flow should occur at the level of the foramen ovale *(FO)*. *PV,* Pulmonary vein. (See Fig. 26-9, *B*.)

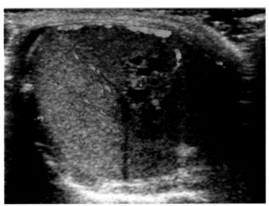

COLOR PLATE 37 Transverse view shows cystic components and internal blood flow. (See Fig. 28-1, *B*.)

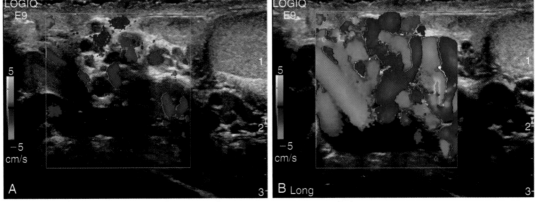

COLOR PLATE 38 A, Longitudinal color Doppler image shows minimal blood flow with normal respiration. **B,** Increased flow with Valsalva maneuver. (See Fig. 28-6, *B* and C.)

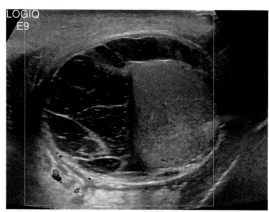

COLOR PLATE 39 Complex septate paratesticular collection in a man 13 days after vasectomy, which was a pyocele at surgical exploration. (See Fig. 28-7.)

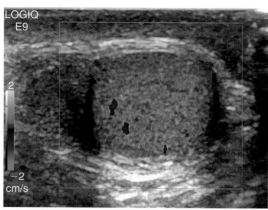

COLOR PLATE 41 An otherwise normal testis and epididymis seen in the inguinal canal of a 5-year-old boy. (See Fig. 28-18.)

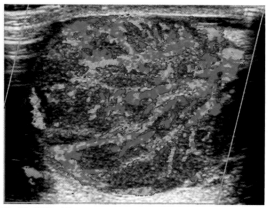

COLOR PLATE 40 Transverse color Doppler view of the same patient demonstrating the typical finding of undistorted vasculature. (See Fig. 28-17, *B*.)

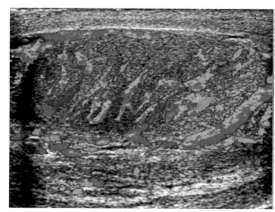

COLOR PLATE 42 Color Doppler image showing hyperemia of epididymo-orchitis, including in the scrotal skin. (See Fig. 28-20.)

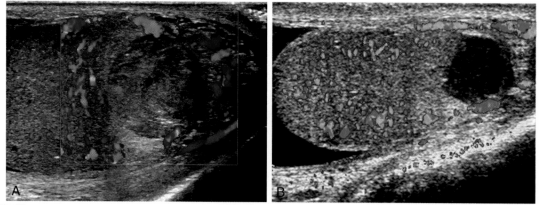

COLOR PLATE 43 A, Rounded complex intratesticular mass in a patient with acute scrotal pain is avascular but surrounded by hyperemia, suggesting epididymo-orchitis abscess instead of neoplasm. **B,** Follow-up examination 2 weeks later shows the mass to be shrinking and with continued avascularity, confirming the diagnosis. (See Fig. 28-21.)

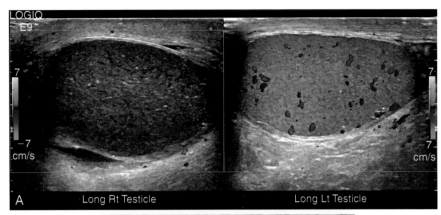

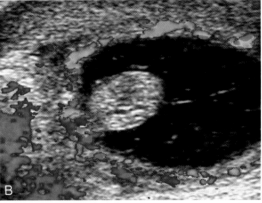

COLOR PLATE 44 **A,** Dual bilateral image of right testicular torsion. The affected testis is enlarged, is hypoechoic, and lacks blood flow, and there is a small hydrocele. **B,** This hyperechoic mass within a complex hydrocele is a torqued appendix testis. Note the hyperemic tissue surrounding the abnormality. The testicle was normal. (See Fig. 28-22.)

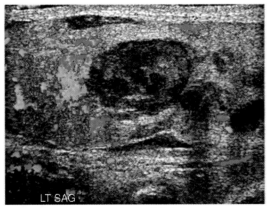

COLOR PLATE 45 Testicular hematoma resulting from a motorcycle straddle injury does not have blood flow within it. (See Fig. 28-23.)

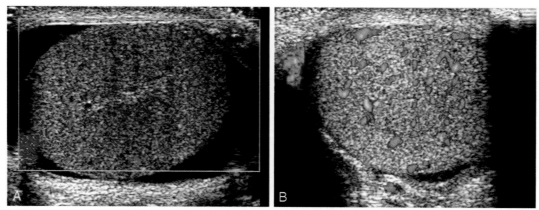

COLOR PLATE 46 A, Longitudinal image of an enlarged and hypoechoic testis was acquired early in the examination. Spectral Doppler at that time showed diminished, high-resistance blood flow. **B,** Image of the same testis at the end of the examination shows normal perfusion. Spectral Doppler measurements at this time showed normal resistive index. (See Fig. 28-27.)

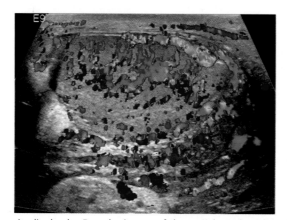

COLOR PLATE 47 Longitudinal color Doppler image of the testicle and epididymis. (See Fig. 28-28, *B*.)

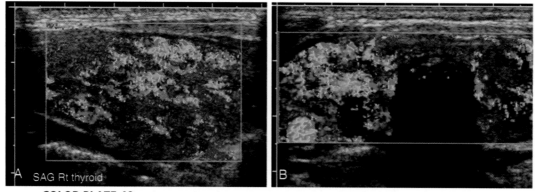

COLOR PLATE 48 Color Doppler of thyroid inferno seen with Graves' disease. (See Fig. 29-2.)

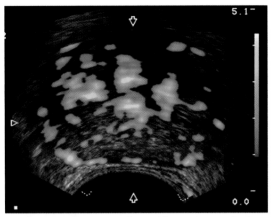

COLOR PLATE 49 Prostatitis. Hyperemia evident with power Doppler imaging. (See Fig. 30-8.)

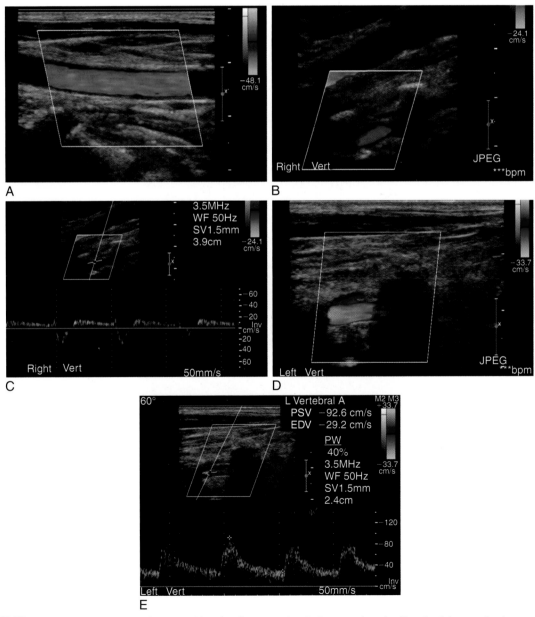

COLOR PLATE 50 A, Right common carotid artery with color flow Doppler. **B,** Retrograde color flow in right vertebral artery. **C,** Retrograde spectral Doppler in right vertebral artery. **D,** Antegrade flow in left vertebral artery. **E,** Antegrade flow in left vertebral artery. (See Fig. 34-1, *A-E.*)

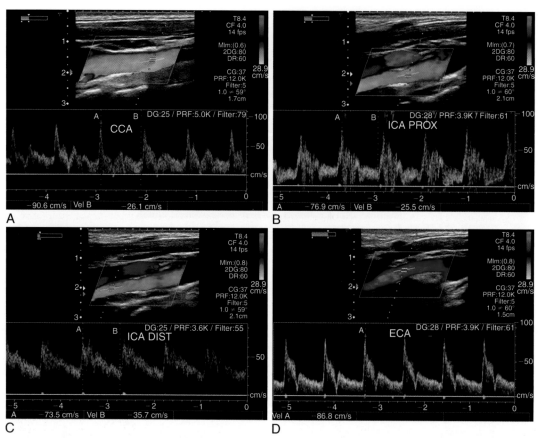

COLOR PLATE 51 Spectral Doppler waveforms taken in CCA **(A)**, proximal ICA **(B)**, distal ICA **(C)**, and ECA **(D)**. PSV and EDV measurements are seen in the common carotid artery and proximal and distal ICA. (See Fig. 34-17, *A-D.*) *(Courtesy Deziree Rada-Brooks, BSHS, RDMS, RVT.)*

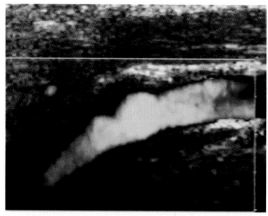

COLOR PLATE 52 Internal carotid artery from a patient with fibromuscular dysplasia. Note peapod appearance of artery. (See Fig. 34-21.) *(Courtesy Doug Marcum, Orlando Ultrasound Associates, Inc., Orlando, Florida.)*

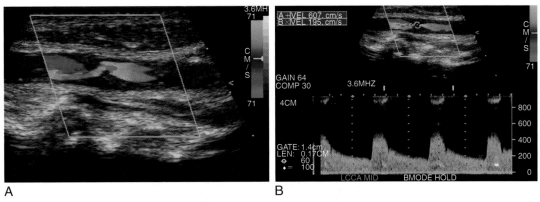

COLOR PLATE 53 Images of left CCA with color with color Doppler **(A)** and spectral analysis **(B)** demonstrating a peak systolic velocity of 607 cm/s and peak diastolic velocity of 195 cm/s. (See Fig. 34-22.)

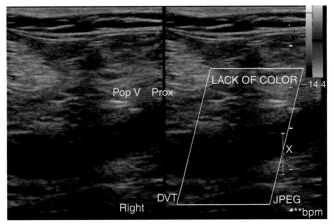

COLOR PLATE 54 Longitudinal image right popliteal vein with lack of color Doppler flow. (See Fig. 35-2.) *(Courtesy Maureen O'Neil DiGiorgio, RDCS, RVT.)*

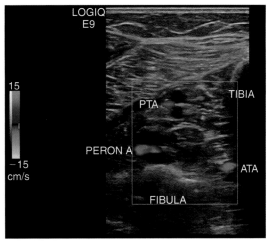

COLOR PLATE 55 Sonographic, cross-sectional (transverse) image of the calf vessels. Note the relationship of the vessels to the tibia and fibula. (See Fig. 36-1, C.)

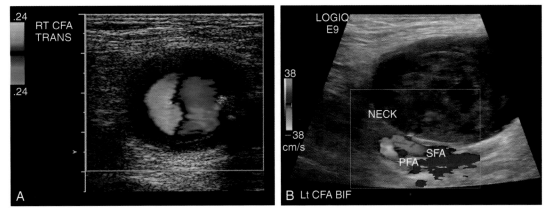

COLOR PLATE 56 A, Yin-yang color Doppler flow pattern seen in aneurysms of the native vessels or within a pseudoaneurysm. **B,** Pseudoaneurysm with evidence of internal thrombus formation and a visible neck connecting to the superficial femoral artery *(SFA).* (See Fig. 36-3.)

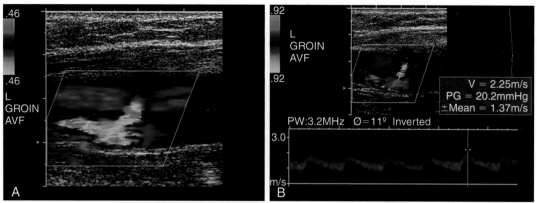

COLOR PLATE 57 A, AVF with clear communication between the artery and vein. Also supporting the diagnosis is the presence of a tissue bruit as is evident by the ghosting, or flash artifact in color Doppler. (See Fig. 36-4.)

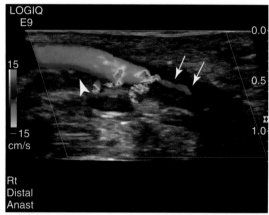

COLOR PLATE 58 Distal anastomosis of a vein graft to the smaller caliber native vessel *(arrows)*. Note the normal finding of backflow into the native vessel *(arrowhead)*. (See Fig. 36-5, *B.*)

Clinical Guide to Sonography

Exercises for Critical Thinking

Second Edition

Charlotte Henningsen, MS, RT(R), RDMS, RVT, FSDMS, FAIUM
Chair & Professor
Sonography Department
Adventist University of Health Sciences
Orlando, Florida

Kathryn (Katie) Kuntz, MEd, RT(R), RDMS, RVT, FSDMS
Clinical Assistant Professor
College of Health Sciences
University of Wisconsin Milwaukee
Milwaukee, Wisconsin

Adjunct Assistant Professor
Mayo Clinic College of Medicine
Rochester, Minnesota

Adjunct Faculty
Sonography Department
Adventist University of Health Sciences
Orlando, Florida

Diane Youngs, MEd, RDMS, RVT
Program Director
Mayo School of Health Sciences Sonography Program
Assistant Professor
Department of Radiology
Mayo Clinic College of Medicine
Rochester, Minnesota

With a foreword by
Lennard D. Greenbaum, MD

With more than 1100 illustrations and 60 color plates

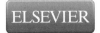

ELSEVIER
MOSBY

3251 Riverport Lane
St. Louis, Missouri 63043

CLINICAL GUIDE TO SONOGRAPHY, EXERCISES
FOR CRITICAL THINKING   ISBN: 978-0-323-09164-0
Copyright © 2014 by Mosby, an imprint of Elsevier Inc.
Copyright © 2004 by Mosby, Inc., an affiliate of Elsevier Inc.

Notices

Knowledge and best practice in this field are constantly changing. As new research and experience broaden our understanding, changes in research methods, professional practices, or medical treatment may become necessary.

Practitioners and researchers must always rely on their own experience and knowledge in evaluating and using any information, methods, compounds, or experiments described herein. In using such information or methods they should be mindful of their own safety and the safety of others, including parties for whom they have a professional responsibility.

With respect to any drug or pharmaceutical products identified, readers are advised to check the most current information provided (i) on procedures featured or (ii) by the manufacturer of each product to be administered, to verify the recommended dose or formula, the method and duration of administration, and contraindications. It is the responsibility of practitioners, relying on their own experience and knowledge of their patients, to make diagnoses, to determine dosages and the best treatment for each individual patient, and to take all appropriate safety precautions.

To the fullest extent of the law, neither the Publisher nor the authors, contributors, or editors, assume any liability for any injury and/or damage to persons or property as a matter of products liability, negligence or otherwise, or from any use or operation of any methods, products, instructions, or ideas contained in the material herein.

ISBN: 978-0-323-09164-0

Content Strategy Director: *Jeanne Olson*
Content Strategist: *Linda Woodard*
Content Coordinator: *Rachel Allen*
Publishing Services Manager: *Julie Eddy*
Senior Project Manager: *Marquita Parker*
Senior Book Designer: *Amy Buxton*

Printed in United States

Last digit is the print number: 9 8 7 6 5 4

Working together
to grow libraries in
developing countries

www.elsevier.com • www.bookaid.org

Holly M. Bostick, BS, RDMS
Sonographer
Orlando Hospital
Orlando, Florida

Daniel Breitkopf, MD
Associate Professor
Department of Obstetrics
    and Gynecology
Mayo Clinic College of Medicine
Rochester, Minnesota

Douglas L. Brown, MD
Professor
Department of Radiology
Mayo Clinic College of Medicine
Rochester, Minnesota

Jane J.K. Burns, AS, RT, RDMS
Senior Perinatal Sonographer
Minnesota Perinatal Physicians
Abbott Northwestern Hospital
Minneapolis, Minnesota

Nancy Chouinard, MAppSc, BS, RDMS, RDCS, RVT
Instructor
Diagnostic Medical Sonography
British Columbia Institute
    of Technology
Burnaby, British Columbia
Canada

Daniel J. Donovan, BS, RDMS, RVT, RT(R)
Sonographer
Radiology-Ultrasound Section
Mayo Clinic
Rochester, Minnesota

Terry J. DuBose, MS, RDMS, FSDMS, FAIUM
Associate Professor Emeritus
Division of Diagnostic Medical
    Sonography
Department of Imaging and
    Radiologic Sciences
University of Arkansas for Medical
    Sciences
College of Health Sciences
Little Rock, Arkansas

Jennie Durant, BS, RDMS, RVT, RDCS
Ultrasound Supervisor
Perinatal Associates of Central
    California
Fresno, California

Armando Fuentes, MD, MBA
Director
Maternal Fetal Medicine
Children's Hospital Central
    California
Madera, California

Catherine F. Fuhs, MS, RDMS, RVT
Clinical Coordinator
Sonography
Mayo School of Health Sciences
Assistant Professor
Department of Radiology
Mayo Clinic College of Medicine
Rochester, Minnesota

Sheryl E. Goss, MS, RT(R)(S), RDMS, RDCS, RVT
Chair and Assistant Professor
Diagnostic Medical Sonography
Misericordia University
Dallas, Pennsylvania

Lennard D. Greenbaum, MD
Co-Director
The Hughes Center for Fetal
    Diagnostics
The Winnie Palmer Hospital for
    Women and Babies
Orlando Health
Past-President
American Institute of Ultrasound
    in Medicine
Orlando, Florida

Joyce Grube, MS, RDMS
Ultrasound Applications Specialist
Toshiba America Medical Systems
Jamestown, Ohio

Joy Guthrie, PhD, RDMS, RDCS, RVT, FSDMS
Program Director/Ultrasound
    Supervisor
Community Regional Medical
    Center
Fresno, California

Sandra Hagen-Ansert, MS, RDCS, FASE, FSDMS
Supervisor
Echo Lab
Scripps Clinic
La Jolla, California

Jennifer J. Kurnal-Herring, BS, RDMS, RDCS, RVT
Faculty
Diagnostic Medical Sonography
Adventist University of Health
    Sciences
Orlando, Florida

John R. Lindsey, RDMS, RVT, RT(R)
Assistant Professor of Radiology
College of Medicine, Mayo Clinic
Rochester, Minnesota

Gregory A. Logsdon, MD
Clinical Assistant Professor
Clinical Sciences
The Florida State University College
    of Medicine
Tallahassee
Pediatric Radiologist
Radiology
The Florida Hospital for Children
Orlando, Florida

Rebecca A. Madery, BS, RDMS, RVT, RT(R)
Academic Coordinator
Mayo School of Health Sciences
Sonography Program
Instructor of Radiology
College of Medicine, Mayo Clinic
Rochester, Minnesota

Kenneth G. Marken, CRGS, RDMS
Instructor
Diagnostic Medical Sonography
British Columbia Institute of
  Technology
Burnaby, British Columbia
Canada
St. Paul's Hospital Radiology
Providence Healthcare
Vancouver, British Columbia
Canada

Duane Meixner, AS, RDMS, RVT
Instructor
Department of Radiology
Mayo Clinic College of Medicine
Education and Innovation
  Sonographer
Radiology Department
Mayo Clinic
Rochester, Minnesota

**Kimberly Michael, MA, RT(R),
  RDMS, RVT**
Assistant Professor and Program
  Director
Diagnostic Medical Sonography
Division of Radiation Sciences
  Technology Education
University of Nebraska Medical
  Center
Omaha, Nebraska

Kelly Mumbert, MBA, RVT, RDCS
Assistant Professor
Sonography
Adventist University of Health
  Sciences
Orlando, Florida

Allan E. Neis, RDMS, RVT
Supervisor
MFM and REI Ultrasound
Obstetrics and Gynecology
Mayo Clinic
Rochester, Minnesota

Susanna Ovel, RT, RDMS, RVT
Sonographer III
Ultrasound Department
Radiological Associates of
  Sacramento
Sacramento, California

Aubrey Rybyinski, BS, RDMS, RVT
Staff Sonographer
Ultrasound Section
Hospital of the University
  of Pennsylvania
Philadelphia, Pennsylvania

**Dana Loveridge Salmons, BS, RT,
  RDMS**
Staff Sonographer
Ultrasound
Florida Hospital
Orlando, Florida

Emily A.B. Smith, BS, RDMS, RVT
Instructor
Department of Radiology
Mayo Clinic College of Medicine
Sonography Educator
Radiology
Mayo Health Systems
Rochester, Minnesota

**Kristy E. Stohlmann, MS, RDMS,
  RVT, RT(R)**
Project Coordinator
GE Oil & Gas
Stavanger, Norway

Nicole L. Strissel, MS, RVT, RDMS
Lead Sonographer
Radiology Department
Mayo Clinic
Rochester, Minnesota

Jenni Taylor, BS, RDCS, RVT
Technical Director
UCF Pegasus Health
Orlando, Florida

**Felicia M. Toreno, PhD, RDMS,
  RDCS, RVT**
Program Director
Diagnostic Medical Sonography
Tidewater Community College
Virginia Beach, Virginia

**Jill D. Trotter, BS, RT(R), RDMS,
  RVT**
Director
Diagnostic Medical Sonography
  Program
Radiology
Vanderbilt University Medical
  Center
Nashville, Tennessee

**Kerry E. Weinberg, MPA, MA,
  RT(R), RDMS, RDCS, FSDMS**
Chair and Associate Professor
Diagnostic Medical Sonography
Long Island University
Brooklyn, New York

Ted Whitten, BA, RDMS, RVT
Ultrasound Practitioner
Ultrasound Department
Elliot Hospital
Manchester, New Hampshire

Sharlette D. Anderson, MHS, RDMS, RVT, RDCS
Clinical Coordinator/Instructor
University of Missouri
Columbia, Missouri

Anthony L. Baker, MEd, RDMS, RVT
Assistant Professor
University of Arkansas for Medical Sciences
College of Health Related Professions
Little Rock, Arkansas

Terrie Ciez, MS, RDMS, RDCS, RT, CNMT
Professor and Program Coordinator
College of DuPage
Glen Ellyn, Illinois

Jann Dolk, MA, RDMS
Adjunct Faculty
Palm Beach State College
Palm Beach, Florida

Ecaterina Mariana Hdeib, MA, RDMS
Clinical Assistant Professor
Diagnostic Medical Ultrasound Program
University of Missouri
Columbia, Missouri

Jacqueline Renee Hopkins, BSRS, RT(R,CT), RDMS, RVS
Sonography Program Director
Weatherford College
Weatherford, Texas

Ellen E. Lauritsen, BS, RDMS, RVT
Sonography Instructor
Asheville-Buncombe Technical Community College
Asheville, North Carolina

Daniel A. Merton, BS, RDMS, FSDMS, FAIUM
Technical Coordinator of Ultrasound Research
Thomas Jefferson University Hospital
Philadelphia, Pennsylvania

Susanna Ovel, RT, RDMS, RVT
Sonographer III
Ultrasound Department
Radiological Associates of Sacramento
Sacramento, California

Kellee Stacks, BS, RT(R), RDMS, RVT
Program Director
Cape Fear Community College
Wilmington, North Carolina

To my husband
PETE
for the love, patience, and understanding that he showed
while I sat at my computer writing for hours on end, again.
And for the encouragement he gives me on a daily basis
to share my passion for my profession.
His unwavering support and timely humor are the reasons
that I dedicate this book to him.
Charlotte Henningsen

To my husband
JOE
for the miles he put on with me, as we walked and talked
about this book. We've shared the imaging profession
for over 30 years and his willingness to listen and make
suggestions are invaluable.
And to my colleagues and sonographers who
make this the best career a person could ever pursue.
Katie Kuntz

To my husband
CHRIS
for his loving support, care, and patience.
And to my children Jessica, Nick, and Cristine
for bringing joy and brightness to my days.
Diane Youngs

It has been 9 years since the publication of the first edition of Charlotte Henningsen's *Clinical Guide to Sonography*. For the second edition, she is joined by coauthors Kathryn Kuntz and Diane Youngs. These three women combined have more than 60 years of ultrasound experience, both as clinical sonographers and ultrasound educators. Their multifaceted experience with sonography makes this book a crucial resource for sonographers, especially those early in their career.

This edition follows the same format as the first edition. The subjects are covered from the clinical perspective. A clinical history is provided, representative ultrasound pictures are displayed, and then the subject matter is presented. If this sounds familiar, it is because this is what sonographers do every time they scan a patient. They take a history from the patient or the chart, start scanning the patient, and then adjust the images that they take, depending on their understanding of what is evolving in front of their eyes.

By having the chapters organized by clinical findings, rather than by organ systems, the *Clinical Guide to Sonography* is a real-world reference book for sonographers that should be kept close by for quick access to information. I know of sonographers whose first edition of this book is "dog-eared" from repeated use.

In conclusion, there is a great deal of new information regarding ultrasound that has come out in the past 9 years. This updated version continues to be a valuable reference for sonographers. Even if you own a first edition, having a copy of the second edition of this book should help improve the quality of your sonograms, which benefits both the patient and the interpreting physician.

Lennard D. Greenbaum, MD
Co-Director
The Hughes Center for Fetal Diagnostics
Winnie Palmer Hospital for Women & Babies
Orlando Health
Past- President
American Institute of Ultrasound in Medicine

Clinical Guide to Sonography is a pathology-focused ultrasound textbook that presents the abnormalities encountered with sonography from a clinical perspective. This text is not intended to replace comprehensive texts, which also focus on basic anatomy and imaging techniques, but to partner with those texts as a ready reference for sonographic pathology or to enhance discussion of clinical case studies. *Clinical Guide to Sonography* is a practical resource for students and sonographers as they consider patient symptoms with possible findings and diagnoses.

CONTENT AND ORGANIZATION

The book is organized into four major parts: abdomen, gynecology, obstetrics, and superficial structures. A few miscellaneous topics are covered in a separate part. Chapters are organized by patient symptom or clinical presentation to correlate with the patient history that the sonographer or sonography student may encounter in the clinical environment.

Hundreds of ultrasound images, including color Doppler, 3D and power imaging, assist the sonographer in visualizing the pathologic conditions described. Many of the chapters are enhanced with illustrations that demonstrate relevant anatomic information. The text also includes pediatric and vascular imaging, subjects that are not always covered in other clinical textbooks.

FEATURES

Every chapter contains an opening clinical scenario that sets up a realistic situation for the student to use as a frame of reference. These clinical scenarios heighten reader interest, facilitate applying information in the clinical setting, and encourage the critical thinking skills necessary for a sonographer to be more than a "picture taker." Normal anatomy is briefly reviewed, with the remainder of the chapter focused on the pathology associated with the titular symptom. Summary tables and a glossary provide quick references to covered material. Additional case studies and study questions close each chapter and are designed to develop and enhance critical thinking skills and measure comprehension of the material. Answers to case studies and study questions are provided in an appendix to provide opportunity for discussion before seeking the answers.

NEW FEATURES

- Three new chapters were added to this new edition of *Clinical Guide to Sonography*. These chapters are "Suspect Appendicitis," "Neonatal Spinal Dimple,"

and "Claudication: Peripheral Arterial Disease." These chapters provide more complete coverage of the pathology sonographers are likely to encounter in practice.
- Completely new case studies and critical thinking questions are included in each chapter to help develop students' critical-thinking skills.
- More than 600 updated images for this edition allow students to see images produced by the latest technology.

INSTRUCTOR RESOURCES

Additional Case Studies

Additional case studies that correspond to each chapter are available on Evolve for instructors teaching with the text. Instructors can use these extra case studies as classroom handouts or as homework to develop students' critical thinking skills further.

Electronic Image Collection

An electronic image collection on Evolve that includes more than 1100 images from the book is available for instructors teaching a course with the text, providing an easy-to-use and cost-effective alternative to traditional pathology slide sets.

EVOLVE—ONLINE COURSE MANAGEMENT

Evolve is an interactive learning environment designed to work in coordination with *Clinical Guide to Sonography*. Instructors may use Evolve to provide an Internet-based course component that reinforces and expands on the concepts delivered in class. Evolve may be used to publish the class syllabus, outlines, and lecture notes; set up "virtual office hours" and e-mail communication; share important dates and information through the online class Calendar; and encourage student participation through Chat Rooms and Discussion Boards. Evolve allows instructors to post examinations and manage their grade book online. For more information, visit http://www.evolve.elsevier.com or contact an Elsevier sales representative.

This textbook is designed to provide realistic clinical applications of sonography to the sonography student and the sonographer. Identification of pathology by the sonographer is the key to a correct diagnosis. I hope this book inspires you to embrace the knowledge necessary to be a valuable member of a diagnostic imaging team.

Charlotte Henningsen

ACKNOWLEDGMENTS

I would like to express my gratitude to my colleagues at Adventist University of Health Sciences who have celebrated this process every step of the way. Thanks to the college administrators, Dr. David Greenlaw and Dr. Don Williams, for allowing me the time and resources I required and for their continuing encouragement; the department student workers, John Polizzi and Britney Shaver, for diligently gathering research; the department administrative assistant, Anita Spry, for being so attentive to my needs; and the faculty of the sonography department, Jennifer Kurnal-Herring, Kelly Mumbert, and Deziree Brooks, for taking on extra tasks with such enthusiasm.

I must also acknowledge Dr. Armando Fuentes, Dr. Lennard Greenbaum, Sandy Hagen-Ansert, Donald Haydon, Dr. Diane Kawamura, Dr. Gregory Logsdon, and Dr. Alfredo Tirado for the unique roles that they have played in my professional development. I thank each of the students that I have taught over the years for inspiring and challenging me. I am especially grateful to Katie Kuntz and Diane Youngs for their willingness to join me on this journey of writing and editing a second edition.

Finally, I thank my many family and friends, who have been extremely supportive, encouraging, and understanding—especially my parents who instilled in me a love of reading and learning.

Charlotte Henningsen

My gratitude goes to all the sonographers, colleagues, physicians, and students who inspired me not only to practice the art and science of sonography, but also to share my knowledge and to teach. I am especially grateful for my career at Mayo Clinic, which spanned more than 30 years. I am grateful to the University of Wisconsin-Milwaukee and Adventist University Health Sciences for allowing me to reinvent myself in my postretirement career as an educator again!

I also want to acknowledge the support of family and friends, who encouraged me to take on this endeavor when Charlotte Henningsen first asked the question, "How would you like to help me write the second edition of the book?" Thanks goes out to all of them for believing that I could do this and always being supportive, as they looked into the office and asked, "Are you working on 'the book'?"

Finally, to the contributors who worked with me on the chapters I coauthored with you, or edited, thank you for sharing your expertise and educating those who will read and use this textbook.

Katie Kuntz

I wish to extend my gratitude to my Mayo Clinic sonography colleagues for their continual quest for knowledge and excellence and their willingness to share their expertise and to Dr. Rusty Brown, who has been a constant source of guidance, support, and encouragement. A special note of gratitude goes to Katie Kuntz for her mentoring and friendship over the last 25 years and to Charlotte Henningsen for giving me the opportunity to share my passion for sonography and education.

Diane Youngs

We acknowledge the contributors who worked diligently to meet their deadlines and produce chapters of excellence in this second edition. We also appreciate the contributors who assisted with the first edition, making the opportunity for a second edition possible.

Finally, we would like to recognize the very supportive and able staff at Elsevier who have guided us through this process: Linda Woodard, for her expertise and friendship, and Rachel Allen, for helping to put it all together in the end. Their encouragement never waned.

CH, KK, DY

PART I

Abdomen

Right Upper Quadrant Pain

Charlotte Henningsen, Gregory Logsdon

CLINICAL SCENARIO

A 72-year-old man with right upper quadrant (RUQ) pain, nausea and vomiting, and unexplained weight loss is seen by his physician. The patient has a positive Murphy's sign on clinical examination, and an RUQ ultrasound is ordered. The sonographic examination results reveal a thick-walled gallbladder with a 3.5-cm cauliflower-shaped mass projecting into the gallbladder in the fundal region (Fig. 1-1, *A* and *B*). A layering of low-level echoes also is identified in the dependent portion of the gallbladder that moves slowly with a change in patient position. The common bile duct (CBD) measures 4 mm. The sonographer also identifies two hyperechoic lesions in the liver (Fig. 1-1, *C*). What is the most likely diagnosis for this patient?

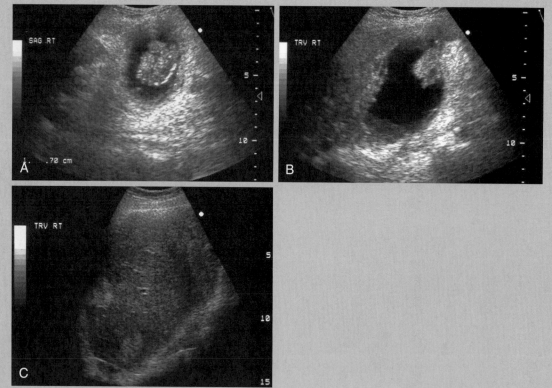

FIGURE 1-1 A cauliflower-shaped mass **(A)** protrudes from the fundus **(B)** of the gallbladder. **(C),** Two hyperechoic lesions are identified in the liver.

OBJECTIVES

- Describe the sonographic appearance of common gallbladder disease.
- List the risk factors associated with gallbladder disease.
- Identify laboratory values specific to gallbladder disease.
- Describe the sonographic appearance of liver cysts and abscesses.

- List the most common causes of abscess development in the liver.
- Describe the sonographic appearance of hematomas of the liver.

Right upper quadrant (RUQ) pain is a common clinical problem. The causes of RUQ pain include cholelithiasis and other gallbladder diseases; however, liver diseases and neoplasms (see Chapters 2 and 3) may manifest with similar symptoms. A thorough clinical examination, laboratory tests, and an RUQ ultrasound may be used to reveal the source of the discomfort. When gallbladder and liver diseases are suspected, the sonographer should take note of specific laboratory findings including bilirubin levels, liver function test results, and white blood cell counts.

In addition to the conditions discussed in this chapter, right-sided pain may be associated with diseases of the kidney (see Chapters 5, 6, and 7), the pancreas (see Chapter 4), and the gastrointestinal (GI) tract.

GALLBLADDER

Normal Sonographic Anatomy

The gallbladder is a teardrop-shaped structure that is responsible for the concentration and storage of bile. The normal gallbladder is 7 to 10 cm in length and 2.5 to 4 cm in diameter. The lumen of the gallbladder is anechoic in normal circumstances, and the gallbladder wall appears thin and smooth, with a measurement of less than 3 mm in thickness (Fig. 1-2).[1] A sonographic evaluation of the gallbladder should also include an evaluation of the bile ducts. The common bile duct (CBD) (Fig. 1-3) should measure 6 mm or less, and the common hepatic duct should measure 4 mm or less. The CBD size may be increased in patients who have undergone a cholecystectomy and in older patients.

Cholelithiasis

Cholelithiasis, also known as gallstones, is the most common disease of the gallbladder. Gallstones are usually composed of cholesterol, although stones may be made up of pigment or have a mixed composition. A predisposition for gallstone formation is seen in patients with impaired gallbladder motility and bile

stasis. The typical patient has the "five f's": fat, female, forty, fertile, and flatulent. Family history, sedentary lifestyle, absence of alcohol use, and inflammatory bowel disease may contribute to gallstone formation; patients with gallstones also show an increased prevalence of heart disease.[2] Other risk factors that predispose a patient to the development of gallstones include diet-induced weight loss, pregnancy (Fig. 1-4), total parenteral nutrition (TPN), diabetes, estrogen use, oral contraceptive use, hemolytic diseases, and white or Hispanic race. Cholelithiasis has also been identified in both genders, in children, and in the fetus.

Most individuals with cholelithiasis are asymptomatic. A symptom of cholelithiasis is RUQ pain, especially after meals; patients may also have increased symptoms after a meal high in fat. Other symptoms include epigastric pain, nausea and vomiting, and pain that radiates to the shoulder.

Sonographic Findings. Gallstones appear sonographically as an echogenic focus (Fig. 1-5) or as multiple echogenic foci that shadow and move. The imaging protocol should include two patient positions (i.e., supine and decubitus) to document the movement of the stones.

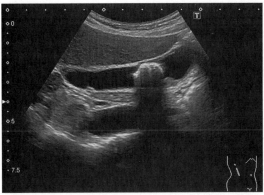

FIGURE 1-3 A 40-year-old woman presents with pain after eating. The gallbladder contains a large gallstone. *(Courtesy Toshiba America Medical Systems.)*

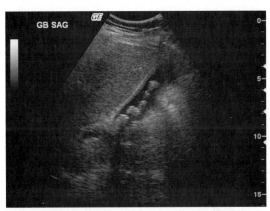

FIGURE 1-4 Multiple gallstones are identified in a pregnant patient with RUQ pain. *(Courtesy Lori Davis and Natalie Cauffman, Florida Hospital Deland.)*

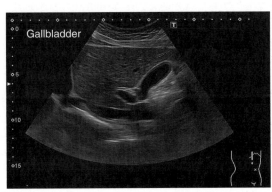

FIGURE 1-2 Normal gallbladder. *(Courtesy Toshiba America Medical Systems.)*

Sludge

Sludge, also referred to as echogenic bile, frequently occurs from bile stasis. This condition can occur with prolonged fasting or hyperalimentation therapy and with obstruction of the gallbladder. The clinical significance of this finding is unclear.

Sonographic Findings. The sonographic appearance of sludge is that of low- to medium-level echoes within the gallbladder (Fig. 1-6) that are nonshadowing, layer, and move slowly with a change in patient position from the viscous nature. Sludge may be identified in conjunction with cholelithiasis, cholecystitis, and other biliary diseases, including gallbladder carcinoma.

Cholecystitis

Cholecystitis is an inflammation of the gallbladder that can have many forms—acute or chronic, calculous or acalculous. In addition, acute cholecystitis may present with severe complications including emphysematous cholecystitis, gangrenous cholecystitis, and gallbladder perforation.

Acute Cholecystitis. The most common cause of acute cholecystitis is cholelithiasis that creates a cystic duct obstruction. Because of the high prevalence of associated cholelithiasis, acute cholecystitis is more common in female patients; however, when cholecystitis develops in male patients, it is usually more severe.[3] Clinical symptoms include RUQ pain, fever, and leukocytosis. Serious complications can occur in patients with acute cholecystitis, including empyema, gangrenous cholecystitis, emphysematous cholecystitis, and gallbladder rupture.

Acalculous cholecystitis (ACC) is an acute inflammation of the gallbladder in the absence of cholelithiasis (Fig. 1-7). The etiology is multifactorial. ACC occurs in patients with TPN, postoperative patients, and trauma and burn patients. ACC is more common in male patients.

Sonographic Findings. The sonographic findings (Fig. 1-8) associated with acute cholecystitis usually include cholelithiasis. Other findings include a thickened

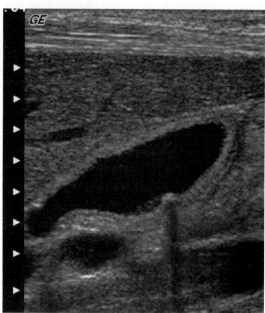

FIGURE 1-5 A small echogenic focus with shadowing is noted in the gallbladder. *(Courtesy GE Medical Systems.)*

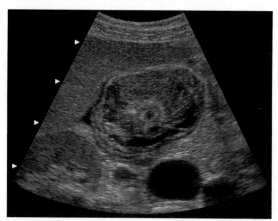

FIGURE 1-7 A patient with acute cholecystitis has a grossly thickened gallbladder wall and pericholecystic fluid. *(Courtesy GE Medical Systems.)*

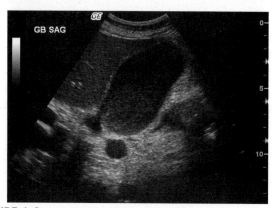

FIGURE 1-6 Gallbladder is filled with sludge. *(Courtesy Lori Davis and Natalie Cauffman, Florida Hospital Deland.)*

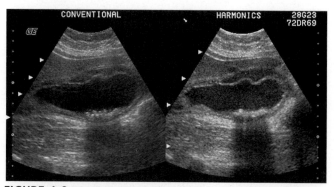

FIGURE 1-8 Thickened gallbladder wall, sludge, and cholelithiasis are identified in a patient with acute cholecystitis. *(Courtesy GE Medical Systems.)*

gallbladder wall, a sonographic Murphy's sign, sludge, pericholecystic fluid, and an enlarged gallbladder.

Chronic Cholecystitis. Chronic cholecystitis occurs from multiple attacks of acute cholecystitis and results in fibrosis across the gallbladder wall. Patients may have transient biliary colic, but usually lack the acute tenderness identified in patients with acute cholecystitis.

Sonographic Findings. The sonographic findings suggestive of chronic cholecystitis include gallbladder wall thickening and cholelithiasis. The WES (wall, echo, shadow) sign is described as a contracted gallbladder and the presence of gallstones (Fig. 1-9) and may be identified in association with chronic cholecystitis, and cholelithiasis.

Emphysematous Cholecystitis. Emphysematous cholecystitis is a complication of acute cholecystitis in which gas invades the gallbladder wall and lumen, and may also be present in the biliary ducts. Emphysematous cholecystitis occurs with ischemia of the gallbladder wall and subsequent bacterial invasion. It is more common in male patients, and is frequently associated with underlying diseases such as diabetes mellitus and peripheral atherosclerotic disease.[4] Complications of emphysematous cholecystitis include the development of gangrene of the gallbladder and gallbladder rupture.

Sonographic Findings. The ultrasound appearance of emphysematous cholecystitis includes air in the gallbladder wall and lumen (Fig. 1-10). Air may be seen as increased echogenicity with or without reverberation artifact.

Gangrenous Cholecystitis. Another complication of acute cholecystitis is gangrenous cholecystitis (Fig. 1-11), which is associated with increased morbidity and mortality and may lead to gallbladder perforation. The gallbladder wall is thickened and edematous, with focal areas of exudate, hemorrhage, and necrosis. Patients more commonly have generalized abdominal pain rather than a positive Murphy's sign.

Sonographic Findings. The sonographic appearance of gangrenous cholecystitis includes focal thickening of the gallbladder wall, striations across the gallbladder wall (Fig. 1-12), intraluminal echoes, and intraluminal membranes. Pericholecystic fluid may be present as well

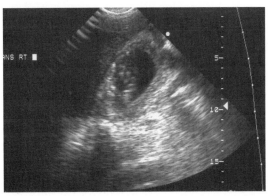

FIGURE 1-10 Comet-tail artifacts emanate from the lumen and wall of an emphysematous gallbladder.

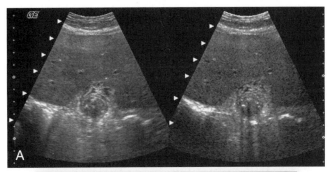

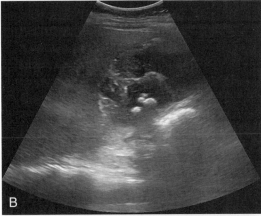

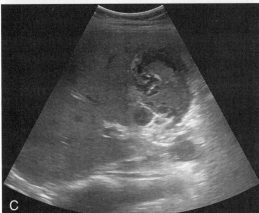

FIGURE 1-11 A, Grossly abnormal gallbladder is seen in a patient with gangrenous cholecystitis. **(B)** and **(C)**, A 45-year-old woman had gangrenous cholecystitis develop after a severe attack of acute cholecystitis precipitated by cholelithiasis. Sonographic evaluation demonstrates a grossly heterogeneous gallbladder. (**A**, *Courtesy GE Medical Systems.*)

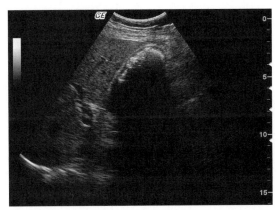

FIGURE 1-9 Contracted gallbladder filled with stones. (*Courtesy Lori Davis and Natalie Cauffman, Florida Hospital Deland.*)

as cholelithiasis, which is often associated with gangrenous cholecystitis.

Gallbladder Perforation. Gallbladder perforation is a complication of acute cholecystitis that may develop within a few days to several weeks after the onset of the symptoms of the acute gallbladder inflammation. Perforation usually occurs in the gallbladder fundus after cystic duct obstruction, gallbladder distention, and resultant ischemia and necrosis.

Risk factors for gallbladder rupture include gallstones, infection, diabetes, trauma, malignant disease, drugs, angiitis, and atherosclerosis. Clinical presentation may include abdominal pain, leukocytosis, and fever. The mortality rate is significant.

Sonographic Findings. The sonographic findings of gallbladder perforation may include cholelithiasis, gallbladder wall thickening, intraluminal debris, and ascites. In addition, sonographic visualization of the gallbladder may reveal the actual perforation site in the gallbladder wall (described as the "hole" sign), pericholecystic abscess, and gallstones free-floating in ascites that surrounds the liver.[5]

Hyperplastic Cholecystosis

Hyperplastic cholecystosis refers to a group of proliferative and degenerative conditions that affect the gallbladder. The incidence of hyperplastic cholecystosis is increased in female patients. These benign conditions include adenomyomatosis and cholesterolosis and may be diffuse, segmental, or localized.

Adenomyomatosis. Adenomyomatosis of the gallbladder occurs with diffuse or localized hyperplasia of the gallbladder mucosa that extends into the muscular layer and results in mucosal diverticula, known as Rokitansky-Aschoff sinuses.[6] Adenomyomatosis may be asymptomatic, or may be seen with symptoms similar to those of gallstones.

Sonographic Findings. Adenomyomatosis may appear sonographically as anechoic or echogenic foci within the gallbladder wall corresponding to the Rokitansky-Aschoff sinuses. Shadowing or comet-tail artifact (Fig. 1-13) may be seen emanating from the diverticula, and gallbladder wall thickening may be noted.[7] Adenomyomatosis may also be seen in association with cholelithiasis.

Cholesterolosis. Cholesterolosis is characterized by the deposition of cholesterol across the gallbladder wall. It is also referred to as a strawberry gallbladder because of the appearance of the cholesterol deposits within the gallbladder mucosa. This condition may be localized or diffuse and is associated with cholelithiasis.

Sonographic Findings. Cholesterolosis may appear sonographically as multiple small cholesterol polyps that arise from the gallbladder wall (Fig. 1-14). These polypoid lesions do not shadow or move with variation in patient position. Comet-tail artifacts may also be identified emanating from the cholesterol polyps and may be indistinguishable sonographically from adenomyomatosis. Gallbladder polyps may also occur in isolation, and when they are small, they are insignificant.

Gallbladder Carcinoma

Carcinoma of the gallbladder is the most common cancer of the biliary tract, and most tumors occur in the gallbladder fundus. Most gallbladder cancers are classified as adenocarcinoma. The etiology is unclear; however, risk factors include gallstones, chronic cholecystitis, porcelain

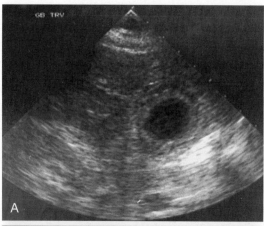

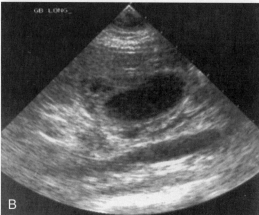

FIGURE 1-12 **(A)** and **(B)**, Striated, thickened gallbladder wall and low-level echoes are shown within the gallbladder lumen.

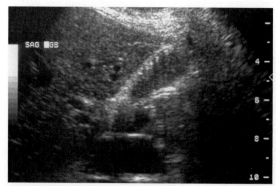

FIGURE 1-13 Comet-tail artifacts are seen emanating from the gallbladder wall. Lack of comet-tail artifact from within lumen differentiates hyperplastic cholecystosis from emphysematous cholecystitis.

gallbladder, exposure to carcinogens, and some blood groups. Gallbladder carcinoma is also more common in female patients and elderly patients.

The clinical symptoms are nonspecific in the early stages and may mimic benign gallbladder disease. Patients may present with weight loss, anorexia, RUQ pain, jaundice, nausea and vomiting, and hepatomegaly. Late diagnosis is common, which is related to the poor prognosis of this malignant disease; the 5-year survival rate is 5% to 12% with advanced disease.[8]

Sonographic Findings. The sonographic findings of gallbladder carcinoma (Fig. 1-15) include an inhomogeneous, polypoid lesion with irregular margins; localized wall thickening; a mass that replaces the gallbladder; and calcification of the gallbladder wall. Gallbladder polyps greater than 10 mm in size suggest malignancy.[8] Associated gallstones as well as metastatic lesions within the liver, ascites, and intraductal biliary dilation may be visualized. Color Doppler imaging may be used to differentiate biliary sludge, which is avascular, from a hypoechoic mass, which would show flow.

Table 1-1 lists gallbladder pathology, symptoms, and sonographic findings.

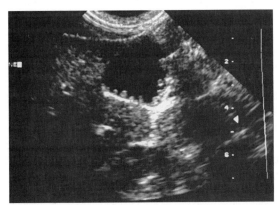

FIGURE 1-14 Multiple polypoid lesions are seen in the gallbladder wall; this was an incidental finding in a patient undergoing renal ultrasound examination.

BILIARY TRACT DISEASE

Choledocholithiasis

Choledocholithiasis refers to stones that are located in the bile ducts. This condition usually occurs with the migration of gallstones into the common duct. When obstruction of the duct occurs, the patient has jaundice and an elevated bilirubin level. Patients may also have RUQ pain.

Sonographic Findings. The sonographic findings of choledocholithiasis include echogenic foci that shadow within the duct (Fig. 1-16, *A*) with or without ductal dilation (Fig. 1-16, *B*).

Cholangiocarcinoma

Cholangiocarcinoma is a rare malignant disease that can occur anywhere along the biliary tract, although it most commonly occurs in the perihilar region (Klatskin's tumor). The incidence of cholangiocarcinoma has increased worldwide with the highest geographic prevalence in northern Cambodia, Laos, and Thailand.[9] Cholangiocarcinoma is predominantly classified as an

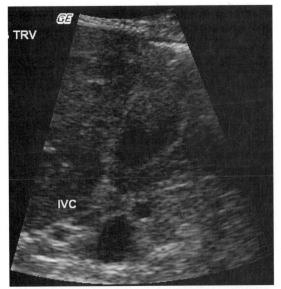

FIGURE 1-15 An irregular mass is seen in the gallbladder fundus. *(Courtesy Lori Davis and Natalie Cauffman, Florida Hospital Deland.)*

TABLE 1-1	Diseases of the Gallbladder	
Pathology	**Symptoms**	**Sonographic Findings**
Cholelithiasis	Asymptomatic, RUQ pain, pain after fatty meals, epigastric pain, nausea and vomiting	Echogenic foci that shadow and move
Cholecystitis	RUQ pain, fever	Thickened gallbladder wall; gallstones and sludge may be seen; WES sign
Adenomyoma-tosis	Asymptomatic, RUQ pain	Anechoic or echogenic foci in gallbladder wall; wall thickening or comet-tail or shadow artifacts may be seen
Cholesterolosis	Asymptomatic, RUQ pain	Multiple polypoid lesions in gallbladder wall; comet-tail artifact may be seen
Adenocarcinoma	RUQ pain, weight loss, anorexia, jaundice, nausea and vomiting, hepatomegaly	Irregular polypoid mass, localized wall thickening, calcification of gallbladder wall

adenocarcinoma. Risk factors include exposure to radio-nuclides and chemical carcinogens and some biliary tract diseases, including sclerosing cholangitis and choledochal cyst.

The clinical manifestations of cholangiocarcinoma include painless jaundice, which is the most common presentation, pruritus, abdominal pain, anorexia, malaise, and weight loss. Gallstones and intrahepatic stones may also be identified with cholangiocarcinoma. Pertinent laboratory findings include elevated bilirubin level, abnormal liver function test results, and a positive carcinoembryonic antigen (CEA). Many patients are not candidates for surgical resection at the time of diagnosis because of extensive vascular involvement, and treatment may be palliative only and may focus on relief of obstruction. The prognosis depends on the stage of the disease at the time of diagnosis, but overall is considered poor with a mean survival rate of 4% for unresectable tumors.[9]

Sonographic Findings. The sonographic evaluation of cholangiocarcinoma may reveal a liver mass or a mass arising from within the ducts (Fig. 1-17). Intrahepatic biliary tract dilation may also be identified in the absence of extrahepatic dilation. Sonographic imaging may show a mass disrupting the union of the right and left hepatic ducts (Fig. 1-18), and the gallbladder may be collapsed.

Cholangitis

Cholangitis is defined as inflammation of the bile ducts. Cholangitis may be classified as Oriental cholangitis, which may be identified in the United States with increasing immigration; sclerosing cholangitis, which may be associated with ulcerative colitis; AIDS cholangitis; and acute obstructive suppurative cholangitis. Depending on the type of cholangitis, the cause may be ductal strictures, parasitic infestation, bacterial infection, stones, or neoplasm. Clinical symptoms include fever, abdominal pain, and jaundice.

Sonographic Findings. The sonographic findings of cholangitis (Fig. 1-19) include biliary duct dilation and thickening of the walls of the ducts.

Table 1-2 lists biliary tract pathology, symptoms, and sonographic findings.

LIVER

Normal Sonographic Anatomy

The liver is located in the RUQ and extends partially into the left upper quadrant. Normal liver parenchyma

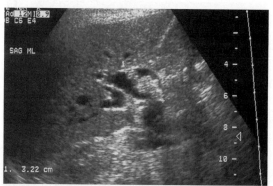

FIGURE 1-17 An irregular, echogenic mass is arising within CBD of a 95-year-old woman with a prior history of cholecystectomy and current history of jaundice. Intrahepatic ductal dilation was also identified.

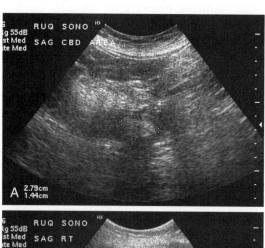

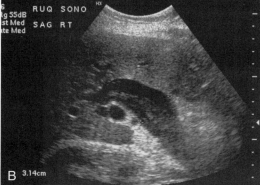

FIGURE 1-16 Echogenic focus with shadowing **(A)** is visualized within dilated CBD **(B)** of a patient with a history of cholecystectomy and RUQ pain. Biliary sludge is also seen layering within dilated CBD.

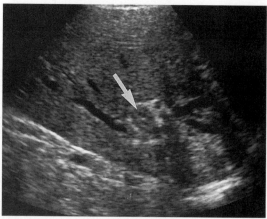

FIGURE 1-18 Cholangiocarcinoma. Transverse scan at level of porta hepatis reveals intrahepatic dilation of the right and left bile ducts. A poorly defined isoechoic mass *(arrow)* is causing obstruction.

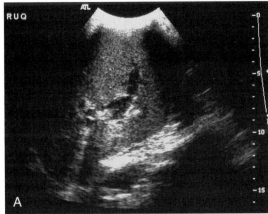

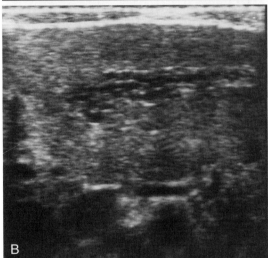

FIGURE 1-19 **(A),** Ultrasound findings of dilated ducts with thickened walls and intraductal stones in a 67-year-old man with a history of sclerosing cholangitis and AIDS cholangitis. **(B),** Transverse scan through the left lobe of the liver shows irregular thickening of walls of intrahepatic bile ducts.

should appear homogeneous and display midlevel echogenicity (Fig. 1-20, *A*). Compared with the renal parenchyma, normal liver parenchyma appears hyperechoic or isoechoic (Fig. 1-20, *B*), and compared with the pancreas, the liver appears hypoechoic or isoechoic. Within the parenchyma, tubular structures corresponding to veins, arteries, and ducts can also be visualized. The normal size of the liver is 15 to 20 cm in length at the midclavicular line.

Abscess

Liver abscess is associated with an increased incidence of morbidity and mortality. Hepatic abscess may be bacterial (pyogenic) in origin or result from a parasite. In addition, the candidal fungus can also affect the liver, especially in patients with immunocompromised conditions.

The liver may also be infected by the *Echinococcus* tapeworm, which is more common where sheep herding is prevalent. Hepatic echinococcosis is an inflammatory cystic reaction that may manifest as a cystic or complex lesion (Fig. 1-21). Some causes of inflammatory reactions of the liver, including amebiasis and echinococcosis, are not endemic to the United States; however, patients who have traveled to affected areas and immigrants from endemic populations may have these uncommon lesions.

Pyogenic Abscess. Pyogenic abscess or bacterial abscess is responsible for 6 to 22 of 100,000 hospitalizations each year.[10] These pus-containing lesions are most commonly the result of biliary tract disease, but are also associated with spread from an infection via the hepatic artery or portal vein and with trauma or surgery. Cirrhosis, neoplasm, and sickle cell anemia can also predispose a patient to abscess formation. The most common

TABLE 1-2	Diseases of the Biliary Tract	
Pathology	**Symptoms**	**Sonographic Findings**
Choledocholithiasis	RUQ pain, jaundice	Echogenic foci that shadow in ducts; with or without ductal dilation
Cholangiocarcinoma	Painless jaundice, pruritus, abdominal pain, anorexia, malaise, weight loss	Liver mass, mass within ducts, intrahepatic ductal dilation
Cholangitis	Fever, abdominal pain, jaundice	Biliary ductal dilation, thickening of ductal walls

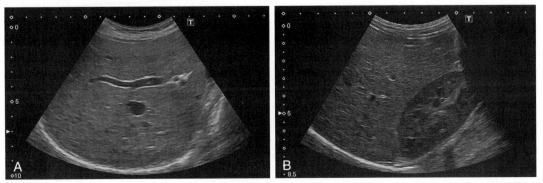

FIGURE 1-20 Normal liver shows typical homogeneous texture **(A)** and comparative echogenicity of liver to kidney **(B),** which may be hyperechoic or isoechoic. *(Courtesy Toshiba America Medical Systems.)*

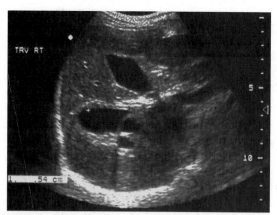

FIGURE 1-21 A thick-walled cyst with daughter cysts is identified in a patient with abdominal pain.

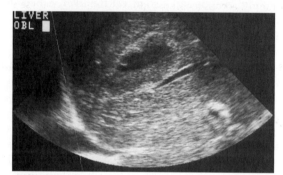

FIGURE 1-22 Thick-walled abscess shows fluid-debris level.

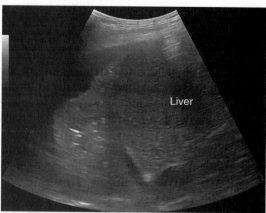

FIGURE 1-23 Large subdiaphragmatic fluid collection consistent with abscess formation secondary to bowel perforation.

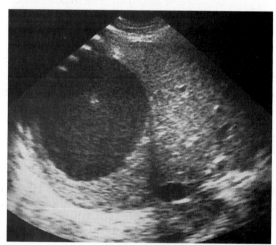

FIGURE 1-24 Amebic liver abscess—classic morphology. Transverse sonogram shows a well-defined oval subdiaphragmatic mass increased through transmission. Uniform low-level internal echoes and absence of a well-defined wall are noted.

organisms identified in pyogenic abscesses are *Escherichia coli, Klebsiella pneumoniae, Proteus, Staphylococcus,* and *Streptococcus.*[11]

Pyogenic abscesses may be singular or multiple. When solitary, pyogenic abscess is more common in the right lobe of the liver, but multiple abscesses may be identified in both lobes. Symptoms include fever, jaundice, and RUQ pain. Patients may also have nausea and vomiting, anorexia, and fatigue. Liver function test results are usually elevated but nonspecific, and most patients have leukocytosis. Diagnostic procedures may include aspiration of the purulent material for microscopic evaluation that may be performed with ultrasound guidance. Prompt diagnosis and treatment are essential because untreated pyogenic abscesses are virtually uniformly lethal.

Sonographic Findings. On sonographic evaluation, abscesses are variable in size, number, and appearance. They can appear complex or hypoechoic and can show a fluid-debris level (Fig. 1-22). They are typically round or ovoid with irregular walls. Artifacts of enhancement or shadowing (if gas is present) may also be identified.

Amebic Abscess. Amebiasis is caused by the protozoan parasite *Entamoeba histolytica,* which is endemic to parts of Mexico, Central America, South America, India, Southeast Asia, and Africa; however, it may be seen in the United States as a result of the increase in worldwide travel and immigration.[12] Amebiasis most commonly involves the GI tract and may be asymptomatic. Dissemination

outside the GI tract most commonly involves the liver through the portal vein, where ischemia and resultant hepatic necrosis lead to abscess formation; however, spreading to the brain and lungs may also occur.

The clinical presentation of hepatic amebic abscess includes RUQ pain, hepatomegaly, fever, weight loss, and diarrhea. Liver function test results are nonspecific, and laboratory test results may also reveal leukocytosis. Amebic abscesses are more common in male patients and are more commonly identified in the right lobe of the liver. Amebiasis is usually treated medically with metronidazole; however, other treatments may also be administered. Aspiration for diagnostic and therapeutic purposes may be done in patients with resistance to medical treatment. The mortality rate without treatment is high because of abscess rupture.

Sonographic Findings. The sonographic evaluation of hepatic amebiasis may reveal multiple, hypoechoic lesions (Fig. 1-23). The lesions may be round or oval with irregular walls (Fig. 1-24). Fluid-debris levels and acoustic enhancement may also be seen. Amebic abscess

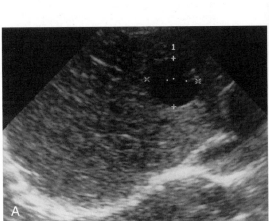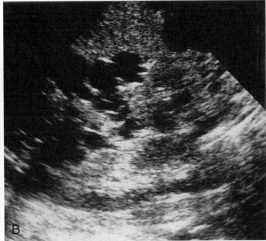

FIGURE 1-25 **(A)**, Simple hepatic cyst shows smooth, uniform borders and no internal echoes (anechoic). **(B)**, Polycystic liver disease shows multiple cysts throughout liver and kidney.

may not be differentiated sonographically from pyogenic abscess, echinococcal cysts, or necrotic neoplasm; therefore clinical correlation is paramount in an accurate diagnosis.

Cysts

Hepatic cysts of the liver may be congenital or acquired. Congenital cysts of the liver are lined with epithelium and are ductal in origin. Autosomal dominant polycystic kidney disease (ADPKD) is an inherited disorder that leads to renal failure. Liver cysts are frequently identified in addition to the renal findings in patients with ADPKD; however, these liver cysts do not affect liver function.

Acquired cysts of the liver are not true cysts and may be the result of trauma, parasitic or pyogenic abscesses, or necrotic neoplasm.

Sonographic Findings. The ultrasound diagnosis of a simple cyst is made based on certain criteria. The cyst should be anechoic, smooth-walled, and round or oval and have posterior enhancement (Fig. 1-25, *A*). Cysts may be solitary or multiple (especially when associated with ADPKD) and vary greatly in size (Fig. 1-25, *B*).

Cysts of the liver are commonly asymptomatic and incidental findings.

Hematoma

Hematomas of the liver may be classified as subcapsular or intrahepatic and are usually the result of trauma. Hematomas may result from hemorrhage within a neoplasm; they may also be a rare complication of pregnancy associated with preeclampsia and hemolysis, elevated liver enzymes, and low platelet count (HELLP) syndrome. Patients with hematomas of the liver may have hepatomegaly and RUQ pain. Hypotension and a decreased hematocrit may indicate a severe hemorrhage.

Sonographic Findings. The ultrasound appearance of hematomas (Fig. 1-26) varies depending on the age of the bleed. An acute process is usually echogenic in appearance and eventually becomes cystic, although septations may be visualized in a resolving hematoma. A subcapsular hematoma may also have varying echogenicity and is usually comma-shaped. Serial ultrasound scans may be used to show resolution of these lesions.

Table 1-3 lists liver lesion pathology, symptoms, and sonographic findings.

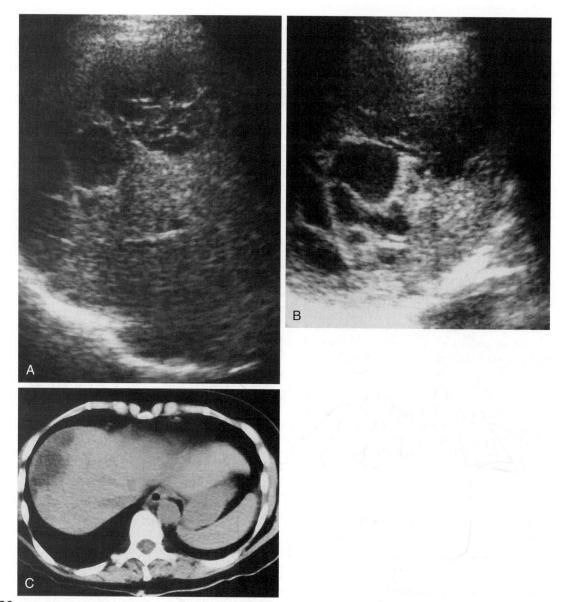

FIGURE 1-26 Hepatic trauma. **(A)** and **(B)**, A complex mass was found in the right lobe of the liver in a patient who had been in a car accident. **(C)**, CT scan of a 54-year-old woman shows collection of blood in the right lateral border of the liver.

TABLE 1-3	Lesions of the Liver	
Pathology	**Symptoms**	**Sonographic Findings**
Abscess	RUQ pain, fever, jaundice, nausea and vomiting, anorexia, fatigue	Round or oval, hypoechoic lesion; fluid-debris level; complex, irregular wall; with or without enhancement
Cysts	Asymptomatic, pain when cysts are large	Round or oval, anechoic, thin-walled; posterior enhancement
Hematoma	RUQ pain, hepatomegaly	Echogenic to cystic, septations

SUMMARY

Multiple causes exist for RUQ pain, including various diseases of the liver and gallbladder. Clinical examination, laboratory tests, and imaging procedures including ultrasound can assist with an accurate diagnosis so that an appropriate treatment plan can be implemented.

CLINICAL SCENARIO—DIAGNOSIS

The large, irregular polypoid mass suggests gallbladder cancer. The echogenic lesions in the liver further confirm the diagnosis and point to metastatic disease. Sludge is also seen within the gallbladder, and the normal CBD confirms that the malignant disease does not obstruct the biliary tract.

CASE STUDIES FOR DISCUSSION

1. A 61-year-old white woman presents with RUQ pain and nausea. An RUQ sonogram reveals a gallbladder with a layering of low-level echoes containing small echogenic foci that shadow (Fig. 1-27, *A*). Additionally, the CBD measures 12.4 mm (Fig. 1-27, *B*). The remainder of the sonographic examination is unremarkable. What is the most likely diagnosis for this patient?

2. A 55-year-old woman underwent an abdominal sonogram because of a feeling of fullness in her abdomen. The liver demonstrated multiple anechoic lesions, some with irregular walls and many with acoustic enhancement (Fig. 1-28, *A* and *B*). A follow-up computed tomography (CT) scan was ordered that confirmed the sonographic findings (Fig. 1-28, *C*). A couple of cystic lesions were also identified arising from the right and left kidneys. What is the most likely diagnosis?

3. A 49-year-old woman is seen in the emergency department with complaints of an attack of RUQ pain following a meal of a cheeseburger and French fries. The sonographic examination reveals layering echoes within the gallbladder with small echogenic foci that shadow. The gallbladder wall and CBD are unremarkable (Fig. 1-29). What is the most likely diagnosis?

4. A 78-year-old man presents with RUQ pain, malaise, and weight loss. An RUQ sonogram reveals irregular echoes within the gallbladder wall and a hypoechoic lesion in the right lobe of the liver (Fig. 1-30). What is the most likely diagnosis?

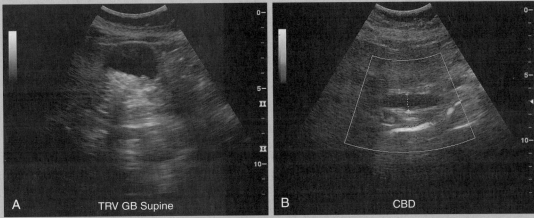

A TRV GB Supine B CBD

FIGURE 1-27 RUQ sonogram. **(A),** Gallbladder in transverse plane demonstrates layering low-level echoes containing small echogenic foci that shadow. **(B),** CBD measures 12.4 mm.

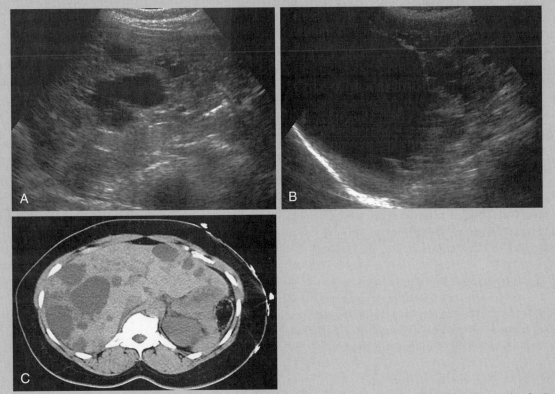

A B C

FIGURE 1-28 Longitudinal images of the liver at the midline **(A)** and right lobe **(B)**. **(C),** CT verifies sonographic findings.

Continued

5. A 36-year-old man presents to the emergency department with significant RUQ pain with nausea and vomiting since the night before. Bedside sonographic evaluation reveals a large echogenic focus with shadowing within the gallbladder, the gallbladder wall measures 5.5 mm, and the CBD measures 3.7 mm. These findings are most consistent with what diagnosis?

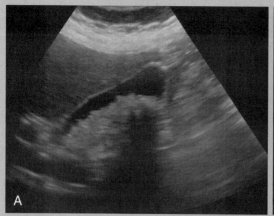 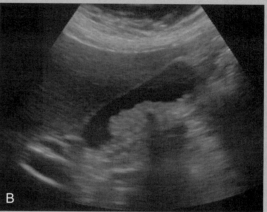

FIGURE 1-29 **(A),** Normal gallbladder wall, layering echoes, and echogenic foci with shadowing are demonstrated. **(B),** Gallbladder findings are again demonstrated with normal CBD noted posterior to the gallbladder.

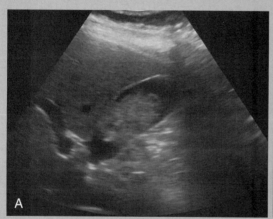 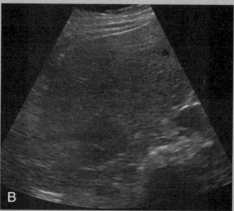

FIGURE 1-30 Sonographic findings in gallbladder **(A)** and liver **(B).**

STUDY QUESTIONS

1. A 42-year-old woman who is morbidly obese undergoes a sonographic evaluation of the RUQ. The patient complains of having RUQ pain after a lunch of pepperoni pizza. Sonographic investigation reveals multiple small echogenic foci within the gallbladder that shadow and are gravity-dependent. What is the most likely diagnosis?
   a. Cholecystitis
   b. Cholelithiasis
   c. Cholesterolosis
   d. Gallbladder carcinoma
   e. Sludge

2. An 82-year-old woman presents with RUQ pain, jaundice, nausea, and vomiting. The physician orders a sonogram of the gallbladder to rule out which of the following?
   a. Amebiasis
   b. Adenomyomatosis
   c. Choledocholithiasis
   d. Cholelithiasis
   e. Gallbladder carcinoma

3. A 57-year-old man with long-standing diabetes presents to the emergency department with signs and symptoms of severe, acute cholecystitis. The sonographic findings include gallbladder wall thickening and multiple comet-tail artifacts emanating from the wall. The gallbladder lumen contains low-level echoes from which comet-tail artifacts are also seen; however, there is no evidence of cholelithiasis. What is the most likely diagnosis?
   a. Acute cholecystitis
   b. Adenomyomatosis
   c. Chronic cholecystitis
   d. Emphysematous cholecystitis
   e. Gallbladder perforation

4. A 35-year-old man with AIDS undergoes a sonogram for abdominal pain, fever, and jaundice. Sonographic findings reveal dilation of the bile ducts and thickening of the bile duct walls. Based on the patient history, what is the most likely diagnosis?
   a. Abscess
   b. Acute cholecystitis
   c. Cholangitis
   d. Gallbladder carcinoma
   e. Hematoma

5. A 60-year-old woman presents with severe RUQ pain, fever, and a history of a recent surgery for cholelithiasis. Laboratory values reveal elevated liver function tests and leukocytosis. An RUQ ultrasound examination reveals a solitary, hypoechoic lesion in the right lobe of the liver that measures 3.7 cm at its largest diameter. The walls of the lesion appear thickened, and acoustic enhancement is identified posterior to the lesion. These findings are most consistent with which of the following?
   a. Amebic abscess
   b. Hemorrhagic cyst
   c. Hematoma
   d. Hepatoma
   e. Pyogenic abscess

6. A 62-year-old man undergoes an RUQ sonogram because of mild epigastric pain after ingestion of spicy foods. A solitary, anechoic lesion is identified in the right lobe measuring 1.5 cm with smooth walls and acoustic enhancement. This lesion most likely represents which of the following?
   a. Abscess
   b. Cholecystitis
   c. Hematoma
   d. Hepatoma
   e. Liver cyst

7. A 34-year-old woman with intermittent pain in the RUQ undergoes an abdominal sonogram. The sonogram reveals a gallbladder with multiple, small polypoid lesions projecting from the gallbladder wall. The lumen of the gallbladder is anechoic, and the remainder of the examination is unremarkable. These findings most likely represent which of the following?
   a. Adenomyomatosis
   b. Cholangitis
   c. Cholecystitis
   d. Cholelithiasis
   e. Carcinoma

8. A patient in the intensive care unit because of a spinal cord injury with a long hospitalization complains of intermittent RUQ pain, and a sonographic evaluation of the RUQ is ordered. Sonography reveals a gallbladder containing low-level echoes that layer and are gravity-dependent. This finding is most consistent with which of the following?
   a. Abscess
   b. Cholecystitis
   c. Cholelithiasis
   d. Emphysematous cholecystitis
   e. Sludge

9. A 42-year-old man with significant RUQ pain, diarrhea, and fever undergoes a sonographic evaluation of the liver. Laboratory test results are pending. The patient reports that he spent 1 month in Africa last year participating in a medical mission trip. The sonogram reveals a hypoechoic lesion measuring 4.8 cm in the right lobe of the liver with acoustic

enhancement. Which of the following diagnoses is most likely?

a. Hematoma
b. Pyogenic abscess
c. Amebic abscess
d. Complex cyst
e. Neoplasm

10. An 82-year-old woman presents with RUQ pain, jaundice, nausea, and vomiting. She also reports unexplained weight loss. Ultrasound of the gallbladder reveals cholelithiasis. In addition, an irregular focal thickening of the gallbladder wall is seen in the fundus. These findings are most suggestive of which of the following?

a. Abscess
b. Cholecystitis
c. Gallbladder carcinoma
d. Gallbladder perforation
e. Gangrenous cholecystitis

REFERENCES

1. Tsung JW, Raio CC, Ramirez-Schrempp D, et al: Point-of-care ultrasound diagnosis of pediatric cholecystitis in the ED, *Am J Emerg Med* 28:338–342, 2010.
2. Sakuta H, Suzuki T: Homocysteine and gallstone diseases: is hyperhomocysteinemia a prerequisite for or secondary to gallstone formation? *J Gastroenterol* 40:1085–1087, 2005.
3. Strasberg SM: Acute calculous cholecystitis, *N Engl J Med* 358:2804–2811, 2008.
4. Grayson DE, Abbott RM, Levy AD, et al: Emphysematous infection of the abdomen and pelvis: a pictorial review, *Radiographics* 22:543–561, 2002.
5. Neimatullah MA, Rasuli P, Ashour M, et al: Sonographic diagnosis of gallbladder perforation, *J Ultrasound Med* 17:389–391, 1998.
6. Cariati A, Cetta F: Rokitansky-Aschoff sinuses of the gallbladder are associated with black pigment gallstone formation: a scanning electron microscopy study, *Ultrastruct Pathol* 27:265–270, 2003.
7. Stunell H, Buckley O, Geoghegan T, et al: Imaging of adenomyomatosis of the gall bladder, *J Med Imaging Radiat Oncol* 52:109–117, 2008.
8. Park JY, et al: Long-term follow up of gallbladder polyps, *J Gastroenterol Hepatol* 24:219–222, 2009.
9. Olnes MJ, Erlich R: A review and update on cholangiocarcinoma, *Oncology* 66:167–179, 2004.
10. Alvarez JA, Baldonedo RF, Bear IG, et al: Anaerobic liver abscesses as initial presentation of silent colonic cancer, *HPB* 6:41–42, 2004.
11. Holzheimer RG, Mannick JA, editors: *Surgical treatment: evidence-based and problem-oriented*, Munich, 2001, Zuckschwerdt.
12. Wells CD, Arguedas M: Amebic liver abscess, *South Med J* 97:673–682, 2004.

Liver Mass

Catherine F. Fuhs

CLINICAL SCENARIO

An 84-year-old woman is seen in the sonography department for a diagnostic paracentesis and biopsy of hepatic masses seen on computed tomography (CT). She has a past history of total hysterectomy and unilateral salpingo-oophorectomy (25 years ago). She was recently found to have a large pelvic mass and markedly elevated cancer antigen 125 (CA 125) level. Multiple small hepatic masses are seen (Fig. 2-1). A core biopsy sample is taken from one of the masses and sent to the pathology laboratory. What is the pathology report most likely to reveal?

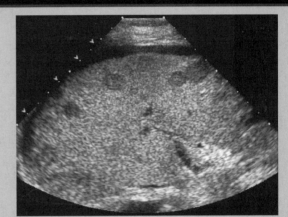

FIGURE 2-1 Multiple hypoechoic masses throughout the liver.

OBJECTIVES

- Describe the sonographic appearance of commonly encountered benign liver neoplasms.
- Describe the sonographic appearance of commonly encountered malignant liver neoplasms.
- Differentiate the Doppler findings in various liver neoplasms.

- List the risk factors associated with specific lesions of the liver.
- Identify pertinent laboratory values associated with specific liver neoplasms.

A sonographic examination of the abdomen that reveals a liver mass may be ordered for many reasons based on patient symptoms and clinical findings. Many benign liver lesions are asymptomatic and are discovered incidentally by the sonographer. The mass may be palpable on clinical examination, or abnormal laboratory values may warrant further investigation of the liver. Patients may have right upper quadrant pain that, when coupled with symptoms such as weight loss and fever, suggests malignant disease.

In addition to neoplasms of the liver, patients with pain or a palpable mass in the right upper quadrant may have biliary disease or pathology of the kidney or adrenal gland. Based on the patient's history and clinical presentation, a thorough sonographic examination of the patient's abdomen should aid in the identification of the origin of the symptoms.

LIVER

Normal Sonographic Anatomy

The liver is located in the right upper quadrant and extends partially into the left upper quadrant. Normal liver parenchyma should appear homogeneous and display midlevel echogenicity (Fig. 2-2). Compared with the renal parenchyma, normal liver parenchyma appears slightly hyperechoic or isoechoic, and compared with the pancreas, the liver appears slightly hypoechoic or isoechoic. Within the parenchyma, tubular structures corresponding to veins, arteries, and ducts can also be visualized. The average size of the liver is less than 15 cm in length at the midclavicular line, but size varies with patient height and weight. The liver is divided into three lobes: right, left, and caudate (Fig. 2-3, *A*). The right lobe

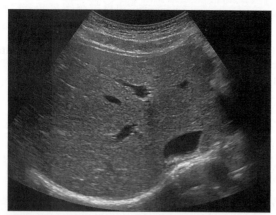

FIGURE 2-2 Transverse image of normal liver shows homogeneous texture interrupted by vascular structures.

is divided into anterior and posterior segments; the left lobe is divided into lateral and medial segments. Couinaud's classification more precisely divides the liver into eight segments (Fig. 2-3, *B*). Accurate documentation of the location of a mass is important for follow-up imaging, surgical excision, and treatment.

BENIGN MASSES

Hepatic Cyst

True cysts of the liver are found with sonography in 2.5% to 10% of the general population.[1] Their exact origin is unclear, although it is thought to be ductal. Generally, hepatic cysts are discovered incidentally. Patients are asymptomatic unless the cyst becomes infected or hemorrhages. The incidence of hepatic cysts increases

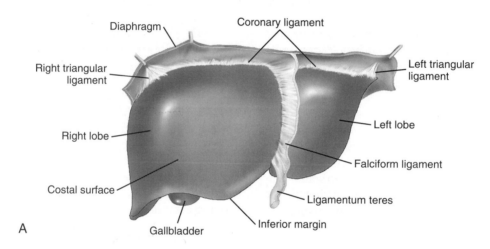

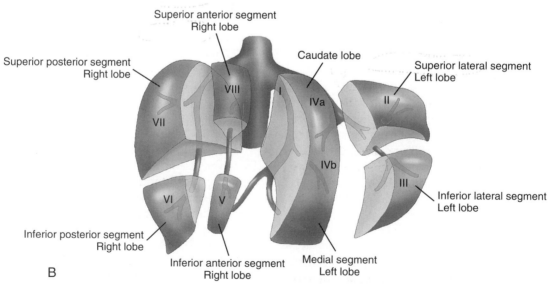

FIGURE 2-3 Liver anatomy. **(A),** Anterior view of the liver. The right lobe is the largest of the lobes; the left lobe lies in the epigastric and left hypochondriacal regions. The caudate lobe is situated on the posterior surface of the liver. **(B),** Couinaud's hepatic segments divide the liver into eight segments. The three hepatic veins are the longitudinal boundaries. The transverse plane is defined by the right and left portal pedicles. Segment I includes the caudate lobe. Segments II and III include the left superior and inferior lateral segments. Segments IVa and IVb include the medial segment of the left lobe. Segments V and VI are caudal to the transverse plane. Segments VII and VIII are cephalad to the transverse plane.

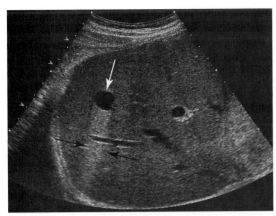

FIGURE 2-4 A simple cyst in the right lobe of the liver *(white arrow)* is anechoic, is round, and displays sharp walls with through transmission *(black arrows)*.

with age. The likelihood that they are clinically relevant is low.

Sonographic Findings. Simple hepatic cysts present as anechoic masses with sharp walls and through transmission. Occasionally, thin septations may be seen within the cyst. Color Doppler reveals absence of flow (Fig. 2-4).

Hemangioma

Cavernous hemangiomas are the most common benign tumors of the liver. Cavernous, blood-filled channels make up these lesions. Hemangiomas are found with sonography in 0.7% to 1.5% of the population, although the incidence at autopsy reaches 20%.[1] Most hemangiomas are small and asymptomatic and are discovered incidentally. They are typically found in adults, and are more common in women than men. Although patients are usually asymptomatic, larger hemangiomas may cause pain because of hemorrhage or rupture.

Sonographic Findings. The most common appearance of a cavernous hemangioma is a well-defined, hyperechoic mass that may be round, oval, or lobulated. Acoustic enhancement may be seen because of the vascular nature of this lesion. The sonographic appearance of hemangiomas may also be of variable echogenicity depending on the size of the lesion and the amount of fibrosis and degeneration. Because of the low flow of blood within a cavernous hemangioma, color Doppler and power Doppler are of little use in the characterization of hemangiomas (Fig. 2-5).

Focal Nodular Hyperplasia

Focal nodular hyperplasia (FNH) is the second most common benign liver mass after hemangioma. FNH is believed to be a hyperplastic area of normal liver cells that is associated with a congenital vascular malformation. A distinguishing feature of FNH is that it has a central stellate scar. Incidence of the scar at autopsy ranges from 0.3% to 3%.[1] Female hormones are believed to play a role in the development of FNH because it is most often seen in women of childbearing age. It is usually asymptomatic and discovered incidentally, as a solitary lesion in the right lobe.

Sonographic Findings. Because FNH is comprised of liver cells, it is often isoechoic to the liver parenchyma and can be very subtle. A change in the contour of the liver or displacement of vascular structures is often a clue to its existence. FNH may also appear hypoechoic or hyperechoic. Color Doppler or power Doppler is useful in identification of the prominent vascularity of the central stellate scar (Fig. 2-6).

Hepatocellular Adenoma

Hepatocellular adenoma occurs much less frequently than FNH; however, it is a more worrisome lesion because of its propensity to hemorrhage and its tendency to transform into hepatocellular carcinoma (HCC). There is a clearly established relationship between hepatocellular adenoma and the use of oral contraceptives. Hepatocellular adenoma has also been associated with type I glycogen storage disease (von Gierke's disease).

Hepatocellular adenoma may be silent, or it may be discovered as a mass on physical examination. The patient may present with pain if the mass has hemorrhaged. Because the incidence of hepatocellular adenoma is greater in women taking oral contraceptives than in women who are not, these masses have been seen to regress with cessation of oral contraceptive therapy and to increase in size during pregnancy.[1] Because of the tendency for hepatocellular adenoma to develop into serious complications, surgical resection is the recommended treatment.

Sonographic Findings. The sonographic appearance for hepatocellular adenoma is varied and nonspecific. Fat content may cause it to be hyperechoic, or it may be hypoechoic. Hemorrhage within the lesion may appear anechoic, hypoechoic, or hyperechoic (Fig. 2-7). Color Doppler imaging may show the significant peripheral vasculature of this lesion.[2]

Lipoma

Lipomas of the liver are rare tumors composed of fat cells. Patients are usually asymptomatic. An association is found between lipomas, renal angiomyolipomas, and tuberous sclerosis.

Sonographic Findings. Lipomas are highly echogenic lesions, most often appearing identical to cavernous hemangiomas. A distinguishing feature is a propagation speed artifact that may be noted because of the slower speed of sound through fatty tissues than through the adjacent liver parenchyma; this feature may be identified by noting that structures deep to the lipoma are displaced (Fig. 2-8).

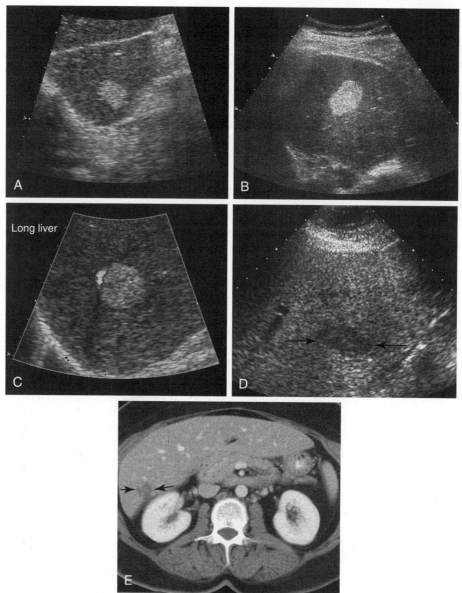

FIGURE 2-5 Hemangiomas. **(A)**, Typical sonographic appearance—well-circumscribed, round, echogenic mass. **(B)**, Enhancement posterior to a hemangioma. **(C)**, Typical lack of color Doppler flow. **(D)**, Hypoechoic hemangioma *(arrows)*. **(E)**, Arterial phase contrast-enhanced CT image *(arrows)*.

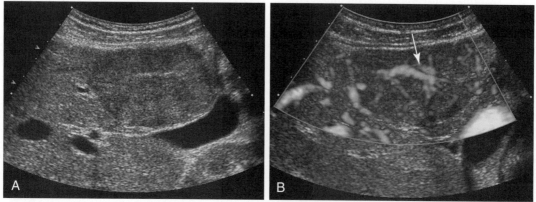

FIGURE 2-6 FNH. **(A)**, Slightly hypoechoic FNH demonstrates slight contour irregularity. **(B)**, Power Doppler shows central stellate vascularity *(arrow)*.

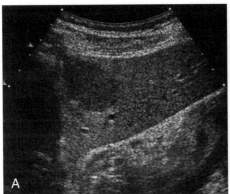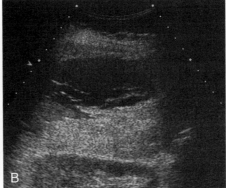

FIGURE 2-7 Hepatocellular adenoma. **(A),** Hypoechoic, well-circumscribed mass in the left lobe. **(B),** Hemorrhagic hepatocellular adenoma in the right lobe.

Other Benign Neoplasms

In addition to the benign masses discussed here, other benign masses infrequently occur in the liver. These include abscess, hydatid cyst, angiomyolipoma, cystadenoma, lymphangioma, and nodular regenerative hyperplasia.

MALIGNANT MASSES

Hepatocellular Carcinoma

HCC is the most common primary malignant neoplasm of the liver. Risk factors include hepatitis B and C, cirrhosis, nonalcoholic steatohepatitis, and aflatoxin exposure. Prevalence varies worldwide depending on predisposing factors, with aflatoxin exposure contributing to the high frequency of HCC in developing countries. It is the third leading cause of cancer death in the world and the ninth leading cause in the United States.[3] HCC has a male predominance, and most cases are seen in patients with preexisting conditions.

Patients with HCC may have a palpable mass, hepatomegaly, fever, and signs of cirrhosis. In addition to abnormal liver function tests related to cirrhosis, patients may have elevated serum alpha fetoprotein levels. The tumor may invade the hepatic veins and cause Budd-Chiari syndrome or may invade the portal venous system. Patients often have advanced stages of the disease at the time of diagnosis, which negatively affect survival.

Sonographic Findings. The sonographic appearance of HCC is variable; lesions may appear hypoechoic, hyperechoic, or complex. HCC may manifest as a solitary mass, multiple masses, or diffuse infiltration. Small discrete lesions are usually hypoechoic, and larger lesions are commonly hyperechoic or heterogeneous owing to fibrosis and necrosis. Posterior acoustic enhancement may be present in as many as half of HCCs.[3] Lesions may have a hypoechoic halo. HCC tends to invade the portal system in 30% to 60% of cases; the hepatic venous system is involved less frequently. Color Doppler is useful in showing tumor invasion in the hepatic veins, inferior vena cava, or portal veins. In addition, color and power Doppler may show flow within and surrounding the tumor (Fig. 2-9).

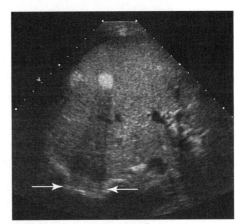

FIGURE 2-8 Hepatic lipoma causing a propagation speed artifact *(arrows)*; diaphragm deep to the lipoma appears displaced.

Metastasis

Metastases are the most common malignant liver tumors. They occur 20 times more frequently than primary hepatic neoplasms. The liver is the second most common site of metastatic disease; 25% to 50% of patients who die of cancer have liver metastases at autopsy.[2] Common primary carcinomas that metastasize to the liver include gallbladder, colon, stomach, and pancreas.

Patients with liver metastasis may have symptoms of jaundice, pain, weight loss, and anorexia. They also have abnormal liver function tests and hepatomegaly. A history of a primary malignant disease may help to confirm the diagnosis of metastatic disease when lesions of the liver are discovered.

Sonographic Findings. Metastatic disease of the liver may have variable appearances, and multiple lesions are more commonly seen than solitary masses. The sonographic appearance of a lesion does not definitively correlate with the type of primary malignant disease. Metastatic lesions may appear hyperechoic, hypoechoic, or isoechoic to the liver parenchyma. A hypoechoic halo surrounding the metastatic lesion is frequently seen. Lesions may have a target or bull's-eye appearance, contain calcifications, and appear heterogeneous or complex. Anechoic lesions are uncommon presentations for metastatic disease and, if discovered, frequently contain

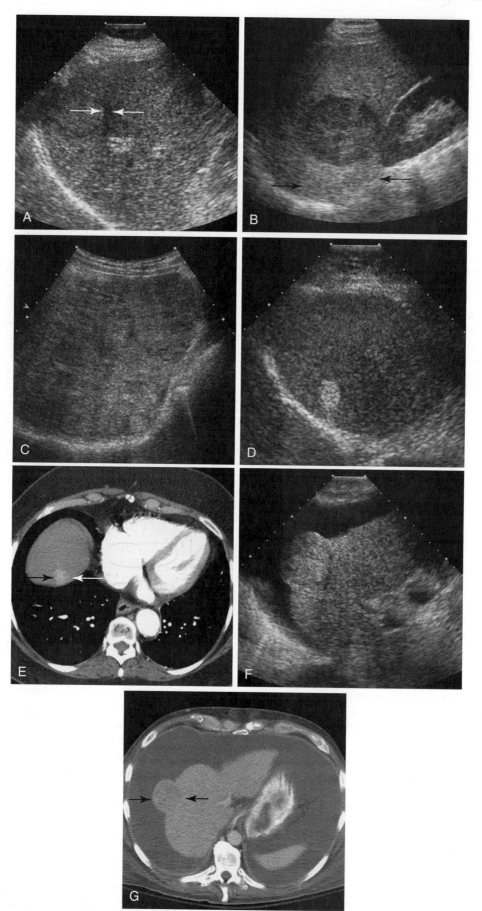

FIGURE 2-9 HCC. **(A)**, HCC displaying a hypoechoic halo *(arrows)*. **(B)**, Heterogeneously hypoechoic HCC displaying posterior enhancement *(arrows)*. **(C)**, Infiltrative presentation of HCC. **(D)** and **(E)**, Echogenic HCC in the dome of the right lobe with correlating CT image *(arrows)*. **(F)** and **(G)**, HCC *(arrows)* in the setting of cirrhosis and ascites with correlating CT image.

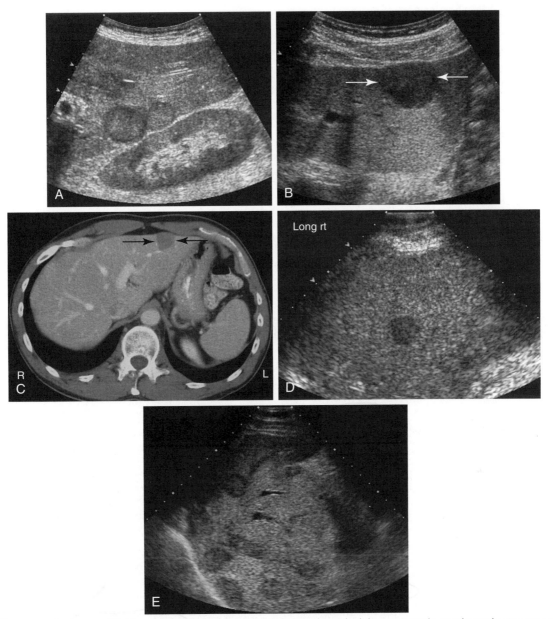

FIGURE 2-10 Metastatic disease. **(A),** Two masses with hypoechoic halos in the right lobe; metastatic gastric carcinoma was confirmed. **(B)** and **(C),** Hypoechoic liver mass *(arrows)* with correlating CT image; biopsy confirmed metastatic small cell lung cancer. **(D),** Single hypoechoic lesion—metastatic breast cancer. **(E),** Multiple lesions with target or bull's-eye appearance—advanced colorectal cancer.

low-level echoes and thick walls. Metastasis to the liver may also present as a diffuse process with an overall inhomogeneous parenchymal pattern (Fig. 2-10).

Other Malignant Neoplasms

In addition to the malignant neoplasms discussed here, other malignant neoplasms infrequently occur in the liver. These include angiosarcoma, cystadenocarcinoma, fibrolamellar carcinoma, epithelioid hemangioendothelioma, and lymphoma.

SUMMARY

Sonographic examination of the liver can assist in the identification of liver masses. Characterization of the

sonographic appearance coupled with patient history and laboratory values can lead to diagnosis and proper patient management (Table 2-1). Using contrast-enhanced sonography it is often possible to distinguish between the hemodynamics in various phases of blood flow. This technique has been shown to improve accuracy in diagnosing liver masses.[4] Biopsy is the most definitive method of tumor diagnosis; however, it may not always be indicated, in which case imaging methods may serve as the final diagnostic tools.

CLINICAL SCENARIO—DIAGNOSIS

The pathology report confirmed metastatic adenocarcinoma, possibly from colon or ovary. The paracentesis was also positive for malignancy.

TABLE 2-1	Lesions of the Liver	
Pathology	**Symptoms/Laboratory Values**	**Sonographic Findings**
Hemangioma	Asymptomatic, right upper quadrant pain	Round or oval, well-defined, hyperechoic; may enhance
Adenoma	Right upper quadrant pain	Encapsulated, well-defined, hyperechoic lesion; peripheral vasculature with Doppler scan
Focal nodular hyperplasia	Usually asymptomatic	Isoechoic, hyperechoic, or hypoechoic lesion; homogeneous, central vascular scar with Doppler scan
Lipoma	Usually asymptomatic	Highly echogenic lesion; propagation speed artifact
Hepatocellular carcinoma	Palpable mass, hepatomegaly, fever, signs of cirrhosis	Hypoechoic mass when small; hyperechoic and inhomogeneous when large; diffuse inhomogeneity; peripheral and intratumoral flow with Doppler scan
	Laboratory values: Elevated serum alpha fetoprotein often present; elevated liver function tests in the setting of cirrhosis	
Metastasis	Jaundice, pain, weight loss, anorexia	Multiple lesions, variable echogenicity; diffuse inhomogeneity
	Laboratory values: Elevated liver function tests possible	

CASE STUDIES FOR DISCUSSION

1. A 38-year-old woman undergoes a sonogram of the liver. She was seen in the emergency department 3 days earlier for severe right upper quadrant pain. At that time, a CT scan was done, which showed a liver lesion that contained fresh blood. The patient had been taking oral contraceptives. Today's examination shows a 6.5 cm × 5.5 cm heterogeneous, complex, solid and cystic-appearing mass (Fig. 2-11). Given the history and clinical presentation, what does this lesion most likely represent?

2. A 77-year-old man undergoes a sonography-guided biopsy after a CT scan. His history includes complete gastrectomy 8 months earlier for grade IV gastric cancer, and the CT scan today shows multiple liver lesions. The sonogram reveals several hypoechoic lesions in both lobes of the liver (Fig. 2-12). What is the biopsy most likely to show?

3. A 64-year-old inpatient with a history of renal failure undergoes a renal sonogram. A large anechoic mass in the right lobe of the liver is incidentally noted. The mass displays through transmission and sharp walls (Fig. 2-13). What is this mass? Should it be considered worrisome?

4. A 77-year-old woman undergoes an abdominal sonogram. She is known to have hepatitis C, presumably contracted from a blood transfusion during coronary artery bypass surgery in the 1970s.

The sonogram reveals a cirrhotic-appearing, heterogeneous liver. A 1.6-cm solid mass is seen at the periphery of the right lobe. A large amount of ascites is present (Fig. 2-14). Given the patient's history of hepatitis C and the cirrhotic appearance of the liver, what is the most likely diagnosis?

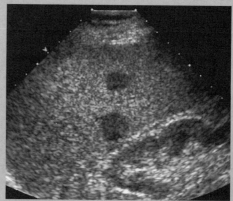

FIGURE 2-12 Two small hypoechoic lesions in the right lobe in a patient with gastric cancer.

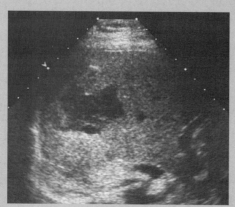

FIGURE 2-11 Ill-defined cystic mass in the right lobe of the liver.

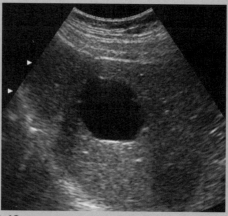

FIGURE 2-13 Large anechoic mass in an asymptomatic patient.

CASE STUDIES FOR DISCUSSION—cont'd

5. A 66-year-old man undergoes a sonography-guided biopsy of a large liver mass previously discovered on CT. He has a history of persistent cough, shortness of breath, unexplained weight loss, low-grade fever, and abdominal wall discomfort. Two large hyper- echoic lesions with peripheral halos are seen in the right lobe, the largest measuring 12.6 cm × 13.2 cm (Fig. 2-15). What is the biopsy likely to confirm?

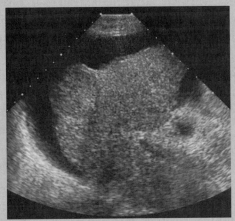

FIGURE 2-14 Mass projecting from the right lobe of a cirrhotic liver.

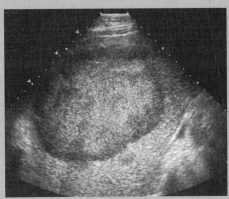

FIGURE 2-15 One of two large masses in a patient with a recent diagnosis of lung cancer.

STUDY QUESTIONS

1. A 22-year-old woman experiencing right upper quadrant pain presents to the emergency department. A sonogram is ordered to rule out gallbladder pathology. A 3-cm mass at the periphery of the right lobe of the liver is incidentally noted. The mass appears solid, homogeneous, and nearly isoechoic to the liver parenchyma. With color Doppler, the mass exhibits central blood flow in a stellate configuration. What is the most likely diagnosis?
   a. Focal nodular hyperplasia
   b. Hemangioma
   c. Hepatocellular carcinoma
   d. Liver cell adenoma
   e. Metastasis

2. A 72-year-old man with a history of alcohol abuse is seen for monitoring of cirrhosis. In addition to elevated liver function tests, his clinician notes elevated serum alpha fetoprotein. On today's sonogram, the liver appears lobulated and coarsened, and a moderate amount of ascites is noted. A 2.5-cm hypoechic solid mass is seen in the medial segment of the left lobe. What is the most likely diagnosis?
   a. Focal nodular hyperplasia
   b. Hemangioma
   c. Hepatocellular carcinoma
   d. Liver cell adenoma
   e. Metastasis

3. A 33-year-old man with tuberous sclerosis undergoes sonographic evaluation of the kidneys. In addition to multiple renal angiomyolipomas, a 2.4-cm hyperechoic mass is noted in the dome of the patient's liver. Deep to this mass, the diaphragm appears to be displaced. What is the most likely diagnosis?
   a. Focal nodular hyperplasia
   b. Hemangioma
   c. Hepatocellular carcinoma
   d. Lipoma
   e. Metastasis

4. A 38-year-old woman with mildly elevated liver function tests undergoes a sonogram of the abdomen. In the right lobe of the liver, three small echogenic masses are noted, which are well circumscribed and display no flow with color Doppler. What is the most likely diagnosis?
   a. Focal nodular hyperplasia
   b. Hemangioma
   c. Hepatocellular carcinoma
   d. Liver cell adenoma
   e. Metastasis

5. A 45-year-old man with a history of colon cancer has increasing abdominal pain, elevated liver function tests, and weight loss. On sonography, the liver has several masses within the right lobe. The masses appear echogenic with a hypoechoic halo. Given the patient's history and the appearance of the hepatic masses, what is the most likely diagnosis?

a. Angiomyolipoma
b. Hemangioma
c. Hepatocellular carcinoma
d. Liver cell adenoma
e. Metastasis

6. A 54-year-old, morbidly obese man with markedly elevated liver function tests undergoes an abdominal sonogram. The patient has a coarsened, highly echogenic liver suggestive of steatohepatitis. There is a single hypoechoic lesion measuring 5 cm in the medial segment of the left lobe. What is the most likely diagnosis for this mass?
a. Angiosarcoma
b. Hemangioma
c. Hepatocellular adenoma
d. Hepatocellular carcinoma
e. Metastatic disease

7. A 62-year-old man who recently moved to the United States from Southeast Asia undergoes an abdominal sonogram. His chief complaint is abdominal discomfort, and his clinician notes low-grade fever and suspicion of hepatomegaly. Recent laboratory tests reveal elevated alpha fetoprotein. The sonogram shows a 6-cm heterogeneous mass occupying the left lobe of the liver. What is the most likely diagnosis for this mass?
a. Focal nodular hyperplasia
b. Hemangioma
c. Liver cell adenoma
d. Hepatocellular carcinoma
e. Solitary metastatic lesion

8. A 59-year-old woman with a past history of breast cancer and recent unintentional weight loss undergoes an abdominal sonogram. The sonogram reveals ascites and multiple, hypoechoic lesions in the right and left lobes of the liver. What is the most likely diagnosis?
a. Angiosarcoma
b. Epithelioid hemangioendothelioma
c. Hepatocellular carcinoma
d. Metastasis
e. Nodular regenerative hyperplasia

9. A 39-year-old woman presents to the emergency department with severe right upper quadrant pain. Sonography shows that the gallbladder is normal, but a 3.8-cm heterogeneous mass is noted in the anterior segment of the right lobe of the liver. The patient reveals that she has been taking oral contraceptives since she was 22 years old. What is the most likely diagnosis?
a. Angiosarcoma
b. Hemorrhagic adenoma
c. Epithelioid hemangioendothelioma
d. Hepatocellular carcinoma
e. Metastasis

10. A 47-year-old woman with a history of renal cancer and elevated liver function tests undergoes an abdominal sonogram to evaluate the liver. The liver appears normal except for a 2-cm anechoic mass in the posterior segment of the right lobe. This mass displays sharp walls, posterior enhancement, and no flow on color Doppler. What is the most likely diagnosis?
a. Hemangioma
b. Metastasis
c. Simple cyst
d. Liver cell adenoma
e. Hepatocellular carcinoma

REFERENCES

1. Shaked O, Siegelman ES, Olthoff K, et al: Biologic and clinical features of benign solid and cystic lesions of the liver, *Clin Gastroenterol Hepatol* 9:547–562, 2011.
2. Gore RM, Newmark GM, Thakrar KH, et al: Hepatic incidentalomas, *Radiol Clin North Am* 49:291–322, 2011.
3. Maturen KE, Wasnik AP, Bailey JE, et al: Posterior acoustic enhancement in hepatocellular carcinoma, *J Ultrasound Med* 30:495–499, 2011.
4. Sugimoto K, Shiraishi J, Moriyasu F, et al: Improved detection of hepatic metastases with contrast-enhanced low mechanical-index pulse inversion ultrasonography during the liver-specific phase of Sonazoid: observer performance study with JAFROC analysis, *Acad Radiol* 16:798–809, 2009.

Diffuse Liver Disease

Felicia Toreno, Kathryn Kuntz

CLINICAL SCENARIO

A 51-year-old man undergoes an abdominal sonogram. He has elevated aspartate aminotransferase (AST) and alanine aminotransferase (ALT) levels and increasing abdominal girth. No previous films are available for comparison. The abdominal sonogram reveals a small, dense liver (Fig. 3-1) with increased echogenicity, surrounding ascites, and an irregular liver surface. A hyperechoic mass is noted anterior to the right portal vein (Fig. 3-2). The hepatic vasculature is difficult to visualize, but no flow within the portal vein is noted (Fig. 3-3; see Color Plate 1). What are the possible diagnoses for this patient?

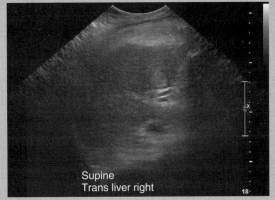

Supine
Trans liver right

18·

FIGURE 3-2 Transverse image of hyperechoic mass anterior to the right portal vein.

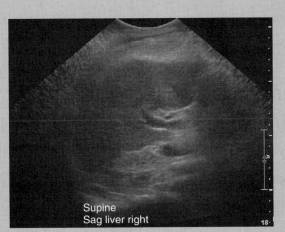

Supine
Sag liver right

18·

FIGURE 3-1 Transverse image of small, dense liver.

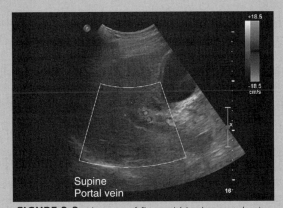

Supine
Portal vein

16·

FIGURE 3-3 Absence of flow within the portal vein.

OBJECTIVES

- Define the processes that cause and affect diffuse liver disease.
- Define and describe hepatocellular diseases and their sonographic findings.
- Compare and contrast the various diffuse liver diseases and their sonographic appearances.
- Understand and describe the changes in laboratory values associated with diffuse liver diseases.
- Describe the changes in portal venous circulation that accompany diffuse liver diseases.
- Define and describe the sonographic findings associated with conditions caused by diffuse liver diseases.

DIFFUSE LIVER DISEASE

Diseases that affect the functional cells of the liver, the hepatocytes, are referred to as diffuse liver diseases. These diseases are treated medically rather than surgically. Diffuse disease occurs as the hepatocytes are damaged and liver function decreases. Disease processes that affect the liver diffusely include infections, fatty infiltration, and liver fibrosis. The sonographic appearance of the liver varies depending on the cause. The sonographic appearance of the liver changes as diffuse disease progresses from the acute phase to long-standing chronic illness.

Patients with diffuse liver diseases often have altered laboratory values for enzymes and proteins essential to liver function. Elevated liver enzyme levels, especially aspartate aminotransferase (AST) and alanine aminotransferase (ALT), elevate as cellular function decreases as a result of the diffuse changes to the hepatocytes. Although both ALT and AST levels are sensitive to liver diseases, AST levels may also elevate in patients with diseases of the skeletal or muscular systems.

Laboratory values for proteins such as γ-glutamyl transpeptidase (GGT) and albumin may be helpful in determining the nature of liver disease. These protein levels are likely to increase in cases of long-standing hepatic cellular damage, although acute damage to liver cells may lead to a decrease in albumin levels. Prothrombin is a blood-clotting protein manufactured in the liver. Prothrombin time (PT) is used to measure how long it takes the prothrombin in blood to merge and form a clot. PT can be impaired by diffuse liver disease.

Bilirubin is produced by the breakdown of hemoglobin; the process begins in the spleen and continues in the liver. The terms "direct" and "indirect" reflect the way the two types of bilirubin chemically react. Bilirubin that has been absorbed by the hepatocytes is referred to as *direct,* or *conjugated,* bilirubin. Levels of direct bilirubin are likely to increase in cases of biliary obstruction and liver cellular diseases. *Indirect,* or *unconjugated,* bilirubin levels may increase in cases of anemia or other diseases that lead to increased breakdown of red blood cells. When there is an excess of bilirubin circulating in the blood (hyperbilirubinemia), it may leak out into surrounding tissues causing jaundice, a yellowish tinge to the skin and sclera (the white part of the eye).

Because many laboratory values are likely to be altered by a wide variety of diseases, other laboratory values in addition to liver function values should be considered in determining a definitive diagnosis. For example, increased white blood cell (WBC) levels may indicate infection or abscess in the liver. When diffuse liver disease is suspected, it is imperative that a good clinical history and laboratory values accompany a thorough assessment with sonography. Table 3-1 provides a guide to laboratory values related to diffuse liver disease.

HEPATOCELLULAR DISEASE

The liver may be enlarged especially in acute stages of hepatocellular disease. In some diseases, such as hepatitis, sonographic findings in the acute stage may be subtle and difficult to detect. The liver often becomes atrophied as pathologic changes become chronic, and the hepatocytes are replaced either by fat cells or by fibrous tissue (Fig. 3-4). Over time, replacement of the hepatocytes by fat and fibrous components leads to decreased liver function and an increase in liver enzymes. Liver cells regenerate, and this process may be accompanied by the development of regenerating liver nodules. The presence of these nodules further complicates the sonographic evaluation of the liver parenchyma and sonographic assessment of the liver for possible masses.

As damage to the hepatocytes increases, liver function decreases, which affects the liver's ability to conjugate bilirubin and to receive blood from the portal venous system. Damage to the liver can lead to jaundice when bilirubin accumulates in the interstitial fluids as it leaks from the damaged hepatocytes. The type of bilirubin, along with patterns of elevated levels, can help determine which disease is present. For example, direct or conjugated bilirubin levels become elevated as the hepatocytes become damaged. Direct bilirubin levels also increase in cases of

TABLE 3-1	Liver-Related Laboratory Values
Test	**Significance of Change**
Alkaline phosphatase	↑ in liver disease
Ammonia	↑ in liver disease and diabetes mellitus
Bile and bilirubin	↑ during obstruction of bile ducts
Glucose	↑ in diabetes mellitus and liver disease
Hematocrit	↓ in cirrhosis of liver
Hemoglobin	↓ in cirrhosis of liver
Iron	↑ in liver disease
Lactic dehydrogenase	↑ in liver disease
Cholesterol	↑ in chronic hepatitis
	↓ in acute hepatitis
Platelet count	↑ in cirrhosis of liver
Transaminase	↑ in liver disease
Urea	↑ in some liver diseases
	↓ during obstruction of bile ducts

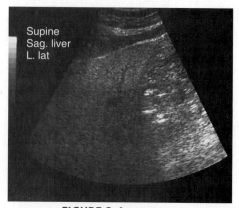

Supine
Sag. liver
L. lat

FIGURE 3-4 Fatty liver.

biliary obstruction. Damage to the hepatocytes can lead to an increase in both direct and indirect bilirubin levels.

The hepatocytes become unable to perform their normal functions because of fibrous and fatty replacement; this can eventually lead to high blood pressure in the portal vein and its tributaries, which is known as portal hypertension. The increased pressure within the portal vein causes it to become enlarged and tortuous. The spleen enlarges as it is forced to store the excess blood that the liver is unable to receive. As this process worsens, varices or collateral channels form to provide a means of bypassing the high pressure in the portal vein.

Ascites, the accumulation of free fluid within the abdominal cavity, may develop as pressure within the liver increases, and serous fluids leak from the hepatocytes into the surrounding peritoneal cavity. This condition may be due to low levels of albumin (hypoalbuminemia) or severe portal hypertension. The increased pressure within the liver causes the fluids to leak from the liver sinuses into the hepatic lymphatics. When the pressure is high enough, some fluids leak directly into the peritoneal cavity (Fig. 3-5).

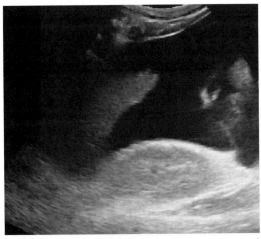

FIGURE 3-5 Ascites surrounding the liver as a result of severe hepatocyte damage and liver failure.

The increasing pressure within the portal venous system may prevent blood from flowing in its normal direction, hepatopetal, which is toward the liver. Patients with suspected diffuse liver disease should undergo evaluation with color or spectral Doppler, which may detect hepatofugal, or reverse, blood flow in the portal-splenic circulatory system (Fig. 3-6; see Color Plate 2). These patients may develop vascular collateral channels to supply the liver with blood. Patients with impaired blood flow may undergo surgical placement of shunts or transjugular intrahepatic portosystemic shunt (TIPS) placement to help return portal blood to the systemic circulation.

Fatty Liver Disease

Fatty liver disease is an acquired, reversible disorder that results from the accumulation of triglycerides (fats) within the hepatocytes. Alcoholism, obesity, and diabetes are the most common causes of fatty liver disease. In most instances, liver function is not permanently impaired. Nonalcoholic steatohepatitis (NASH) is a form of fatty liver that occurs in a few patients with fatty liver. NASH may impair the ability of the liver to function and lead to complications.

Sonographic Findings. The appearance of diffuse fatty infiltration of the liver varies from mild to severe. The fatty replaced liver has increased echogenicity because of increased attenuation of the sound beam, as seen in Figure 3-4. As fatty replacement becomes more severe, the liver is difficult to penetrate, and the vascular structures are poorly visualized, especially the hepatic veins (Fig. 3-7). In some instances, the entire liver is not affected, and areas of the liver may be spared from fatty infiltration. These fat-spared areas appear as localized regions of decreased echogenicity within the fatty echogenic liver (Fig. 3-8). This fat sparing is often seen anterior to the gallbladder and the right portal vein, or within the left lobe.

Because fat increases the attenuation of the liver parenchyma, use of a lower frequency transducer may be

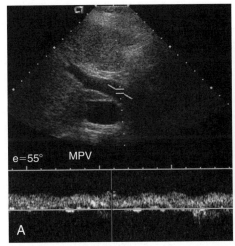

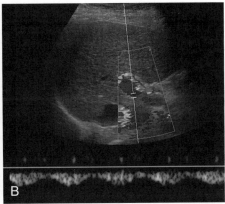

FIGURE 3-6 (A), Hepatopetal (normal) flow in the main portal vein. **(B),** Hepatofugal (reversed) flow in the main portal vein.

helpful in imaging of the liver anatomy. The sonographer must keep in mind the loss of resolution that accompanies a lower frequency transducer. Harmonic imaging, if available, can be another useful tool in evaluation of the dense liver. The frame rate of the image may become degraded on certain machines when using this option.

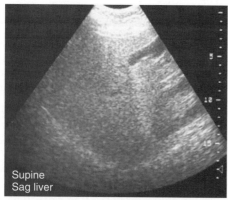

FIGURE 3-7 Transverse image of fatty replaced liver with increased echogenicity. Vascular structures are difficult to visualize.

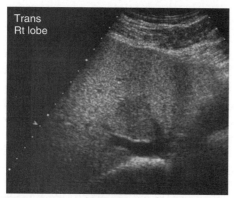

FIGURE 3-8 Transverse image. Area of localized fat-spared liver parenchyma is anterior to IVC and hepatic vein. The focal normal area is surrounded by more echogenic fatty replaced liver.

Hepatitis

The multiple variations of hepatitis (hepatitis A to G) vary in severity and sonographic findings (Table 3-2). The most common forms of hepatitis are A, B, and C. Hepatitis A is a contagious liver disease that results from infection with the hepatitis A virus. It can range in severity from a mild illness lasting a few weeks to a severe illness lasting several months. Hepatitis A is usually spread when a person ingests fecal matter (even in microscopic amounts) from contact with objects, food, or drinks contaminated by the feces or stool of an infected person.

Hepatitis B is usually spread when blood, semen, or another body fluid from a person infected with the hepatitis B virus enters the body of someone who is not infected. This can happen through sexual contact with an infected person or sharing needles, syringes, or other drug-injection equipment. Hepatitis B can also be passed from an infected mother to her infant at birth. Acute infection can, but does not always, lead to chronic infection. Chronic hepatitis B is a serious disease that can result in long-term health problems and death.

Hepatitis C is usually spread when blood from a person infected with the hepatitis C virus enters the body of someone who is not infected. Hepatitis C is a rapidly growing concern to health care workers. Hepatitis C can be either acute or chronic. Acute hepatitis C is a short-term illness that occurs within the first 6 months after someone is exposed to the hepatitis C virus. For most people, acute infection leads to chronic infection. Chronic hepatitis C is a serious disease that can result in long-term health problems or death and is now the leading indication for liver transplantation in the United States.

TABLE 3-2	**Types of Hepatitis**						
	Hepatitis A	**Hepatitis B**	**Hepatitis C**	**Hepatitis D**	**Hepatitis E**	**Hepatitis F**	**Hepatitis G**
Facts and findings		Increased risk for development of cirrhosis and HCC	Increased risk for development of cirrhosis and HCC; leading cause of liver failure and transplantation	Occurs only in patients with hepatitis B infection	Mostly found in Asia and South America	Similar to hepatitis C; uncertain whether it is a separate virus	Similar to hepatitis C
Acute vs. chronic	Mostly acute and resolves	Acute and chronic forms; acute can become chronic	Acute and chronic forms; acute converts to chronic in most infected people	See hepatitis B; severity of infection worsens with coinfection	Mostly acute and resolves within 6 mo	Similar to hepatitis C; uncertain whether it is a separate virus	Similar to hepatitis C
Mechanisms of contraction	Infected food or drinking water	Blood and body fluid contact	Blood and body fluid contact	Blood and body fluid contact	Infected food or drinking water	Blood and body fluid contact	Blood and body fluid contact
Vaccine available	Yes	Yes	No	See hepatitis B	Being developed	No	No

Damage to the liver from hepatitis may vary from mild to severe. Liver cells are damaged, healed by the reticuloendothelial system, and then regenerated. Patients develop flulike symptoms, including nausea, vomiting, and fatigue, and progression to liver failure can occur depending on the patients' immune response. The liver is often slightly enlarged, and splenomegaly may be present. AST and ALT levels are usually markedly elevated.

Sonographic Findings. The liver may be enlarged and may show decreased echogenicity (Fig. 3-9), although it often appears normal in echo texture. Because of an accumulation of fluid within the hepatocytes, the walls of the gallbladder may thicken and appear prominent. Periportal cuffing, or thickening of the portal vein walls, may be noted, and the walls of the portal veins may appear more hyperechoic than normal, which is referred to as the "starry sky" appearance.

Hepatitis that persists for more than 6 months is considered chronic. Most often this occurs with hepatitis B and hepatitis C. In chronic hepatitis, the liver texture becomes coarse and hyperechoic. Chronic hepatitis is difficult to distinguish from fatty infiltration of the liver on the basis of sonographic appearances only. The walls of the portal veins may become more difficult to assess and appear hypoechoic because of fibrosis.

Cirrhosis

Cirrhosis is an abnormal liver condition in which there is irreversible scarring of the liver. Chronic liver disease and cirrhosis result in about 35,000 deaths each year in the United States. Cirrhosis is the ninth leading cause of death in the United States.[1] The main causes of cirrhosis are sustained excessive alcohol consumption and viral hepatitis B and C; however, there are many possible causes, including the use of certain drugs, chemical reactions, biliary obstruction, and cardiac disease. Cirrhosis leads to liver necrosis, fibrosis, and regeneration. The liver becomes atrophied and dense. Cirrhotic liver changes often start and are associated with fatty liver replacement, but that is not always the case. Patients with cirrhosis have hepatomegaly, jaundice, and ascites.

Sonographic Findings. The diagnosis of cirrhosis is traditionally established with biopsy results, but it can often be suggested at imaging. The cirrhotic liver is described as coarse with a nodular surface. With the presence of ascites, the surface of the liver can appear scalloped (Fig. 3-10). Regenerating nodules form on a micronodular or macronodular level, depending on the severity of the disease. However, these nodules are not often seen sonographically because of their small size. If seen sonographically, regenerating nodules are hypoechoic compared with the surrounding liver (Fig. 3-11). Hypertrophy of the caudate lobe and atrophy of the right lobe, thought to be caused by changes to their blood supply, may also be identified on a sonogram, and ratios comparing the size or volume of the caudate lobe with the shrunken right lobe have been used to diagnose cirrhosis. The caudate lobe and the lateral segment of the left lobe are most commonly hypertrophied (Fig. 3-12), with a caudate-to-right lobe ratio greater than 0.65 considered abnormal.

Because of the replacement of hepatocytes by fibrotic tissues, the cirrhotic liver is often described as "bright," and the hepatic vasculature is difficult to visualize sonographically. The caudate lobe is often spared from this process and may appear normal in echogenicity. The

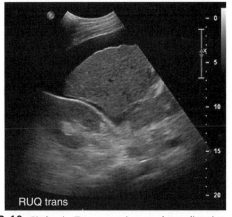

FIGURE 3-10 Cirrhosis. Transverse image shows liver is surrounded by ascites and displays a nodular surface.

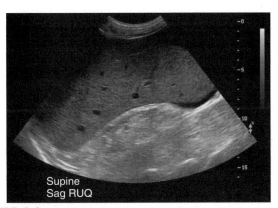

FIGURE 3-9 Hepatitis. Liver is enlarged with slightly decreased echogenicity.

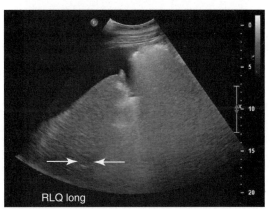

FIGURE 3-11 Regenerating nodule. Transverse image shows small hypoechoic nodule, posterior aspect *(arrows)*.

changes associated with liver fibrosis from cirrhosis are irreversible, and patient symptoms include nausea, anorexia, weight loss, and development of portal-splenic varicosities secondary to impaired venous blood flow to the liver. Patients with cirrhosis are at increased risk to develop portal hypertension and hepatocellular carcinoma (HCC), also called hepatoma. Eventually, cirrhosis progresses to liver failure. Table 3-3 compares laboratory values that are present with hepatitis, cirrhosis, and HCC.

Portal Hypertension

The most common cause of portal hypertension in North America is cirrhosis. Portal hypertension is defined as an increase in portal venous pressure exceeding 12 mmHg. Damaged hepatocytes impede the flow of blood into the liver and cause an increase in portal vein pressure.

Patients with portal hypertension have enlarged portal veins (main portal vein >13 mm in diameter) that show decreasing respiratory variations with steady, monophasic spectral Doppler tracings. Normal blood flow within the liver is hepatopetal (Fig. 3-13, *A*). Hepatofugal blood flow (reversed) may be present as venous collateral flow and splenomegaly develop (Fig. 3-13, *B*). Color and spectral Doppler are used to evaluate portal blood flow in patients with suspected portal hypertension. Additionally, contrast-enhanced sonography may be helpful

in detecting collateral and low-velocity portal vein flow by increasing the reflectivity of the red blood cells within the circulation.[3]

Portal Vein Thrombosis and Collateral Pathways

As blood pools and is unable to enter the hepatic circulation, the risk of portal vein thrombosis increases. Thrombi vary in appearance with age. New thrombus is hyperechoic, and older thrombus is hypoechoic (Fig. 3-14). The formation of venous channels within or around a thrombosed portal vein is referred to as cavernous transformation of the portal vein.

Varices are veins that dilate because of increased pressure in the portal venous system (Fig. 3-15; see Color Plate 3). Collateral veins redirect blood to alternative pathways to reenter the main venous circulation. Not all collateral pathways are visualized sonographically.

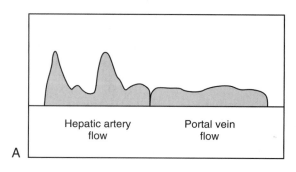

A

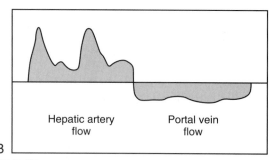

B

FIGURE 3-13 (A), Hepatopetal portal vein blood flow. **(B)**, Hepatofugal portal vein blood flow.

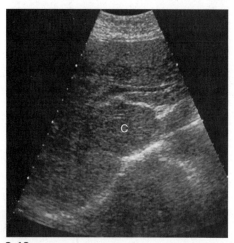

FIGURE 3-12 Transverse image shows hypertrophied caudate lobe.

TABLE 3-3	Liver Function Tests for Diffuse Liver Diseases				
	ALT	**AST**	**ALP**	**Direct Bilirubin**	**AFP**
Hepatitis	↑↑↑	↑↑	↑	↑↑↑	
Cirrhosis	↑	↑	↑	↑↑↑	
HCC	↑	↑	↑↑		↑↑↑

ALP, Alkaline phosphatase.

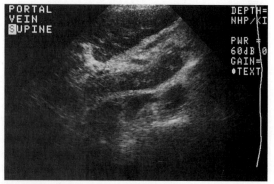

FIGURE 3-14 Portal vein is enlarged and filled with hypoechoic echoes indicative of portal vein thrombosis.

Examples of portal venous collateral pathways can be seen in Fig. 3-16.

A common collateral pathway that forms is via the splenorenal route. Blood is diverted from the splenic vein into the left renal vein. From there blood enters the inferior vena cava (IVC). Another pathway that is seen sonographically is through the paraumbilical vein and is referred to as a recanalized umbilical vein. The remnant of the fetal umbilical vein lies in the space occupied by the ligament of teres in the left lobe of the liver and becomes patent when the pressure in the liver increases to allow for a collateral pathway of blood to bypass the damaged hepatocytes. As the umbilical vein becomes patent again, it can be visualized sonographically within the space occupied by the ligament of teres (Fig. 3-17; see Color Plate 4). The development of collaterals via this pathway is referred to as Cruveilhier-Baumgarten syndrome, and some research indicates that

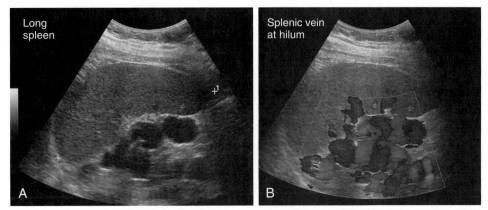

FIGURE 3-15 **(A)**, Splenic varices. **(B)**, Color Doppler.

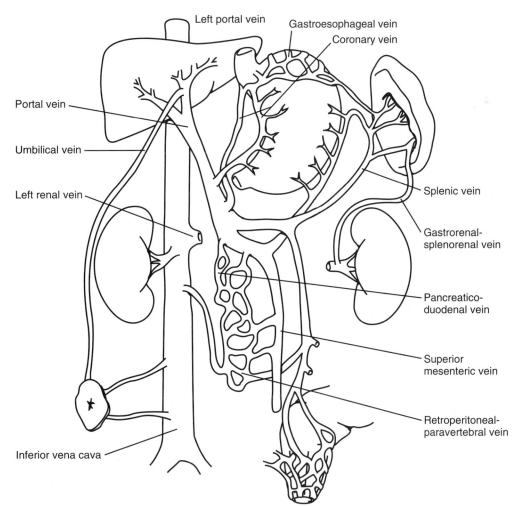

FIGURE 3-16 Portal venous collateral blood flow pathways resulting from portal hypertension.

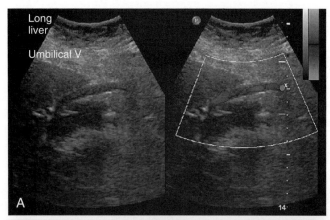

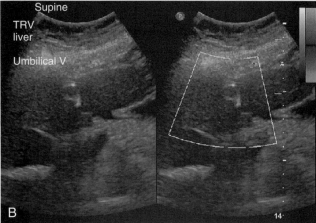

FIGURE 3-17 (A), Longitudinal image of patent, recanalized umbilical vein. **(B),** Transverse image of patent umbilical vein in the ligament of teres.

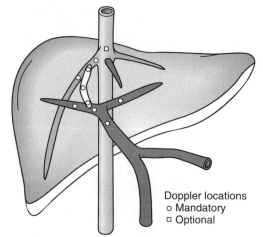

FIGURE 3-18 TIPS. Diagram of the placement of the hepatic vein-to-portal vein shunt.

these patients are at less risk of developing esophageal vein varices (see Fig. 3-16) and gastrointestinal bleeding, which can be fatal.

A third pathway is through the left gastric (also called coronary) vein. Blood is diverted from the portal vein to the esophagus. This pathway may be present in 80% of patients with cirrhosis and puts a patient at great risk because the varices in the distal esophagus are fragile and subject to hemorrhage. These patients may develop gastrointestinal bleeding and are at risk for fatal hemorrhaging.

When collateral pathways form, shunts may be placed surgically to reduce the buildup of pressure within the portal venous system and reduce the risk for hemorrhage. Common shunts include the portacaval shunt, in which blood is redirected from the main portal vein at the confluence of the superior mesenteric vein directly into the IVC; the splenorenal shunt, in which blood is shunted from the splenic vein into the left renal vein; and the mesocaval shunt, in which blood is shunted from the superior mesenteric vein directly into the IVC.

The TIPS procedure is a less invasive alternative to surgical shunt placement. Typically performed as an interventional radiologic procedure, a TIPS catheter is placed via the jugular vein into the right atrium of the heart. From the right atrium, the catheter enters a hepatic vein

(Fig. 3-18), usually the right hepatic vein. The shunt is forced into the nearby portal vein, usually the right portal vein. This shunt establishes a pathway through which blood can bypass the liver and return directly to the IVC. **Sonographic Findings.** A TIPS has strong echogenic walls and an anechoic lumen (Fig. 3-19, *A*). Color Doppler can confirm patency and direction of flow (Fig. 3-19, *B*; see Color Plate 5). Pulsed Doppler examination of a normal functioning TIPS should demonstrate flow toward the IVC with an average velocity of 100 to 190 cm/s. Flow with a velocity of less than 90 cm/s indicates decreased flow through the stent (shunt) and may be the result of thrombosis in the shunt. Flow velocities of more than 190 cm/s indicate high-grade stenosis within the shunt.

Hepatocellular Carcinoma

Hepatocellular carcinoma (also called malignant hepatoma) is the most common type of primary liver cancer. Patients with a history of long-standing hepatitis or cirrhosis are at a greater risk to develop HCC, and as many as 80% of patients with cirrhosis may develop this cancer. The presence of HCC rarely affects liver enzymes, although it may produce an increase in alpha fetoprotein (AFP), which is a protein normally made by the immature liver cells in the fetus. Postnatally, high blood levels of AFP are seen with liver cancer (see Table 3-3). **Sonographic Findings.** HCC can appear as diffuse texture changes throughout the liver or as focal masses. Masses can be either hypoechoic or hyperechoic (Fig. 3-20) and often have a peripheral halo surrounding them. Distinguishing between HCC and liver metastases or focal fatty liver changes without biopsy results and a strong patient history may be impossible. Portal veins or hepatic veins may be invaded by tumor infiltration from HCC. Spectral and color flow Doppler can be used to help rule out tumor invasion of these vessels.

Contrast-enhanced ultrasound imaging has been shown to be effective in documenting small lesions

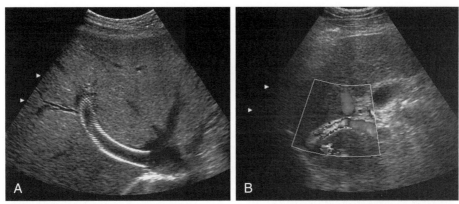

FIGURE 3-19 TIPS. **(A),** Bright, echogenic walls and anechoic lumen. **(B),** Color Doppler of TIPS demonstrating blood flow toward IVC.

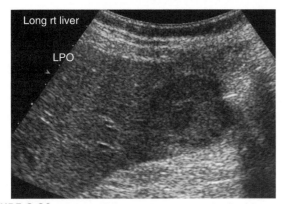

FIGURE 3-20 Hepatocellular carcinoma. Longitudinal image of a hypoechoic, heterogeneous mass in the right lobe of the liver.

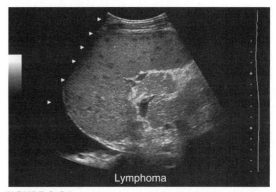

FIGURE 3-21 Lymphoma. Multiple hypoechoic masses.

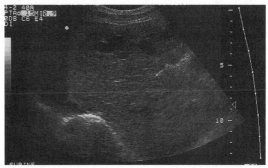

FIGURE 3-22 Lymphoma. Anechoic appearance; this can be mistaken for cystic masses.

within the liver. Contrast agents are administered intravenously before sonographic examination and enhance the detection of blood flow and parenchymal variations. Contrast-enhanced harmonic imaging with microbubble contrast agents generally causes hepatic lesions to appear hypervascular. Small hypoechoic lesions, such as hepatomas, show enhanced borders and parenchymal differentiation after contrast agent administration.

Contrast agents detect these changes with enhancement of the acoustic properties of the parenchyma. The contrast agents are eventually removed from the body by the reticuloendothelial system. Hepatic imaging must occur within 15 minutes after contrast agent administration, but effects of the agent may last longer. The ability of contrast-enhanced sonography to detect small lesions may enable patients to avoid undergoing more expensive imaging procedures such as computed tomography (CT) or magnetic resonance imaging (MRI).[2] Another advantage to contrast-enhanced ultrasound is that, in comparison to CT contrast agents, sonographic contrast agents do not cause adjacent tissues to resonate and can be administered to patients with renal failure.[3]

Lymphoma

Although lymphoma is not a disease related directly to the hepatocytes and their function, it may diffusely affect the echo texture of the liver. When multiple organs contain lymphoma, the disease is referred to as lymphosarcoma, or sarcoma. When just the lymph nodes are affected pathologically, the disease is referred to as lymphadenopathy.

Sonographic Findings. Patients with lymphoma that affects the liver have hepatomegaly and possibly splenomegaly. Hodgkin's lymphoma in the liver may appear as heterogeneous parenchyma or focal hypoechoic masses (Fig. 3-21). Non-Hodgkin's lymphoma tends to be more echogenic in sonographic appearance. Lymphomas are often anechoic and may be mistaken for cystic masses (Fig. 3-22). To distinguish lymphoma from a true cyst, the sonographer should search for true cysts to display well-defined borders, good posterior enhancement, and

TABLE 3-4	Summary of Diffuse Liver Disease Pathologies	
Pathology	**Symptoms**	**Sonographic Findings**
Fatty liver	Usually asymptomatic; may progress (see cirrhosis)	Increased echogenicity, increased attenuation, decreased penetration, difficulty visualizing vascular structures, decreased penetration
Fat sparing	Usually asymptomatic	Regions of decreased echogenicity within hyperechoic liver, often anterior to right portal vein or within left lobe
Hepatitis, acute	Flulike symptoms; nausea, vomiting, fatigue	Normal appearance or enlarged liver with decreased echogenicity, prominent periportal echoes
Hepatitis, chronic	Flulike symptoms; nausea, vomiting, fatigue; possible symptoms of cirrhosis	Coarse and hyperechoic liver parenchyma, poorly visualized vasculature
Cirrhosis, initial	Asymptomatic; peripheral edema, ascites, fatigue	Normal appearance of caudate lobe and left lateral lobe hypertrophy (caudate-to right-lobe ratio >0.65), right and left medial lobes often atrophy
Cirrhosis, long-standing	Possible nausea, anorexia, weight loss, tremors, jaundice, dark urine, fatigue, varicosities; may have symptoms of portal hypertension	Coarse parenchyma, decreased size, nodular surface, ascites
Portal hypertension	Asymptomatic; possible symptoms of cirrhosis	Enlarged portal veins, monophasic spectral tracings, hepatofugal blood flow, portal-splenic varices, ascites, splenomegaly
Hepatocellular carcinoma	Possible abdominal pain, weight loss, palpable mass, fever, jaundice and possible symptoms of chronic hepatitis or cirrhosis	Diffuse parenchymal changes, focal mass (hypoechoic or hyperechoic) with possible peripheral hypoechoic halo
Lymphoma	Enlarged, nontender lymph nodes; fever, fatigue, night sweats, weight loss, bone pain, abdominal mass	Diffuse parenchymal changes, focal hypoechoic masses with or without posterior enhancement, focal hyperechoic masses (more commonly associated with non-Hodgkin's lymphomas)
HIV	May be associated with symptoms of hepatitis B or C	Normal or similar to hepatitis

no internal echoes. Cystic masses from lymphoma usually lack well-defined borders.

Human Immunodeficiency Virus

Patients with human immunodeficiency virus (HIV) may have many organs of the body affected, and changes may be noted on sonograms. The liver may be normal in sonographic appearance, or diffuse parenchymal changes are possible. Because many patients with HIV have concurrent hepatitis B or C infection, the liver may have the same sonographic appearance as previously discussed. An increased incidence of cholangitis and biliary duct pathologies (see Chapter 1) is also noted in patients with HIV.[4]

Table 3-4 summarizes the pathology, symptoms, and sonographic findings of diffuse liver disease.

SUMMARY

Sonographic evaluation of liver parenchyma and the portal venous circulation can help in the diagnosis and follow-up of diffuse liver diseases. Patient history and laboratory values are important in developing a differential diagnosis. A definitive diagnosis is often not possible without a biopsy.

CLINICAL SCENARIO—DIAGNOSIS

Based on the elevated laboratory values, the change in liver echogenicity, and the lack of flow within the portal vein, advanced hepatocellular disease is the most likely diagnosis. Cirrhosis is a form of hepatocellular disease. Cirrhosis develops as a result of long-term continuous damage to the liver. There can be many causes for hepatocellular disease. In this patient, hepatitis was proven histologically (with biopsy) to be the cause. When healthy liver tissue is destroyed and replaced by scar tissue, hepatocellular disease becomes serious. It may lead to portal hypertension or portal vein thrombosis, which is present in this patient.

The echogenic, vascular mass is also significant in this patient. This mass could represent focal fatty liver infiltration, if the patient were obese and other findings were lacking. A liver mass found in a patient with long-standing cirrhosis makes this mass highly suspicious for HCC. Another possible cause for this mass is a regenerating nodule. After biopsy, this mass was proven to be HCC. A parenchymal biopsy of the liver tissue and a CT scan supported and confirmed the diagnosis of cirrhosis caused by chronic hepatitis.

CASE STUDIES FOR DISCUSSION

1. A 34-year-old man undergoes sonographic evaluation of the right upper quadrant. The patient presents with slightly elevated AST, ALT, and direct bilirubin. Initial imaging (Fig. 3-23) demonstrates ascites and irregularity of the surface of the liver. What do the presence of ascites and this appearance of the liver surface most likely indicate? What other images should the sonographer obtain to help confirm the diagnosis for this patient?

2. A 51-year-old man is referred for sonography of the abdomen because of vague upper abdominal fullness. The patient reports a history of moderate alcohol use. AST and ALT are mildly elevated. The sonogram reveals the findings seen in Figure 3-24. What diagnosis is supported by the sonographic findings? What role does the patient's history play in this case?

3. A 47-year-old woman with hepatitis C virus was admitted to the hospital because of increasing abdominal girth. Laboratory values showed a typical pattern of elevated liver enzymes seen with cirrhosis. Sonography of the liver was requested, and the findings are shown in Figure 3-25 (see Color Plate 6). What finding does this represent, and what additional images should the sonographer obtain in this examination?

4. A moderately overweight woman undergoes sonographic examination. A hypoechoic mass is noted anterior to the right portal vein (Fig. 3-26). All liver-related laboratory values are within normal limits. Discuss the diagnostic options and reasoning for your opinion.

5. A 63-year-old man presents with symptoms related to cirrhotic liver disease and possible portal hypertension. While assessing his liver, you note blood flow in a vessel between the left lateral and medial lobes of the liver (Fig. 3-27). What does this region of flow likely represent? What other sonographic changes might you expect to encounter?

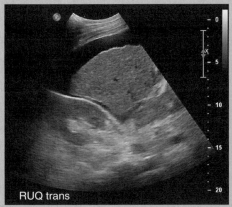

FIGURE 3-23 Right upper quadrant image shows ascites and scalloped surface of the liver.

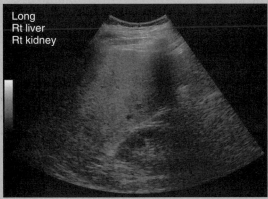

FIGURE 3-24 Longitudinal image of echogenic liver; vascular structures are poorly visualized.

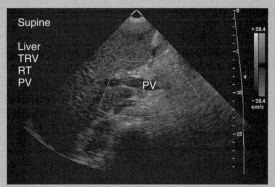

FIGURE 3-25 Transverse midline image.

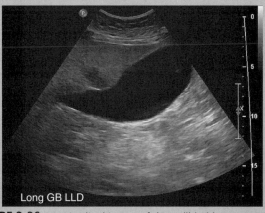

FIGURE 3-26 Longitudinal image of the gallbladder. Hypoechoic mass effect is anterior to the gallbladder. *(Courtesy Elizabeth Jacob.)*

Continued

CASE STUDIES FOR DISCUSSION—cont'd

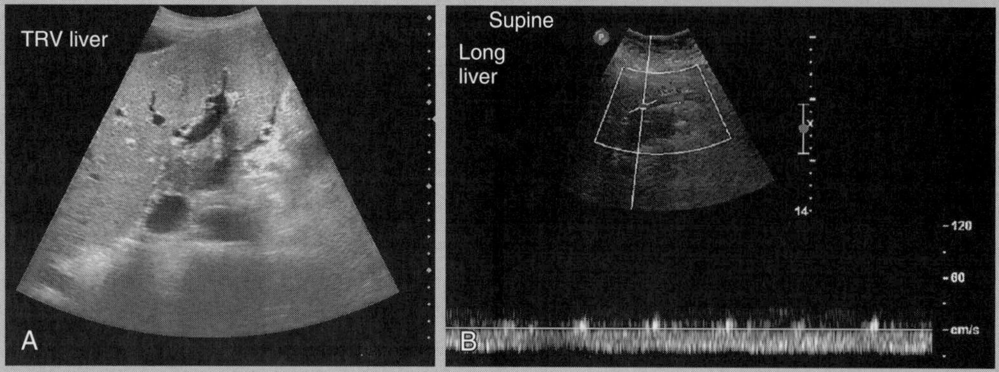

FIGURE 3-27 (A), Transverse image of the liver at the level of the ligament of teres. **(B),** Flow is noted in the region between the left medial and left lateral lobes of the liver.

STUDY QUESTIONS

1. A right upper quadrant sonogram has been ordered to rule out gallbladder disease in an obese 47-year-old woman. The right upper quadrant organs appear mostly normal; however, the liver is hyperechoic, with a 5.4 cm × 3.5 cm × 3.0 cm, poorly defined, hypoechoic area in the right lobe, anterior to the gallbladder. All laboratory values are within normal ranges. Which of the following diagnoses is most likely?
   a. Lymphoma
   b. Hepatocellular carcinoma
   c. Focal fatty infiltration
   d. Focal fat sparing

2. The liver is evaluated with a high-frequency transducer. Ascites and significant scalloping of the surface of the liver are noted. These findings most likely represent:
   a. A regenerating nodule
   b. Cirrhosis
   c. Lymphoma
   d. Fat sparing

3. The liver is evaluated with color Doppler through the right intercostal spaces. The color Doppler images show flow in the main portal vein to be "away from" the transducer. This finding indicates:
   a. Stenosis
   b. Hepatofugal flow
   c. A normal venous finding
   d. The presence of varices

4. A patient presents with elevated AST and ALT. She has a history of colon carcinoma. The liver sonogram demonstrates a liver of normal size and echogenicity. No liver masses are noted. What is the most likely explanation for the elevated enzymes?
   a. Metastatic bone disease
   b. Hepatocellular carcinoma
   c. Lymphoma
   d. Fat sparing

5. A moderately obese patient with slightly elevated AST, ALT, and direct bilirubin is referred for liver sonography. The patient has no previous significant medical history. The liver sonogram demonstrates an overall hyperechoic appearance. The hepatic vasculature was difficult to visualize. What is the most likely explanation for these findings?
   a. Cirrhosis
   b. Fatty liver disease
   c. Chronic hepatitis
   d. Portal hypertension

6. A patient presents with moderately elevated AST and markedly elevated ALT. The patient has a history of drug abuse and needle-sharing. A liver sonogram reveals an overall hypoechoic appearance. The smaller portal veins appear more echogenic than normal. The liver is enlarged, measuring 19 cm from superior to inferior border. What is the most likely explanation for these findings?
   a. Cirrhosis
   b. Fatty liver disease
   c. Acute hepatitis
   d. Fat sparing

7. A patient with a history of chronic hepatitis C presents with two hypoechoic liver masses, one in the left lobe and one in the right lobe. The masses display halos. A likely conclusion is the presence of:
   a. Metastatic liver disease
   b. Hepatocellular carcinoma
   c. Lymphoma
   d. Fat sparing

8. A patient with biopsy-proven cirrhosis is referred for sonographic evaluation of the liver. Which lobe of the liver should the sonographer expect to demonstrate hypertrophy?
   a. Right medial segment
   b. Left lateral segment
   c. Caudate
   d. Right

9. A TIPS evaluation with pulsed-wave Doppler demonstrates a peak systolic velocity in the shunt of 216 cm/s. This finding suggests:
   a. The presence of varices
   b. Normal-functioning TIPS
   c. Occlusion of the shunt
   d. TIPS stenosis

10. A patient with cirrhosis and portal hypertension is referred for sonographic evaluation. A hypoechoic, tubular structure in the region of the ligament of teres is noted. Within this structure, pulsed-wave and color Doppler demonstrate blood flow exiting the liver. This finding most likely represents:
    a. A regenerating nodule
    b. A failed TIPS
    c. Esophageal varices
    d. Recanalization of the umbilical vein

REFERENCES

1. Wolf DC: *Cirrhosis*. Emedicine.medscape.com. http://emedicine.medscape.com/article/185856-overview. Retrieved February 18, 2012.
2. Numata K, et al: Contrast-enhanced wide-band harmonic gray scale imaging of hepatocellular carcinoma: correlation with helical computed tomographic findings, *J Diag Med Sonogr* 20:89–97, 2001.
3. Merton DA: Contrast enhanced hepatic sonography, *J Ultrasound Med* 18:5–15, 2002.
4. Mortelé K, Segatto E, Ross P: The infected liver: radiologic-pathologic correlation, *Radiographics* 32:937–955, 2004.

Epigastric Pain

Joyce Grube, Kathryn Kuntz

CLINICAL SCENARIO

A 69-year-old man presents with moderate to severe epigastric pain that he describes as "gnawing." He also reports a recent 15-lb weight loss and a slight "yellow tinge to his eyeballs." He is a heavy smoker and uses alcohol in moderation. Electrocardiogram results are normal, and an acute cardiac event is ruled out. Laboratory results reveal elevated direct bilirubin. An abdominal sonogram is ordered and reveals the findings shown in Figure 4-1.

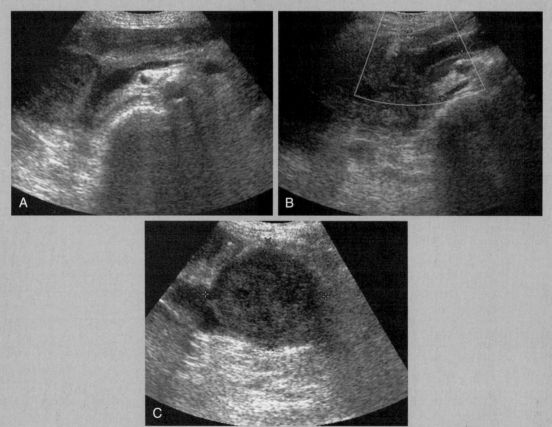

FIGURE 4-1 **(A),** Transverse image shows a hypoechoic mass in the head of pancreas. **(B),** Color Doppler demonstrates absence of flow in dilated pancreatic duct. **(C),** Longitudinal image shows mass with dilated common bile duct.

OBJECTIVES

- List several causes of epigastric pain not associated with pancreatic disease.
- Describe the normal sonographic appearance of the pancreas and surrounding structures.
- Describe the sonographic appearance of common inflammations of the pancreas.
- Describe the sonographic appearance of common benign and malignant neoplasms of the pancreas.
- List the risk factors associated with various diseases of the pancreas.
- Identify pertinent laboratory values associated with specific diseases of the pancreas.

Initial sonographic evaluation of a patient with epigastric pain may reveal a broad spectrum of findings. If the pancreas appears normal, the clinician must include inflammation of the pancreas and other pathology not related to the pancreas among the differential diagnoses. Diagnoses not specific to the pancreas may include gastric or duodenal ulcer disease, gastric reflux disease or esophagitis, diverticulitis of the transverse colon, biliary disease, liver abscess, heart disease, or aortic dissection. Diseases that cause epigastric pain specific to the pancreas are discussed in this chapter.

Although computed tomography (CT) plays a primary role in evaluation of the pancreas for disease, sonography is more readily available, is more cost-effective, and offers a nonradiation alternative for the evaluation of epigastric pain. The pancreas is often thought of as the most difficult organ in the abdomen to image. Sonographers may improve visualization of the pancreas by employing (1) a complete understanding of the surrounding anatomy and gastrointestinal structures, (2)

persistence while scanning, (3) image optimization, and (4) oral contrast agents.

Nonetheless, sonography plays a significant role in the evaluation of patients with jaundice, serial examination of inflammatory processes, and needle guidance for interventional procedures of the pancreas.

PANCREAS

Normal Sonographic Anatomy

The pancreas is a retroperitoneal organ that lies in the anterior pararenal space of the epigastrium. The entire pancreas is contained between the C-loop of the duodenum and the splenic hilum. The parts of the pancreas include the head, uncinate process, neck, body, and tail (Fig. 4-2). A normal adult pancreas is approximately 12 to 15 cm in length. A normal pancreatic duct may be visualized at a measurement of 2 mm or less.

The echogenicity of the pancreas is isoechoic to hyperechoic compared with the liver and may increase with age and obesity because of fatty infiltration. In children, the pancreas may appear proportionally larger and more hypoechoic to isoechoic compared with the liver because of less fat composition.

The lie of the pancreas in the epigastrium is transverse yet slightly oblique, with the head located more inferior than the tail. The pancreas is a nonencapsulated organ, so the borders are indistinct on sonography. The sonographer must have a thorough understanding of the surrounding vasculature to aid in the detection of the pancreatic boundaries (Fig. 4-3).

The sonographer must also appreciate the portions of the gastrointestinal tract that surround the pancreas

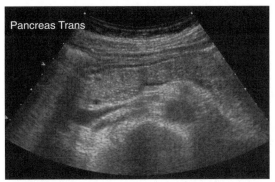

FIGURE 4-2 Transverse image of normal pancreas.

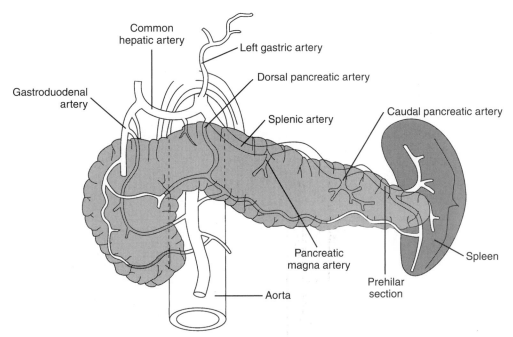

FIGURE 4-3 Pancreatic vasculature.

and make visualization difficult. The fundus of the stomach lies superior to the pancreatic tail. The body of the stomach lies anterior to the pancreatic tail. The pylorus lies anterior to the pancreatic body and neck. The superior duodenum (first portion) lies anterior to the pancreatic neck and superior to the head of the pancreas. The descending duodenum (second portion) lies lateral to the head. The horizontal duodenum (third portion) lies inferior to the pancreatic head. The ascending duodenum (fourth portion) lies inferior to the body of the pancreas. The transverse colon lies anterior and inferior to the entire length of the pancreas (Fig. 4-4). Identification of the various portions of the gastrointestinal tract during scanning allows the sonographer to change the patient position to move obscuring bowel away from the pancreas.

Harmonics may enable the sonographer to optimize visualization of the pancreas, especially in technically difficult cases. Harmonic imaging is based on the concept that an ultrasound pulse interacts with tissue, and echoes are created at the original or fundamental frequency along with echoes at multiples of the original frequency (i.e., a 2-MHz pulse generates echoes at 2 MHz, 4 MHz [second harmonic], 6 MHz, [third harmonic], 8 MHz [fourth harmonic]). Conventional ultrasound listens to the fundamental frequency and ignores the harmonic frequencies. Tissue harmonic

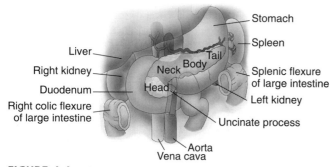

FIGURE 4-4 Relationship of the stomach, duodenum, and transverse colon with the pancreas.

imaging typically uses the second harmonic frequency for improved image clarity. Harmonic imaging in the abdomen may also reduce image artifacts, haze, and clutter, and significantly improve contrast resolution (Fig. 4-5).

If the pancreatic tail is the primary area of interest, the sonographer or physician may elect to use an oral contrast agent to complement the study. A cellulose suspension should remain in the stomach for an adequate period to provide an acoustic window for better visualization of the pancreatic tail. Alternatively, distilled water can be used to enhance visualization (Fig. 4-6). Although oral contrast agents are not yet used consistently in day-to-day practice, the use of intravenous ultrasound contrast agents shows significant potential.

PANCREATITIS

Acute Pancreatitis

Acute pancreatitis is characterized by the escape of toxic pancreatic juices into the parenchymal tissues of the gland. These digestive enzymes cause destruction of the acini, ducts, small blood vessels, and fat and may extend beyond the gland to peripancreatic tissues. Acute inflammation of the pancreas is generally caused by one of two factors: biliary disease and alcoholism. Other sources of inflammation may include trauma, pregnancy, peptic ulcer disease, medications, hereditary factors, systemic infections, posttransplant complications, and iatrogenic causes (e.g., endoscopic retrograde cholangiopancreatogram [ERCP] endoscopy). Patients with acute pancreatitis have a sudden onset of persistent midepigastric pain that may be moderate to severe and often radiates to the midback. Fever and leukocytosis accompany the attack. Classically, serum amylase levels increase within 24 hours of onset, and lipase levels increase within 72 hours. **Sonographic Findings.** The pancreas may appear normal in the early stage of acute pancreatitis, with no noticeable change in the size or echogenicity of the gland.

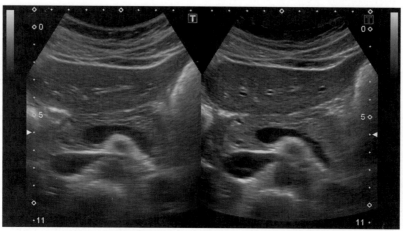

FIGURE 4-5 Harmonic imaging.

Once changes become evident, acute pancreatitis may have a diffuse or focal appearance on sonographic examination. The pancreatic duct may be enlarged in either presentation. Diffuse disease causes an increase in size and a decrease in echogenicity from swelling and congestion (Fig. 4-7). The borders of the pancreas may appear irregular. Focal inflammation may be seen as enlargement and a hypoechoic appearance to a specific region of the gland. If focal pancreatitis is present in the pancreatic head, biliary dilation and a Courvoisier's gallbladder may also be appreciated. The sonographer must carefully evaluate the pancreatic head for adenocarcinoma and the biliary tree for the presence of cholelithiasis and choledocholithiasis as possible causes of pancreatitis.

Chronic Pancreatitis

Chronic pancreatitis is defined as recurrent attacks of acute inflammation of the pancreas. Further destruction of the pancreatic parenchyma results in atrophy, fibrosis, scarring, and calcification of the gland. Stone formation within the pancreatic duct is common, and pancreatic pseudocysts develop in 25% to 40% of patients.[1,2] Patients generally have progressing epigastric pain. Jaundice may also be seen in patients with a distal biliary duct obstruction.

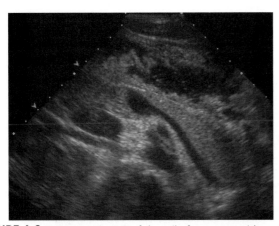

FIGURE 4-6 Transverse image of the tail of pancreas with water as an oral contrast agent.

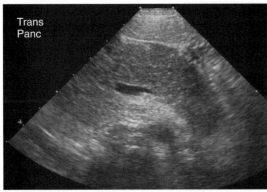

FIGURE 4-7 Acute pancreatitis. Transverse image shows increase in size and decrease in echogenicity from swelling and congestion.

Sonographic Findings. On sonography, the pancreas generally appears smaller than normal and hyperechoic because of scarring and fibrosis. Diffuse calcifications are the classic sonographic feature of chronic pancreatitis and are usually noted throughout the parenchyma, causing a coarse echotexture (Fig. 4-8, *A*). Stones may also be visualized within a dilated pancreatic duct (Fig. 4-8, *B* and *C*). Associated findings include pseudocyst formation, cholelithiasis, choledocholithiasis, and portal-splenic thrombosis.

Pseudocysts

Pseudocysts are composed of extravasated pancreatic enzymes that escape into the peripancreatic soft tissues. The fluid begins to collect, and eventually a thickened wall of collagen and granulation tissue develops (different from the thin, epithelial cell wall of a true cyst). Pseudocysts may result from acute and chronic pancreatitis or from trauma to the pancreas. Pseudocysts can be singular or multiple. Most often, they arise from the tail of the pancreas and are located in the lesser sac. Less often, they may be located in the right and left anterior pararenal spaces, peritoneum, mesentery, pelvis, groin, or mediastinum. Pseudocysts may be large on initial diagnosis because of late symptoms from compression effects. Aspiration or surgery is necessary in 80% of pancreatic pseudocysts, and 20% resolve spontaneously.[3]

Sonographic Findings. Pancreatic pseudocysts are generally well defined and internally anechoic with posterior acoustic enhancement (Fig. 4-9). Occasionally, they may appear complex with internal echoes from inflammation, hemorrhage, or necrosis. They may also have internal septations or calcified walls. Serial sonographic examination is an excellent method for following spontaneous regression of pseudocysts. Sonography also plays a useful role in guiding percutaneous aspiration of pseudocysts.

PANCREATIC NEOPLASMS

Adenocarcinoma

The most common form of pancreatic cancer is adenocarcinoma. It is a highly aggressive cancer. Adenocarcinoma arises from the pancreatic ductal epithelium and rarely from the acini. Men are more often affected than women, and peak incidence is between 60 and 80 years of age. Mortality from pancreatic cancer increased in high-income countries between the 1950s and the 1980s and has been leveling off since, particularly in men.[1] In men, carcinoma of the pancreas is the fourth most common cause of cancer death after lung, prostate, and colorectal cancer. In women, it is the fifth most common cause of cancer death. Risk factors for pancreatic cancer include high-fat diet, smoking, chronic pancreatitis, primary sclerosing cholangitis, hereditary

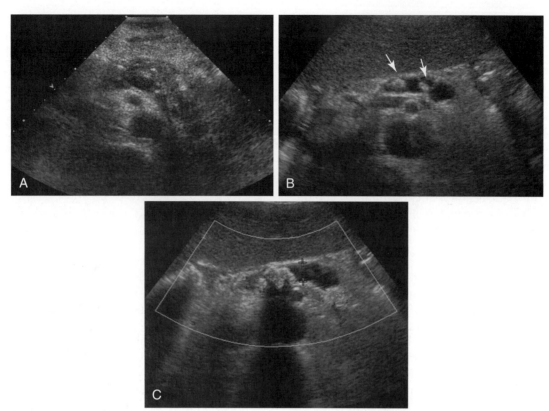

FIGURE 4-8 Chronic pancreatitis. **(A)**, Transverse image shows diffuse calcifications throughout the parenchyma, causing a coarse echotexture. **(B)** and **(C)**, Calcifications within dilated pancreatic duct.

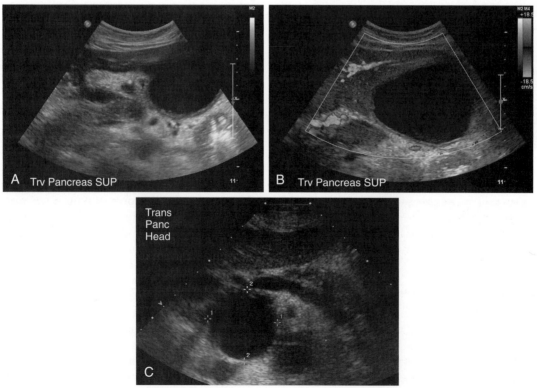

FIGURE 4-9 Pseudocysts. A well-defined mass is demonstrated in the tail **(A)** and **(B)**, and typical location in the head is demonstrated **(C)**. Pseudocysts are internally anechoic with posterior acoustic enhancement.

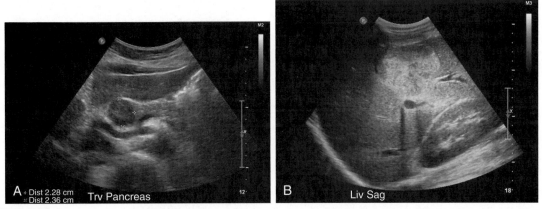

FIGURE 4-10 Adenocarcinoma. **(A)**, Irregular, hypoechoic mass in the head of pancreas. **(B)**, Associated liver metastasis.

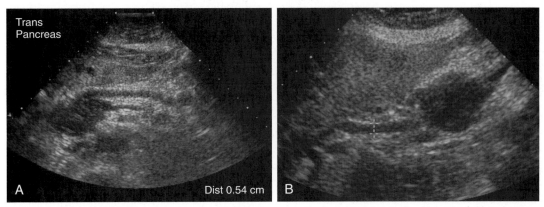

FIGURE 4-11 Double duct sign. **(A)**, Transverse image of dilated pancreatic duct. **(B)**, Longitudinal image of dilated common bile duct.

pancreatitis, family history of pancreatic cancer, and diabetes mellitus.[2]

Adenocarcinoma is most commonly found in the head of the pancreas and least commonly in the tail. The most frequently recognized symptom is a persistent, aching pain in the midepigastrium or midback. The type and onset of symptoms are also related to the location of the tumor. Tumors that arise from the pancreatic head cause constriction of the distal biliary duct, and symptoms are seen fairly early. Patients typically have a palpable gallbladder and obstructive jaundice. If the tumor arises from the pancreatic body or tail, symptoms tend to manifest later in the disease, and metastasis is likely. Patients may have weight loss, nausea and vomiting, diabetes, and intestinal malabsorption.

Other malignant tumors that affect the pancreas include cystadenocarcinoma, malignant islet cell tumors, ampullary carcinoma, squamous cell carcinoma, and lymphoma.

Sonographic Findings. The most common sonographic appearance of adenocarcinoma is an irregular hypoechoic mass in the pancreas (Fig. 4-10, *A*). Isoechoic tumors may simply be seen as enlargement or an irregular contour of a specific region of the pancreas. If the tumor is large on initial diagnosis, compression or deviation of adjacent structures may be evident. Sonographers must also rely on indirect sonographic features

of adenocarcinoma, which may include pancreatic duct dilation, displacement of vasculature surrounding the pancreas, Courvoisier's gallbladder, dilated extrahepatic and intrahepatic bile ducts, biliary sludge, lymphadenopathy, and liver metastasis (Fig. 4-10, *B*). The double duct sign of a dilated pancreatic duct (Fig. 4-11, *A*) and dilated bile duct (Fig. 4-11, *B*) has been described as the hallmark feature of periampullary pancreatic cancer.

Cystadenoma

Cystadenoma of the pancreas is a rare cystic tumor that arises from the pancreatic duct tissues and typically affects women more often than men. Cystadenoma may be microcystic serous type (cysts measure <2 cm) (Fig. 4-12) or macrocystic mucinous type (cysts measure >2 cm) (Fig. 4-13). The microcystic form is always benign, and the macrocystic form is associated with suspicion of malignant disease (cystadenocarcinoma). Cystadenoma occurs more frequently in the body and tail of the pancreas. It may be unilocular or multilocular and may have internal echoes, septations, papillary projections, and calcifications. Patients may be asymptomatic or have epigastric pain, weight loss, palpable abdominal mass, or jaundice.

Sonographic Findings. Cystadenoma has various sonographic appearances. It generally appears as a

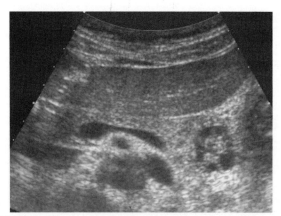

FIGURE 4-12 Microcystic cystadenoma in the tail of pancreas.

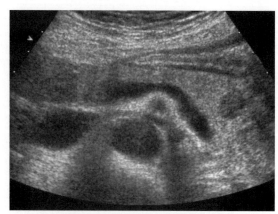

FIGURE 4-14 Functioning islet cell tumor.

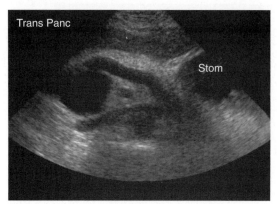

FIGURE 4-13 Macrocystic cystadenoma in the head of pancreas.

single or lobulated anechoic mass with posterior acoustic enhancement. It may have internal septations, thick walls, internal echoes, papillary projections, calcifications, or an overall solid appearance. Differentiation between benign and malignant tumors is impossible without histopathology. Cystadenoma may also appear similar to pseudocysts, polycystic disease, cystic fibrosis, and von Hippel-Lindau disease.[4]

Islet Cell Tumors

Islet cell tumors of the pancreas are primary tumors that arise from the islets of Langerhans. They are classified as functioning or nonfunctioning based on their potential to secrete hormones. Nonfunctioning islet cell tumors constitute approximately 30% of all islet cell tumors and have a tendency to be malignant. Functioning islet cell tumors are more often benign, with the two most common known as insulinomas and gastrinomas. Patients with insulinomas may have obesity and hypoglycemic episodes. Islet cell tumors are slow-growing small tumors that are generally found in the body and tail of the pancreas. Multiple islet cell tumors may be present on diagnosis.

Sonographic Findings. Most islet cell tumors are hypoechoic compared with the surrounding pancreas tissues (Fig. 4-14). Visualization of these tumors is difficult

because of their small size. Intraoperative ultrasound has been extremely valuable in identifying and localizing islet cell tumors. Harmonic imaging, as part of image optimization techniques, may also improve the detection of small tumors.[5]

Table 4-1 summarizes the pathology, location, and sonographic findings of pancreatic masses.

SUMMARY

Sonographic assessment of a patient with epigastric pain may be performed to help determine the initial diagnosis or as a follow-up examination of pancreatic disease. New techniques are being applied to imaging of the pancreas. Contrast-enhanced ultrasound is gaining influence in Europe and Asia. This technique uses the combination of microbubbles of gas that enhance the echogenicity of blood flow and tissue harmonic imaging that uses an ultrasound frequency twice as high as standard sonography to improve the assessment of vascularity of lesions. PET/CT scans, which allow image fusion from positron emission tomography (PET) and CT, have improved tumor identification.[6] Sonography provides valuable information in differentiation of solid and cystic tumors, assessment of tumor extent, provision of serial evaluation, and performance of interventional treatments of pancreatic diseases. Clinicians should recognize the feasibility of sonography for precise diagnosis and avoidance of unnecessary and costly examinations for the patient.

CLINICAL SCENARIO—DIAGNOSIS

This patient has an adenocarcinoma in the head of the pancreas. The clinical history details of being male, smoking, abdominal pain, weight loss, and jaundice also support the diagnosis. The sonogram reveals an irregular, ill-defined, solid mass in the head of the pancreas (see Fig. 4-1, *A* and *B*). Because of its location, the mass is obstructing the common bile duct (see Fig. 4-1, *C*) and causing obstructive jaundice and elevated direct bilirubin on laboratory tests.

TABLE 4-1	Pancreatic Masses	
Pathology	**Typical Location**	**Sonographic Findings**
Pseudocyst	Tail	Anechoic, posterior enhancement; may also appear complex with internal septations or calcified walls
Adenocarcinoma	Head	Irregular, hypoechoic mass; may have secondary pancreatic duct dilation, biliary dilation, lymphadenopathy, and liver metastasis
Cystadenoma	Body and tail	Single or lobulated anechoic mass, posterior enhancement; may have internal septations, thick walls, internal echoes, papillary projections, calcifications, or solid appearance
Microcystic		
Macrocystic		
Cystadenocarcinoma		
Islet cell tumor	Body and tail	Hypoechoic, small
Malignant islet cell tumor		
Insulinoma		
Gastrinoma		

CASE STUDIES FOR DISCUSSION

1. A 33-year-old man with a history of alcoholism presents with acute onset of epigastric pain, nausea and vomiting, elevated white blood cell (WBC) count, elevated serum amylase, and increasing lipase level. The entire pancreas appears enlarged and hypoechoic, with well-defined borders (Fig. 4-15). What is the most likely diagnosis?

2. A 55-year-old, moderately obese woman with previous cholelithiasis returns to her physician for a 6-month follow-up examination after cholecystectomy. She now has mild to moderate, intermittent epigastric pain and occasional fever. Sonographic results show choledocholithiasis, a dilated pancreatic duct, and fluid collection anterior to the tail of the pancreas (Fig. 4-16). Discuss the most likely cause for the sonographic findings.

3. A 41-year-old obese woman presents in acute distress. The family member accompanying her reports that her initial symptoms were mild and included anxiety and hunger. Earlier in the day, she began to have what appears to have been a seizure. Imaging studies are ordered, and the sonogram reveals a small hypoechoic lesion (Fig. 4-17) that measures approximately 1 cm. Discuss the patient history and likely reason for the sonographic finding.

4. A 50-year-old woman undergoes a sonogram for nonspecific abdominal pain and a feeling of general malaise. While scanning the upper abdomen, the sonographer notices a multicystic mass in the tail of the pancreas (Fig. 4-18). The patient denies any history of smoking or alcohol abuse. Laboratory tests are unremarkable. A CT scan was performed and confirmed that the multicystic lesion was arising from the pancreas. Discuss the diagnostic possibilities for this mass.

5. A 75-year-old man is referred for an abdominal sonogram to rule out gallstones and biliary disease. He reports recent significant epigastric pain and recent weight loss. The sonogram reveals the findings shown in Figure 4-19. What is the most likely cause for these findings?

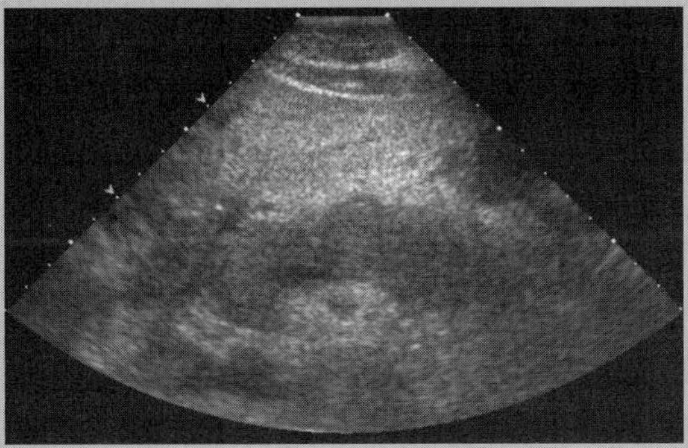

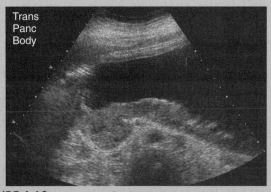

FIGURE 4-16 Large cystic fluid collection, anterior to pancreas.

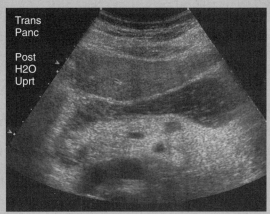

FIGURE 4-17 Small (<1 cm) hypoechoic mass in the body of pancreas.

FIGURE 4-15 Transverse, diffusely enlarged, hypoechoic pancreas.

Continued

CASE STUDIES FOR DISCUSSION—cont'd

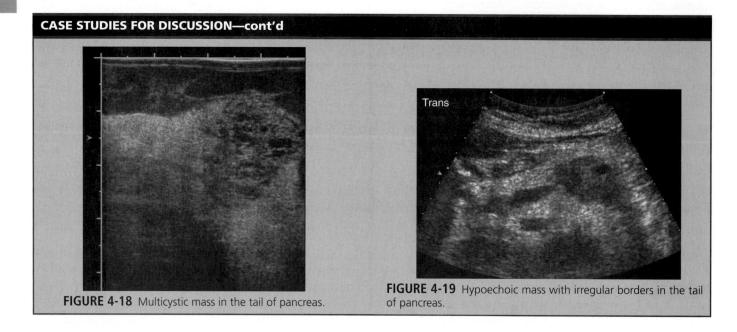

FIGURE 4-18 Multicystic mass in the tail of pancreas.

FIGURE 4-19 Hypoechoic mass with irregular borders in the tail of pancreas.

STUDY QUESTIONS

1. Pancreatic tumors that have the potential to secrete hormones are known as:
   a. Adenocarcinoma
   b. Microcystic cystadenomas
   c. Functioning islet cell tumors
   d. von Hippel-Lindau disease

2. A history of previous biliary surgery, intermittent epigastric pain, and occasional fever and the sonographic finding of a fluid collection anterior to the tail of the pancreas support which of the following entities?
   a. Acute focal pancreatitis
   b. Acute diffuse pancreatitis
   c. Chronic pancreatitis
   d. Pseudocyst

3. Acute pancreatitis often manifests with which of the following clinical signs or symptoms?
   a. Obstructive jaundice
   b. Palpable gallbladder
   c. Sudden, severe onset of epigastric pain
   d. Elevated direct bilirubin
   e. Decreasing hematocrit

4. Adenocarcinoma of the pancreas has a high mortality rate and occurs most often in:
   a. Women younger than age 60
   b. Women older than age 60
   c. Men older than age 60
   d. Men younger than age 60

5. Courvoisier's gallbladder, pancreatic duct dilation, liver metastasis, and a dilated biliary tract all are considered:
   a. Signs of pseudocyst formation
   b. Suspicious for functioning islet cell tumor
   c. Direct signs of pancreatic neoplasm
   d. Indirect signs of pancreatic adenocarcinoma

6. Which of the following pancreatic neoplasms occurs more frequently in the body and tail and is associated with a suspicion for malignant conversion?
   a. Pseudocyst
   b. Microcystic cystadenoma
   c. Macrocystic cystadenoma
   d. Islet cell tumor
   e. von Hippel-Lindau disease

7. A technique that uses microbubbles of gas to enhance the echogenicity of blood flow and improve the assessment of vascularity of lesions is known as:
   a. Variable focusing capability
   b. Power Doppler
   c. Harmonic imaging
   d. Contrast-enhanced ultrasound

8. Pseudocyst formation in the pancreas is associated with all of the following except:
   a. Acute pancreatitis
   b. Chronic pancreatitis
   c. von Hippel-Lindau disease
   d. Trauma

9. An oral contrast agent is used during pancreatic sonography to improve visualization of which of the following structures?
   a. Head of the pancreas
   b. Tail of the pancreas
   c. Peripancreatic tissues
   d. Uncinate process of the pancreas

10. Atrophy, fibrosis, scarring, and calcification of the pancreas are consistent with which of the following pancreatic pathologies?
    a. Chronic pancreatitis
    b. Acute pancreatitis
    c. Functioning islet cell tumor
    d. Nonfunctioning islet cell tumor

REFERENCES

1. Bosetti C, et al: Pancreatic cancer: overview of descriptive epidemiology, *Mol Carcinog* 51:3–13, 2012.
2. Krejs GJ: Pancreatic cancer: epidemiology and risk factors, *Dig Dis* 28:355–358, 2010.
3. Habashi S, Draganov PV: Pancreatic pseudocyst, *World J Gastroenterol* 15:38–47, 2009.
4. Scott J, et al: Mucinous cystic neoplasms of the pancreas: imaging features and diagnostic difficulties, *Clin Radiol* 55:187–192, 2000.
5. Ding H, et al: Sonographic diagnosis of pancreatic islet cell tumor: value of intermittent harmonic imaging, *J Clin Ultrasound* 29:411–416, 2001.
6. Kwon RS, Brugge WR: New advances in pancreatic imaging, *Curr Opin Gastroenterol* 21:561–567, 2005.

5

Hematuria

Kerry Weinberg, Kathryn Kuntz

CLINICAL SCENARIO

A 65-year-old man is referred for an abdominal sonogram following an episode of right upper quadrant pain. During the physical examination and interview, the patient reports that he also has painless hematuria. His physician suspects gallstones. The patient is mildly obese, is mildly hypertensive, and smokes. The sonogram reveals a normal gallbladder, an incidental finding of a small aortic aneurysm, and a 5-cm mass arising from the midlateral aspect of the right kidney (Fig. 5-1). What does the renal mass most likely represent?

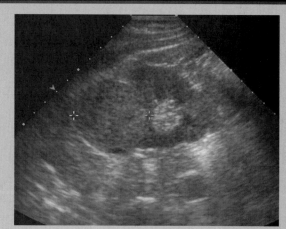

FIGURE 5-1 Solid mass arising from the kidney.

OBJECTIVES

- Describe the sonographic appearance of the genitourinary system.
- List the causes of hematuria.
- Describe the sonographic appearance of urolithiasis.
- Describe the sonographic appearance of common benign neoplasms of the kidney.
- Describe the sonographic appearance of common malignant neoplasms of the kidney.
- Describe the clinical signs and symptoms and laboratory tests associated with hematuria.

Hematuria is often the first sign of a urinary tract problem. The cause of hematuria may be anywhere within the urinary system (kidney, ureters, bladder, or urethra) or outside the urinary system (enlarged prostate or gynecologic problem). The amount of blood in the urine can vary from gross (visible) hematuria to microscopic hematuria. Problems of the lower urinary tract (i.e., ureter or bladder) are more likely to have gross hematuria than are problems of the upper urinary tract (i.e., kidney). Patients presenting with gross hematuria are at a higher risk of having a malignancy than patients with microscopic hematuria.[1]

Hematuria is a nonspecific finding, and the most common causes are acute infection (see Chapter 6), stones within the urinary tract, or tumor. Other, less common causes include trauma, congenital anomaly, renal vein thrombosis, renal cysts, renal infarction, sickle cell disease, enlarged prostate (see Chapter 30), and bleeding disorders, or the cause may be unknown or undetected. In children, blunt or penetrating trauma is the most common cause of urinary tract injury. Hematuria in children may also be caused by nephroblastomas (see Chapter 9). In most cases of microscopic hematuria, imaging is not necessary unless there are associated injuries.

Urinary tract diseases may not be diagnosed during the early stages, when many patients are asymptomatic and do not have urine discoloration, unless the amount of red blood cells is significant. The symptoms are primarily related to the cause of the hematuria. Patients with a bladder or kidney tumor, polycystic renal disease, hydronephrosis, benign prostatic hyperplasia, or urolithiasis may not have pain. Patients passing a stone have

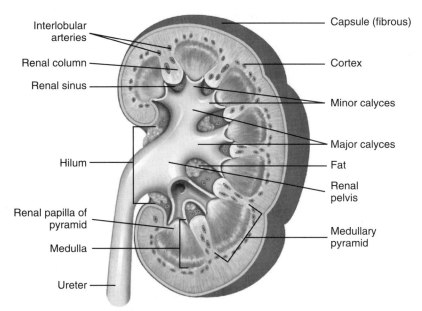

FIGURE 5-2 Internal anatomy of the kidney.

pain or renal colic. Other symptoms include flank pain, fever, vomiting, nausea, fatigue, and dysuria.

Urinalysis is performed to confirm the presence of blood in the urine. A culture may also be performed to detect whether bacteria or tumor cells are present in the urine. Patients who are at high risk for significant renal disease have a history of smoking, have a history of occupational exposure to toxic chemicals and dyes, are older than age 40, have had prior urinary tract infections or symptoms of irritative voiding, or have had prior urinary tract disease. Patients who have abused analgesics or have had pelvic irradiation are also at a higher risk for microscopic hematuria. When hematuria is detected, a urologic consultation, cystoscopy, intravenous pyelogram (IVP) or excretory urography, computed tomography (CT), magnetic resonance imaging (MRI), renal sonographic examination, or transurethral sonography may be performed to determine the pathology. The use of three-dimensional sonography and three-dimensional contrast-enhanced sonographic examinations has shown promise in differentiating between noninvasive and invasive tumors, especially in the case of bladder tumors.[2] This chapter presents some conditions responsible for hematuria that can be evaluated sonographically.

GENITOURINARY SYSTEM

Normal Sonographic Anatomy

The kidneys are oval or bean-shaped organs that measure approximately 11 cm × 7 cm × 3 cm. They are retroperitoneal and lie anterior to the psoas muscles in the paralumbar region at the level of the twelfth thoracic vertebra (T12) and the third lumbar vertebra (L3). The upper poles lie more medial than the lower poles. The liver usually causes the right kidney to be situated slightly lower than the left kidney.

The kidneys have a well-defined border with three layers of protective tissue. The inner or true layer is a fibrous capsule that is continuous with the outer layer of the ureters. It protects the kidney from infection. The middle layer is called the perinephric capsule and is composed of adipose tissue. It helps hold the kidney in place and protects the kidney from trauma. The outer layer, which surrounds the kidney and adrenal gland, is called Gerota's fascia. It consists of fibrous connective tissues that protect and anchor the kidney.

The inner anatomy of the kidney consists of the following three distinct sections: the renal parenchyma (cortex), medullary pyramids (which collect and transport urine to the collecting system), and renal sinus (which contains the collecting system, vessels, fat, and lymphatic tissue) (Fig. 5-2).

Sonographically, the renal sinus is the echogenic oval region in the midportion of the kidney, the renal cortex has a midlevel echogenicity, and the medullary pyramids are less echogenic than the cortex. When the renal cortex is compared with the liver, it is hypoechoic (Fig. 5-3).

The ureters are not usually imaged on a sonogram unless they are dilated. The ureters exit from the medial aspect of the kidneys and follow a vertical course anterior to the psoas muscle to the posterior-lateral aspect of the urinary bladder. When the ureter is dilated, it appears as a linear anechoic or sonolucent structure on a sagittal view (Fig. 5-4) and a round anechoic structure on a transverse view.

The urinary bladder is visualized only when it is distended, and then it appears as a fluid-filled, anechoic, thin-walled, symmetric structure. Reverberations may be seen in the anterior portion of the fluid-filled urinary bladder. The urethra is a tubular structure that extends from the base of the urinary bladder to the outside of the body. The urethra in women is much shorter than in men. It is typically not imaged unless an obstruction

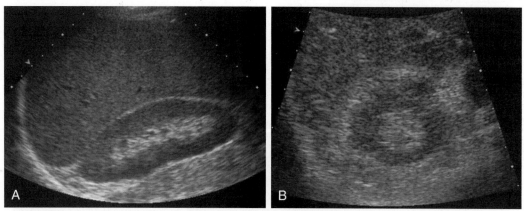

FIGURE 5-3 (A), Sagittal image of normal right kidney. **(B)**, Transverse image of normal right kidney.

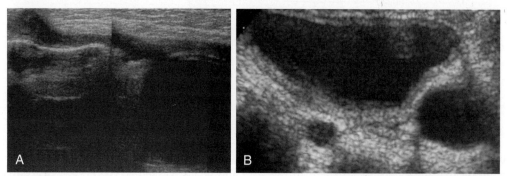

FIGURE 5-4 Dilated ureter. **(A)**, Longitudinal image. **(B)**, Transverse image at the level of the bladder.

exists at the urethral level. With sonographic imaging, the urethra appears as a short anechoic or sonolucent tubular structure (Fig. 5-5).

UROLITHIASIS

Nephrolithiasis

Calculi, or stones, can form anywhere within the urinary tract. Most stones originate within the kidney (nephrolithiasis). The development of calculi is influenced by heredity, familial predisposition, geographic location (living in a dry, hot climate), high concentrations of stone constituents (uric acid, calcium salts, or a combination of calcium oxalate and calcium phosphate), changes in urine pH, or the presence of bacteria. Development may also be idiopathic. Stones are more commonly found in men. The clinical presentation varies depending on the size or location of the stone or whether the stone is being passed. Calculi located in the kidney or proximal portion of the ureter may cause either no pain or dull flank pain, whereas stones in the distal ureter or bladder may cause lower back pain radiating down the pelvis. Severe, sharp pain (renal colic) is usually caused by the passage of a stone down the urinary tract. Other clinical symptoms may include nausea, vomiting, fever, chills, or painful urination. Depending on the presence of obstruction, oliguria may also be present. If the hematuria is due to infection, the laboratory findings may consist of increased white blood cell count and bacteria in the urine and bloodstream.

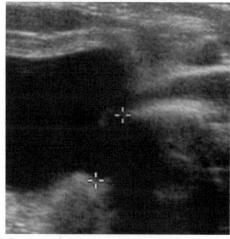

FIGURE 5-5 Dilated urethra caused by posterior urethral valves (PUV).

Stones can cause obstruction of the renal collecting system, or they may pass into the ureter and obstruct it, causing a hydroureter. The two most common sites of obstruction are the ureteropelvic junction and the ureterovesical junction. Sonographic documentation of a ureteral stone may be difficult to obtain because of the small size of the calculi, posterior location of the ureter (where the area of interest may not be in the focal zone), lack of fluid surrounding the stone, and adjacent bowel gas. A staghorn calculus is a stone that fills the renal pelvis and extends into the infundibulum and calyces, causing dilation of the calyces. Stones may also pass into the urinary bladder or, in rare cases, obstruct the urethra.

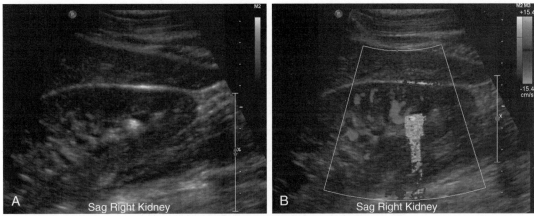

FIGURE 5-6 Renal calculi. **(A),** Calculi in the kidney—no shadowing. **(B),** Multiple colors are seen posterior to renal stone (twinkle sign). *(Courtesy Aubrey Rybyinski, BS, RDMS, RVT, Department of Radiology Ultrasound Section, Hospital of the University of Pennsylvania, Philadelphia, Pennsylvania.)*

Sonographic Findings. Calculi appear sonographically as crescent-shaped, echogenic foci. The presence of posterior acoustic shadowing varies according to the size and composition of the stone. Very small stones may not have posterior acoustic shadowing, or shadowing may be difficult to demonstrate (Fig. 5-6, A). The use of tissue harmonics when small calculi are suspected increases the chance of seeing posterior acoustic shadowing. A color Doppler artifact, the twinkle sign (Fig 5-6, B; see Color Plate 7), may be seen with small stones and may be helpful when shadowing cannot be demonstrated. When seen, this artifact appears as rapidly changing color with a comet tail posterior to the stone.

A calculus in the kidney may cause obstructive hydronephrosis (see Chapter 6). Stones that pass into the ureter may obstruct it, leading to ureteral dilation proximal to the site of the obstruction. A stone that causes a complete unilateral obstruction results in absence of a ureteral jet on the affected side (Fig. 5-7, A). A stone causing a partial ureteral obstruction may cause a weak ureteral jet (Fig. 5-7, B) or powerful jets of urine flow into the bladder, which has a color Doppler pattern that resembles a burning candle (candle sign) (Fig. 5-7, C).

Stones in the urinary bladder appear as echogenic foci that move when patient position is changed. An abdominal radiograph, intravenous urogram, or antegrade or retrograde study may be used in the diagnosis of small stones that are not imaged on a sonographic study.

BLADDER NEOPLASMS

Malignant bladder neoplasms are more common than benign neoplasms. Bladder malignancy has a higher incidence of occurrence than other urinary tract malignancies. The most common bladder neoplasm is transitional cell carcinoma (TCC). Squamous cell neoplasms, adenocarcinomas, lymphomas, and rhabdomyosarcomas in children are rare.

In advanced cases of malignancy, patients present with lower back pain, swelling of the legs, suprapubic pain, **dysuria,** urinary frequency with a small amount of

urine being passed, and blood or blood clots in the urine. Bladder cancer occurs more frequently in men with a peak incidence at age 60 to 70 years. Most masses are superficial and located at the trigone and along the lateral and posterior walls of the bladder.

Sonographic Findings

The sonographic appearance of bladder cancer varies and may have the same echogenicity as a benign neoplasm. Malignant neoplasms tend to appear as an echogenic, irregularly shaped mass projecting into the bladder lumen (Fig. 5-8). Hypervascular bladder wall thickness may also be present. The use of three-dimensional ultrasound imaging increases the distinction of the layers of the bladder wall to differentiate between noninvasive and invasive tumors.[3]

MALIGNANT NEOPLASMS

Renal Cell Carcinoma

Renal cell carcinoma (RCC) is also referred to as hypernephroma or adenocarcinoma. RCC accounts for most clinically relevant renal tumors. There is a significant predominance of men over women, with peak incidence occurring between age 60 and 70.[4] Etiologic factors include lifestyle factors, such as smoking, obesity, and hypertension. Cigarette smoking is a definite risk factor for RCC. The roles of obesity and hypertension as risk factors for RCC have not been as definitively clarified. Chemical exposure (e.g., asbestos, cadmium), long-term kidney dialysis, and von Hippel-Lindau disease are also linked to the development of RCC.

Some patients with RCC have hematuria. Other clinical signs include a palpable mass, flank pain, weight loss, fever, or hypertension. Because of the increased detection of tumors with the use of imaging, a growing number of incidentally diagnosed RCCs are found. These tumors are more often smaller and of lower stage. Today, more than 50% of RCCs are detected incidentally using noninvasive imaging for the evaluation of various nonspecific

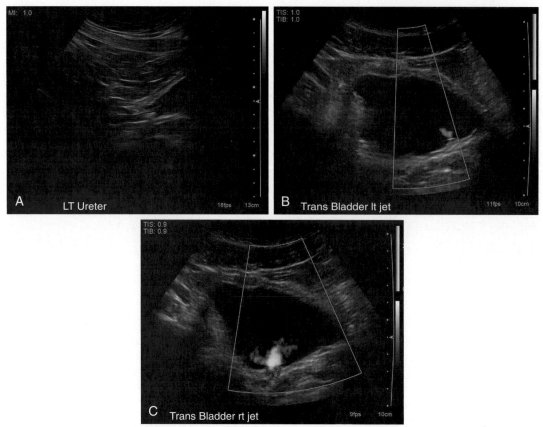

FIGURE 5-7 Partial ureteral obstruction of the ureter at the ureterovesical junction. **(A),** Stone in lower ureter. **(B),** Weak ureteral jet. **(C),** Powerful ureteral jet—color Doppler burning candle sign.

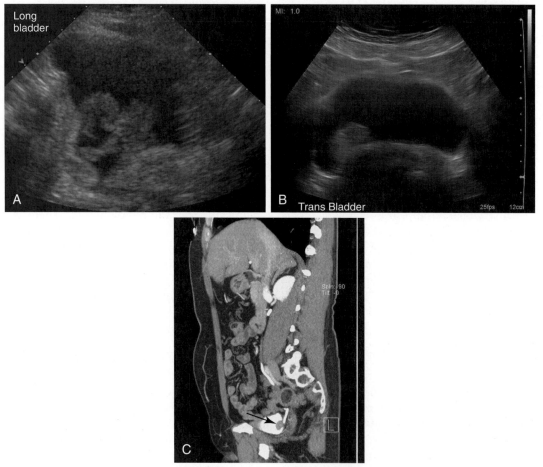

FIGURE 5-8 **(A),** Irregular-shaped mass projecting into the bladder lumen. **(B),** Echogenic mass projecting into the bladder lumen. **(C),** MRI of bladder tumor projecting into the bladder lumen.

symptoms.[4] The previously reported classic triad of flank pain, gross hematuria, and palpable abdominal mass is now rarely found. In addition, abnormal laboratory findings may be seen, such as erythropoietin blood level; red blood cells, white blood cells, and bacteria in the urine; and elevated creatinine and blood urea nitrogen (BUN) levels. The tumor may spread throughout the kidney and perinephric fat, invade the renal vein, and travel to the inferior vena cava (IVC). Approximately one-third of patients have metastasis at the time of diagnosis. Metastasis to the regional lymph nodes, lungs, bone, contralateral kidney, liver, adrenal glands, and brain may occur. At the time of diagnosis, a very small percentage of RCCs are bilateral. Prognosis depends on the stage of the disease at diagnosis. RCCs can be staged using the American Joint Committee on Cancer TNM (tumor, node, metastases) classification, as follows:

- Stage 1 RCCs are 7 cm or smaller and confined to the kidney.
- Stage 2 RCCs are larger than 7 cm but still confined to the kidney.
- Stage 3 tumors extend into the renal vein or vena cava, involve the ipsilateral adrenal gland or perinephric fat or both, or have spread to one local lymph node.

- Stage 4 tumors extend beyond Gerota's fascia to more than one local node or have distant metastases.

More recent literature has questioned whether the cutoff in size for stage 1 and 2 tumors should be 5 cm instead of 7 cm.[6]

Sonographic Findings. Sonography is frequently used to differentiate solid masses from simple cysts and to visualize the internal architecture of lesions more effectively than CT or MRI. The sonographic appearance of RCC is variable. On sonograms, RCC can be isoechoic, hypoechoic, or hyperechoic relative to the remainder of the renal parenchyma (Fig. 5-9). A smaller lesion with less necrosis is more likely to be hyperechoic and may be confused with an angiomyolipoma (AML). Larger lesions usually are more heterogeneous and more often hypoechoic.[6]

RCC may have calcifications or appear complex, with tumor necrosis or hemorrhage. Spectral Doppler and color flow imaging are useful in the identification of invasion of the IVC and renal vein (Fig. 5-10), with renal vein blood flow demonstrating low velocity, if the renal vein obstruction is severe. Research studies using three-dimensional contrast-enhanced sonography have increased the ability to differentiate between noninvasive and invasive tumors.[3,5]

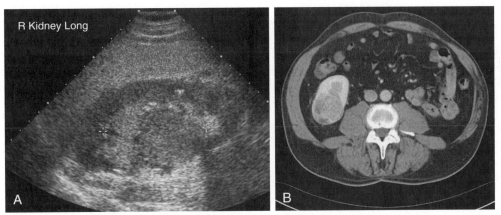

FIGURE 5-9 RCC. **(A),** Echogenic mass. **(B),** Corresponding CT scan.

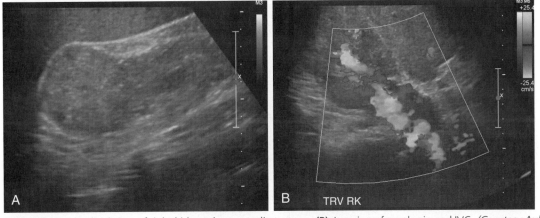

FIGURE 5-10 RCC. **(A),** Longitudinal view of right kidney shows a solitary mass. **(B),** Invasion of renal vein and IVC. *(Courtesy Aubrey Rybyinski, BS, RDMS, RVT, Department of Radiology Ultrasound Section, Hospital of the University of Pennsylvania, Philadelphia, Pennsylvania.)*

Transitional Cell Carcinoma

In the United States, more than 90% of malignant diseases that involve the bladder are TCCs. TCCs most often involve the urinary bladder. In a small percentage of cases, involvement of the kidneys and ureters is seen.

Patients with TCC typically have painless hematuria, but if the lesion involves the renal collecting system, the patient may have pain and hydronephrosis. Bladder lesions may cause hematuria and blood clots. TCC occurs more often in men, and an increased incidence is seen with advancing age.
Sonographic Findings. The most common sonographic appearance of TCC is a bulky, hypoechoic mass in the bladder (see Fig. 5-8). TCC lesions in the kidney found within the renal sinus (Fig. 5-11) may cause separation and dilation of the renal collecting system. The renal contour is preserved and the internal renal architecture becomes distorted with malignant invasion. Calcifications are rare.

Squamous Cell Carcinoma

In the United States, only about 5% of bladder cancers are squamous cell carcinomas (SCCs). Worldwide, SCC is the most common form of bladder cancer, accounting

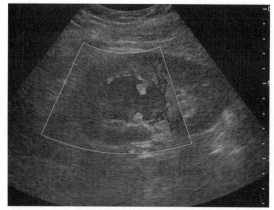

FIGURE 5-11 TCC. A renal mass in the renal sinus is a less common presentation.

for 75% of cases in developing nations.[7] In the United States, the development of SCC is associated with persistent inflammation from long-term indwelling Foley catheters, bladder stones, and possibly infections. In underdeveloped nations, SCC is often associated with bladder infection by *Schistosoma haematobium*.[7]
Sonographic Findings. The most common appearance of SCC is a large, bulky mass in the renal pelvis (Fig. 5-12). CT and IVP are typically used to make a preoperative diagnosis.

BENIGN NEOPLASMS

Benign neoplasms of the kidney are rare. Any neoplasm of the kidney seen with sonography is assumed to be malignant unless it is proved otherwise.

Angiomyolipoma (Hamartoma)

AML is a common renal cortex mass that consists mostly of fat and muscle cells and arterial vessels. Most small AML lesions are asymptomatic and are found incidentally on imaging studies. When lesions are symptomatic, there may be a palpable abdominal mass, and they may cause hematuria or flank pain. Solitary sporadic tumors may cause acute abdomen and shock as a result of spontaneous hemorrhage in the tumor. Two types are described: isolated AML and AML that is associated with tuberous sclerosis; 80% are of the solitary type. Isolated lesions are more common in women 40 to 60 years old and in the right kidney. When associated with tuberous sclerosis, the lesions are typically larger than isolated AMLs, and they are often bilateral and multiple.[8]
Sonographic Findings. The most characteristic sonographic feature of an AML is its echogenicity (Fig. 5-13). Renal AMLs are intensely echogenic and may cause acoustic shadowing. AMLs are located in the renal cortex and are hyperechoic even at low gain settings. Because of their intense echogenicity, AMLs only a few millimeters in diameter may be identified.

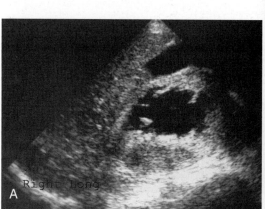
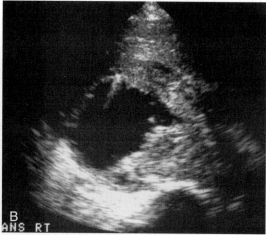

FIGURE 5-12 SCC (atypical, low-echogenicity appearance) in a 60-year-old patient with metastatic disease. **(A),** Sagittal image of right kidney shows an irregular-shaped mass filling the renal sinus. **(B),** Transverse image of SCC.

Oncocytoma

Oncocytoma is a benign renal cell neoplasm that accounts for a small percentage of all adult primary renal epithelial neoplasms. Men are reported to be affected more than women. The epidemiology of oncocytoma is similar to RCC, and the main clinical importance of this lesion is the difficulty in distinguishing it from RCC with preoperative imaging. Most patients with a renal oncocytoma are asymptomatic. In cases in which the mass is large, a flank or abdominal mass may be present. Occasionally, hypertension, hematuria, or pain may be the complaint. The imaging characteristics of oncocytomas and RCCs overlap, and differentiating an oncocytoma from an RCC and other solid renal neoplasms is not always possible with sonography,

CT scanning, or MRI. The presence of a central scar on CT or MRI and a spoke-wheel pattern of vessels on angiogram may be suggestive of oncocytoma but are not entirely specific.[7-10]

Sonographic Findings. On a sonogram, oncocytoma appears as a well-defined, homogeneous, and hypoechoic to isoechoic mass (Fig. 5-14).[7,9,10] The central scar cannot be confidently identified on sonograms; however, when the scar is seen, especially in large lesions, it may appear echogenic.[9] Color Doppler sonography may show central radiating vessels.

Hemangiomas

Hemangiomas of the kidneys are rare benign neoplasms that consist of a mass of blood vessels and usually occur

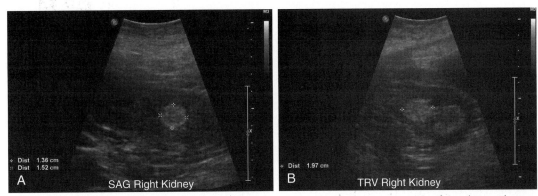

FIGURE 5-13 AML. **(A),** Longitudinal view of right kidney shows a solitary, highly echogenic mass arising from the renal cortex. **(B),** Transverse image of AML. *(Courtesy Aubrey Rybyinski, BS, RDMS, RVT, Department of Radiology Ultrasound Section, Hospital of the University of Pennsylvania, Philadelphia, Pennsylvania.)*

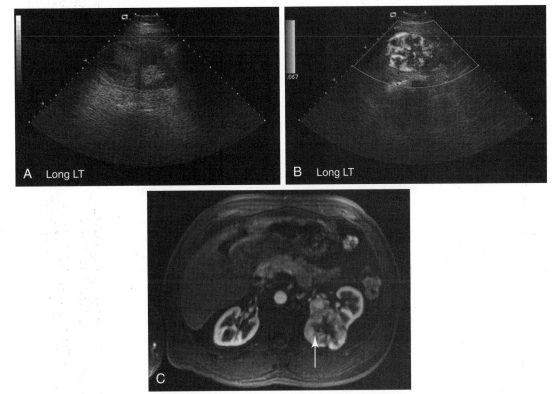

FIGURE 5-14 Oncocytoma. **(A),** Longitudinal image shows echogenic mass. **(B),** Transverse image demonstrates hypervascularity. **(C),** MRI demonstrates a central scar *(arrow),* which is characteristically used in diagnosis of oncocytoma.

TABLE 5-1	Causes of Hematuria	
Pathology	**Symptoms**	**Sonographic Findings**
Nephrolithiasis	Pain (renal colic), nausea, vomiting, fever, chills, painful urination, increased white blood cell count, and bacteriuria	Echogenic foci with shadow (dependent on size of calculi), possible hydronephrosis or dilated ureter, decreased ureteral jets, color Doppler twinkle sign, color Doppler candle sign (partial ureteral obstruction)
Hemangioma	Pain (renal colic), hematuria	Variable echogenicity, located near renal sinus
Hematoma	Mild abdominal or flank pain to intense pain, low hematocrit if severe	Variable; acute stage is echogenic followed by possible hypoechoic, complex, calcification
Lipoma	Small—asymptomatic; large—abdominal, flank pain, or both may have hematuria	Echogenic, well-defined mass
Oncocytoma	Asymptomatic, possible flank or abdominal mass, occasionally hypertension and hematuria	Well-defined homogeneous, hypoechoic to isoechoic; central scar or stellate scar seldom seen with sonography
Angiomyolipoma (hamartoma)	Small lesions are asymptomatic; possible palpable abdominal mass, hematuria, or flank pain; solitary tumors may cause acute abdomen and shock as a result of spontaneous hemorrhage	Intensely echogenic; may cause acoustic shadowing
Renal cell carcinoma (hypernephroma, adenocarcinoma)	Hematuria; possible palpable mass, flank pain, weight loss, fever, or hypertension	Variable; smaller more likely to be hyperechoic; larger lesions more heterogeneous and hypoechoic; may invade the renal vein and inferior vena cava
Transitional cell carcinoma	Painless hematuria, possible pain and hydronephrosis if involving the renal collecting system	Bladder—bulky, hypoechoic mass; kidney—separation of collecting system, dilation of collecting system
Squamous cell carcinoma	Painless gross hematuria, possible pain and hydronephrosis if involving the renal collecting system	Bladder—bulky, hypoechoic mass; kidney—separation of collecting system, dilation of collecting system
Bladder mass	Suprapubic pain, frequent urination with small amounts of urine (oliguria)	Echogenic, irregularly shaped mass; hypervascular wall; thickened bladder wall

in young adults. Recurrent episodes of hematuria and renal colic are typical presenting symptoms; however, incidental diagnosis in asymptomatic patients is also common.[7]

Sonographic Findings. Renal hemangiomas are usually of variable echogenicity.[7] They are frequently located at the pelvocalyceal junction or in the inner medulla.

Hematoma

The possible causes for hematoma are extensive and include post–renal biopsy, trauma, RCC, AML, segmental renal infarction, arteriovenous malformation, hemorrhagic cyst, abscess, extracorporeal shock wave lithotripsy (ESWL) for the treatment of symptomatic renal and ureteral stones, or idiopathic. Blood tends to collect either in the perinephric space or below the renal capsule (subcapsular hematoma). Symptoms range from mild abdominal or flank pain to intense pain, depending on the amount of blood that has undergone extravasation. Hematocrit levels decrease in cases with severe blood loss.

Sonographic Findings. Hematoma varies in sonographic appearance, depending on the age of the hematoma. Fresh blood (<24 hours) may appear anechoic. With a high-resolution transducer, swirling internal echoes may be seen. Hematomas in the acute stages are echogenic. As a clot forms, the hematoma becomes complex, with hypoechoic and echogenic areas. As the blood clot liquefies, the sonographic appearance may become anechoic. A chronic hematoma may display areas of calcification with posterior acoustic shadowing. Spectral Doppler and color flow imaging can be used to determine whether a hematoma is actively bleeding. A subcapsular hematoma is located between the renal capsule and the cortex and may flatten the cortex. Subcapsular hematomas are difficult to visualize sonographically during the acute phase; they may have the same sonographic echogenicity as the renal cortex. A perinephric hematoma may have an elongated shape that follows the contour of the kidney.

Lipoma

Primary renal lipoma is a very rare neoplasm of the kidney, exclusively composed of adipose tissue with very few cases reported in published literature.[10] Reported lesions were predominant in middle-aged women. Small lesions were asymptomatic, but large neoplasms were usually present with abdominal or flank pain, or both, and occasionally with hematuria.[7,11]

Sonographic Findings. The imaging feature of a lipoma is a well-marginated mass with entirely fatty components appearing sonographically as echogenic.

Table 5-1 summarizes the pathology, symptoms, and sonographic findings in hematuria.

SUMMARY

Hematuria is a nonspecific finding, but it may be an early sign of a serious renal disease. Causes of hematuria include tumor, stones, and trauma. In older men, benign prostatic hyperplasia is a common cause of hematuria. Sonographic examination of the urinary system can aid in the identification of the cause of hematuria. Patients commonly present with a history of hematuria and no other clinical symptoms, and depending on the amount of red blood cells in the urine, an imaging work-up may be unnecessary.[12] Characterization of the sonographic appearance of the urinary tract coupled with the patient history and other tests, including urinalysis, cystoscopy, IVP, CT, or MRI, can lead to diagnosis and proper patient management.

CLINICAL SCENARIO—DIAGNOSIS

This patient is a male cigarette smoker who also has the lifestyle risk of obesity. This history, along with hypertension and hematuria, puts the patient at risk for the development of RCC. Sonography frequently discovers a renal mass when a sonogram is requested for other indications. In these instances, sonography is able to differentiate a solid mass from a simple cyst by visualizing the internal architecture of a lesion. This mass appears slightly hyperechoic and must be considered highly suspicious for RCC. Spectral Doppler and color flow evaluation should be performed to rule out invasion of the IVC and renal vein. A survey of the remainder of the abdomen and contralateral kidney (for metastasis) should also be completed.

CASE STUDIES FOR DISCUSSION

1. A 60-year-old man is seen by his physician for a routine examination. A routine laboratory work-up is performed, and microscopic hematuria is found. The patient has mild hypertension and a history of cigarette smoking. A urinary tract sonogram is requested to help find the cause of the hematuria. The findings are seen in Figure 5-15. What is the most likely diagnosis? How does the patient history contribute?

2. A middle-aged woman presents to the emergency department with flank pain, nausea and vomiting, and a low-grade fever. Urinalysis reveals microscopic hematuria, and she is referred for a urinary tract sonogram. The findings are seen in Figure 5-16. What is the most likely diagnosis consistent with the sonographic findings? What scanning techniques should the sonographer employ in completing this examination?

3. A 40-year-old man with a clinical history of gross hematuria is seen for a urinary tract sonogram. No prior imaging examinations of the urinary tract are available for comparison. A mass is seen in Figure 5-17. Where is this mass located? Discuss the likely type of mass. What is the prognosis for this patient?

4. A 45-year-old, mildly obese woman sees her physician with complaints of right upper quadrant pain and nausea and vomiting after eating. Laboratory analysis reveals elevated cholesterol levels and microscopic hematuria. She is referred for sonography to rule out gallstones. The examination is positive for gallstones. During the course of the right upper quadrant examination, the sonographer discovers an incidental solid, well-defined isoechoic to hyperechoic mass (Fig. 5-18). A follow-up CT scan (not shown here) suggests a central scar within the mass. What is the likely cause of this mass?

5. A 65-year-old man with a history of painless hematuria is referred for renal sonography. A solid mass is identified (Fig. 5-19). What possible neoplasms might this mass represent? What stage is this mass?

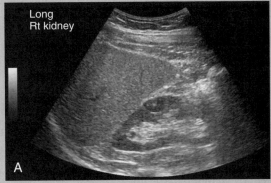
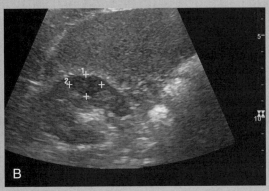

FIGURE 5-15 **(A)** and **(B)**, Small solid renal mass.

Continued

CASE STUDIES FOR DISCUSSION—cont'd

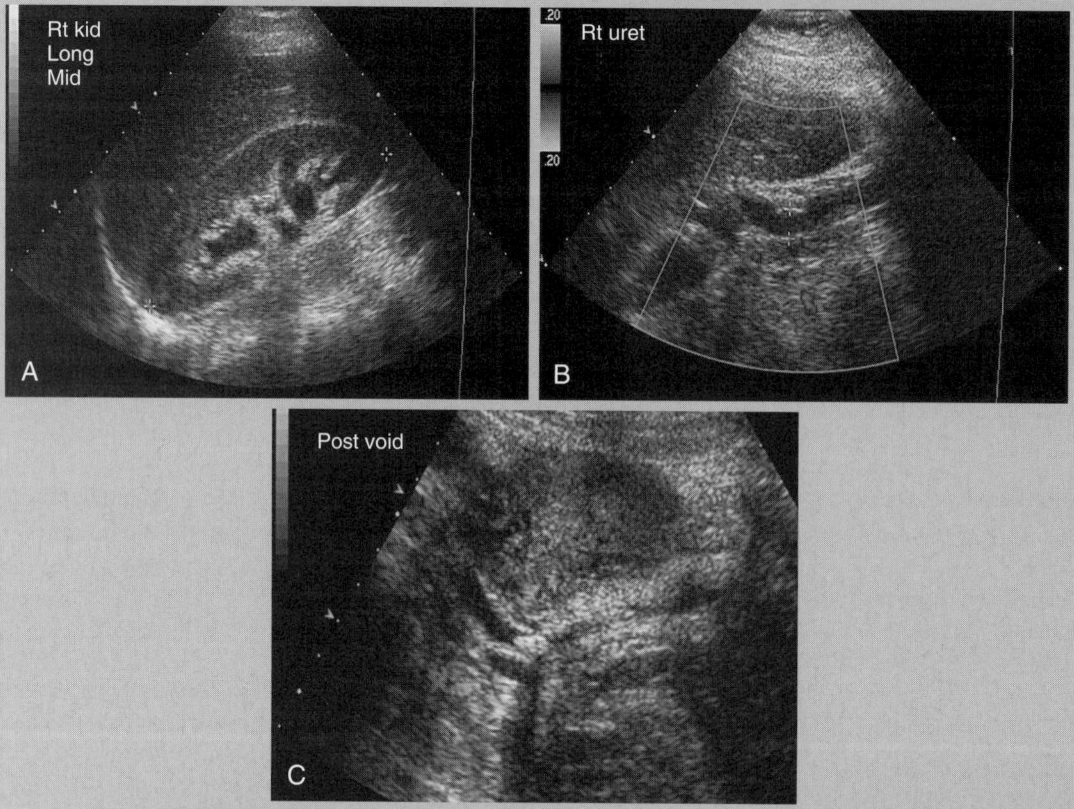

FIGURE 5-16 (A-C), Mild hydronephrosis—echogenic foci near the bladder.

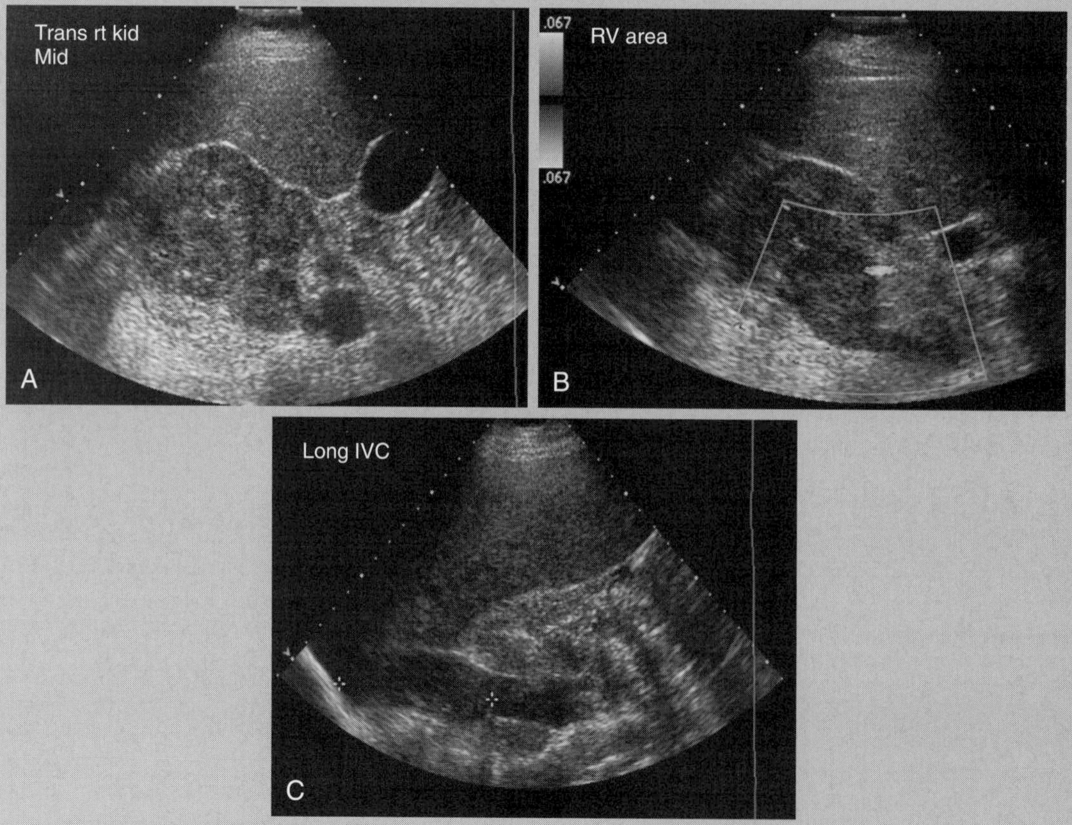

FIGURE 5-17 (A-C), Solid mass in the region of the renal sinus.

CASE STUDIES FOR DISCUSSION—cont'd

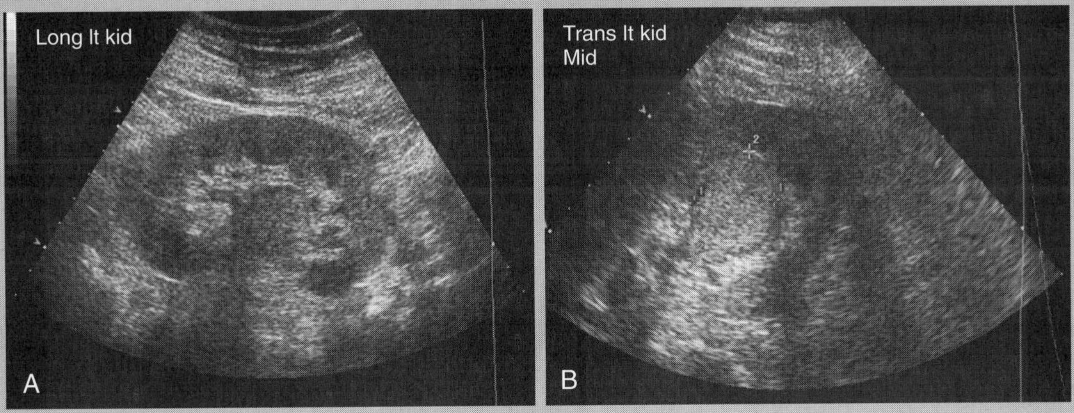

FIGURE 5-18 **(A)** and **(B),** Isoechoic to hyperechoic mass in midportion of the right kidney.

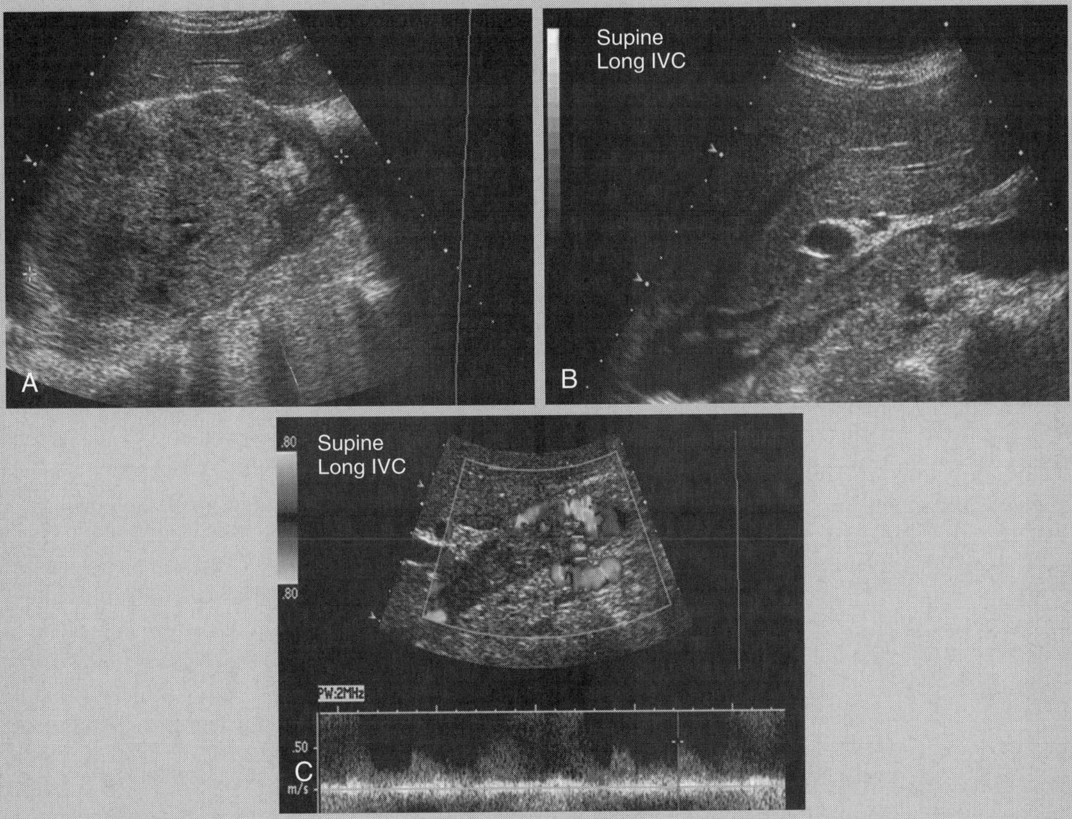

FIGURE 5-19 **(A),** Solid renal mass arising from the renal cortex. **(B)** and **(C),** Echogenic material in IVC.

STUDY QUESTIONS

1. A 51-year-old man presents with severe left flank pain and hematuria and is referred for an abdominal sonogram. A dilated left renal collecting system and proximally dilated ureter are identified. The right kidney appears normal. The bladder is also scanned, and no ureteral jet can be identified on the left. These findings are most consistent with:
   a. Bladder hematoma
   b. Ureteral stone
   c. Kidney stone
   d. Bladder stone

2. A young patient with right flank pain, hematuria, and nausea and vomiting undergoes a renal sonogram. The left kidney appears mildly hydronephrotic. Small, echogenic foci with posterior acoustic shadowing are seen at the base of the bladder at the insertion site of the ureter; color Doppler reveals a "twinkle sign." What is the most likely diagnosis?
   a. Hematoma with candle sign
   b. Calculi with partial ureteral obstruction
   c. Transitional cell carcinoma of the renal sinus and urinary bladder
   d. Renal cell carcinoma with venous invasion

3. A 40-year-old woman is referred for a renal sonogram after discovery of microscopic hematuria. The sonogram is unremarkable except for a 3-cm, well-defined mass with a central scar in the left kidney. Despite the fact that all solid renal masses must be considered suspicious for RCC, what mass is suggested by the presence of the central scar?
   a. Hematoma
   b. Angiomyolipoma
   c. Adenoma
   d. Oncocytoma

4. A middle-aged woman who has recently undergone a kidney biopsy for renal disease developed microscopic hematuria and a decreasing hematocrit level. A renal sonogram is ordered. The left kidney is normal. The right kidney appears normal with the suggestion of a sonolucent crescent at the kidney's edge. This is most consistent with:
   a. Ruptured cyst
   b. Perinephric hematoma
   c. Angiomyolipoma
   d. Hemangioma

5. A 55-year-old man presents for his annual medical evaluation. He is mildly obese and has been a smoker for more than 20 years. He reports some shortness of breath and a new symptom of intermittent, gross hematuria. He is referred for renal sonography. A solid, hypoechoic mass is identified in the renal cortex of the right kidney. What is the most likely diagnosis?
   a. Renal cell carcinoma
   b. Renal calculi
   c. Complex renal cyst
   d. Transitional cell carcinoma

6. A patient with a history of smoking presents with painful frequent urination and gross hematuria. A sonogram of the urinary tract demonstrates mild hydronephrosis and an irregular echogenic mass in the bladder. This is most consistent with:
   a. Bladder stone
   b. Cystitis
   c. Angiomyolipoma
   d. Transitional cell carcinoma

7. A 75-year-old man with microscopic hematuria and no pain undergoes renal imaging. The sonogram reveals a small solid left renal mass. The sonographer notes echogenic material in the left renal vein. This is most suggestive of:
   a. Renal cell carcinoma with renal vein invasion
   b. Oncocytoma with renal vein invasion
   c. Transitional cell carcinoma with metastasis to the renal veins
   d. Hemangioma with clot formation in the renal vein

8. A middle-aged woman with microscopic hematuria is referred for renal sonography. She has no significant symptoms or laboratory findings. The abdominal sonogram reveals an intensely echogenic mass in the cortex of the left kidney. The echogenicity of the mass is equal to that of the renal sinus fat. What is this mass most likely to represent?
   a. Angiomyolipoma
   b. Hemangioma
   c. Transitional cell carcinoma abutting the renal sinus
   d. Hematoma

9. A 55-year-old woman with a history of tuberous sclerosis, recent onset of hematuria, and pain is referred for renal sonography. The sonographer is asked to evaluate for the presence of angiomyolipoma. Given the patient history, what is the most likely appearance if a mass is discovered?
   a. Bilateral, well-defined, small echogenic renal cortex masses
   b. Unilateral, well-defined, hypoechoic renal cortex masses
   c. Bilateral, poorly defined, echogenic renal cortex masses
   d. Unilateral, poorly defined, hypoechoic renal cortex masses

10. A 65-year-old man with known RCC is referred for sonography to evaluate the extent of the tumor. The mass is found to be 4 cm and confined to the kidney. What stage is this tumor?
a. Stage 1
b. Stage 2
c. Stage 3
d. Stage 4

REFERENCES

1. Choyke PL: Radiologic evaluation of hematuria: guidelines from the American College of Radiology's Appropriateness Criteria, *Am Fam Physician* 78:347–352, 2008.
2. Helck A, et al: Improved visualization of renal lesions using three-dimensional ultrasound—a feasibility study, *Clin Hemorheol Microcirc* 49:537–550, 2011.
3. Li Q-Y, et al: Clinical utility of three-dimensional contrast-enhanced ultrasound in the differentiation between noninvasive and invasive neoplasms of urinary bladder. *Eur J Radiol* http://dx.doi.org/10.1016/j.ejrad.2011.12.024. Retrieved February 5, 2012.
4. Ljungberg B, et al: Renal cell carcinoma guideline, *Eur Urol* 51:1502–1510, 2007.
5. Nicolau C, Bunesch L, Peri L, et al: Accuracy of contrast-enhanced ultrasound in the detection of bladder cancer, *Br J Radiol* 84:1091–1099, 2011.
6. Baumgarten DA: *Renal cell carcinoma imaging*Emedicine. medscape.com.http://emedicine.medscape.com/article/380543-overview. Retrieved February 5, 2012, .
7. Steinberg GD: *Bladder cancer*. Emedicine.medscape.com.http://emedicine.medscape.com/article/438262-overview. Retrieved February 5, 2012.
8. Pradad SR, et al: Benign renal neoplasms in adults: cross-sectional imaging findings, *AJR Am J Roentgenol* 190:158–160, 2008.
9. Kalva SP, et al: *Renal oncocytoma imaging*. Emedicine. medscape.com.http://emedicine.medscape.com/article/379653-overview. Retrieved February 3, 2012.
10. De Carli P, Vidiri A, Lamanna L, et al: Renal oncocytoma: image diagnosis and therapeutic aspects, *J Exp Clin Cancer Res* 19:287–289, 2000.
11. Chang IC, et al: Case report. Huge renal lipoma with prominent hypervascular non-adipose elements. *Br J Radiol* 79:148–151, 2006.
12. Grossfeld GD, et al: Evaluation of asymptomatic microscopic hematuria in adults: the American Urological Association best practice policy—part II: patient evaluation, cytology, voided markers, imaging, cystoscopy, nephrology evaluation, and follow-up, *Urology* 57:604–610, 2001.

6

Rule Out Renal Failure

Aubrey Rybyinski

CLINICAL SCENARIO

A 21-year-old woman is sent from the emergency department for a renal sonogram. She complains of right flank pain with urinary urgency for the last day and has a fever. Laboratory findings reveal elevated white blood cells (WBCs), and urinalysis is positive for protein, blood, and WBCs. This is the first occurrence of these symptoms, and the patient reports otherwise being healthy.

A bilateral renal sonogram shows the right kidney exhibiting a decrease in corticomedullary echogenicity with a loss of differentiation (Fig. 6-1). The renal sinus appears prominent but compressed on the right. The left kidney is normal-appearing (Fig. 6-2). What is the possible diagnosis for these findings?

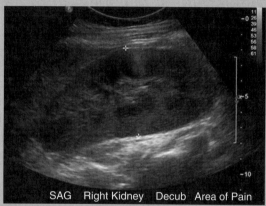

FIGURE 6-1 Sagittal image of right kidney. *(Courtesy Lisa Jones, MD, PhD, Department of Radiology, University of Pennsylvania, Philadelphia, Pennsylvania.)*

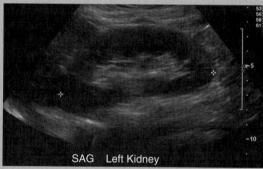

FIGURE 6-2 Sagittal image of left kidney. *(Courtesy Lisa Jones, MD, PhD, Department of Radiology, University of Pennsylvania, Philadelphia, Pennsylvania.)*

OBJECTIVES

- Describe the typical causes and sonographic appearance of hydronephrosis.
- List the common causes and characteristics of acute glomerulonephritis.
- Describe the etiology and sonographic appearance of papillary necrosis.
- Differentiate between acute and chronic renal failure sonographically.
- Describe the Doppler characteristics typically found with renal artery stenosis.

- Describe what may cause acute tubular necrosis.
- Describe the sonographic appearance of pyonephrosis.
- Differentiate between acute, chronic, emphysematous, and xanthogranulomatous pyelonephritis sonographically.
- Describe possible causes and sonographic appearances of renal abscesses.
- Describe the sonographic appearance of a typical fungal infection.

A renal sonogram may be ordered for assessment of the kidneys when renal failure is suspected. Renal decline and failure are associated with significant morbidity and mortality. Renal failure results when the kidneys are no longer able to remove waste products from the bloodstream. Depending on the cause and the stage of the renal failure, patients present with a variety of symptoms. Initial symptoms may be nonspecific, but the symptoms eventually progress to flank pain; nausea; vomiting; anemia; headaches; and increased (polyuria), decreased (oliguria), or absent (anuria) urine production. Laboratory values may show pyuria, hematuria, WBCs or bacteria in the urine (suggestive of inflammation or infection), and elevated blood urea nitrogen (BUN) and creatinine levels.

Renal failure may be caused by obstruction of urine flow, decreased renal blood flow, or renal parenchymal disease. Disease processes within the kidney that may be precursors to renal failure include hydronephrosis, acute glomerulonephritis, papillary necrosis, renal artery stenosis, acute tubular necrosis, and various renal infections. Lower genitourinary tract diseases within the ureter, bladder, or urethra causing obstruction may lead to renal failure. In most cases, bilateral obstruction is necessary for renal insufficiency to develop.

Sonographic assessment for renal failure should include a thorough investigation of the genitourinary system with a search for signs of obstruction, tumors, anatomic abnormalities, calculi, infection, stenosis, and decreased renal vascular flow. The sonogram should be initiated with B-mode technology for assessment of kidney size and sonographic characteristics. Next, a Doppler evaluation (color and pulsed-wave) of the renal vascular system should be performed for determination of patency. Abnormal Doppler signals that suggest decreased vascular flow include high systolic peak velocities, low or no diastolic flow, turbulence, and the tardus parvus effect (dampening of the waveform).[1]

HYDRONEPHROSIS

Hydronephrosis occurs when the renal collecting system of one or both kidneys becomes dilated from the obstruction of urine outflow. Hydronephrosis is caused by calculi, tumor, infection, previous obstruction, overdistended bladder, anatomic or congenital abnormalities, and pregnancy. Infection may occur with an extended period of urinary stasis. Prolonged hydronephrosis destroys the tubules in the cortex resulting in renal parenchymal atrophy, scarring, or irreversible renal damage. This condition progressively leads to the loss of renal function. With long-standing hydronephrosis, the renal collecting system remains dilated after the obstruction is relieved. Patients with hydronephrosis may be asymptomatic, but this condition can also manifest with pain in the kidney region, infection, nausea, dysuria, fever, chills, vomiting, uremia, and microscopic hematuria.

Sonographic Findings

The distention of the renal pelvis and calyces found in patients with significant hydronephrosis causes overall renal enlargement. Sonographically, a hydronephrotic kidney manifests with a group of anechoic, fluid-filled spaces within the renal sinus (Figs. 6-3 and 6-4). Acute obstruction may initially cause the kidney to cease to excrete urine, which delays the onset of any renal dilation. Echogenic calculi (with or without shadowing) may be located throughout the genitourinary system. Smaller stones blend into the echogenic renal sinus. Previous

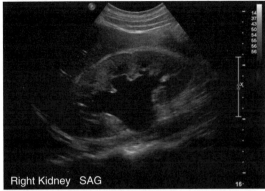

FIGURE 6-3 Sagittal image of right kidney shows hydronephrosis. *(Courtesy Lisa Jones, MD, PhD, Department of Radiology, University of Pennsylvania, Philadelphia, Pennsylvania.)*

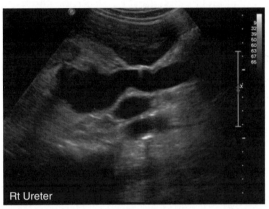

FIGURE 6-4 Transverse image of right kidney shows hydronephrosis with hydroureter. *(Courtesy Lisa Jones, MD, PhD, Department of Radiology, University of Pennsylvania, Philadelphia, Pennsylvania.)*

obstruction, pregnancy, megaureter, or an extremely full bladder also causes normal calyceal dilation. Chronic obstruction causes atrophy of the renal parenchyma.

Hydronephrosis manifests with a slight distention of the collecting system displaying a small separation of the calyceal pattern (splaying).[2] As hydronephrosis progresses, the collecting system dilates with fluid extending into the major and minor calyceal systems (bear-claw effect).[2] Severe hydronephrosis manifests with massive dilation including the renal pelvis. It is associated with cortical thinning or loss of the renal parenchyma. With assessment for hydronephrosis, parapelvic cysts should be ruled out. Generally, dilated calyces have a more echogenic margin than a parapelvic cyst. An extra renal pelvis should also be considered because it can be confused with hydronephrosis owing to its large cystic appearance within the renal hilum.

Doppler examination is important in the evaluation for hydronephrosis. Doppler examination reveals prominent renal vasculature that may be confused with a dilated renal collecting system. Increased intrarenal pressure caused by urinary obstruction leads to a decline in renal blood flow and a thinning of the parenchyma. The resistance index on the affected side is increased compared with the healthy kidney. In normal conditions, a relatively low renal vascular resistance is found. With partial obstruction, the resistive index may be unaffected. Ureteral jets, detectable with color Doppler examination, may be absent or decreased in frequency in acute obstruction.

ACUTE GLOMERULONEPHRITIS

Acute glomerulonephritis is an inflammation of the renal glomeruli that frequently occurs as a late complication of an infection, typically of the throat (pharyngitis).[3] Glomerulonephritis is characterized by bilateral inflammatory changes in the glomeruli that are not the result of infection of the kidneys. It is more common in males than in females and is more common in children than in adults.[4] Symptoms are variable and include foggy urine, history of recent fever, sore throat, joint pains, peripheral edema (e.g., face, ankles), nausea, oliguria, anemia, azotemia, and hypertension. Laboratory findings may include hematuria, proteinuria, decreased glomerular filtration rate (GFR), increased BUN value, and increased serum creatinine level.[5]

Inflammation and scarring of the glomeruli result in an inability to filter the blood properly to make urine.[6] The inflammation and scarring lead to poor kidney function and ultimately renal failure. Acute glomerulonephritis commonly leads to chronic glomerulonephritis. Chronic glomerulonephritis develops slowly and may not be detected until the kidneys fail, which could take 20 to 30 years.[3]

Chronic glomerulonephritis is characterized by irreversible and progressive glomerular fibrosis that leads to a reduction in the GFR and a retention of uremic toxins.[7] Chronic glomerulonephritis leads to chronic renal failure, end-stage renal disease, and eventually death. It requires long-term treatment with dialysis or transplantation.

Sonographic Findings

Acute glomerulonephritis may not have any differentiating sonographic features. An irregular cortical echo pattern may be seen. When evident, the acute form of glomerulonephritis may cause an increase in the cortical echogenicity. The renal pyramids are well visualized. Bilateral renal enlargement is also a common sonographic finding. Chronic glomerulonephritis initially shows an increase in cortical echotexture without an increase in the medullary echotexture. It progresses to increase both echodensities. Sonography of chronic glomerulonephritis shows small, smooth, echogenic kidneys.

PAPILLARY NECROSIS

The renal papillae are the rounded tips at the apex of each renal medullary pyramid. The renal papillae face toward the renal hilum and represent the confluence of the collecting ducts from each nephron within that pyramid. Necrosis of the renal papillae causes hydronephrosis from the sloughed papillae obstructing the calyces. Hydronephrosis is also caused by sloughed papillae obstructing the ureters. Any narrowed area can make a nesting spot for sloughed papillae, leading to obstruction.

The sloughed papillae calcify, further increasing the potential for obstructive hydronephrosis. The actual sloughing of the renal papilla is the result of vascular ischemia, which leads to necrosis of the renal medullary pyramids.[8] Papillary necrosis is the result of medullary vasculature being compressed with inflammation.

Papillary necrosis is typically a bilateral process and generally more common in women than men. Focal papillary necrosis involves only the tip of the papilla. Diffuse papillary necrosis involves the whole papilla and areas of the medulla. Papillary necrosis can affect a single papilla, or the entire kidney may be involved. Renal papillary necrosis is limited to the inner, more distal zone of the medulla and the papilla.

Patients with diabetes and females are more prone to papillary necrosis.[8] Patients have fever from infection, flank or abdominal pain, hypertension (from renal ischemia), dysuria, and hematuria. Laboratory results typically show a positive urine culture (from passage of sloughed papillae), proteinuria, pyuria, bacteriuria, and low urine-specific gravity. Papillary necrosis can be a complication of severe pyelonephritis. Infection is also a complication of papillary necrosis because the necrotic papillae act as an origin for infection and the formation of stones. Papillary necrosis has the potential to lead to renal failure and ultimately death.

Sonographic Findings

Papillary necrosis is visualized sonographically as clubbing of the calyces as a result of obstruction caused by sloughed papillae.[5] Obstruction caused by sloughed papillae manifests sonographically with signs of hydronephrosis. The sonographic evaluation should include a search for calculi or obstruction, including an evaluation for stones large enough to produce a shadow and hydronephrosis resulting from papillary necrosis. Round or triangular cystic collections within the medullary pyramids may be visible. A sloughed papilla, when visualized, appears as an echogenic, nonshadowing structure within the renal collecting system. If the papillae calcify, acoustic shadowing would be shown (Fig. 6-5). Severe papillary necrosis may cause the papillae to be replaced with urine-filled sacs.[9] Papillary necrosis would then appear as multiple cystic structures in the renal pyramid region that do not communicate with the renal pelvis.

RENAL FAILURE

Renal failure can be categorized as either acute or chronic. Acute symptoms are sudden and severe, whereas chronic symptoms are slow and irreversible. In both acute and chronic forms of renal failure, the excretory and regulatory functions of the kidneys are decreased. Obstructive causes of renal failure are treatable and are an important diagnosis during patient evaluation. Renal disease is considered end-stage when the kidneys are unable to fulfill more than 10% of their normal function.[3] At this point, dialysis may be necessary.

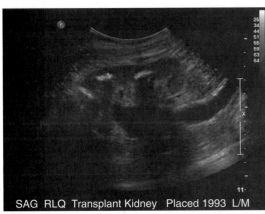

FIGURE 6-5 Sagittal image of a transplant kidney with hydronephrosis from the sloughed papillae obstructing the calyces.

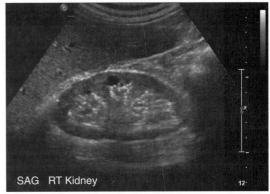

FIGURE 6-6 Right kidney with chronic renal failure. There is increased echogenicity of the kidney compared with the liver and thin renal parenchyma.

Acute Kidney Injury (Acute Renal Failure)

The term "acute kidney injury" represents the entire spectrum of acute renal failure (risk, injury, and then failure).[10] Acute kidney injury is the generic term used to define an abrupt decrease in renal function resulting in retention of nitrogenous waste (BUN and creatinine). An acute kidney injury may cause a decrease in renal blood flow and produce renal parenchymal insult or obstruction. Reduction of renal blood flow causes a decrease in the GFR, which leads to retention of water and salts. This retention causes oliguria, concentrated urine, and a progressive inability to excrete nitrogenous wastes. Decreased renal blood flow leads to ischemia and eventually to cell death. Recovery from an acute kidney injury depends on restoration of normal renal blood flow. Earlier blood flow normalization leads to a better prognosis for recovery of renal function. Patients with an acute kidney injury may have symptoms of hypovolemia, hypertension, edema, oliguria, and hematuria.[11] Laboratory results may include increased WBCs, increased creatinine levels, and increased BUN values.

An acute kidney injury may have different causes depending on the stage of the disease. Prerenal causes of acute renal failure are the result of hypoperfusion of the kidney. Renal causes result from parenchymal diseases, such as acute glomerulonephritis, renal vein thrombosis, and acute tubular necrosis.[11] Postrenal causes of acute renal failure are the result of obstruction.
Sonographic Findings. Acute renal failure may manifest sonographically with normal-sized or enlarged kidneys. The parenchymal echogenicity is increased compared with the liver.

Chronic Renal Failure

Chronic renal failure that necessitates dialysis or transplantation is referred to as end-stage renal disease. Failed kidneys are unable to regulate electrolyte, fluid, and acid-base balances.[12] In chronic renal failure, dialysis is necessary until a kidney transplant is performed. Chronic renal failure has many different causes, including infection, diabetes, hypertensive vascular disease, congenital and hereditary disorders, toxic nephropathy, and obstructive nephropathy.[12]

Renal failure produces no symptoms early in the course of the disease. The most common cause of chronic renal failure is diabetes mellitus.[5] Glomerulonephritis, interstitial nephritis, and chronic upper urinary tract infection are also causes of chronic renal failure. Patients with chronic renal failure may have malaise, increased concentration of urea in blood, fatigue, anorexia, nausea, hypotension, and hyperkalemia. Laboratory findings include decreased GFR, hyperkalemia, elevated BUN and serum creatinine levels, and anemia (from loss of erythropoietin production).
Sonographic Findings. Initially, the kidneys are enlarged; but over time, patients with chronic renal disease have a progressive decrease in renal size bilaterally. With unilateral involvement, the affected kidney is almost impossible to visualize. Sonographically, patients with chronic renal disease have increased cortical echogenicity with poor corticomedullary differentiation. With end-stage renal disease, the kidneys continue to become smaller and more echogenic, and the renal parenchyma becomes thinned (Fig. 6-6).

RENAL ARTERY STENOSIS

Renal artery stenosis is a common cause of renovascular hypertension. Renal artery stenosis also causes chronic renal insufficiency and end-stage renal disease. Atherosclerosis is a common cause of renal artery stenosis in older patients. As the renal artery lumen progressively narrows, renal blood flow decreases and eventually compromises renal function and structure. In patients with renal artery stenosis, chronic ischemia causes atrophy with decreased tubular cell size, patchy inflammation and fibrosis, and intrarenal arterial medial thickening.[13]

Renal artery stenosis causes a decrease in GFR when arterial luminal narrowing exceeds 50%.[13] Renal artery stenosis results in hypertension and a progressive loss of renal function; when bilateral, renal artery stenosis causes renal failure. Renal artery stenosis is a common vascular complication of transplantation, and it affects the renal function.

Sonographic Findings

Sonographically, a patient with renal artery stenosis has significant asymmetry in kidney size. The affected kidney initially increases in size and then ultimately decreases significantly in size, although the renal structures appear normal. Early renal artery stenosis and severe long-standing renal artery stenosis do not show a reduced kidney size.

Spectral Doppler and color flow evaluations are helpful in showing reduced or no flow to the involved kidney or renal area. Duplex evaluation combines B-mode sonography with pulsed Doppler to obtain flow velocity data. In healthy patients, a steep systolic upstroke is seen with a second small peak in early systole and significant diastolic flow. Patients with renal artery stenosis have abnormal Doppler waveforms. Specifically, Doppler analysis in patients with renal artery stenosis shows high systolic peak velocities (Fig. 6-7) with little or no diastolic flow at the site of stenosis. Flow disturbances can occur 1 cm distal to the stenosis.[1] The stenotic area is typically at the junction of the renal artery and the aorta. The tardus parvus effect (seen distal to the stenosis) is apparent in the intrarenal vasculature of patients with renal artery stenosis. The tardus parvus effect is the dampening of the distal waveform–lengthened systolic rise time or slow systolic acceleration (tardus)/lowering and rounding of the systolic peak (parvus).[1]

ACUTE TUBULAR NECROSIS

Acute tubular necrosis results from the lack of blood being supplied to kidneys. This condition may be caused by trauma, surgery, or hypotension and leads to necrosis of the renal tubular epithelium. Acute tubular necrosis is a type of inherent renal failure that cannot be attributed to glomerular, vascular, or interstitial causes. Acute tubular necrosis is caused by the deposit of cellular debris within the renal collecting tubules. Both ischemic and toxic insults cause tubular damage. Acute tubular necrosis is a common cause of acute transplant failure. Acute tubular necrosis may have different causes: prerenal (normal kidney responding to hypoperfusion), renal (pathology is within the kidney itself), or postrenal (caused by urinary tract obstruction).

Patients with acute tubular necrosis may have hypertension, oliguria, edema, hypotension, intermittent flank pain (if caused by calculi), nausea, vomiting, hematuria, infection, sepsis, decreased consciousness, and muscle necrosis. Laboratory findings show an acute decrease in GFR to very low levels and a sudden increase in serum creatinine and BUN concentrations.

Sonographic Findings

Acute tubular necrosis is difficult to diagnose with sonography alone. The sonographic appearance of acute tubular necrosis depends on its cause. When hypotension is the cause, no sonographic abnormalities are apparent. Drugs, metal, and solvent exposures that result in acute tubular necrosis cause enlarged echogenic kidneys. Severe cases of

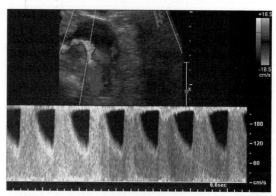

RRA Origin

FIGURE 6-7 Spectral Doppler of right renal artery origin. Note elevated velocities and spectral broadening caused by renal artery stenosis. *(Courtesy Lisa Jones, MD, PhD, Department of Radiology, University of Pennsylvania, Philadelphia, Pennsylvania.)*

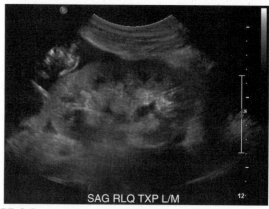

FIGURE 6-8 Sagittal image of a transplant kidney. Note markedly increased echogenicity and enlarged renal pyramids. The diagnosis in this patient was acute tubular necrosis.

acute tubular necrosis also show bilateral renal enlargement. The increase is more apparent in the cross-sectional area than in the length. Less severe cases of acute tubular necrosis may not have any noticeable renal enlargement. The renal parenchymal pattern typically appears normal. Some patients may have an increase in the cortical echodensity with no increase in medullary echodensity. Enlarged renal pyramids may also be visualized (Fig. 6-8). In patients with acute tubular necrosis severe enough to cause renal failure, the Doppler patterns show reduced diastolic flow.

RENAL INFECTION

Many renal diseases involve infection. The spectrum of severity varies depending on the type of renal infection. Renal infection can progress from pyelonephritis to focal nephritis to renal abscess. Most renal infections are contained in the kidney and may be treated with antibiotics. "Nephritis" is a general term for any inflammation of the kidney. It may involve the glomeruli (glomerulonephritis), the spaces within the kidney (interstitial nephritis), or the main tissue of the kidney and pelvis (pyelonephritis). Nephritis may be acute (sudden onset) or chronic (slow onset).

Pyonephrosis

Pyonephrosis refers to distention of the renal collecting system with pus or infected urine. It usually occurs as a result of long-standing ureteral obstruction from calculus disease, stricture, or a congenital anomaly. Pyonephrosis may develop from a broad variety of conditions ranging from an ascending urinary tract infection to the spread of a bacterial pathogen throughout the bloodstream. Upper urinary tract infection in combination with obstruction and hydronephrosis may lead to pyonephrosis. It may be caused by urinary obstruction in the presence of pyelonephritis; this would lead to a collection of WBCs, bacteria, and debris in the collecting system that would cause pyonephrosis. A hydronephrotic kidney filled with stagnant urine may become infected and filled with pus. This pus collects and eventually forms an abscess. Without early recognition, patients with pyonephrosis may have rapid deterioration and develop septic shock. Delayed diagnosis and treatment lead to irreversible kidney parenchymal damage and loss of renal function, ultimately requiring nephrectomy. Death results from excessively delayed diagnosis.

Pyonephrosis is uncommon. It typically is associated with fever, chills, urinary tract infection, obstruction, hydronephrosis, and flank pain, although some patients are asymptomatic. Laboratory results may include **leukocytosis, pyuria, and bacteriuria**.

Sonographic Findings. Sonographic findings suggestive of pyonephrosis include the presence of hydronephrosis in conjunction with debris in the collecting system. The presence of debris and the layering of low-amplitude echoes in a hydronephrotic kidney are indicators of pyonephrosis. These low-level echoes in the collecting system are the most consistent finding in pyonephrosis. In some cases, echogenic pus can be seen filling the collecting system or layering in the dependent portion of the collecting system. Sometimes a kidney with pyonephrosis is indistinguishable from ordinary, noninfected hydronephrosis.

Pyelonephritis

Pyelonephritis is an inflammation of the renal collecting system and renal parenchyma, particularly from local bacterial infection. It is categorized as acute or chronic. Pyelonephritis may localize and intensify to form a renal cortical abscess. It usually stems from retrograde migration of bacteria up the ureter and into the kidney. Generally, pyelonephritis extends from the tip of the papilla to the periphery of the cortex, involving the kidney in a patchy manner. Differentiation between infected and normal parenchyma is usually noticeable.

Pyelonephritis is a common cause of flank pain (mild and dull). Fever, chills, nausea, dysuria, and vomiting are the most common symptoms. Leukocytosis, bacteriuria, and pyuria are typical findings in pyelonephritis.

Sonographic Findings. A renal sonogram to identify hydronephrosis may be helpful in some cases because pyelonephritis should not show any renal pelvic or

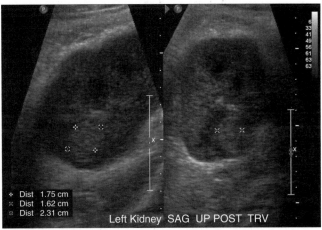

FIGURE 6-9 Transverse image of left kidney with calipers measuring area of altered cortical echogenicity in a patient with acute pyelonephritis.

ureteral dilation. If collecting system dilation is found, pyonephrosis should be suspected. Pyelonephritis shows isolated increases in medullary echogenicity and renal enlargement. Focal pyelonephritis causes increased or decreased areas of echogenicity in the kidney that may bulge outside of the renal outline. Often there are no sonographic findings in cases of pyelonephritis.

Acute Pyelonephritis

Acute pyelonephritis is acute inflammation of the renal parenchyma and pelvis. It is characterized by small cortical abscesses in the medulla from pus in the collecting tubules and interstitial tissue. Acute pyelonephritis is usually the result of a bladder infection (cystitis) that has spread to the kidney.

Acute pyelonephritis is more common in females than in males.[4] Patients with acute pyelonephritis have sudden onset of pain in the lower back, fever with chills, nausea, dysuria, and frequent urination. Laboratory tests show leukocytosis, pyuria, and bacteriuria.

Sonographic Findings. Sonographically, most cases of acute pyelonephritis appear normal. With unilateral involvement, renal enlargement with decreased cortical echogenicity may be apparent. Renal echogenicity varies from a normal appearance to generalized changes to focal decreases in the parenchyma (Fig. 6-9). This decrease in corticomedullary echogenicity causes the renal sinus to appear more prominent. The renal sinus also appears compressed. A loss of corticomedullary differentiation and poorly marginated masses are also apparent in cases of pyelonephritis. Severe cases of acute pyelonephritis show an enlarged kidney (both in length and in cross-sectional area). Severe, prolonged, or multiple episodes of pyelonephritis cause calyceal clubbing and cortical scarring.[1]

Chronic Pyelonephritis

Chronic pyelonephritis refers to recurrent or persistent inflammation of the renal parenchyma and pelvis resulting from bacterial infection. It is characterized by calyceal deformities and large renal scars with patchy distribution. Chronic pyelonephritis is caused by destruction and scarring of the kidney tissue from untreated bacterial infections. It occurs mostly in patients with major anatomic anomalies, including urinary tract obstruction, calculi, renal dysplasia, or vesicoureteral reflux. Chronic pyelonephritis is associated with parenchymal narrowing and progressive renal scarring. If the condition is left untreated, renal failure occurs, requiring dialysis or transplantation.

If symptomatic, patients with chronic pyelonephritis have a high fever, malaise, progressive kidney dysfunction, anemia, lethargy, nausea, vomiting, intense flank pain, dysuria, and hypertension. Chronic pyelonephritis is more common in females than in males.[5] Laboratory findings may include pyuria, proteinuria, bacteriuria, increased serum creatinine levels, and increased BUN values.

Sonographic Findings. Chronic pyelonephritis may show sonographic evidence of calculi. Renal changes are either unilateral or bilateral. Sonographically, a dilated blunt calyx may be visualized with an overlying cortical scar or atrophy. Chronic pyelonephritis shows an increase in cortical and medullary echodensity. Islands of normal tissue are visualized and are potentially confused with tumor formation. Patients with chronic pyelonephritis have clubbing of calyces, irregular renal outline, and thinning of the parenchymal tissue. The pelvis and calyces appear distorted, which causes difficult visualization of the renal boarders. A small, shrunken, misshapen kidney is a common sonographic finding of chronic pyelonephritis.

Emphysematous Pyelonephritis

Emphysematous pyelonephritis is an uncommon, severe, life-threatening infection that results in gas formation in the renal parenchyma. It is caused by vascular disease, elevated glucose levels, and necrotizing infection with a gas-forming organism.[9] Patients with emphysematous pyelonephritis usually need emergency nephrectomy. Generally, emphysematous pyelonephritis affects only one kidney. Emphysematous pyelitis is a less serious condition in which the gas forms in the collecting system (not in the renal parenchyma as in cases of emphysematous pyelonephritis).

Emphysematous pyelonephritis is more common in females than in males and is more common in patients with diabetes.[5] Patients are extremely ill with a fever of unknown origin, flank pain, dehydration, and electrolyte imbalance. Laboratory results include presence of *Escherichia coli* bacteria, hyperglycemia, and acidosis.[9]

Sonographic Findings. Emphysematous pyelonephritis rarely shows echogenic gas. Sonographically, intrarenal gas appears as dirty shadows. Sonographic evaluation is made more difficult because of the gas-producing echogenic foci with distal dirty shadows (Fig. 6-10). Bright reflectors with dirty shadows or ring-down artifacts are

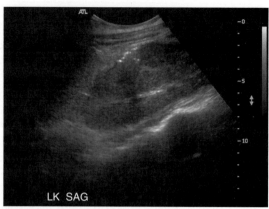

FIGURE 6-10 Left kidney in a patient with emphysematous pyelonephritis. Echogenic foci are causing dirty shadows from intrarenal gas. *(Courtesy Lisa Jones, MD, PhD, Department of Radiology, University of Pennsylvania, Philadelphia, Pennsylvania.)*

also demonstrated. Emphysematous pyelonephritis manifests as a unilateral, enlarged, hypoechoic, inflamed kidney.

Xanthogranulomatous Pyelonephritis

Xanthogranulomatous pyelonephritis is a serious, long-term, debilitating illness characterized by an infectious renal phlegmon. It is a chronic inflammatory disorder of the kidney characterized by a mass originating in the renal parenchyma. A kidney affected with xanthogranulomatous pyelonephritis is usually nonfunctional, and nephrectomy typically is required. It is usually a unilateral disease. Xanthogranulomatous pyelonephritis results from long-term renal obstruction and infection. Frequently, xanthogranulomatous pyelonephritis manifests with stones. Xanthogranulomatous pyelonephritis displays neoplasm-like properties, capable of local tissue invasion and destruction. Xanthogranulomatous pyelonephritis may be contained in the kidney, spread to the perinephric fat, or infiltrate the adjacent retroperitoneal structures. Xanthogranulomatous pyelonephritis has been known to fistulize (either in the renal parenchyma or in the gastrointestinal tract).

Patients with xanthogranulomatous pyelonephritis often are immunocompromised in some manner. Xanthogranulomatous pyelonephritis is more common in females than in males and is more common in patients with diabetes.[5] Patients with xanthogranulomatous pyelonephritis often appear chronically ill. Symptoms include anorexia; fever; weight loss; urinary tract infection; and dull, persistent flank pain. Laboratory findings include leukocytosis, anemia, and bacteria in the urine.

Sonographic Findings. Sonographically, a patient with xanthogranulomatous pyelonephritis has a moderately enlarged kidney. Focal abscesses are also demonstrated. Xanthogranulomatous pyelonephritis may be sonographically indistinguishable from renal cell carcinoma. Most patients have renal calculi, often in the form of a large, echogenic, shadowing staghorn calculus within the collecting system. A staghorn calculus is a calculus that takes the shape of the renal pelvis and sometimes the major caly-ces. These stones do not pass through the ureter and may require lithotripsy. A heterogeneous, inflammatory paren-chymal mass and hydronephrosis may be apparent in the affected kidney. The mass has through transmission and could appear to involve adjacent organs. Xanthogranulo-matous pyelonephritis may show multiple areas of variable echogenicity. Multiple hypoechoic areas corresponding to dilated calyces are apparent. Xanthogranulomatous pyelo-nephritis causes a general decrease in echodensity with some areas of increased echogenicity. Perinephric fluid collections, inflammatory tissues, and dilated calyces are also seen.

Renal Abscess

An abscess is defined as a collection of pus. Renal abscesses tend to cause more intense pain than pyelonephritis, pos-sibly because of the increased edema and inflammation stretching the renal capsule. Renal abscesses are corti-comedullary or cortical. Corticomedullary abscesses are derived from an ascending urinary infection and are associated with obstruction. Severe renal parenchymal involvement is observed with corticomedullary abscesses. Cortical abscesses develop from the spread of bacteria from elsewhere in the body through the vascular system. Renal abscesses result from acute focal bacterial nephri-tis, acute multifocal bacterial nephritis, emphysematous pyelonephritis, and xanthogranulomatous pyelonephri-tis. Without adequate treatment, acute pyelonephritis leads to parenchymal necrosis with abscess formation.

Patients with renal abscesses may have intense flank or abdominal pain, palpable flank mass, fever, chills, dysuria, fatigue, nausea, vomiting, weight loss, and his-tory of a recent urinary tract infection or renal calculi. Patients with diabetes are at an increased risk for renal abscesses. Laboratory findings include urinary infection, leukocytosis, positive urine and blood cultures, hematu-ria, elevated BUN value, elevated creatinine level, bacte-riuria, anemia, proteinuria, and pyuria.

Sonographic Findings. An intrarenal abscess manifests sonographically as an ill-defined renal mass with low-amplitude internal echoes and disruption of the corticome-dullary junction. Renal abscesses appear as thick-walled, hypoechoic, complex cystic masses (Fig. 6-11). Internal mobile debris, gas with dirty shadowing, and septations are occasionally visualized within the abscess. Renal abscesses have irregular borders. Bowel loops filled with air and stool may mimic abscesses when the bowel is lying in close prox-imity to the kidney. Abscess formation generally appears as a complex fluid collection with varying degrees of internal echogenicity and a moderate increase in through transmis-sion of sound. Renal abscesses tend to be solitary.

Fungal Infection

Fungal infections are diseases caused by the growth of fungi in or on the body. Fungal bezoars (fungus balls) are

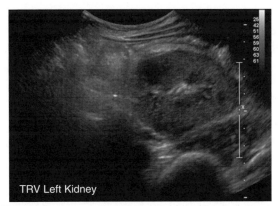

FIGURE 6-11 Transverse image of left kidney with a renal abscess. *(Courtesy Lisa Jones, MD, PhD, Department of Radiology, University of Pennsylvania, Philadelphia, Pennsylvania.)*

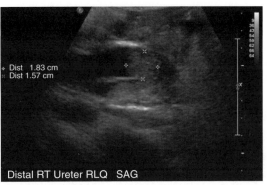

FIGURE 6-12 Sagittal image of distal right ureter demonstrates obstruction by *Candida albicans* (fungal balls). *(Courtesy Lisa Jones, MD, PhD, Department of Radiology, University of Pennsylvania, Philadelphia, Pennsylvania.)*

rare. When fungus balls are present, they can obstruct the renal pelvis or the ureters, resulting in pyonephrosis. Fungal infections diffusely involve the renal parenchyma. Multiple small focal parenchymal abscesses occur that may calcify over time. Fungal infections extend into the perinephric space. Fungal balls result from fungal infec-tions invading the collecting system. Fungus balls are mobile and cause obstruction, leading to development of hydronephrosis. These fungus balls must be differenti-ated from other disorders such as blood clots, radiolucent stones, transitional cell tumors, and sloughed papillae.

Fungal infections of the urinary tract are more often found in diabetic and immunocompromised patients.[9] They are also found in patients with indwelling catheters, malignant diseases, hematopoietic disorders, histories of long-term antibiotic or steroid therapy, and intravenous drug abuse. Laboratory findings include hematuria, bac-teriuria, and pyuria.

Sonographic Findings. A fungal infection appears sonographically as a medium echodensity, nonshadow-ing, mobile defect. Fungus balls are visualized as echo-genic, nonshadowing, soft tissue masses within the renal collecting system (Fig. 6-12). Fungal infections also appear as small, hypoechoic parenchymal masses.

TABLE 6-1	**Pathology Associated with Renal Failure**	
Pathology	**Symptoms**	**Sonographic Findings**
Hydronephrosis	Asymptomatic, pain, infection, nausea, dysuria, fever, chills, vomiting, uremia, microscopic hematuria	Fluid-filled spaces that connect, increased resistance index; when severe, cortical thinning, renal enlargement
Acute glomerulonephritis	Foggy urine, recent fever, sore throat, joint pains, peripheral edema, nausea, oliguria, anemia, azotemia, hypertension	Irregular cortical echo pattern, increased cortical echogenicity, prominent pyramids, bilateral renal enlargement; when chronic, small, smooth, echogenic kidneys
Papillary necrosis	Fever, hematuria, hypertension, dysuria, pain	Hydronephrosis, clubbing of calyces, shadows from calculi, round or triangular anechoic collections in medullary pyramids; when severe, multiple anechoic noncommunicating structures in pyramid area
Acute kidney injury	Hypovolemia, hypertension, edema, oliguria, hematuria	Normal or enlarged kidneys, increased parenchymal echogenicity
Chronic renal failure	Malaise, increased concentration of urea in blood, fatigue, anorexia, nausea, hypotension, hyperkalemia	Decreased renal size, increased cortical echogenicity, poor corticomedullary differentiation; when end-stage, small, echogenic kidney with thin parenchyma
Renal artery stenosis	Hypertension	Initially increased size progressing to decreased size, high systolic peak velocities, little or no diastolic flow at stenosis site, tardus parvus effect distal to stenosis
Acute tubular necrosis	Hypertension, oliguria, edema, hypotension, pain, vomiting, increased cortical echogenicity, hematuria, infection, sepsis, muscle necrosis	Normal appearance, enlarged echogenic kidneys, enlarged and hyperechoic pyramids; when severe, reduced diastolic flow

TABLE 6-2	**Pathology Associated with Renal Infections**	
Pathology	**Symptoms**	**Sonographic Findings**
Pyonephrosis	Asymptomatic, fever, hydronephrosis, urinary tract infection, pain, chills, obstruction	Hydronephrosis with layering of low-amplitude echoes or decreased through transmission
Acute pyelonephritis	Lower back pain, fever, chills, nausea, dysuria, frequent urination	Normal appearance, renal enlargement, decreased cortical echogenicity, focal decreased echogenicity in parenchyma, prominent renal sinus; when severe, cortical scarring, calyceal clubbing
Chronic pyelonephritis	Asymptomatic, high fever, lethargy, nausea, vomiting, intense flank pain, dysuria, hypertension	Shadowing from calculi, dilated blunt calyces, increased parenchymal echodensity, islands of normal tissue, irregular outline, thin parenchyma, decreased kidney size
Emphysematous pyelonephritis	Extreme illness, fever, flank pain, dehydration, electrolyte imbalance, presence of *E. coli* bacteria	Rarely demonstrable, dirty shadows, echogenic foci with distal dirty shadows, ring-down artifacts, unilateral enlarged and hypoechoic kidney
Xanthogranulomatous pyelonephritis	Chronic illness, anorexia, fever, weight loss, urinary tract infection, dull flank pain	Moderately enlarged kidney, focal abscesses, indistinguishable from renal cell carcinoma, large shadowing calculi, areas of variable echogenicity, hydronephrosis, dilated calyces, heterogeneous mass in parenchyma with through transmission, perinephric fluid
Renal abscess	Intense pain, palpable flank mass, fever, chills, dysuria, fatigue, nausea, vomiting, weight loss, recent urinary tract infection, renal calculi	Ill-defined renal mass with low-amplitude internal echoes, internal mobile debris, gas with dirty shadowing, septations, thick-walled, hypoechoic complex cystic mass, irregular borders, moderately increased through transmission
Fungal infection	Found in patients with diabetes, intravenous drug use, immune and hematopoietic disorders, indwelling catheters, malignant disease	Medium echodensity, nonshadowing, mobile defect within renal collecting system, small hypoechoic parenchymal masses

Tables 6-1 and 6-2 provide summaries of the pathology, symptoms, and sonographic findings of renal failure and infections.

SUMMARY

Many precursors to renal failure must be considered in ruling out renal failure. Renal failure is caused by obstruction of urine flow, decreased renal blood flow, or renal parenchymal disease. Hydronephrosis is caused by numerous obstructive processes, including papillary necrosis, pyonephrosis, acute pyelonephritis, xanthogranulomatous pyelonephritis, and fungal infections. Any long-term obstructive process has the potential to lead to renal failure. In addition, any disease that reduces renal function is associated with the ultimate risk of renal failure. Renal function may be ultimately reduced by any of the renal diseases discussed in this chapter. The cause and degree of renal function loss determine the medical path the patient follows (e.g., percutaneous drainage, antibiotics, focal nephrectomy, nephrectomy, dialysis). Sonographically, a thorough B-mode assessment for hydronephrosis, masses, pyonephrosis, and calculi should be done. Color Doppler evaluation should be used to distinguish between pathology and prominent vasculature and to determine patent renal blood flow. Finally, pulsed Doppler evaluation should be used in assessment of renal blood flow for stenosis or thrombosis.

CLINICAL SCENARIO—DIAGNOSIS

The right kidney demonstrates an increase in corticomedullary area with nonvisualization of the pyramids (see Fig. 6-1) compared with the left kidney (see Fig. 6-2). The abnormal laboratory values and patient symptoms are associated with pyelonephritis. Pyelonephritis is a kidney infection that is usually bacterial in origin and stems from an infection in another part of the urinary tract, such as the bladder. Severe cases of pyelonephritis can lead to pyonephrosis. Pyelonephritis requires antibiotic therapy and treatment of any underlying causes to prevent its recurrence. If left untreated, pyelonephritis may localize and intensify to form a renal abscess. Severe, prolonged, or multiple episodes cause cortical scarring. Right pyelonephritis is the only finding in this case study.

CASE STUDIES FOR DISCUSSION

1. A 50-year-old man is sent from the emergency department for a renal sonogram. He complains of "not feeling well" and says his hands and feet are swollen and urine was smoky colored. He recently was treated for strep throat. Vital signs are normal with a blood pressure of 150/110 mm Hg. The renal sonogram reveals prominent pyramids with an increase in the cortical echogenicity (Fig. 6-13). What is the likely diagnosis for this patient?

2. A 65-year-old man undergoes a renal sonogram because of proteinuria and hematuria. He was diagnosed with diabetes 12 years ago and has a 15-year history of hypertension. He admits not taking his medications like he should and complains of being overly tired. Sonographically, the kidneys have a thinned cortex and demonstrate a slight increase in cortical echogenicity (Fig. 6-14). What is the likely diagnosis for this patient?

3. A 30-year-old woman arrives from the emergency department for a renal sonogram. She presents with fever, nausea, and a sudden sharp pain on the right side and back. This is the first time she has ever experienced this type of pain and reports being otherwise healthy. The renal sonogram shows an echogenic calculus with posterior acoustic shadowing in the proximal right ureter causing obstructive hydronephrosis. Within the dilated, primarily anechoic collecting system are low-level echoes that show a layering effect (Fig. 6-15). What are the most likely diagnoses?

4. A 25-year-old man who was admitted after a serious automobile accident has a portable renal sonogram performed in the surgical intensive care unit. He is recovering after surgery for repair of a fractured pelvis and femur. The patient has remained hypotensive with decreased urine output despite being given fluid and medications. The renal sonogram reveals appropriately sized but echogenic kidneys bilaterally (Fig. 6-16). What is the likely diagnosis for this patient?

5. A 62-year-old man with a history of hypertension and increased BUN and creatinine presents for a renal sonogram. He has a 40-pack per year history of tobacco use and complains of pain in his buttocks with walking. Sonographically, there is no evidence of stone, cyst, mass, or hydronephrosis bilaterally. The right kidney measures 8 cm in length, and the left measures 12 cm in length. Doppler evaluation reveals a velocity too high to measure accurately at the origin of the right renal artery (Fig. 6-17). There is a lengthened systolic rise and blunting of the systolic peak in the right intrarenal segmental arteries (Fig. 6-18). What is the likely diagnosis?

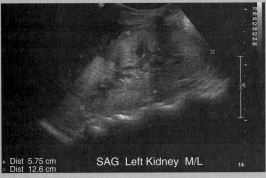

FIGURE 6-13 Sagittal image of right kidney. *(Courtesy Lisa Jones, MD, PhD, Department of Radiology, University of Pennsylvania, Philadelphia, Pennsylvania.)*

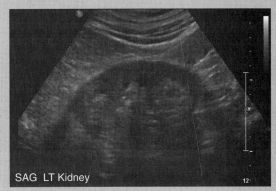

FIGURE 6-14 Sagittal image of left kidney.

Continued

CASE STUDIES FOR DISCUSSION—cont'd

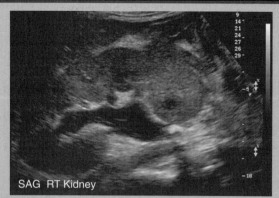

FIGURE 6-15 Sagittal image of right kidney. (*Courtesy Lisa Jones, MD, PhD, Department of Radiology, University of Pennsylvania, Philadelphia, Pennsylvania.*)

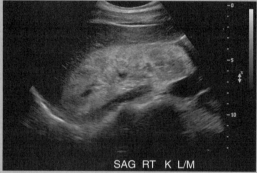

FIGURE 6-16 Sagittal image of right kidney. (*Courtesy Lisa Jones, MD, PhD, Department of Radiology, University of Pennsylvania, Philadelphia, Pennsylvania.*)

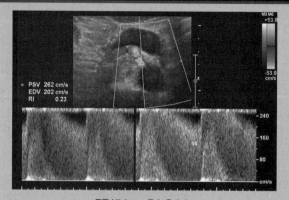

RT Kidney RA Origin

FIGURE 6-17 Spectral Doppler of right renal artery origin.

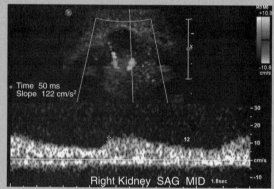

FIGURE 6-18 Spectral Doppler of right segmental artery.

STUDY QUESTIONS

1. A 69-year-old man with a history of an enlarged prostate presents with left flank pain and painful urination. He claims to drink large amounts of milk every day. Laboratory findings include microscopic hematuria. An abdominal sonogram shows normal anatomy except for the left kidney. It displays a hypoechoic, dilated renal collecting system to include the ureter with no echogenic foci. This finding is most consistent with which of the following?
   a. Hydronephrosis caused by the enlarged prostate obstructing flow
   b. Pyonephrosis caused by prolonged obstruction from staghorn calculi
   c. Pyelonephritis caused by infection spreading from the enlarged prostate
   d. Pyonephrosis caused by calcium deposits from excessive milk consumption
   e. Hydronephrosis caused by calcium deposits from excessive milk consumption

2. A 55-year-old man with fatigue, pruritus, and nausea undergoes a renal sonogram. He has a history of diabetes mellitus. Laboratory test results show a decrease in GFR, increased BUN level, elevated creatinine value of 5.1, and anemia. Sonographically, the kidneys are echogenic and decreased in size bilaterally compared with previous sonograms, and the renal parenchyma appears thin. These findings are most consistent with which of the following?
   a. Acute kidney injury
   b. Chronic kidney disease
   c. Papillary necrosis
   d. Renal artery stenosis
   e. Renal infection

3. An 8-year-old boy undergoes a renal sonogram. The patient has recent fever, sore throat, foggy appearance to urine, joint pains, and costovertebral tenderness. Laboratory test results show increased BUN and creatinine levels, hematuria, and proteinuria. Sonographically, the kidneys appear enlarged bilaterally. The left kidney shows irregular cortical echotexture. These findings are most consistent with which of the following?
   a. Papillary necrosis
   b. Hydronephrosis
   c. Acute glomerulonephritis
   d. Fungal infection
   e. Acute tubular necrosis

4. A 23-year-old man presents to the emergency department complaining of severe sharp pain in the left side and back. The pain was of sudden onset. He reports that he also feels nauseated. His urine is positive for blood. There is an echogenic shadowing focus in the lower pole of the left kidney. These findings are most suggestive of which of the following?
   a. Renal abscess
   b. Calcium stone
   c. Pyelonephritis
   d. Pyonephritis
   e. Papillary necrosis

5. A morbidly obese, 51-year-old man is seen for a renal sonogram. He has a history of hypertension, difficulty breathing, and lower back pain. Laboratory test results show a decrease in GFR. The kidneys have a normal sonographic appearance and measure within normal limits bilaterally. Doppler analysis of the left kidney appears normal. The right kidney shows a lengthened systolic rise time, slow systolic acceleration, and rounding of the systolic peak on Doppler analysis. What is a possible diagnosis from these sonographic findings?
   a. Early papillary necrosis
   b. Acute tubular necrosis on right
   c. Renal artery stenosis
   d. Normal findings
   e. Chronic pyelonephritis

6. A 24-year-old female opera singer presents with pharyngitis and decreased volume and frequency of urination. Laboratory test results reveal hematuria. The only sonographic findings are enlarged kidneys with increased echogenicity of the parenchymal cortex. Which of the following diagnoses may result from these limited findings?
   a. Pyonephrosis
   b. Acute glomerulonephritis
   c. Hydronephrosis
   d. Papillary necrosis
   e. Renal abscess

7. A 39-year-old woman undergoes a renal sonogram for hematuria. She has a history of long-term antibiotic use for chronic renal infections. Sonographically, the right kidney is normal, whereas the left kidney shows a hypoechoic, dilated renal pelvis with medium echodensity and round, mobile, nonshadowing soft tissue masses throughout the collecting system. These findings are most suggestive of which of the following?
   a. Renal abscess
   b. Chronic pyelonephritis
   c. Fungal infection
   d. Artifact
   e. Chronic renal failure

8. A 29-year-old woman arrives for renal sonogram. She had a renal sonogram last week in the emergency department but left against medical advice because of long wait time for results. The prior sonogram revealed an enlarged right kidney with decreased cortical echogenicity that was diagnosed as pyelonephritis. She presents today in the emergency department with worsened symptoms. Today's sonogram reveals an ill-defined anechoic mass with internal echoes and faint dirty shadowing. These findings are most suggestive of which of the following?
   a. Renal abscess
   b. Chronic pyelonephritis
   c. Acute tubular necrosis
   d. Papillary necrosis
   e. Prominent pyramid

9. A 33-year-old man with a history of tobacco use is sent for a renal sonogram. The patient has a history of a urinary tract obstruction. He now has reduced urine output and hematuria. Laboratory test results reveal increased creatinine levels, increased BUN values, and a decrease in the GFR. Sonographically, the kidneys are enlarged and show increased echogenicity compared with the liver. What might be the cause of these findings?
   a. Papillary necrosis
   b. Xanthogranulomatous pyelonephritis
   c. Chronic renal failure
   d. Acute renal failure
   e. Emphysematous pyelonephritis

10. A 50-year-old woman who was involved in a motor vehicle accident has a portable renal sonogram performed in the surgical intensive care unit. She was in the operating room 2 days previously, where 3 units of blood were transfused. In the recovery room, it was discovered the patient had a transfusion reaction. Urine output has steadily declined since. Today's sonogram shows an increase in cortical echodensity with a normal-appearing medulla. What is the most likely diagnosis?
    a. Emphysematous pyelonephritis
    b. Acute tubular necrosis
    c. Acute pyelonephritis
    d. Renal abscess
    e. Papillary necrosis

REFERENCES

1. McGahan J, Goldberg B, et al: *Diagnostic ultrasound: a logical approach*, Philadelphia, 1998, Lippincott-Raven.
2. Hagen-Ansert SL: *Textbook of diagnostic ultrasonography*, vol 1, ed 6, St Louis, 2006, Mosby.
3. Cheers G: *Anatomica: the complete home medical reference*, Willoughby, 2000, Global Book Publishing Pty Ltd.
4. Hall R: *The ultrasound handbook: clinical, etiologic, pathologic, implications of sonographic findings*, ed 2, Philadelphia, 1993, JB Lippincott.

5. Rumack C, Wilson S, Charboneau J, et al: *Diagnostic ultrasound*, vol 1, ed 2, St Louis, 2006, Mosby.

6. Parmar MS: *Acute glomerulonephritis*. Emedicine.medscape. comhttp://www.emedicine.com/med/topic879.htm. Retrieved July 9, 2003.

7. Salifu MO, Delano BG: *Chronic glomerulonephritis*. Emedicine. medscape.com.http://www.emedicine.com/med/topic880.htm. Retrieved July 9, 2003.

8. Donohoe JM, Mydlo JH: *Papillary necrosis*. Emedicine. medscape.com.http://www.emedicine.com/med/topic2839. htm. Retrieved July 9, 2003.

9. Kurtz A, Middleton W: *Ultrasound: the requisites*, St Louis, 2003, Mosby.

10. Lewington A, Kanagasundaram S: *Acute kidney injury* http://www.renal.org/Clinical/GuidelinesSection/Acute KidneyInjury.aspx. Retrieved September 2, 2011.

11. Workeneh BT, Agraharkar M, Gupta R: *Acute renal failure*,Emedicine.medscape.com.http://www.emedicine.com/med/ topic1595.htm. Retrieved September 2, 2011.

12. Verrelli M: *Chronic renal failure*. Emedicine.medscape. com.http://www.emedicine.com/med/topic374.htm. Retrieved July 9, 2003.

13. Spinowitz BS, Rodriguez J: *Renal artery stenosis*. Emedicine. medscape.com.http://www.emedicine.com/med/topic2001. htm. Retrieved July 9, 2003.

Renal Mass: Cystic versus Solid

Nancy Chouinard, Ken Marken

CLINICAL SCENARIO

A 55-year-old man presented to the emergency department with left upper quadrant pain and hypertension. The initial sonogram demonstrated a left upper quadrant cystic mass of uncertain origin (Fig. 7-1, A). A computed tomography (CT) scan was ordered to establish the organ of origin (Fig. 7-1, B).

What is the most likely diagnosis for this mass? What finding on the CT scan is helpful to confirm the diagnosis?

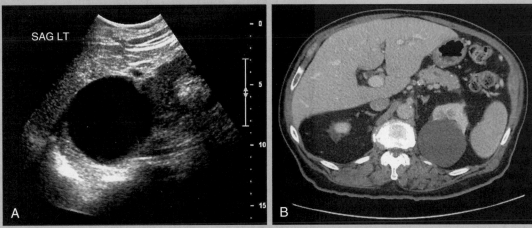

FIGURE 7-1 (A), Sonogram demonstrating cyst adjacent to upper pole left kidney (LK). **(B)**, Axial CT image demonstrating cyst arising from upper pole LK.

OBJECTIVES

- Describe and differentiate cystic renal lesions that can be identified sonographically.
- Differentiate the sonographic findings of various cystic renal lesions.
- Describe the Bosniak renal cyst classifications.
- Describe hereditary diseases associated with renal cysts.
- List anomalies associated with cystic renal diseases.
- Identify Doppler findings associated with cystic lesions.
- List symptoms associated with specific renal cystic lesions.

A renal sonogram may be ordered to identify a mass or characterize the nature of a known mass. The task of the sonographer is to define whether the mass is cystic or solid. When the mass is cystic, it must be further defined sonographically to determine whether alternative imaging or other diagnostic procedures are necessary.

The sonographer must take particular care to demonstrate accurately whether the cyst is simple or contains features such as thick walls, septations, or nodules. The Bosniak Renal Cyst Classification System is a rubric for determining patient management based on these features.[1] Although the system also includes contrast enhancement on CT, the remaining criteria can be helpful in determining appropriate follow-up of a renal cyst demonstrated on a sonogram (Table 7-1).

When cystic lesions are associated with decreasing renal function or other symptoms, such as hematuria

TABLE 7-1	Bosniak Renal Cyst Classification System
Classification	**Description**
1	Simple cysts, 100% benign; no follow-up warranted
2	<3 cm cyst with thin septa or small calcifications; no follow-up warranted
2F	Minimally complicated cyst with suspicious features; follow-up scan recommended, most likely benign
3	Moderately complicated, possible wall nodularity or multiseptated cyst, 50% malignant; surgery recommended because malignancy cannot be ruled out
4	Clearly malignant lesion; surgery recommended

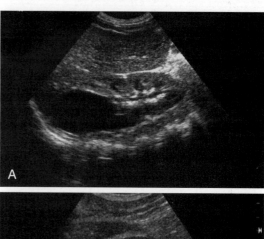
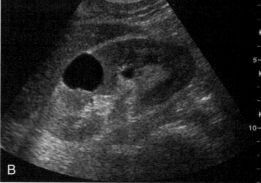

FIGURE 7-2 **(A)** and **(B)**, Simple renal cysts. (**B**, *Courtesy GE Medical Systems.*)

or hypertension, a treatment plan must be developed to avoid other complications. The sonographic examination may assist in defining whether or not the renal cysts are part of a genetic disease.

This chapter explores numerous cystic lesions and cystic diseases of the kidneys. Descriptions of renal neoplasms and the normal sonographic appearance of the kidneys are provided in Chapter 5.

SIMPLE RENAL CYSTS

Cortical Renal Cysts

Cortical renal cysts are common and have been identified in patients of all ages, although they are seen with increasing frequency with increased age. The exact origin of cortical renal cysts is unknown, but they are thought to be acquired. Cysts may be unilateral or bilateral, solitary or multiple. Simple cysts are usually asymptomatic and considered benign, although pain or hematuria may be present.

Sonographic Findings. The sonographic appearance of a renal cyst should meet the criteria of a simple cyst. The cyst should be anechoic, thin-walled, and round or oval, and the sonogram should show acoustic enhancement posterior to the cyst (Fig. 7-2). Edge shadowing is frequently shown along the lateral margins of the cyst. Doppler analysis of the cyst shows the absence of flow (Fig. 7-3, *A*). In addition, aside from recognition of a simple cyst, sonography can examine for renal contour or relational anatomy changes. The claw sign is a concavity in the renal contour where the parenchyma appears to be cupping the cyst or mass, indicating that the cyst or mass has a renal origin.[2] A renal cyst or mass can cause distortion of the perirenal fat outline or displace adjacent structures (Fig. 7-3, *B*).

Parapelvic Cyst

Parapelvic cysts are located in the renal sinus and are thought to be of lymphatic origin. These cysts do not communicate with the renal collecting system, although they may mimic hydronephrosis on sonographic examination. Parapelvic cysts are usually asymptomatic.

Sonographic Findings. Sonographically, a parapelvic cyst appears as a cystic structure arising from the renal sinus. If multiple cysts exist, they may be confused with hydronephrosis. Sonographic differentiation may be made by demonstrating the lack of communication with the cyst or cysts and the collecting system (Fig. 7-4).

COMPLEX RENAL CYSTS

When a cyst does not meet the criteria of a simple cyst, it may be classified as a complex cyst. Complex cysts may exist within the cortex, medulla, or pelvis. A complex cyst may have one or all of the following findings: a perceptible wall, internal echoes, and variable enhancement. A perceptible wall may include wall (mural) calcification, irregularity, nodularity, or thickening. Internal echoes may include thick viscous fluid, debris, or septations. Septations may result from material aggregating within the fluid or possibly from the inner lining of a cyst separating from its wall (see Table 7-1). These cysts can be hemorrhagic cysts, infected cysts, multilocular or septated cysts, cystic malignancies, or calcified cysts (Fig. 7-5). The diagnosis may be made based on the patient's symptoms or may require additional imaging with CT or needle aspiration and histologic examination.

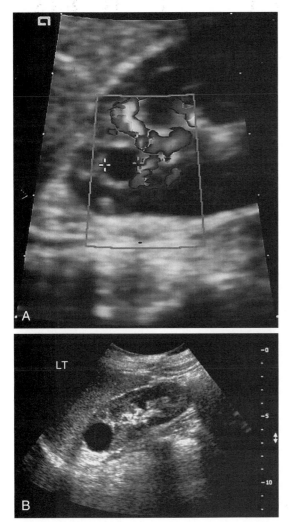

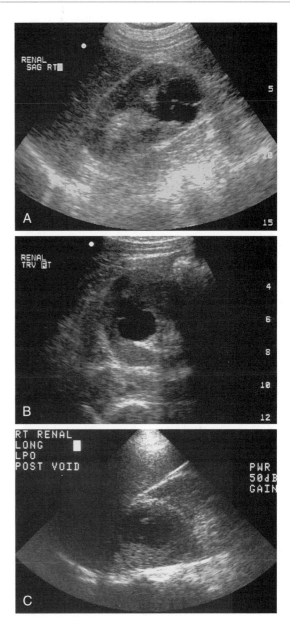

FIGURE 7-3 (A), Upper pole renal cyst with no blood flow to cyst. **(B)**, Simple cyst demonstrating claw sign. (**A**, *Courtesy Shpetim Telegrafi, New York University.*)

FIGURE 7-5 Variable appearances of atypical cysts. **(A)** and **(B)**, Septate cyst. **(C)**, Infected cyst.

Hemorrhagic Cyst

Hemorrhage may occur in simple cysts or in cysts associated with cystic diseases. Patients may have flank pain and hematuria.

Sonographic Findings. Blood has a variable appearance on sonography depending on whether the process is acute or chronic. The cyst may appear anechoic, contain low-level echoes, or have a complex appearance. A hemorrhagic cyst may or may not show acoustic enhancement. A retracted clot may have a similar appearance to a mass, and Doppler may assist in documenting the lack of flow in a hemorrhagic cyst.

Infected Cyst

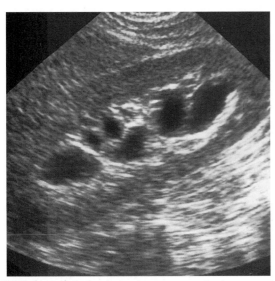

FIGURE 7-4 Multiple, haphazard noncommunicating central cystic spaces represent parapelvic cysts.

When a cyst becomes infected, the patient may have flank pain, fever, hematuria, and white blood cells in the urine.

Sonography can be useful in the diagnosis and treatment of these cysts through guided aspiration and drainage.

Sonographic Findings. Infected cysts can have a variable appearance. Debris may appear as low-level echoes within the cyst and may show a layering effect that moves with a shift in the patient's position. In addition, the cyst wall may be thickened.

Multilocular Cyst

Cysts may contain septations or loculations and may be the result of resolved hemorrhage or infection. Thin septations typically are of no clinical significance, although aspiration may be used to exclude malignant disease.

Sonographic Findings. A septated or multilocular cyst shows thin linear echoes within the cyst or an infolding of the cyst wall. If the septation is thick or shows papillary projections, it is suspicious for malignant disease.

Calcification in Cyst

Calcifications within a cyst wall may be identified in a cyst that has been previously infected or hemorrhagic. A small amount of calcification may be clinically insignificant; however, thick calcifications are worrisome for malignant disease and should be investigated further.

Sonographic Findings. Calcifications appear echogenic and should display shadowing. If the calcification is significant in size, attenuation of the sound beam may prevent adequate visualization of the characteristics of the cyst.

Milk of Calcium Cysts

Milk of calcium cysts occur in patients with a calyceal diverticulum. Urine stasis in the diverticulum leads to formation of the milk of calcium, which is composed primarily of calcium carbonate crystals. Milk of calcium cysts are usually asymptomatic and clinically insignificant. Hematuria, or flank pain, or infection is present in a few patients.[3]

Sonographic Findings. Sonographically, a milk of calcium cyst shows a well-defined cystic lesion with echogenic milk of calcium that layers in the dependent portion of the cyst (Fig. 7-6) and shifts with changes in the patient's position.

Cystic Malignancy

Cystic malignancies include rare cystic neoplasms such as cystic nephroma or cystic renal cell carcinoma.

Sonographic Findings. Malignant masses may appear as unilocular or multilocular cystic masses possibly containing solid nodules, wall irregularity, or calcifications. Large tumors have a heterogeneous appearance because of intratumoral hemorrhage or necrosis. Renal malignancies are often highly vascular. The use of color

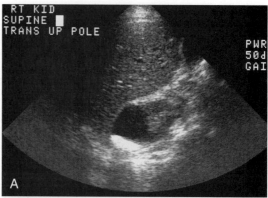

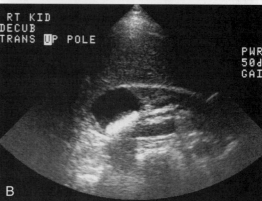

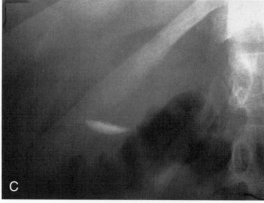

FIGURE 7-6 Shift in position of milk of calcium is noted in cyst as the patient is moved from supine position **(A)** to decubitus position **(B)**. **(C)**, Radiograph taken with patient standing also shows layering effect.

Doppler can determine if blood flow is evident within septa, intra-mass nodules, or the walls of the mass. The sonographer must also evaluate for metastatic spread to the inferior vena cava, local nodes, or the contralateral kidney.

RENAL CYSTIC DISEASE

Autosomal Dominant Polycystic Kidney Disease

Autosomal dominant polycystic kidney disease (ADPKD) is a progressive hereditary disorder that leads to renal failure. ADPKD affects 1:1000 individuals; three genotypes

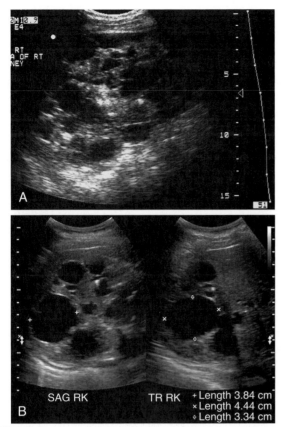

FIGURE 7-7 Possible variations in size of renal cysts seen in two different patients with a history of ADPKD.

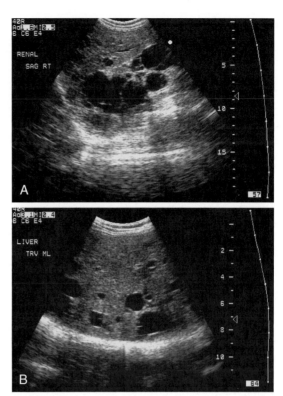

FIGURE 7-8 Multiple cysts are identified in kidneys bilaterally (A) in a 50-year-old woman in whom a polycystic liver is also seen (B).

have been identified with a range of severity.[4] Some cystic renal diseases are seen more frequently in pediatric patients, such as autosomal recessive polycystic kidney disease (ARPKD) and multicystic dysplastic kidney (MCDK). These conditions are discussed in more detail in Chapter 9.

Patients with ADPKD present clinically in the third to fourth decades of life.[5] Patients may have decreasing renal function and hypertension. ADPKD may also affect other organs, and cysts may be found in the liver, pancreas, and spleen. In addition, patients may present with abnormalities of heart valves, colonic diverticula, and cerebral aneurysms. Symptoms may include flank pain and hematuria because cysts associated with ADPKD are prone to hemorrhage or become infected. Renal calculi may also be associated with ADPKD.

Sonographic Findings. Patients with ADPKD have multiple cysts of varying sizes noted bilaterally (Fig. 7-7). The identification of multiple cysts noted bilaterally aids in distinguishing ADPKD from multicystic dysplastic kidney (MCDK) (Fig. 7-8, A). As the disease progresses, the kidneys become markedly enlarged, and the presence of nephromegaly has been directly correlated with decreasing renal function.[4] The liver (Fig. 7-8, B), pancreas, and spleen should also be surveyed for the presence of cysts, although they generally appear later in the disease process.

Sonography is a sensitive screening method for patients with a family history of ADPKD. DNA analysis is also available but is expensive and not as widely available as sonographic screening. The sonographic criteria for diagnosis of the disease should be adjusted according to the patient's age. Findings suggestive of ADPKD include the identification of two renal cysts, unilateral or bilateral, in patients younger than 30 years old; two cysts in each kidney in patients 30 to 59 years old; and four cysts in each kidney in patients 60 years old or older.[5,6] These criteria are discussed in the Unified Criteria for ADPKD.[7]

Acquired Cystic Kidney Disease

Acquired cystic kidney disease (ACKD), or acquired cystic renal disease, is a progressive disorder that results in chronic renal failure from a noncystic renal disorder. It is characterized by the development of multiple cysts in the kidneys and is seen frequently in patients on long-term dialysis.[6,8,9]

ACKD is usually asymptomatic; however, patients may present with clinical symptoms secondary to complications of ACKD, which include hemorrhage and the development of renal cell carcinoma.[6,8,9] When ACKD is associated with renal cell carcinoma, the patient may have hematuria, flank pain, and fever.

Sonographic Findings. The diagnosis of ACKD can be made sonographically when three or more cysts are identified in each kidney (Figs. 7-9 and 7-10). The kidneys

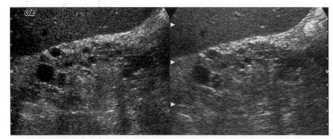

FIGURE 7-9 Multiple cysts are identified in this patient consistent with ACKD. *(Courtesy GE Medical Systems.)*

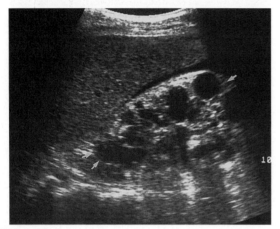

FIGURE 7-10 ACKD. Sagittal sonogram shows echogenic kidney *(arrows)* with parenchymal loss and multiple cysts.

TABLE 7-2	Cystic Lesions of Kidneys	
Pathology	**Symptoms**	**Sonographic Findings**
Simple cyst	Usually asymptomatic	Round or oval, anechoic, thin-walled, posterior enhancement
Hemorrhagic cyst or complex cystic mass	Flank pain, hematuria	Anechoic, low-level echogenicity lesion; with or without posterior enhancement
Infected cyst	Flank pain, fever, hematuria	Cyst with low-level echoes or fluid-debris level; cyst wall thickening
Milk of calcium cyst	Usually asymptomatic	Cystic lesion with layering of echogenic material in dependent portion
Parapelvic cyst	Usually asymptomatic	Cyst or cysts arising in renal sinus
Autosomal dominant polycystic kidney disease	Decreasing renal function, hypertension, flank pain, hematuria	Multiple cysts of variable size, enlargement
Acquired cystic kidney disease	Usually asymptomatic	Three or more cysts in each kidney

are usually decreased in size, but nephromegaly may also be identified.[5] Sonography may also be performed in patients with known ACKD to monitor for the development of malignant neoplasm.

Medullary Cystic Disease

Medullary cystic disease is a rare inherited condition in which tubular atrophy leads to cyst formation in the medulla or at the corticomedullary junction that can occur in children or adults.

Sonographic Findings. Sonography shows small or normal-size kidneys with medullary cysts, as opposed to more common cortical or parapelvic cysts.

Hereditary Conditions Associated with Renal Neoplasia

Von Hippel-Lindau disease and tuberous sclerosis are rare autosomal dominant conditions that affect multiple organ systems. Both conditions produce multiple cortical renal cysts and benign or malignant renal masses. Care should be taken to assess the kidneys to rule out renal masses.

Table 7-2 summarizes the pathology, symptoms, and sonographic findings of cystic lesions of the kidney.

SUMMARY

Sonography is an effective tool for characterizing, differentiating, and documenting renal cystic pathology. Recognizing a complex cyst is paramount and may affect patient follow-up or management.

CLINICAL SCENARIO—DIAGNOSIS

The sonogram demonstrated a roughly 7-cm-diameter simple cyst adjacent to the upper pole of the left kidney. Given the symptom of hypertension and the location of the cystic mass, an adrenal cystic mass should also be considered. The CT scan demonstrated a claw sign, confirming the renal nature of the cyst.

CASE STUDIES FOR DISCUSSION

1. A 50-year-old man presents to his family physician with bilateral flank pain and decreasing renal function. A renal sonogram is ordered. What is the most likely diagnosis based on these images (Fig. 7-11)? Why has the sonographer imaged the liver, and what significance does this image have relative to the diagnosis?

2. A 45-year-old woman presents to the emergency department with severe back pain. The requisition states "abnormal renal function—R/O [rule out] obstruction." What findings indicate an acute rather than a chronic condition? Are these findings consistent with an obstructive cause of the renal impairment? What do the fluid-filled structures (Fig. 7-12) in the kidney likely represent? Are they related to the renal function?

3. A 56-year-old woman is referred for a sonogram for right upper quadrant pain. A previous scan performed in the emergency department determined the presence of a large right upper quadrant cystic mass of indeterminate origin. In what organ or structure does the cyst originate? What sonographic "sign" in these images (Fig. 7-13) suggests this?

4. A 36-year-old woman is referred for a follow-up sonogram of a right renal mass seen on CT scan. The student starting the study is delighted to find this mass and proudly presents the image shown in Figure 7-14, *A*, to her supervising sonographer who then rescans the area, producing the image shown in Figure 7-14, *B*. What differences in technique are displayed between the two images? How might this affect patient management?

5. A 62-year-old man presents with right upper quadrant pain. The sonogram is essentially normal other than the finding shown in the image (Fig. 7-15) of the left kidney. In which Bosniak category does this mass belong? What is the most appropriate follow-up plan for this patient based on this mass?

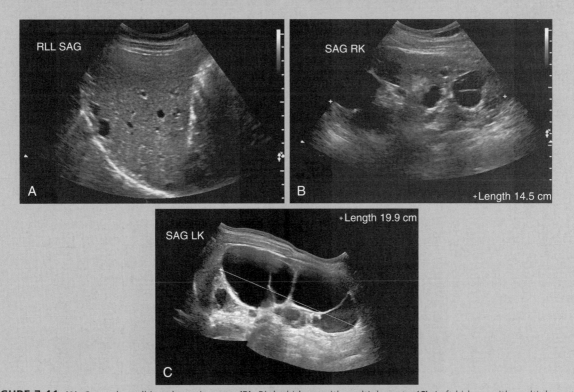

FIGURE 7-11 **(A),** Several small intrahepatic cysts. **(B),** Right kidney with multiple cysts. **(C),** Left kidney with multiple cysts.

Continued

CASE STUDIES FOR DISCUSSION—cont'd

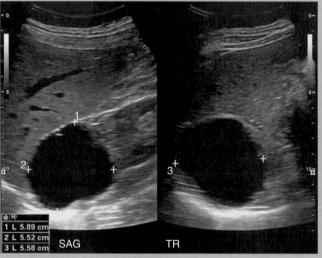

FIGURE 7-12 (A), Perinephric fluid around upper pole of left kidney. **(B),** Longitudinal image of echogenic left kidney with cystic areas in sinus. **(C),** Transverse image of echogenic left kidney with cystic areas in sinus.

FIGURE 7-13 Large right upper quadrant cystic mass.

CASE STUDIES FOR DISCUSSION—cont'd

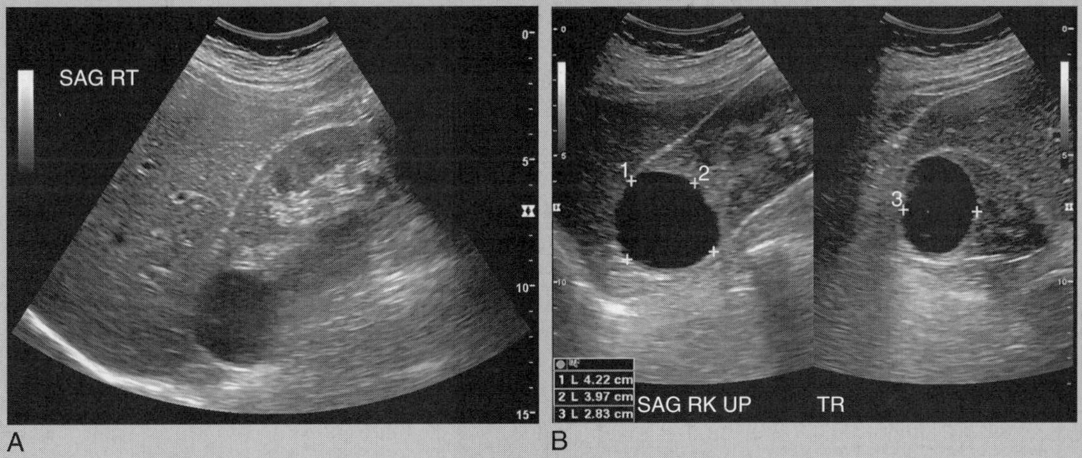

FIGURE 7-14 **(A),** Poorly seen upper pole right kidney. **(B),** Well-seen upper pole right kidney.

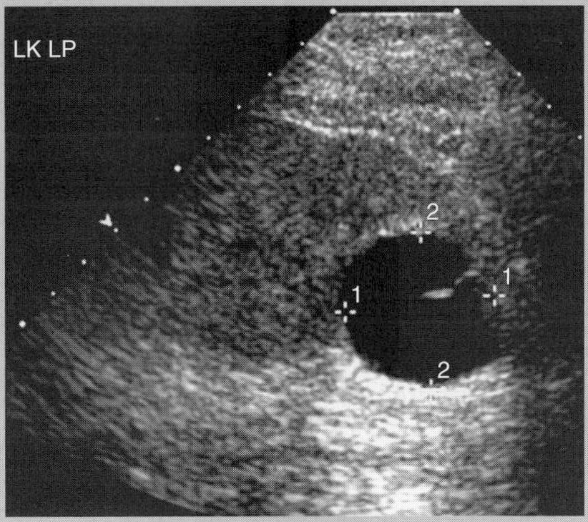

FIGURE 7-15 Longitudinal lower pole left kidney.

STUDY QUESTIONS

1. A 62-year-old woman is sent for an abdominal sonogram for abdominal pain. The sonogram shows normal renal size bilaterally with three cortical cysts on the right kidney and two on the left kidney. This is most likely to be:
   a. MCDK
   b. ACKD
   c. Multiple simple cysts
   d. ADPKD
   e. Multilocular nephroma

2. A 49-year-old asymptomatic man is sent for a follow-up sonogram of a right renal cyst seen on a CT scan performed at another facility. A solitary 2.5-cm right renal cyst with thin septations is seen on the sonogram. This is most consistent with what Bosniak category?
   a. 1
   b. 2
   c. 2F
   d. 3
   e. 4

3. A 48-year-old woman presents with right flank pain. The left kidney is normal. A sagittal view of the right kidney shows multiple centrally located cystic regions. A coronal view of the kidney demonstrates connection between the cysts. This is most consistent with:
   a. Multilocular renal cell carcinoma
   b. MCDK
   c. ADPKD
   d. Hydronephrosis
   e. Medullary cystic disease

4. A 12-year-old, developmentally delayed boy with multiple small facial bumps is referred for a renal sonogram. The sonogram reveals multiple cysts in addition to small echogenic masses in both kidneys. This is consistent with:
   a. Milk of calcium cyst
   b. ARPKD
   c. ADPKD
   d. Medullary cystic disease
   e. Tuberous sclerosis

5. A 30-year-old woman is referred for a renal sonogram for back pain. The sole finding is a 3-cm right renal cyst that is categorized as Bosniak type 1. The most appropriate follow-up to this finding is:
   a. Follow-up sonogram
   b. Contrast-enhanced CT
   c. Magnetic resonance imaging (MRI)
   d. Biopsy
   e. Partial nephrectomy

6. An 88-year-old man is referred for an abdominal sonogram. The requisition is nonspecific, and the patient is a poor historian, but he points to a raised area on his right arm that displays a palpable thrill from a hemodialysis access graft (treatment for renal failure). The sonogram reveals gallstones and bilaterally small kidneys with multiple small cysts. This is consistent with:
   a. MCDK
   b. ADPKD
   c. Multicystic nephroma
   d. Simple cysts
   e. ACKD

7. A 38-year-old woman is referred for a sonogram because of a family history of "kidney problems." The kidneys appear enlarged with five cysts on the right kidney and four on the left kidney. Each cyst measures 2 to 3 cm in diameter. These findings are consistent with:
   a. ARPKD
   b. ADPKD
   c. Simple cysts
   d. MCDK
   e. Tuberous sclerosis

8. A 55-year-old woman with a history of urinary tract infections, an elevated white blood cell count, and right flank pain is referred for a sonogram. Two simple renal cysts are seen on the right kidney. In addition, there is a third cyst that is slightly echogenic. This is consistent with:
   a. Parapelvic cyst
   b. Necrotic renal cell carcinoma
   c. Cystic renal cell carcinoma
   d. ADPKD
   e. Infected cyst

9. A 65-year-old woman has an incidental finding of three irregularly shaped, noncommunicating cystic regions within the right renal sinus that is seen in both longitudinal and transverse scan planes. Which of the following describes the most likely condition seen in this patient?
   a. Right kidney hydronephrosis
   b. Parapelvic cysts left kidney
   c. Multicystic dysplastic right kidney
   d. Parapelvic cysts right kidney
   e. Normal right kidney

10. An asymptomatic patient has a small cyst within the upper pole of the right kidney demonstrating an internal echogenic layer that layers posteriorly. This finding is consistent with:
    a. Simple cyst
    b. Milk of calcium cyst
    c. Parapelvic cyst
    d. Normal medullary pyramid
    e. Angiomyolipoma

REFERENCES

1. Israel GM, Bosniak MA: How I do it: evaluating renal masses, *Radiology* 236:441–450, 2005.
2. Minor TX, Yeh BM, Horval AE, et al: Symptomatic perirenal serous cysts of Mullerian origin mimicking renal cysts on CT, *AJR Am J Roentgenol* 183:1393–1396, 2004.
3. Almeida A, Cavalcanti F, Medeiros A: Milk of calcium in a renal cyst, *Brazilian J Urol* 27:557–559, 2001.
4. Nicolau C, et al: Abdominal sonographic study of autosomal dominant polycystic kidney disease, *J Clin Ultrasound* 22:277–282, 2000.
5. Nicolau C, et al: Autosomal dominant polycystic kidney disease types 1 and 2: assessment of US sensitivity for diagnosis, *Radiology* 213:273–276, 1999.
6. Levine E, et al: Current concepts and controversies in imaging of renal cystic diseases, *Urol Clin North Am* 24:523–543, 1997.
7. Pei Y, et al: Unified criteria for ultrasonographic diagnosis of ADPKD, *J Am Soc Nephrol* 20:205–212, 2009.
8. de Bruyn R, Gordon I: Imaging in cystic renal disease, *Arch Dis Child* 83:401–407, 2000.
9. Choyke PL: Acquired cystic kidney disease, *Eur Radiol* 10:1716–1721, 2000.

8

Left Upper Quadrant Pain

Sheryl E. Goss

CLINICAL SCENARIO

An African American infant was recently hospitalized for hemolytic disease and right hemiparesis secondary to cerebral infarctions, ischemia, and clinical enlargement of the liver and spleen. Computed tomography (CT) scan of the abdomen performed 3 days before the sonogram revealed significant hepatosplenomegaly with heterogene-

ity of the spleen (Fig. 8-1, *A*). The sonogram demonstrates hypoechogenicity of the posterolateral aspect of the spleen compared with the anteromedial aspect (Fig. 8-1, *B*). Color Doppler shows flow in the anteromedial tissue and absence of flow in the posterolateral aspect (Fig. 8-1, *C*; see Color Plate 8). What is the most likely diagnosis?

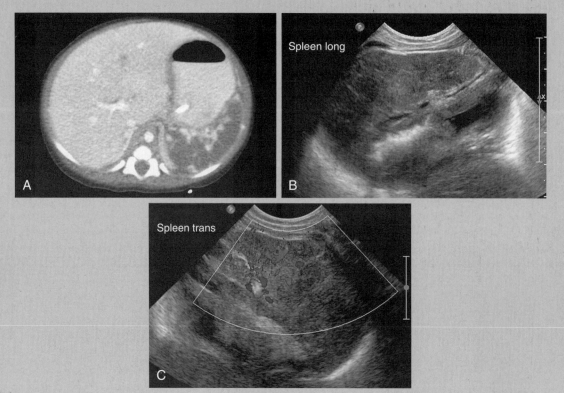

FIGURE 8-1 (A), CT image demonstrates hepatosplenomegaly with irregularity of the spleen. Heterogeneity of spleen **(B)** and absence of color flow in the regions of hypoechogenicity **(C)**.

OBJECTIVES

- List the basic anatomy and physiology of the spleen.
- Describe the sonographic appearance of a normal spleen.
- List the congenital variants of the spleen that may occur, and describe the associated sonographic appearances.
- List the causes of splenomegaly.
- Describe the most common benign splenic neoplasms.

- Identify the sonographic findings associated with blunt trauma to the spleen.
- Define the most common malignant splenic neoplasms.
- Differentiate between the sonographic appearances of benign and malignant neoplasms.
- List the causes of splenic infarct.
- Identify Doppler findings associated with specific splenic anomalies.

Sonography of the spleen is not commonly requested as a focused examination, but rather the spleen is visualized with abdominal sonography, or a splenic sonogram is ordered as a follow-up from other imaging modalities, such as CT or magnetic resonance imaging (MRI). The advantages of sonography include cost-effectiveness, safety because of nonionizing imaging, and portability. The spleen is less often a site for primary disease. Pathologic processes such as portal hypertension, hematologic disorders, and infectious disorders are more commonly encountered. This chapter explores a variety of variants and congenital anomalies, neoplasms, and diseases that may affect the spleen, in conjunction with the clinical significance and sonographic findings.

ANATOMY AND PHYSIOLOGY

The spleen, an intraperitoneal organ, is located in the left upper quadrant (LUQ), with fixation to the greater curvature of the stomach by the gastrosplenic ligament and fixation inferiorly to the left kidney by the splenorenal ligament. Additional ligaments include the phrenicosplenic, providing support from the diaphragm, and splenocolic, providing support from the colic flexure. The shape of the spleen is often described as being convex on its smooth outer surface with close proximity to the diaphragm and pleural cavity. The medial surface is concave, containing the splenic hilum where the splenic artery, vein, and lymphatic vessels enter and exit.

The splenic artery, a branch of the celiac trunk, gives rise to the superior and inferior terminal branches on entering the hilum. Each of these vessels divides further into four to six segmental arteries. The intrasplenic arterial supply is unique in that the branch arteries do not anastomose or communicate with each other, and there is an increased risk for infarction because collateral flow does not occur. The central arterioles, small branches from the segmental arteries, provide blood to the white pulp, terminating in small sinuses. From these sinuses, blood is picked up by the pulp veins and ultimately flows into the portal venous system through the splenic vein. Splenic circulation along with the lymphatics aids the spleen in its physiologic functions.

Physiology of the spleen is complex because the spleen has multiple functions. It is the largest organ of the reticuloendothelial system. The spleen is responsible for filtering aged or damaged blood cells and assists in the body's immune response to blood-borne pathogens. Although the spleen is not vital for life, it provides several key functions, including phagocytosis, antibody production, production of lymph cells, and a reservoir for erythrocytes and plasma cells. The composition of white and red pulp directs splenic function. The white pulp is responsible for immunity through production of antibodies, lymphocytes, and plasma cells. The red pulp comprises the reticuloendothelial tissue, which is responsible for phagocytosis, filtration of aged blood cells, and removal of misshapen or abnormal cells (referred to as culling and pitting).

SPLEEN

Normal Sonographic Anatomy

Lying between the ninth and eleventh left rib, the spleen is best visualized with the patient lying supine or in the left lateral decubitus position and scanning from the coronal plane. A midfrequency small footprint transducer is used. The normal sonographic appearance of the spleen is a homogeneous, comma-shaped or bean-shaped organ, with an echogenicity similar or slightly hyperechoic to the liver and equal to or slightly hyperechoic to the renal parenchyma (Fig. 8-2). Splenic size varies based on age,

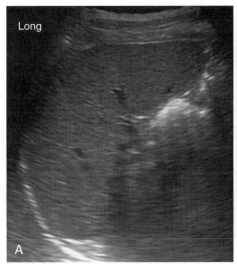
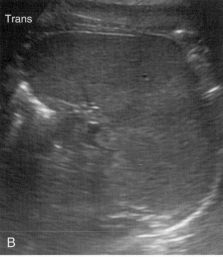

FIGURE 8-2 Normal-appearing spleen on longitudinal **(A)** and transverse **(B)** images.

gender, and height; however, a length of 12 cm is considered to be at the upper limit of normal.[1]

VARIANTS AND CONGENITAL ANOMALIES

Accessory Spleen

Accessory spleen, or splenunculus, is the most common congenital anomaly affecting the spleen, occurring in approximately 10% of the population.[2] This variant is most commonly singular and located in the splenic hilum, although it may be located elsewhere in the abdomen, with a small percentage being multiple (spleniculi). The presence of an accessory spleen is usually insignificant, but accessory spleens may rarely undergo torsion or infarction; affected patients present with acute LUQ pain. Clinical symptoms should also be considered in differentiating between probable accessory spleens, neoplasms, and lymphadenopathy, which may have a similar sonographic appearance.

Sonographic Findings. Accessory spleens are usually round and have an echogenicity and homogeneity equal to the normal spleen (Fig. 8-3). Demonstration of the vascular connection from the accessory spleen to the normal spleen assists in confirmation of the diagnosis.

Ectopic Spleen

Ectopic spleen, a rare entity, may also be referred to as splenia ectopia or wandering spleen. The term "wandering spleen" describes an anomaly in which the spleen migrates from its normal position because of congenital or acquired laxity of the suspensory ligaments. Because of the mobility of the wandering spleen, it may also undergo torsion, resulting in acute abdominal pain and infarction.

Sonographic Findings. The main sonographic finding of an ectopic spleen is the absence of a normal spleen in the LUQ. An ectopic spleen appears as a homogeneous structure consistent with the appearance of a spleen but located outside the LUQ of the abdomen or in the pelvis. It may initially be confused with a mass or neoplasm. The use of power Doppler to show the presence or absence of blood flow in the structure may aid in the diagnosis of torsion or infarction.

Asplenia and Polysplenia

Asplenia and polysplenia are rare congenital anomalies most often associated with visceral heterotaxy, situs ambiguus complexes, or cardiopulmonary abnormalities. Asplenia is the absence of splenic tissue and a bilateral right-sidedness morphology of the heart and lungs. Other anomalies include a reversed aorta and inferior vena cava position or abdominal structures oriented in the midline, such as horseshoe kidney.

Polysplenia is characterized by the development of multiple small splenic nodules. Polysplenia is often associated with a left-sided dominance of lung and cardiac morphology and anomalous development of abdominal structures.

Sonographic Findings. Asplenia is diagnosed through the absence of the splenic tissue after careful evaluation of the entire abdomen to exclude wandering spleen. The diagnosis of polysplenia can be made when multiple small spleens are identified in the LUQ (Fig. 8-4). Additional imaging of the abdomen, heart, and lungs aids in the diagnosis of asplenia or polysplenia-associated complex.

SPLENOMEGALY

Splenomegaly, or enlargement of the spleen, is one of the most common anomalies of the spleen encountered by sonographers. Numerous causes of splenomegaly exist; congestive etiologies associated with portal hypertension are the most common (Fig. 8-5, *A* and *B*). Other causes

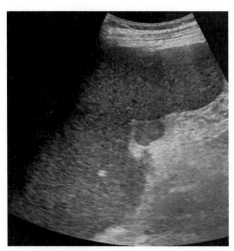

FIGURE 8-3 Accessory spleen is identified in the region of splenic hilum.

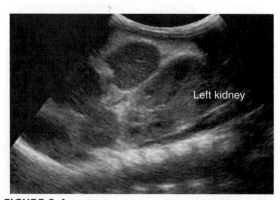

FIGURE 8-4 Multiple spleens noted in LUQ of an infant.

include infection, hematologic disorders, immunologic disorders, trauma, neoplasia, vascular anomalies, and storage diseases. In addition to clinical symptoms associated with the underlying disease, patients with splenomegaly may have LUQ pain.

Sonographic Findings

A diagnosis of splenomegaly (Fig. 8-5, C) may be made when the length of the spleen is greater than 12 cm.[1] A subjective diagnosis of splenomegaly may also be made when the inferior tip of the spleen covers or extends beyond the inferior pole of the left kidney.

HYPOSPLENISM

Hyposplenism, or decreased physiologic function of the spleen, is associated with impaired function or absence of the spleen. Spleen size is not directly in correlation to function; however, autoinfarction associated with sickle cell anemia, celiac disease, autoimmune diseases,

hematologic disorders, or graft bone marrow transplantation can result in diminishing organ volume. Diagnosis is based on a decreased filtration function and compromised immune status.

Sonographic Findings

Hyposplenism cannot be diagnosed with sonography. Absence of the spleen or diminished organ size on the sonogram can assist in confirming clinical associations.

CYSTS

With the detection of a cyst in the LUQ, sonographic examination can be useful in identifying the origin of the cyst—arising in the spleen or arising from adjacent organs such as the adrenal gland, gastrointestinal tract, or a pancreatic pseudocyst extending into the spleen (see Chapter 4). Laboratory tests and patient history may also aid in the differentiation of cyst origin. Cysts arising

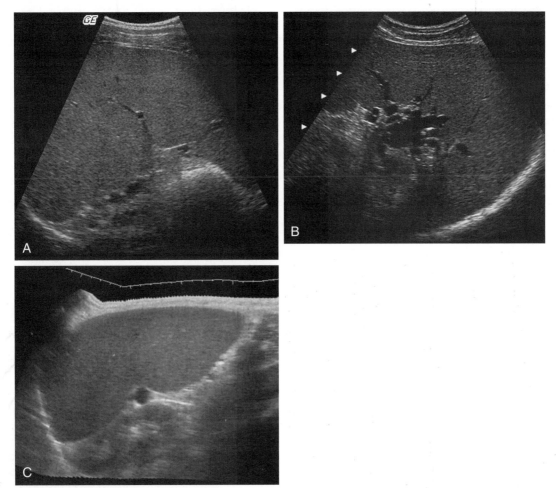

FIGURE 8-5 Longitudinal **(A)** and transverse **(B)** images show enlargement of the spleen with hilar vessel dilation associated with portal hypertension. **(C)**, Extended field-of-view technique demonstrates enlarged spleen extending beyond the lower pole of the kidney. *(**A** and **B**, Courtesy GE Medical Systems.)*

in the spleen may be classified as primary or true cysts, when they have an epithelial or endothelial lining, or secondary (pseudocysts), resulting from trauma, infection, or degeneration. Cysts in the spleen are uncommon and are usually benign. Splenic cysts may be identified on sonograms in asymptomatic patients as an incidental finding, although patients may have symptoms related to the cyst size or origin and may have LUQ pain.

Sonographic Findings

Sonographically, a cyst should appear as a well-defined, round or ovoid, thin-walled, anechoic lesion that shows acoustic enhancement (Fig. 8-6, *A*). Cysts associated with infection or trauma may show calcification of the cyst wall (Fig. 8-6, *B*). Cysts may also show fluid-debris levels from purulent material or hemorrhage. Splenic cysts are rare; in the absence of the classic sonographic features of a cyst, additional imaging or clinical follow-up is indicated to exclude neoplasm.

ABSCESS

Abscess formation in the spleen is considered rare. It is associated with various origins, including hematologic spread of infection, trauma, and endocarditis, which is considered to be the most common predisposition.[3] Abscess formation may manifest as a solitary lesion or multiple masses. Patient symptoms may be silent or subtle, or patients may exhibit LUQ pain, fever, or referred pain to the chest or shoulder. Additional clinical associations include splenomegaly, nausea and vomiting, and leukocytosis. Abscesses may rupture; ruptured splenic abscess is associated with a high mortality rate. Sonography-guided aspiration may be used in combination with appropriate antibiotics to treat this disease; however, splenectomy may be necessary if there is an insufficient response to antibiotic therapy.

Sonographic Findings

The sonographic appearance of a splenic abscess is variable. Lesions may be solitary or multiple and are characterized by an ovoid or round shape, with irregular walls (Fig. 8-7). Hypoechoic or anechoic lesions may be identified, and acoustic enhancement may be noted. If gas is present, dirty shadowing may be seen.

INFARCT

Splenic infarction may occur secondary to an embolic event, a hematologic disorder, vascular or pancreatic disease, congenital abnormalities, or neoplasm. Infarction of the spleen, although uncommon, is one of the more common causes of focal splenic lesions and should be considered when patients have LUQ pain.

Sonographic Findings

The most specific sonographic finding of a splenic infarct is a wedge-shaped, hypoechoic lesion (Fig. 8-8); the echogenicity may increase over time. An infarct may appear round or be of variable echogenicity and shape

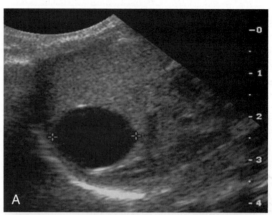
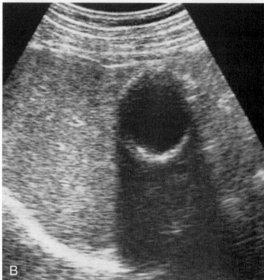

FIGURE 8-6 (A), Coronal scan of spleen shows a 1.5-cm diameter cyst. **(B),** Calcified splenic cyst.

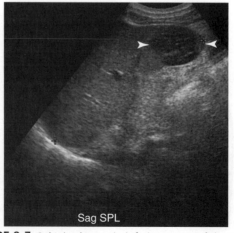

FIGURE 8-7 Splenic abscess in inferior aspect of the spleen.

and indistinguishable from other splenic lesions, including neoplasms, abscesses, and hematomas.

CALCIFICATIONS

Calcifications in the spleen (Fig. 8-9) are usually an incidental finding and a remnant of a previous disease process. Resolution of hematoma, infarction, infection, abscess, or necrosis of a neoplasm may generate calcifications. Granulomas are the most common disseminated calcifications. They can develop from a variety of causes, including tuberculosis, histoplasmosis, sarcoidosis, or brucellosis. Gamna-Gandy bodies (siderotic nodules) represent organized foci of hemorrhage in the spleen caused by portal hypertension. Gamna-Gandy bodies contain hemosiderin, fibrous tissue, and calcium. MRI is the most sensitive imaging modality for the detection of these nodules because of their iron content. CT and sonography also help in detection and characterization of nodules. Linear calcifications are associated with vascular wall calcification. The clinical history can assist in establishing the potential cause of splenic calcifications.

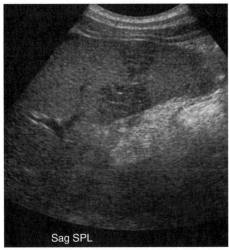

FIGURE 8-8 Two hypoechoic wedge-shaped regions consistent with splenic infarcts.

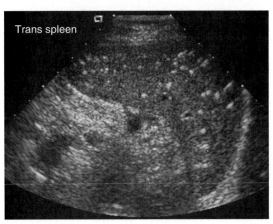

FIGURE 8-9 Multiple echogenic foci resulting from histoplasmosis.

Without the presence of neoplasm, splenic calcifications are considered to be benign.

Sonographic Findings

Calcification can be singular or multiple with variable size depending on the etiology. Posterior shadowing may or may not be present. Color Doppler may demonstrate the twinkle artifact.

BENIGN NEOPLASMS

Hemangioma

Hemangiomas may be identified in the spleen and in the liver. Although benign neoplasms of the spleen are rare, hemangioma is the most common benign tumor of the spleen. They are usually isolated, are insignificant, and measure less than 2 cm. Large lesions are at risk for rupture and hemorrhage, causing LUQ pain. Splenic hemangioma may also occur in association with Klippel-Trénaunay-Weber syndrome.

Sonographic Findings. The sonographic appearance of a splenic hemangioma may be similar to a hemangioma identified in the liver—a well-defined, homogeneous, echogenic mass (Fig. 8-10). Larger hemangiomas may appear heterogeneous or complex or contain calcifications.

Hamartoma

Splenic hamartoma, also termed splenoma or splenadenoma, is a benign rare vascular proliferation tumor that is typically an incidental finding because it is usually asymptomatic. Incidence in male and female patients is equal. The median size is 5 cm; however, the average size of a hamartoma in female patients is reported to be larger, suggesting influence by hormones.[4] When clinical symptoms are present, they may include pancytopenia, anemia, and thrombocytopenia. This lesion can become greatly enlarged, compressing surrounding splenic tissues. Splenic hamartomas can also spontaneously rupture, causing acute pain.

Sonographic Findings. The most common sonographic appearance of a splenic hamartoma is a homogeneous, solid lesion of variable echogenicity. Hamartomas may also appear heterogeneous and complex and contain calcifications. This tumor may also show hypervascularity within the lesion with color Doppler, although this may not always be present.

Lymphangioma

Splenic lymphangioma is a rare vascular tumor that occurs most commonly in childhood. The disease may be isolated to the spleen or involve multiple organs, referred to as lymphangiomatosis. Clinical presentation includes

LUQ pain, nausea, or abdominal distention. Symptoms are related to the developing splenomegaly and the subsequent compression of surrounding structures that occurs as the tumor grows. Large tumors can result in bleeding, coagulopathy, hypersplenism, or portal hypertension, requiring surgical intervention.

Sonographic Findings. Lymphangiomas manifest sonographically as cystic lesions arising within the spleen, with associated splenomegaly. They may demonstrate occasional presence of internal septations or intralocular debris or manifest as multicystic lesions.

Other Benign Neoplasms

Benign splenic neoplasms that may be listed as a differential diagnosis include hemangioendothelioma, angiomyoli-

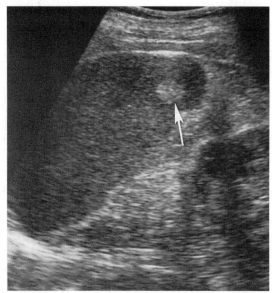

FIGURE 8-10 Splenic hemangioma. Small, well-defined, rounded, echogenic lesion *(arrow)* in the spleen measures 1.4 cm in diameter.

poma, littoral cell angioma, hemangiopericytoma, lipoma, and peliosis. These benign neoplasms are rarely identified.

MALIGNANT NEOPLASMS

Lymphoma

The most common malignant disease that affects the spleen is lymphoma (Hodgkin's disease and non-Hodgkin's lymphoma). Lymphoma may manifest as a primary splenic neoplasm or as a component of a disseminated disease process. Primary splenic lymphoma is more commonly identified in older patients.

Sonographic Findings. Sonographic examination of lymphoma of the spleen may reveal a diffuse, nodular spleen. Hypoechoic lesions or diffuse inhomogeneity have been described (Fig. 8-11).

Angiosarcoma

Angiosarcoma is a primary nonhematolymphoid neoplasm that usually arises in the spleen or liver and may also be termed hemangiosarcoma (Fig. 8-12). It is more prevalent in older patients. Clinical symptoms include LUQ pain, malaise, fever, and weight loss. This tumor has a high incidence of splenic rupture and may cause acute abdominal pain, hemoperitoneum, and death. Hemangiosarcoma is a highly aggressive tumor with a dismal prognosis because of a high incidence of metastasis to bone, bone marrow, the lymphatic system, liver, or lungs.

Sonographic Findings. The sonographic appearance of angiosarcoma may be a heterogeneous, complex mass, overall inhomogeneity, multiple hypoechoic masses, or complex lesions. Associated splenomegaly is also a typical finding. Doppler evaluation may show blood flow in the echogenic solid tissue component of the neoplasm.

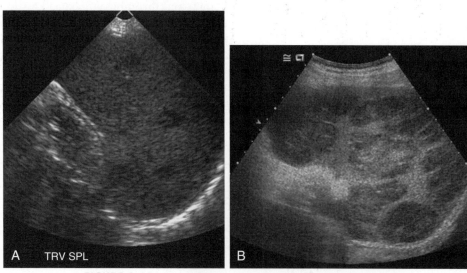

FIGURE 8-11 (A) and **(B)**, Two variable presentations of lymphoma.

Metastasis

Metastasis to the spleen is uncommon and is usually a feature of widespread disease. Organs more frequently associated with splenic metastasis are the ovary, prostate, lung, and breast. It is also seen with colorectal tumors, gastric tumors, and melanoma.

Sonographic Findings. Most metastatic lesions in the spleen appear similar to metastatic liver lesions and exhibit a target or bull's-eye appearance, with a hypoechoic halo. A less common appearance is a cystic, hyperechoic, or complex mass (Fig. 8-13).

Other Malignant Neoplasms

Other malignant neoplasms may arise in the spleen and are rarely identified. Depending on the patient history and symptoms, malignant diseases that may be suggested

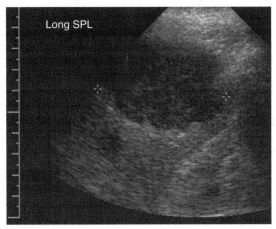

FIGURE 8-12 Hypoechoic lobular lesion measuring 6.1 cm. Biopsy indicated angiosarcoma.

in the differential diagnosis include Kaposi's sarcoma, leiomyosarcoma, fibrosarcoma, littoral cell angiosarcoma, malignant fibrous histiocytoma, cystadenocarcinoma, and teratoma.

TRAUMA

Hematoma, with or without Rupture

Blunt trauma to the LUQ can cause a splenic hematoma, or subcapsular hematoma with or without rupture of the splenic capsule. Clinical symptoms include severe LUQ pain, falling hematocrit, syncope, and hypotension. Complications of nonsurgical management of blunt splenic injuries, although rare, include delayed splenic rupture, pseudocyst formation, and pseudoaneurysm formation. Spontaneous splenic rupture has been identified in patients with infectious diseases, including mononucleosis, HIV, hepatitis A, malaria, and cytomegalovirus.

A consequence of splenic rupture is splenosis, an autotransplantation of splenic tissue deposits. The peritoneal cavity is the most common location for deposits, but cases have been reported with deposits in the retroperitoneum and thorax.

Sonography may be used as a prompt and cost-effective imaging method to diagnose the extent of trauma, to assist in determining the method of treatment, and to follow patients with a history of splenic injuries.

Sonographic Findings. The appearance of a hematoma varies based on the age of the hematoma. Blood may initially appear similar in echogenicity to the spleen, becoming more anechoic over time. A subcapsular hematoma (Fig. 8-14) conforms to the shape of the spleen. When it appears isoechoic to splenic

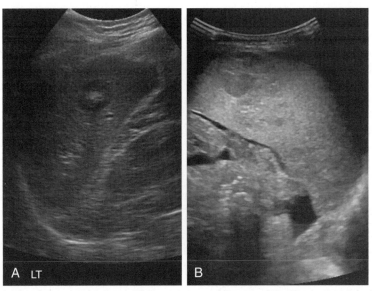

FIGURE 8-13 Variable presentation of metastatic disease from primary melanoma. **(A)**, Classic target lesion. **(B)**, Free fluid and multiple hypoechoic lesions within the spleen.

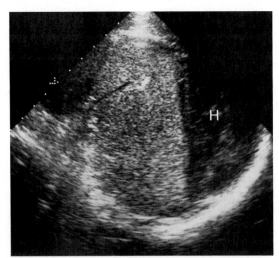

FIGURE 8-14 Subcapsular hematoma of the spleen. Transverse scan shows fluid-filled and debris-filled crescentic hematoma *(H)* in lateral aspect of spleen.

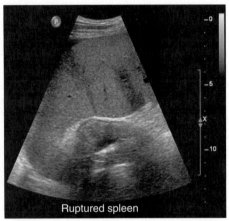

Ruptured spleen

FIGURE 8-15 Rupture of spleen resulting in an inhomogeneous texture with fluid superiorly. *(Courtesy Philips Healthcare.)*

parenchyma, it may mimic splenomegaly. Likewise, a hematoma within the spleen contains echoes initially but may appear inhomogeneous compared with the homogeneous splenic parenchyma. Rupture of the splenic capsule demonstrates fluid within the peritoneal cavity (Fig. 8-15). Color Doppler of anechoic lesions should be used to rule out splenic pseudoaneurysm in a patient with splenic trauma. Splenic deposits from splenosis have the echogenicity of normal spleen; however, because of their small size and locations, nuclear medicine is useful in making this diagnosis.

Table 8-1 summarizes the pathology, symptoms, and sonographic findings of lesions of the spleen.

TABLE 8-1	Lesions of Spleen	
Pathology	**Symptoms**	**Sonographic Findings**
Simple cyst	Usually asymptomatic	Round or oval, anechoic, thin-walled, posterior enhancement
Abscess	LUQ pain, fever, nausea and vomiting	Round or oval lesion with irregular wall, hypoechoic or anechoic, with or without enhancement
Infarct	LUQ pain	Wedge-shaped hypoechoic lesion; may be round with variable echogenicity
Hemangioma	Usually asymptomatic	Well-defined, homogeneous, echogenic lesion
Hamartoma	Usually asymptomatic	Homogeneous, solid lesion of variable echogenicity; may appear inhomogeneous or complex
Lymphangioma	LUQ fullness or pain	Cystic or multicystic lesion
Angiosarcoma	LUQ pain, malaise, fever, weight loss	Inhomogeneous spleen with multiple, hypoechoic lesions and splenomegaly

SUMMARY

The sonographer must understand and be able to differentiate pathology that may be identified in the spleen. Although the spleen is rarely the focus of a sonographic examination, the sonographer may identify pathology as an incidental finding. Sonography also may be used in patients who cannot be transported or for follow-up of pathology previously identified with another imaging method. A thorough understanding of the sonographic appearance of splenic pathology, acquiring a detailed clinical history, and knowledge of associated risk factors and symptoms ensure that the sonographer will provide the physician with images and information necessary to make an accurate diagnosis.

CLINICAL SCENARIO—DIAGNOSIS

This infant has a clinical diagnosis of sickle cell disease, which is associated with a high risk for splenic infarction. Sickle cell anemia, the most common form of sickle cell disease, is characterized by the body manufacturing misshapen or crescent-shaped red blood cells. Sickle-shaped cells create a slower and more difficult flow within vessels, increasing the risk for thrombus, infarction, and infection. Sonographic images demonstrate inhomogeneity of the spleen and absence of color flow consistent with infarction. Cerebral infarction explains the right-sided hemiparesis.

CASE STUDIES FOR DISCUSSION

1. A 22-year-old man with a history of multiple sclerosis and neurogenic bladder has undergone multiple CT scans and sonograms over the years. Figure 8-16 demonstrates a solitary splenic lesion that has been stable in size and appearance across the patient's imaging history. What is the most likely nature of this finding?

2. A 44-year-old woman presents with right upper quadrant discomfort and is referred for an abdominal sonogram. Laboratory values were normal for hematocrit, red blood cell, white blood cell, and platelet values. The patient reported absence of pain or discomfort on the left side. Figure 8-17 demonstrates heterogeneity of the spleen owing to multiple hyperechoic lesions. What are the sonographic appearances and clinical history most suggestive of for this patient?

3. A 16-year-old patient presents to the emergency department with a gunshot wound to the LUQ. A focused assessment by sonography for trauma (FAST) sonogram performed in the emergency department did not reveal peritoneal fluid or bleeding. A complete blood count indicated normal values with the exception of a decreased hematocrit. The blood pressure was stable. The patient was referred for a CT scan, which demonstrated a subcapsular splenic abnormality (Fig. 8-18, *A*); the remainder of the study was

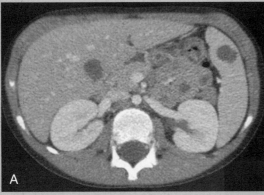 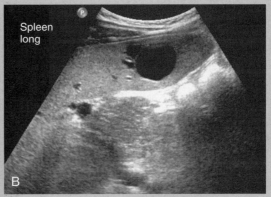

FIGURE 8-16 **(A)**, CT image of the abdomen demonstrates solitary lesions in liver and spleen. **(B)**, Corresponding mass in the spleen.

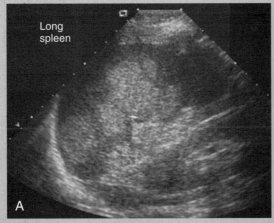 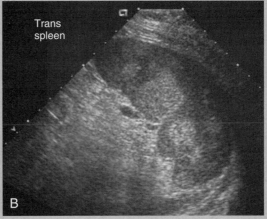

FIGURE 8-17 Longitudinal **(A)** and transverse **(B)** images demonstrate heterogeneity with multiple echogenic lesions.

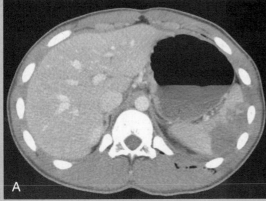 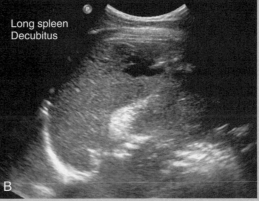

FIGURE 8-18 **(A)**, CT image demonstrates abnormality of lateral aspect of the spleen. **(B)**, Sonogram reveals irregular hypoechoic area on lateral aspect of the spleen.

Continued

CASE STUDIES FOR DISCUSSION—cont'd

normal. The sonogram identified the findings in Figure 8-18, *B,* and the absence of free peritoneal fluid. Discuss these findings.

4. A 62-year-old woman with increasing abdominal girth is referred for an abdominal sonogram before performance of a paracentesis to relieve her shortness of breath. She relayed a clinical history of abnormal liver function tests and chronic hepatitis C, which resulted in cirrhosis and portal hypertension. Sonographic imaging history revealed hepatofugal flow before placement of a transjugular intrahepatic portosystemic shunt (TIPS) 2 years ago and, more recently, TIPS failure. Compared with the sonogram performed 2 years ago, the current sonogram reveals multiple echogenic, punctate calcifications throughout the spleen that were not present 2 years ago. What is the cause of the echogenic foci?

5. A 5-month-old girl with clinical suspicion of splenomegaly undergoes an abdominal sonogram. Her clinical history included an echocardiogram reporting an atrioventricular canal defect, chest x-ray illustrating an interrupted inferior vena cava, and possible situs ambiguus. The sonogram revealed the liver to be located more central in the midline and the spleen to be abnormal in location and appearance. Figure 8-19 was obtained from a trans-

verse scan plane to the left of midline in the region of the spleen. Describe the sonographic findings and congenital associations for this appearance.

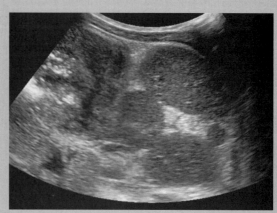

FIGURE 8-19 Transverse image at the region of the spleen.

STUDY QUESTIONS

1. A patient presents with a history of alcohol abuse and ascites. Images of the spleen reveal enlargement with dilation of the vessels at the hilum. This is most likely consistent with which of the following?
   a. Metastasis
   b. Splenic rupture
   c. Splenic aneurysm
   d. Portal hypertension
   e. Trauma

2. A 19-year-old woman presents with enlarged cervical lymph nodes, fatigue, and leukopenia. Before her scheduled bone marrow biopsy, an abdominal sonogram was performed, which revealed diffuse, hypoechoic lesions within the spleen. This describes:
   a. Infarct
   b. Lymphoma
   c. Hamartoma
   d. Metastasis
   e. Hemangioma

3. In what way does the vascular system of the spleen differ from other organ circulation?
   a. The spleen lacks a venous return
   b. Arteries are found only in the periphery
   c. Intrasplenic arteries do not anastomose or communicate
   d. Arteries and veins directly connect with each other

4. An asymptomatic patient undergoes sonography for possible enlargement of the spleen on physical

examination. The sonogram reveals a splenic length of 11.6 cm and a 1.5-cm round hyperechoic nodule in the superior aspect. These findings are most likely consistent with which of the following?
   a. Accessory spleen
   b. Hemangioma
   c. Angiosarcoma
   d. Hamartoma
   e. Splenomegaly

5. An elderly patient who is a poor clinical historian presents for an abdominal sonogram. Splenic images reveal multiple diffuse, small, echogenic foci without posterior shadowing. Which of the following illnesses may the patient have had in the past?
   a. Lymphoma
   b. Malignancy
   c. Pyogenic abscess
   d. Tuberculosis
   e. Portal hypertension

6. A 43-year-old woman presented with abdominopelvic pain. Imaging of the abdomen revealed normal liver and kidneys. The spleen was absent in the LUQ. Sonographic images of the abdomen and pelvis revealed a homogeneous, medium gray, mass-like lesion in the superior left adnexa. This finding is consistent with:
   a. Wandering spleen
   b. Asplenia
   c. Spleniculi
   d. Hyposplenism
   e. Angiosarcoma

7. A 35-year-old man with a history of HIV presents with severe LUQ pain, decreased hematocrit, and hypotension. Clinical assessment and CT imaging confirmed rupture of the spleen. A consequence of splenic rupture is:
   a. Granuloma
   b. Infection
   c. Splenosis
   d. Malignancy
   e. Histoplasmosis

8. A patient with a history of celiac disease and a compromised immune system presents to the sonography department for evaluation of the spleen. The clinical concern is hyposplenism. What sonographic findings might be expected?
   a. Normal size spleen or splenomegaly
   b. Decreased or normal size
   c. Always a decreased volume
   d. Always an increased volume

9. A neonate is referred for echocardiography and abdominal sonogram. The echocardiogram revealed both atria to have features of the right atrium. The abdominal sonogram revealed a partial situs inversus of the abdominal organs. What would the expectation be for the spleen?

   a. Located on the right side
   b. Located normally on the left side
   c. Absence of splenic tissue
   d. Multiple spleens
   e. Accessory spleens

10. An adult patient presents with mild left-sided pain. On a sonogram, the spleen appeared to be of normal echogenicity. In a normal patient, what is the expected echogenicity of the spleen compared with the liver?
    a. Anechoic
    b. Sonolucent
    c. Slightly increased
    d. Slightly decreased
    e. Heterogeneous

REFERENCES

1. Benter T, Kluhs L, Teichgraber U: Sonography of the spleen, *J Ultrasound Med* 30:1281–1293, 2011.
2. Robertson F, Leander P, Ekberg O: Radiology of the spleen, *Eur Radiol* 11:80–95, 2001.
3. Wang CC, Lee CH, Chan CY, et al: Splenic infarction and abscess complicating infective endocarditis, *Am J Emerg Med* 27:1021, 2009.
4. Hwajeong L, Koichi M: Hamartoma of the spleen, *Arch Pathol Lab Med* 133:147–151, 2009.

9

Pediatric Mass

Joy Guthrie, Kathryn Kuntz

CLINICAL SCENARIO

A 2-month-old boy undergoes a renal sonogram to evaluate a palpable abdominal mass and wrinkled abdominal wall skin. The sonogram reveals an enlarged kidney with hydroureteronephrosis, thin renal cortex, and normal bladder dimension (Fig. 9-1). The contralateral kidney is normal. What is the most likely diagnosis?

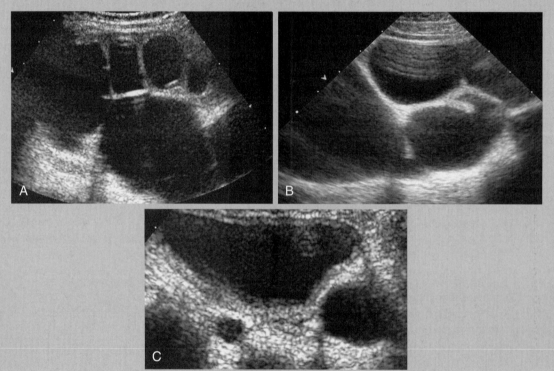

FIGURE 9-1 (A), Longitudinal image demonstrates marked hydronephrosis. **(B),** Markedly dilated, serpiginous ureter. **(C),** Transverse image of normal urinary bladder and bilateral dilated ureters.

OBJECTIVES

- Describe the sonographic appearance of biliary tract anomalies that are common in the pediatric abdomen.
- Differentiate abdominal neoplasms that occur in pediatric patients.
- Identify pertinent laboratory values associated with neoplasms in the pediatric abdomen.

- Describe Doppler findings of pediatric neoplasms.
- Differentiate the causes and sonographic findings of congenital hydronephrosis.
- Describe the sonographic appearances of pediatric renal cystic diseases.

A sonographic examination of the abdomen in a pediatric patient may be based on the patient's symptoms, findings during a clinical examination of an enlarged girth or a palpable mass, or follow-up of an anomaly identified during a prenatal sonogram. Symptoms may be nonspecific, and laboratory data, which may aid in the diagnosis, may be unavailable at the time of the sonogram.

A clinical finding of a palpable mass in a pediatric patient precipitates a search for the origin of the mass. Pediatric abdominal masses commonly arise from the kidney or adrenal gland and less commonly may be associated with a liver, biliary, or gastrointestinal anomaly. Alternatively, a palpable mass may not be directly related to a specific neoplasm but may reflect enlargement of an organ. Organ enlargement may occur with renal cystic diseases and some liver diseases. This chapter focuses on abnormalities of the biliary tract, liver, adrenal gland, and kidneys that occur more commonly in pediatric patients. Anomalies of the gastrointestinal tract and appendicitis are discussed in Chapters 11 and 12.

BILIARY TRACT

Biliary Atresia

Biliary atresia is the most significant life-threatening hepatobiliary disorder in children and is the most common indication for liver transplantation in pediatric patients.[1] Biliary atresia is a serious progressive disease that is the result of narrowing or obliteration of the bile ducts. The different classifications of biliary atresia depend on which portion of the biliary tree is affected. Biliary atresia may affect intrahepatic or extrahepatic ducts and may or may not involve the gallbladder. The most common form of biliary atresia involves the extrahepatic portion of the biliary tree, including the gallbladder. The cause of biliary atresia is unknown, although studies have suggested that biliary atresia may be the result of a congenital maldevelopment of the biliary tree or may be an acquired condition. The association of biliary atresia resulting from a viral infection has also been explored, and hereditary factors have been suggested. Biliary atresia may also be associated with polysplenia syndrome (Fig. 9-2).

The clinical features of biliary atresia include persistent jaundice in the neonatal period, acholic stools, dark urine, and enlarged girth from hepatomegaly. If biliary atresia is left untreated, the prognosis is poor; it leads to either liver transplantation or death from complications of liver failure. The commonly accepted treatment for biliary atresia is restitution of the bile flow via hepatoportoenterostomy (Kasai procedure). A successful hepatoportoenterostomy can delay or decrease the need for a liver transplant.[1] Outcomes are better with surgery performed at less than 45 to 60 days of life and worse after 90 days of age.[2]

Sonographic Findings. The triangular cord sign and an abnormal gallbladder in a fasting infant are widely accepted as the diagnostic criteria for biliary atresia.[3]

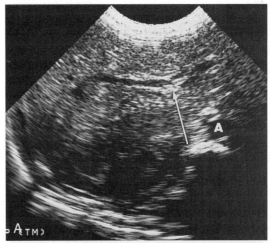

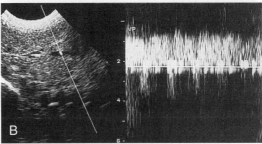

FIGURE 9-2 (A), Transverse liver sonogram in a 3-month-old girl with polysplenia syndrome. Bifurcation of portal vein *(arrow)* is more anterior than usual. **(B),** Right sagittal sonogram. Doppler cursor in portal vein shows normal hepatopetal flow. IVC is missing on both views. Polysplenia is associated with biliary atresia.

The triangular cord sign, which appears as an echogenic area superior to the portal vein bifurcation, represents the obliterated bile duct. A small or absent gallbladder in a fasting infant should be confirmed with postprandial images.

Choledochal Cyst

Choledochal cyst is a cystic dilation of the biliary tree that most commonly affects the common bile duct (CBD). It is estimated to occur in 1 in 5000 live births, with a higher frequency in Asians.[4] Common symptoms include abdominal pain and vomiting, but these are nonspecific making the condition difficult to diagnose during infancy. Jaundice is a more specific symptom, and the diagnosis is usually made early if the jaundice is prolonged during the neonatal period.

Five types of choledochal cysts are described using the Todani modification of the Alonso-Lej classification.[4,5] Type I is characterized by a fusiform dilation of the CBD and is the most common type. Type II manifests as one or more diverticula of the CBD. Type III, known as a choledochocele, is a dilation of the intraduodenal portion of the CBD. Type IV consists of dilation of intrahepatic and extrahepatic ducts. Type V is classified as Caroli's disease and manifests with dilation of the intrahepatic ducts.

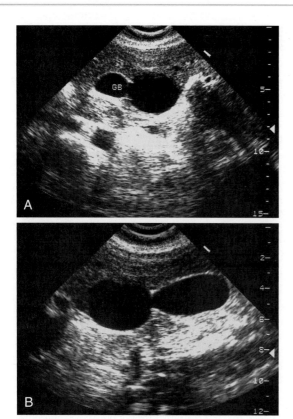

FIGURE 9-3 (A) and **(B),** Choledochal cyst may have the appearance of a cyst adjacent to gallbladder *(GB).*

The clinical presentation of choledochal cyst includes jaundice and pain. A palpable mass may also be present. Sonography is useful to differentiate choledochal cyst from other causes of jaundice in infancy, including biliary atresia and hepatitis. Early surgery greatly decreases the occurrence of disease-related complications, such as acute cholangitis, acute pancreatitis, early formation of biliary stone disease, biliary cirrhosis, liver cirrhosis, and malignancy.[4]

Sonographic Findings. Sonographic investigation of a choledochal cyst most commonly shows fusiform dilation of the CBD (Fig. 9-3), with associated intrahepatic ductal dilation. Depending on the type of choledochal cyst, multiple cysts in the area of the porta hepatis that are separate from the gallbladder may also be identified.

LIVER

Infantile Hemangioendothelioma

Infantile hepatic hemangioendothelioma, also known as infantile hepatic hemangioma, is the third most common hepatic tumor in children, accounting for 12% of all pediatric liver tumors. It is the most common vascular liver tumor of infancy that occurs within the first year of life.[6,7] A gender prevalence is seen, with most cases occurring in girls. This condition is a benign tumor, although it can be associated with serious complications, including congestive heart failure resulting from intratumoral high-flow arteriovenous shunts, anemia, thrombocytopenia, jaundice, and bleeding.[6]

Infants with hemangioendothelioma present with hepatomegaly, which may be accompanied by associated congestive heart failure and cutaneous hemangioma. The serum alpha fetoprotein level is usually within normal range but may be elevated. Because clinical and laboratory findings of infantile hepatic hemangioendothelioma are nonspecific, imaging plays an important role in diagnosis and assessment. Hemangioendothelioma spontaneously regresses by 12 to 18 months of age, but complications may lead to significant morbidity and mortality.[6,7]

Sonographic Findings. Sonographically, infantile hemangioendotheliomas are well-circumscribed, hypoechoic or hyperechoic masses (Fig. 9-4), which may show flow in vascular structures on Doppler (Fig. 9-5). Extensive arteriovenous shunting can lead to high-output congestive heart failure. Calcifications may be seen in 40% of cases.[6,7]

Hepatoblastoma

Hepatoblastomas are the most common primary liver tumors in young children, with a peak presentation at 1 to 2 years of age and a male-to-female ratio of 2:1. Less frequently, hepatoblastomas may also occur in older children, up to 15 years of age.[7] Predisposing conditions include Beckwith-Wiedemann syndrome; hemihypertrophy; familial polyposis coli or familial adenomatous polyposis, which can present with its variant known as Gardner's syndrome; fetal alcohol syndrome; and Wilms' tumor. It has also been reported to be present more commonly in premature infants and infants with low birth weight. The tumor has a tendency to invade hepatic and portal veins.

Clinical findings for hepatoblastoma include palpable abdominal mass, and an elevated serum alpha fetoprotein level may be present in 90% of patients.[7] Patients may also have fever, pain, anorexia, and weight loss. The prognosis for this tumor depends on the resectability of the mass. Many patients are in the advanced stages at the time of diagnosis, so the prognosis is poor.

Sonographic Findings. Sonographically, hepatoblastomas are solid masses with similar echogenicity compared with surrounding liver parenchyma (Fig. 9-6). The spoke-wheel appearance as a result of fibrous septa is rarely appreciated. Calcification is seen in 55% of cases and may cause acoustic shadowing.[7] Additional intralesional necroses or tumor thrombi in the portal vein or hepatic veins may be seen.

ADRENAL GLAND

Hemorrhage

Adrenal glands in the fetus and neonate are prone to hemorrhage because of their large size and increased

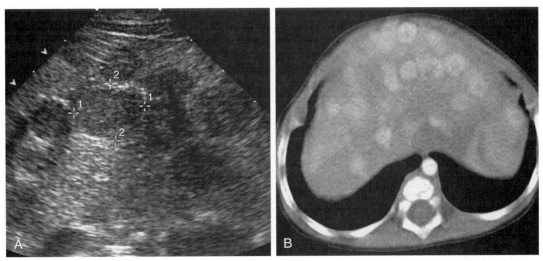

FIGURE 9-4 Hemangioendothelioma. **(A),** Well-circumscribed, hypoechoic masses. **(B),** Associated CT image.

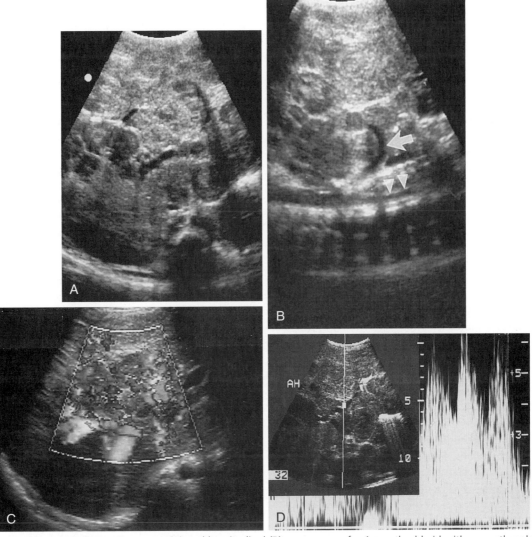

FIGURE 9-5 Hemangioendothelioma. Transverse **(A)** and longitudinal **(B)** sonograms of a 4-month-old girl with a greatly enlarged liver containing multiple nodules. Celiac axis is dilated *(arrow)*, and aorta distal to its origin is narrow *(arrowheads)*. **(C),** Hepatic artery within liver is dilated. **(D),** Low-resistance flow of great velocity is noted in hepatic artery, resembling malignant tumor flow. Cursor is in hepatic artery.

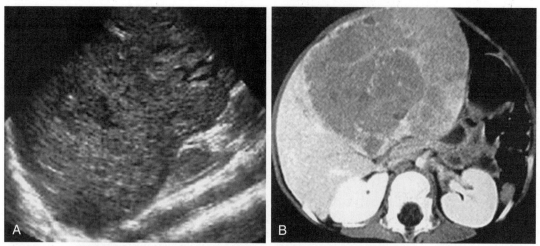

FIGURE 9-6 Hepatoblastoma. **(A),** Large, solid mass. **(B),** Associated CT image.

vascularity. Adrenal hemorrhage is a common cause of an adrenal mass in neonates and occurs most commonly on the right side but may involve both glands. The list of causes for adrenal hemorrhage is extensive and includes anticoagulation, stress caused by overwhelming sepsis, burns, surgery, hypotension, pregnancy and birth, and exogenous steroids or adrenocorticotropic hormone administration.[8,9] Extensive, bilateral adrenal hemorrhage is more common in male infants (male-to-female ratio of 2:1); this probably reflects a male predilection for several of the underlying conditions associated with adrenal hemorrhage.[10] Adrenal hemorrhage in healthy infants has been associated with preterm delivery, prolonged labor, breech delivery, large birth weight, infection, birth trauma, or anoxia. There has also been an association with Beckwith-Wiedemann syndrome.

Signs and symptoms of adrenal hemorrhage are variable and nonspecific. Adrenal hemorrhage may be accompanied by anemia, persistent jaundice, abdominal mass, painful swelling or bluish discoloration of the scrotum, acute adrenal crisis, or shock.[8,11]

Sonographic Findings. Increased use and sophistication of imaging technology have led to adrenal hemorrhage being diagnosed with increased frequency in hospitalized patients. Distinguishing adrenal hemorrhage from adrenal tumors, such as neuroblastoma, is important because identification of a malignant neoplasm requires surgical intervention, and adrenal hemorrhage usually resolves spontaneously. Adrenal hemorrhage initially appears echogenic and becomes hypoechoic over time. Follow-up sonograms (Fig. 9-7) show involution of the hemorrhage that may resolve to calcification or a residual cyst.

Neuroblastoma

Neuroblastoma is a tumor that arises in sympathetic neural crest tissues. It is the most common cancer diagnosed during the first year of life.[12,13] Tumors can arise anywhere along the sympathetic nervous system, with

most occurring in the adrenal medulla. Other locations include the neck, mediastinum, retroperitoneum, and pelvis. The cause of neuroblastoma is unclear. Studies have been conducted to determine potential risk factors for neuroblastoma, but further investigation is still needed to evaluate potential risk factors, including pregnancy and birth factors, certain environmental exposures, and medications. Heredity is the only known risk factor for neuroblastoma; however, it accounts for only 1% to 2% of all neuroblastomas.[13]

Diagnosis of neuroblastoma may be made during the perinatal period based on obstetric sonography. The clinical presentation of neuroblastoma depends on the location of the tumor. The postnatal clinical presentation is highly variable, ranging from a mass that causes no symptoms to a primary tumor that causes critical illness as a result of local invasion, widely disseminated disease, or both.[12] Infants may have an abdominal mass, hypertension, diarrhea, and bone pain with metastasis. Most patients with neuroblastoma have increased catecholamine levels.

Sonographic Findings. The sonographic appearance of neuroblastoma is variable, with small tumors appearing more homogeneous and hyperechoic and large tumors appearing more heterogeneous or complex (Fig. 9-8). Tumors may contain calcifications or may appear cystic. Doppler evaluation may aid in differentiation of neuroblastoma from adrenal hemorrhage because neuroblastoma reveals vascularity within the neoplasm, whereas adrenal hemorrhage does not have flow patterns within the area of hemorrhage.

KIDNEYS

Hydronephrosis

Hydronephrosis is characterized by dilation of the renal collecting system. The role of the sonographic examination is to identify the severity of the dilation and the location of the obstruction. The most common cause of

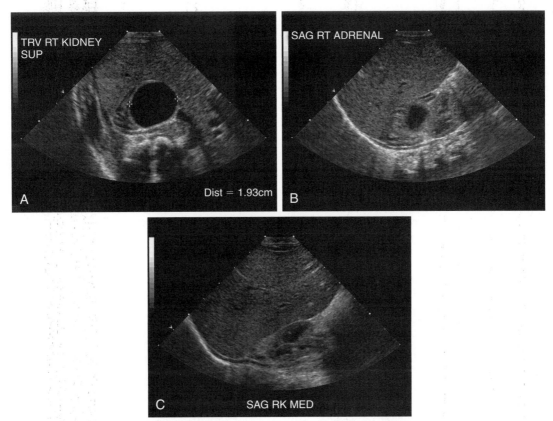

FIGURE 9-7 **(A)**, Cystic suprarenal mass represents adrenal hemorrhage. **(B)**, Mass is smaller 15 days later. **(C)**, Resolving hemorrhage.

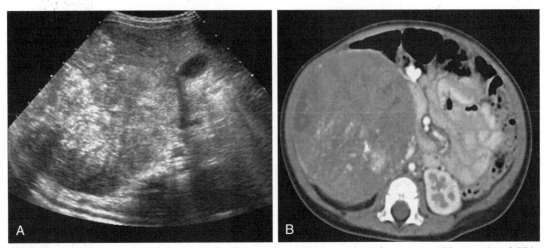

FIGURE 9-8 Neuroblastoma. Renal tissue is difficult to discern. **(A)**, Hyperechoic, large tumor. **(B)**, Associated CT image.

hydronephrosis in a pediatric patient is ureteropelvic junction (UPJ) obstruction. UPJ obstruction may be the result of abnormal development of the muscle fibers of the UPJ, fibrosis and narrowing of the UPJ, compression of fetal vessels, an arrest in the normal development, or a failure of the recanalization of the proximal ureter. UPJ obstruction is usually unilateral, but associated contralateral renal anomalies may be present, including multicystic dysplastic kidney (MCDK), renal duplication, and agenesis.

Hydronephrosis may also be the result of ureterovesical junction (UVJ) obstruction. UVJ obstruction may be the result of an abnormal insertion of the ureter into the bladder wall. This condition is usually part of a renal duplication anomaly, with the ureter arising from the upper pole of the kidney inserting into an ectopic ureterocele in the bladder. UVJ obstruction is more commonly unilateral but may also be bilateral. Other causes of hydronephrosis include posterior urethral valves and megaureter, urethral atresia, prune-belly (Eagle-Barrett) syndrome, and neoplasm. Clinical symptoms depend on the cause of hydronephrosis and include palpable abdominal mass, oliguria, and anuria. Follow-up of findings on an obstetric sonogram also lead to diagnosis of hydronephrosis.

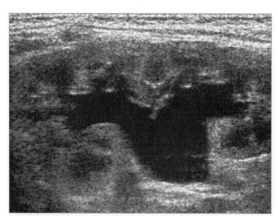

FIGURE 9-9 Moderate hydronephrosis, with dilated renal pelvis and calyces. Dilation ends abruptly at UPJ.

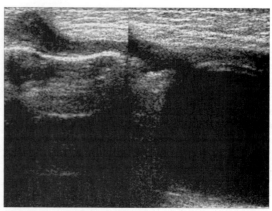

FIGURE 9-11 Dilated ureter (traced to bladder), associated with UVJ obstruction.

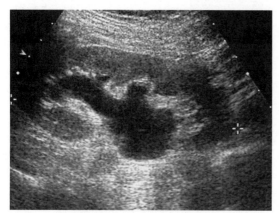

FIGURE 9-10 Longitudinal image demonstrates dilation of the renal pelvis and calyces (pelvicaliectasis) without evidence of dilated ureter consistent with UPJ obstruction.

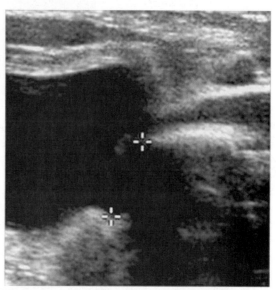

FIGURE 9-12 Characteristic keyhole bladder of UVJ obstruction represents the dilated proximal urethra.

Sonographic Findings. Hydronephrosis (Fig. 9-9) is identified when the renal pelvis is dilated with or without dilation of the renal calyces. Mild hydronephrosis is classified as a dilated renal pelvis (pyelectasis); moderate hydronephrosis is defined as dilation of the renal pelvis and calyces (pelvicaliectasis); and severe hydronephrosis is identified with significant pelvicaliectasis and thinning of the renal parenchyma.

Sonographic identification of the level of obstruction facilitates proper treatment and surgical management and predicts morbidity and mortality. UPJ obstruction can be diagnosed with obstruction of the kidney (Fig. 9-10) without dilation of the ureter or bladder. UVJ obstruction is identified sonographically when the kidney is hydronephrotic and the ureter is dilated (Fig. 9-11). Sonography may also identify the ectopic ureterocele in the bladder that is associated with UVJ obstruction. Posterior urethral valve obstruction is evident when bilateral hydronephrosis and hydroureter are identified with an enlarged bladder. A thickened bladder wall may also be identified with posterior urethral valve obstruction, in addition to the characteristic keyhole bladder (Fig. 9-12) that represents the dilated proximal urethra.

Renal Cystic Disease

Multiple types of cystic diseases of the kidney exist. This chapter focuses on the diseases most commonly seen in the pediatric patient. Cystic diseases that more commonly affect adult patients are discussed in Chapter 7.

Multicystic Dysplastic Kidney

Multicystic dysplastic kidney (MCDK) is an anomaly characterized by multiple cysts in a nonfunctioning kidney. MCDK occurs in 1 in 4300 live births.[14] The cause is poorly understood, but MCDK may be the result of an obstructive process in utero or a cessation of the embryologic development into the metanephros. MCDK is usually unilateral but may be associated with a contralateral renal anomaly, the most common of which is UPJ obstruction. Drugs that may cause kidney dysplasia include prescription medicines, such as antiseizure medication and angiotensin-converting enzyme inhibitors and

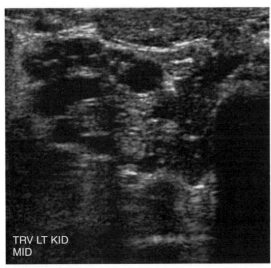

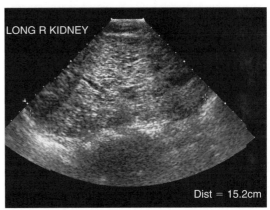

FIGURE 9-14 ARPKD. Enlarged kidney in a newborn, with loss of corticomedullary junction. Kidney measures 15.12 cm in length.

FIGURE 9-13 MCDK. Noncommunicating cysts in the renal bed, characteristic of MCDK.

angiotensin receptor blockers. A mother's use of illegal drugs, such as cocaine, and genetic causes have also been implicated. The disorder appears to be an autosomal dominant trait. Several genetic syndromes that affect other body systems have also been reported to be associated with kidney dysplasia.[15]

MCDK may manifest as a palpable abdominal mass, or a sonographic evaluation of an infant may follow obstetric sonographic findings. Infants with bilateral MCDK or a severe contralateral renal anomaly may have respiratory distress from the lack of amniotic fluid in utero. The prognosis for MCDK is poor when bilateral or associated with a syndrome. Patients with a unilateral MCDK are at increased risk for hypertension and the development of Wilms' tumor.

Sonographic Findings. Sonographic evaluation of the abdomen reveals multiple noncommunicating cysts in the renal bed (Fig. 9-13). Because affected kidneys are generally nonfunctioning, bilateral MCDK also manifests with an empty bladder. The sonographic evaluation should include imaging of the contralateral kidney for associated anomalies such as UPJ obstruction, UVJ obstruction, and agenesis.

Autosomal Recessive Polycystic Kidney Disease

Autosomal recessive polycystic kidney disease (ARPKD) is an inherited disorder involving cystic dilation of the renal collecting ducts and varying degrees of hepatic abnormalities consisting of cysts, fibrosis, and portal hypertension. Both kidney and liver disease are progressive. ARPKD with congenital hepatic fibrosis has an estimated frequency of 1 in 20,000 live births.[16,17] Most affected patients present in the neonatal period; a few present as older children or young adults with evidence of hepatic dysfunction. With modern obstetric sonography, the diagnosis may be suspected when abnormalities are detected by prenatal sonographic examination. Patients with ARPKD and with congenital hepatic fibrosis may present prenatally with oligohydramnios caused by decreased fetal urine, but others present later in life when the clinical symptoms are dominated by renal failure or hepatic dysfunction or both.

ARPKD, also known as infantile polycystic kidney disease, can manifest in various forms depending on severity from perinatal (most severe), to neonatal, to infantile, to juvenile. As stated, most patients with ARPKD present in the neonatal period with enlarged echogenic kidneys. Large bilateral flank masses are invariably present on physical examination. At initial presentation, approximately 45% of infants have liver abnormalities. Pulmonary hypoplasia resulting from oligohydramnios occurs in many affected infants. Approximately 30% die in the neonatal period or in the first year of life primarily of respiratory insufficiency or superimposed pulmonary infections. More than 50% of affected children progress to end-stage renal disease, usually in the first decade of life. With neonatal respiratory support and renal transplant, the 10-year survival of patients who live beyond the first year of life has improved; 15-year survival is estimated to be 67% to 79% and may be improving. A few patients present in older childhood or young adulthood with hepatosplenomegaly and evidence of portal hypertension.[16,17]

Sonographic Findings. The diagnostic criteria for ARPKD on a prenatal sonogram are the presence of bilateral enlarged kidneys with a loss of corticomedullary differentiation (Fig. 9-14). The bladder may appear empty or small in size. Infants display the same characteristic large echogenic kidneys with poor corticomedullary differentiation. Macrocysts are usually not present; however, they may be seen, particularly with worsening disease. Although the kidneys may be markedly enlarged in these infants, over time, most show stable to decreased renal size relative to body growth. With progressive disease, the sonographic appearance of the kidneys may more closely resemble that seen in autosomal

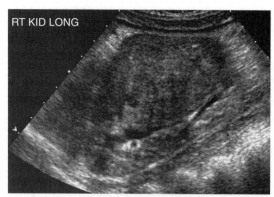

FIGURE 9-15 Wilms' tumor. Large, spherical heterogeneous mass arising from mid–lower pole of right kidney.

dominant polycystic kidney disease (ADPKD). In childhood and young adulthood, the kidneys are echogenic and large, but massive enlargement is usually not seen. Macrocysts, more typical of ADPKD, are often seen in older children. Hepatic findings on prenatal sonography reveal hepatomegaly, mildly increased echogenicity, dilated intrahepatic (and occasionally extrahepatic) biliary ducts, and poorly visualized peripheral portal veins. However, these findings may not be evident at birth.[16,17]

Wilms' Tumor (Nephroblastoma)

Wilms' tumor, also known as nephroblastoma, is the most common renal tumor in children. More than 80% of cases are diagnosed before 5 years of age, with a median age of 3.5 years.[18] Several recognized syndromes are associated with an increased predisposition toward developing Wilms' tumor, including Beckwith-Wiedemann syndrome and isolated hemihypertrophy, WAGR (Wilms' tumor, aniridia, genitourinary anomalies, mental retardation) syndrome, and Denys-Drash syndrome. Wilms' tumor is usually unilateral, but bilateral tumors may occur. With current treatment modalities, the overall survival exceeds 90% for most patients.[18]

The most typical clinical presentation of Wilms' tumor is a palpable abdominal mass. Presenting symptoms include abdominal pain that may be a sign of rupture and bleeding. Gross hematuria may be a sign of tumor extension into the collecting system or ureter. Atypical presentations occur in less than 10% of patients and may result in compression of surrounding organs or vascular invasion into the renal vein or inferior vena cava (IVC).[18] Patients with vascular extension can present with ascites, congestive heart failure, hepatomegaly, and varicocele.

Sonographic Findings. The sonographic appearance of Wilms' tumor is variable. It manifests as a large spherical mass, with a mainly intrarenal location (Fig. 9-15). The tumor can be solid and homogeneous, but it is usually heterogeneous (Fig. 9-16), with areas of hemorrhage,

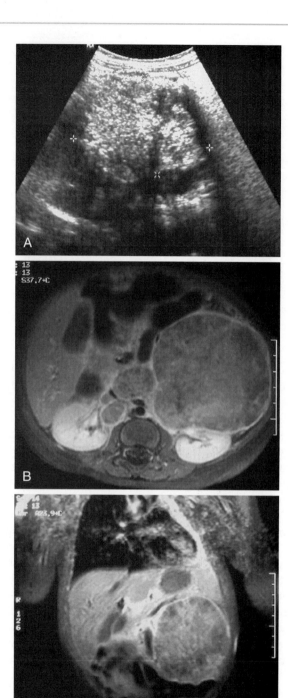

FIGURE 9-16 Wilms' tumor. **(A),** Transverse image demonstrates large complex mass. **(B),** Magnetic resonance imaging. **(C),** Coronal view shows extensiveness of lesion.

necrosis, or cysts. In less than 15% of patients, the tumor contains calcifications.[19] The borders are usually well defined. The remaining normal kidney tissue can be difficult to detect, but is often stretched and visible at the periphery of the tumor. Depending on the size and location of the mass, hydronephrosis may also be identified. The sonographic examination should include imaging of the renal vein and IVC for tumor thrombus. Whenever Wilms' tumor is detected, the contralateral kidney

TABLE 9-1	Pediatric Neoplasms	
Pathology	Symptoms	Sonographic Findings
Hemangioendothelioma	Hepatomegaly, congestive heart failure	Multiple, hypoechoic lesions; arteriovenous shunting with Doppler, hepatomegaly
Hepatoblastoma	Palpable mass, fever, pain, anorexia, weight loss	Solitary mass or multiple lesions, increased vascularity with Doppler
Neuroblastoma	Abdominal mass, hypertension, diarrhea, bone pain	Homogeneous to complex, hyperechoic, calcifications, intratumoral flow with Doppler
Nephroblastoma	Palpable mass, hematuria, hypertension, malaise	Homogeneous or complex, calcifications; associated hydronephrosis may be identified
Mesoblastic nephroma	Palpable mass	Large, solid, homogeneous mass, complex appearance with necrosis

should be examined for synchronous bilateral disease, which occurs in 5% of children.[19]

Mesoblastic Nephroma

Mesoblastic nephroma is the most common renal tumor identified in the neonatal period and the most frequent benign renal tumor in childhood. It represents 3% to 10% of all pediatric renal tumors.[20]

The mass may be first diagnosed when the detailed fetal anatomy scan is performed at 18 to 20 weeks of gestation. These tumors may manifest in utero as a lateral abdominal mass with polyhydramnios. Differentiation between a solid and a cystic mass can easily be made. If the mass is very large, it may be difficult to determine the organ of origin in some cases. When associated with hydrops, the prognosis is grave. Sonography is usually the first imaging study performed when the abdominal mass is palpated in the neonatal period. When identified in the neonatal period, the renal mass may grow through the renal capsule into the retroperitoneum; however, the prognosis is good because of the benign nature of this tumor.

Sonographic Findings. The most common sonographic appearance of a mesoblastic nephroma is a large, solid, homogeneous mass, but there also may be cystic areas because of hemorrhage and necrosis. In utero, mesoblastic nephroma has been described as a solid or complex mass that may replace the kidney.

Table 9-1 summarizes the pathology, symptoms, and sonographic findings of pediatric neoplasms.

SUMMARY

In addition to the diseases that were described previously, sonographic examination of a pediatric patient with abdominal pain or a palpable mass may aid in the diagnosis of a mesenteric cyst, duplication cyst, ovarian cyst, teratoma, cholecystitis, and other benign and malignant neoplasms that are more rarely seen in pediatric patients. When an abdominal sonogram fails to locate a mass in the liver, kidneys, or adrenal glands, the sonographer should also survey the lower quadrants of the abdomen to look for masses that may be associated with the retroperitoneum, gastrointestinal tract, and lower genitourinary system.

CLINICAL SCENARIO—DIAGNOSIS

This is a case of prune-belly syndrome with associated UVJ obstruction. This type of obstruction is usually unilateral but may also be bilateral. UVJ obstruction can be caused by various pathologies. It is often associated with renal duplication anomaly, with the ureter arising from the upper pole of the kidney inserting into an ectopic ureterocele in the bladder. However, in this clinical scenario, the wrinkled abdominal skin points toward prune-belly syndrome as the cause.

CASE STUDIES FOR DISCUSSION

1. A 10-year-old child presented with history of enlarged echogenic kidneys (Fig. 9-17), hepatosplenomegaly, and evidence of portal hypertension. Renal function tests reveal the child is in moderate renal failure. Discuss the clinical findings and significance of the appearance of the kidney and the associated liver abnormalities.

2. A 3-day-old infant presents with a palpable abdominal mass that was also noted on a prenatal sonogram; the origin of the mass could not be determined. Postnatal sonography reveals a large heterogeneous mass (Fig. 9-18). The child had no other symptoms. What are the differential diagnoses for this mass? What laboratory values could aid in making a more definitive diagnosis?

3. A 6-year-old child with fever, chills, and back pain was seen for a renal sonogram. The kidneys were markedly enlarged, and the findings in Figure 9-19 were noted. What is the most likely diagnosis?

4. A 4-year-old girl is seen by the pediatrician for an abdominal mass discovered by the parent. The child is in no physical distress, and the mother reports no recent illness. On questioning the family history, the physician learns that the mother has epilepsy and has been on long-term antiseizure medication. The child is referred for abdominal sonography, which reveals a large, complex cystic mass in the right upper quadrant (Fig. 9-20). The right kidney was not identified. Discuss the probable nature of this mass and how the family history may be significant.

Continued

CASE STUDIES FOR DISCUSSION—cont'd

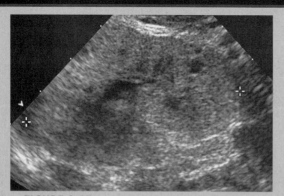

FIGURE 9-17 Enlarged kidney, with macrocysts.

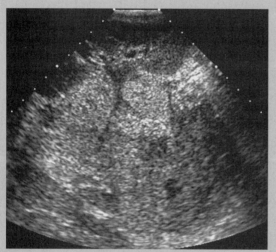

FIGURE 9-18 Large heterogeneous mass occupies right midabdomen. Organ of origin could not be determined.

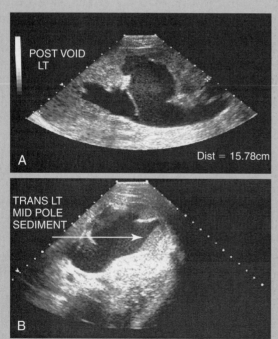

A

Dist = 15.78cm

POST VOID
LT

TRANS LT
MID POLE
SEDIMENT

B

FIGURE 9-19 Debris in dilated renal pelvis. Debris swirls with real-time observation.

5. A 6-month-old boy of Asian ethnicity is seen by the pediatrician for abdominal pain and vomiting. The physician notes physical signs of jaundice, and on questioning, the parent reports this has been present since birth. The physician is also able to palpate a right upper quadrant mass. A sonogram is performed, and a balloon-like dilation of the CBD (Fig. 9-21) and mild intrahepatic ductal dilation are seen. Discuss the likely cause of this mass and the significance of the clinical findings and patient history.

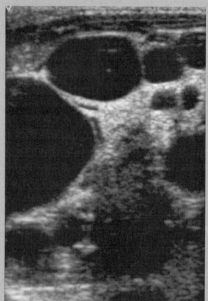

FIGURE 9-20 Reniform-shaped mass in right renal bed, represented non-communicating cysts.

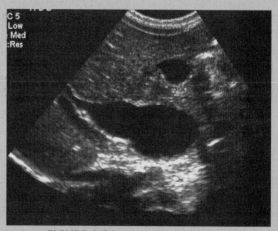

C 5
Low
Med
Res

FIGURE 9-21 Cystic dilation of CBD.

STUDY QUESTIONS

1. A newborn boy is seen for a renal sonogram as follow-up of an obstetric sonogram that showed a markedly distended bladder, hydronephrosis, dilated and tortuous ureters, and keyhole appearance of the proximal urethra. These findings are most consistent with which of the following congenital obstructive disorders?
   a. UPJ obstruction
   b. Posterior urethral valves
   c. Renal agenesis
   d. Eagle-Barrett syndrome

2. A 2-day-old infant is referred for an abdominal sonogram because of an echogenic liver nodule seen on the prenatal obstetric sonogram. Additionally, the infant has a strawberry-colored mass on the right side of her neck. The sonogram is most likely to reveal which type of liver mass?
   a. Hepatoblastoma
   b. Choledochal cyst
   c. Congenital hepatic fibrosis
   d. Hemangioendothelioma

3. A newborn boy born after a prolonged labor and breech delivery presents with a questionable right upper quadrant mass. At physical examination, a swollen and bluish discolored scrotum is noted. Laboratory analysis reveals anemia. A sonogram of the right upper quadrant and scrotum is requested. The abdominal sonogram reveals a crescent-shaped, slightly hyperechoic right suprarenal mass. What is the most likely cause for this finding?
   a. Unilateral adrenal hemorrhage
   b. MCDK
   c. Wilms' tumor
   d. Mesoblastic nephroma

4. A prenatal sonogram reveals the presence of bilateral enlarged kidneys with a loss of corticomedullary differentiation. Hepatomegaly, mildly increased hepatic echogenicity, dilated intrahepatic biliary ducts, and poorly visualized peripheral portal veins are also noted. After delivery, the infant is referred for renal sonography, which displays the same characteristic large echogenic kidneys with poor corticomedullary differentiation; macrocysts are not present. The liver abnormalities noted on prenatal sonogram are no longer evident. What is the most likely cause for these findings?
   a. Unilateral renal agenesis
   b. Neuroblastoma
   c. ARPKD
   d. MCDK

5. A 3-year-old boy with abdominal pain is seen with a large, firm, palpable mass in the left upper quadrant.

He is referred for abdominal sonography. A large, spherical, heterogeneous left upper quadrant mass is identified. The sonographer is able to identify the organ of origin as the kidney. Evaluation of the IVC and left renal vein reveals the presence of tumor thrombus. Based on the clinical presentation and findings, what does this mass most likely represent?
   a. Neuroblastoma
   b. Wilms' tumor
   c. MCDK
   d. Mesoblastic nephroma

6. A 1-year-old girl is referred for abdominal sonography after a palpable mass is noted on the right side. The child has no significant clinical signs or symptoms of disease. The sonogram reveals multiple, noncommunicating cysts in the right renal bed. What is the most likely cause for this sonographic appearance?
   a. UPJ obstruction
   b. UVJ obstruction
   c. MCDK
   d. ARPKD

7. A 3-week-old infant presents with persistent jaundice, dark urine, and enlarged girth. A fasting sonogram is requested. An enlarged liver with an echogenic area superior to the portal vein bifurcation is demonstrated in the right upper quadrant. No gallbladder is identified. What is the likely diagnosis for this patient?
   a. Hemangioendothelioma
   b. Hepatoblastoma
   c. Choledochal cyst
   d. Biliary atresia

8. A 1-month old infant is referred for sonographic evaluation of a palpable abdominal mass. No other clinical signs or symptoms have been noted. Laboratory tests reveal elevated catecholamine levels. The sonogram reveals a 5-cm homogeneous left suprarenal mass; calcifications within the mass are noted. Doppler reveals moderate blood flow within the mass. What does this mass likely represent?
   a. Neuroblastoma
   b. Adrenal hemorrhage
   c. Wilms' tumor
   d. MCDK

9. A 1-year-old boy is referred for an abdominal sonogram. The history reveals that he was delivered prematurely. He presented with hepatomegaly and elevated alpha fetoprotein levels. A 9-cm hepatic mass with calcification is noted. The mass appears to have invaded the adjacent portal vein. What do the clinical history and features of this mass suggest?

a. Neuroblastoma
b. Hepatoblastoma
c. Hemangioendothelioma
d. Biliary atresia

10. A 3-year-old girl is referred for renal sonography following a 6-month history of recurrent urinary tract infections. The sonogram reveals a duplicated collecting system on the right kidney. Mild to moderate hydronephrosis is evident. A mildly dilated right ureter can be followed to its insertion into the bladder where a ureterocele is noted. What condition does this describe?
a. UPJ obstruction
b. UVJ obstruction
c. Posterior urethral valves
d. MCDK

REFERENCES

1. Neimark E, LeLeiko NS: Early detection of biliary atresia raises questions about etiology and screening, *Pediatrics* 128:1598–1599, 2011.
2. Shneider BL, Brown MB, Haber B, et al: Biliary atresia research consortium: a multicenter study of the outcome of biliary atresia in the United States, 1997 to 2000, *J Pediatr* 148:467–474, 2006.
3. Lee MS, Kim MJ, Lee MJ, et al: Biliary atresia: color Doppler US findings in neonates and infants, *Radiology* 252:282–289, 2009.
4. Wong-Hoi S, et al: Management of choledochal cyst: 30 years of experience and results in a single center, *J Pediatr Surg* 44:2307–2311, 2009.
5. Edil BH, Cameron JL, et al: Choledochal cyst disease in children and adults: a 30-year single-institution experience, *J Am Coll Surg* 205:100–1005, 2008.
6. Feng S, Chan T, et al: CT and MR imaging characteristics of infantile hepatic hemangioendothelioma, *Eur J Radiol* 76:24–29, 2010.
7. Jha P, Tavri S, Patel C, et al: Pediatric liver tumors—a pictorial review, *Eur Radiol* 19:209–219, 2009.
8. Simon DR, Palese MA: Clinical update on the management of adrenal hemorrhage, *Curr Urol Rep* 10:78–83, 2009.
9. Nadler EP, Barksdale EM Jr: Adrenal masses in the newborn, *Semin Pediatr Surg* 9:156–164, 2000.
10. Tritos NA: *Adrenal hemorrhage*Emedicine.medscape.com http://emedicine.medscape.com/article/126806-overview#a0199. Retrieved January 19, 2012.
11. Mutlu M, et al: Adrenal hemorrhage in newborns: a retrospective study, *World J Pediatr* 7:355–357, 2011.
12. Maris JM: Recent advances in neuroblastoma, *N Engl J Med* 362:2202–2211, 2010.
13. Perry CL: Sonographic evaluation of neuroblastoma, *J Diag Med Sonogr* 25:101–107, 2009.
14. Schreuder MF, Westland R, van Wijk JA: Unilateral multicystic dysplastic kidney: a meta-analysis of observational studies on the incidence, associated urinary tract malformations and the contralateral kidney, *Nephrol Dial Transplant* 24:1810–1818, 2009.
15. National Kidney and Urologic Disease Clearinghouse: *National Institute of Diabetes and Digestive and Kidney Diseases (NIDDK), National Institutes of Health (NIH)* http://kidney.niddk.nih.gov/kudiseases/pubs/kidneydysplasia/. Retrieved January 29, 2012.
16. Turkbey B, et al: Autosomal recessive polycystic kidney disease and congenital hepatic fibrosis (ARPKD/CHF), *Pediatr Radiol* 39:100–111, 2009.
17. U.S. National Library of Medicine National Institutes of Health: *Polycystic kidney disease, autosomal recessive* http://www.ncbi.nlm.nih.gov/books/NBK1326/. Retrieved January 3, 2012.
18. Ko EY, Ritchey ML: Current management of Wilms' tumor in children, *J Pediatr Urol* 5:56–65, 2009.
19. Smets AM, de Kraker J: Malignant tumours of the kidney: imaging strategy, *Pediatr Radiol* 40:1010–1018, 2010.
20. Singh SP: *Mesoblastic nephroma imaging.* Emedicine. medscape.comhttp://emedicine.medscape.com/article/411147-overview. Retrieved January 31, 2012.

Suspect Abdominal Aortic Aneurysm

Kathryn Kuntz, John Lindsey

CLINICAL SCENARIO

An elderly woman presents to the family medicine department complaining of severe back pain. The patient has a 40-year history of high blood pressure and cigarette smoking. On physical examination, a large, pulsatile midline abdominal mass is felt. During the course of the examination, she suddenly becomes hypotensive and goes into cardiac arrest, at which time her abdomen begins to swell. The sonography department is nearby, and she is rushed there for an emergency sonogram. Sonography revealed the finding in Figure 10-1 and free fluid in the abdomen. This is suggestive of what diagnosis?

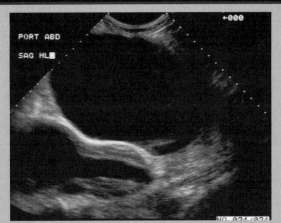

FIGURE 10-1 Large cystic mass is identified anterior to aorta in longitudinal image.

OBJECTIVES

- List the risk factors associated with abdominal aortic aneurysm, dissection, and rupture.
- Describe the techniques for sonographic imaging of the abdominal aorta.
- Identify the sonographic findings associated with abdominal aortic aneurysm, dissection, and rupture.

- Describe the symptoms associated with abdominal aortic aneurysm, dissection, and rupture.
- List the classifications used to characterize the various types of aortic dissections.
- State the recommendations for aortic aneurysm surveillance and screening.

Most abdominal aortic aneurysms (AAAs) are asymptomatic. They are typically not detected on physical examination and remain silent until discovered during radiologic testing for other reasons. Symptomatic aneurysms manifest with back, abdominal, buttock, groin, testicular, or leg pain and require urgent surgical attention. AAAs may be clinically silent, but the risk of rupture and the associated increased mortality rate show the importance of early detection and elective repair. Sonography is the preferred method of evaluation and screening.[1]

The aorta is the largest artery of the human body and is responsible for supplying the body with blood through its many branches. The ascending aorta serves the head, neck, and upper extremities; the descending aorta serves the abdomen, pelvis, and lower extremities by transporting gases, nutrients, and other substances to the tissues and transporting wastes to appropriate sites for excretion. Because of the large size of the aorta and the volume of blood transported through it, disruption of normal aortic flow can be catastrophic. The diagnosis of an aortic aneurysm should precipitate periodic follow-up to monitor for the potential life-threatening complications of rupture and dissection. This chapter explains the clinical symptoms and sonographic findings associated with aneurysm, rupture, and dissection.

ABDOMINAL AORTA

Normal Sonographic Anatomy

Sonographic examination of the abdominal aorta should include longitudinal and transverse images that show the proximal, middle, and distal segments (Fig. 10-2) and the iliac artery bifurcation. A normal aorta gradually tapers toward the distal segment (Fig. 10-2, *B*). The anteroposterior (AP) diameter should be measured in the longitudinal plane (Fig 10-2, *A*). The renal and iliac arteries (Fig. 10-2, *C*) should also be documented. The imaging challenge of overlying bowel gas can be diminished or alleviated with gentle transducer pressure and a patient preparation of an overnight fast. In addition, obese patients or patients with excessive bowel gas may benefit from various imaging techniques, including scanning the patient in a left posterior oblique or decubitus position.

ABDOMINAL AORTIC ANEURYSM

AAA is a common and potentially fatal condition that primarily affects older patients. Ruptured AAAs are a leading cause of death in the United States.[1,2]

The aortic wall comprises an inner layer, the tunica intima; a middle layer, the tunica media; and an outer layer, the tunica adventitia (Fig. 10-3). An aneurysm is a permanent focal dilation of an artery to 1.5 times its normal diameter. Normal infrarenal aortic diameters in patients older than 50 years are 1.5 cm in women and 1.7 cm in men. By convention, an infrarenal aorta 3 cm in diameter or larger is considered aneurysmal.[3] AAAs develop as the tunica media, which is composed largely of smooth muscle cells, collagen, and elastin, thins. Tobacco use, hypertension, a family history of AAA, and male gender are clinical risk factors for the development of an aneurysm.

AAA may be suspected when clinical examination reveals a pulsatile abdominal mass located at the level

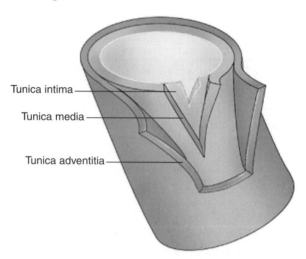

Tunica intima

Tunica media

Tunica adventitia

Artery

FIGURE 10-3 Layers of arterial wall.

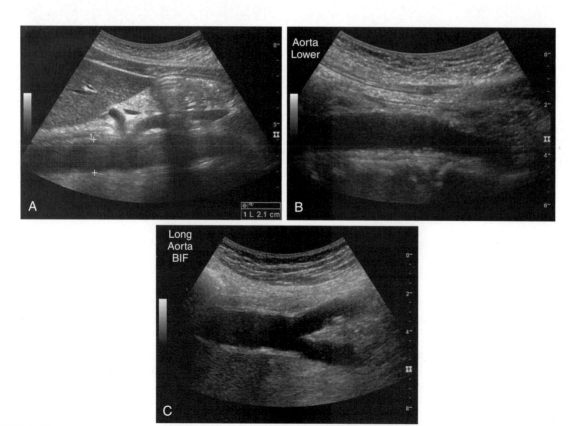

FIGURE 10-2 Longitudinal images. **(A)**, Proximal aorta. **(B)**, Distal aorta showing tapering in a healthy patient. **(C)**, Bifurcation.

of the umbilicus or slightly cephalic to the umbilicus, although a large girth may limit the sensitivity of clinical palpation. In addition, AAA may be suspected when a tortuous calcified aorta is identified on a radiograph that may have been ordered for an unrelated condition or disease. Patients may have abdominal pain or back pain, which may indicate that the aneurysm is enlarging or, with severe symptoms, that rupture has occurred. Repair is indicated when the aneurysm becomes greater than 5.5 cm in diameter or grows more than 0.6 to 0.8 cm per year.[1]

Sonographic Findings

Sonographic imaging of the aorta for detection of aneurysm is the preferred test because of the high sensitivity and specificity of this examination, although results may be limited by obesity, prior abdominal surgery, and overlying bowel gas. Sonography may be more effective when the patient has had nothing by mouth 8 hours before the examination. Sonographically, diagnosis of AAA can be made when the AP diameter is 3 cm or greater in the longitudinal plane. Aortic aneurysms may be fusiform (uniform dilation) or saccular (asymmetric saclike dilation) in appearance, or the aorta may have a gradual widening, referred to as aortic ectasia. Thrombus within the dilation may also be noted (Fig. 10-4) and most commonly appears as low-level echoes, although calcifications and liquefaction may also appear within thrombus. The

absence of flow associated with thrombus in an aneurysm may be confirmed with color Doppler. Also, an important part of the protocol is documentation of the location of the aneurysm relative to the renal arteries—although in practice, the origins of superior mesenteric and celiac arteries are more commonly used to indicate the likelihood of infrarenal status (Fig. 10-2, A).

The recommended sonographic surveillance is no further testing for patients with AAA less than 3 cm and annual sonography for AAAs measuring 3 to 4 cm. When an aneurysm reaches a diameter of 4 cm to 4.5 cm, screening should be performed every 6 months.[1,4,5] Sonography is used in patient follow-up for assessment of an expanding aneurysm for planning of elective surgery. Patients with an aneurysm measuring greater than 4.5 cm should be referred to counseling for elective surgical options.[1,4,5] If repair is undertaken, the walls of an aortic graft appear echogenic on sonogram (Fig. 10-5).

AORTIC ENDOGRAFTS

The latest advance in the treatment of AAA is the placement of endoluminal grafts. These grafts are inserted into the aorta rather than exposing the aneurysm surgically. The advantage of the aortic endograft is that no abdominal incision is required, making recovery time considerably shorter than open resection. Most devices are configured as a metallic, self-expanding framework

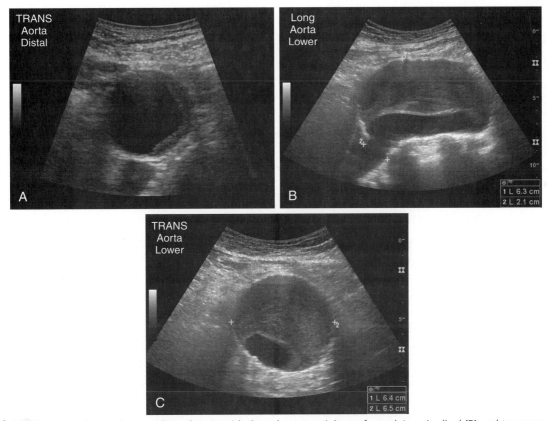

FIGURE 10-4 (A), Transverse image shows enlarged aorta with thrombus at periphery of vessel. Longitudinal **(B)** and transverse **(C)** images of aneurysm, showing thrombus within aneurysm.

covered with various nonporous materials. (Fig. 10-6) The stents may be a straight tube or bifurcated. Blood flow is routed through the endograft depriving the aneurysm sac of blood.

The technique of endovascular AAA exclusion (repair) is a safe and effective method for treating AAAs. Reports have shown a reduction in morbidity and decreased mortality. Despite reduction in overall complications, endoleak is a frequent occurrence after stent-graft deployment. The overall endoleak rate ranges from 7% to 47%, and it is estimated at 21% during the perioperative interval and up to 9% at 1 month after repair.[7] The complication can be due to device failure during placement, changes over time, or failure to control blood flow within the aneurysm sac.[7]

An endoleak occurs when blood is allowed to flow into the aneurysm sac. Endoleaks are classified as one of four types, as follows:[7-9]

- Type 1: An attachment site leak, caused when the device is improperly sealed at the proximal or distal endpoint.
- Type 2: Retrograde flow through collateral branches (i.e., lumbar branches or inferior mesenteric artery).

- Type 3: Flow into the aneurysm secondary to an inadequate seal between components of the device or a tear in the fabric of the graft.
- Type 4: Flow through the fabric of the graft secondary to graft porosity.

In addition to the identification of endoleak, sonographic evaluation is performed to identify an increase in the diameter of the aneurysm; detect graft migration or evidence of iatrogenic injuries; and define hemodynamic abnormalities within the graft, the graft limbs, and the native circulation proximal and distal to the graft. Over time, the aneurysm sac should decrease in size.

Aortic endografts are interrogated sonographically in the perioperative period, at 3- to 6-month intervals during the first year, and at 6- to 12-month intervals thereafter. Long-term surveillance is necessary to ensure that the graft remains in the correct position. Traditionally, computed tomography (CT) angiography has been used for surveillance; however, sonography can be used when aneurysm sac size is the primary concern. Although CT angiography may be used periodically as an alternative to sonographic evaluation, sonographic assessment of aortic endografts plays an important role in lifelong surveillance.[8,9]

RUPTURED ANEURYSM

Rupture of AAA carries a significantly high mortality rate. The risk of rupture sharply increases with aneurysms more than 6 cm in diameter; high blood pressure and current smoking increase the growth rate of aneurysms and resultant rupture.[8] In a study of 116 patients with ruptured AAAs, 45% were hypotensive, 72% had pain, and 83% had a pulsatile abdominal mass.[1,10] Patients with rapidly increasing aneurysms may be offered elective repair to decrease the mortality associated with rupture, and if the patient is a current smoker, smoking cessation should be encouraged. Blood pressure monitoring and control are also important in management for these patients.

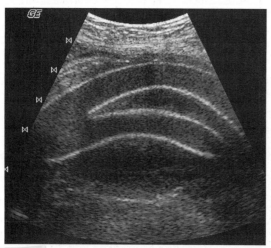

FIGURE 10-5 Echogenic walls of aortic graft. *(Courtesy GE Medical Systems.)*

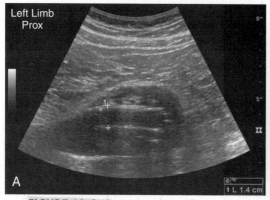
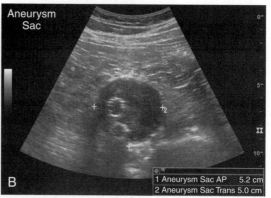

FIGURE 10-6 (A), Longitudinal image of aortic endograft. **(B)**, Transverse image of aortic endograft.

The classic presentation of a ruptured AAA includes the triad of hypotension, abdominal or back pain, and a pulsatile abdominal mass. Pain may also radiate to the back, groin, or scrotum. Patients may present in shock and be unable to communicate, or they may not have a known history of AAA. Patients with ruptured AAAs need immediate intervention to prevent death. Despite advances in perioperative care leading to significant decreases in mortality after AAA repair in asymptomatic patients, postoperative mortality after ruptured AAA repair is still more than 40% in patients who survive the operation.[11,12]

Traditionally, if the AAA expands by more than 0.6 to 0.8 cm per year, the patient should be offered repair.[1,5,10] All patients with AAAs should be educated about the signs of symptomatic and ruptured aneurysms. If they experience new or unusual pain in the back, groin, testicles, legs, or buttocks, emergent medical attention should be sought.[1]

Sonographic Findings

Sonographic examination of the abdomen to rule out rupture (Fig. 10-7) should include a survey of the aorta to confirm the aneurysmal aorta, although the aorta may appear normal in size. The abdomen should

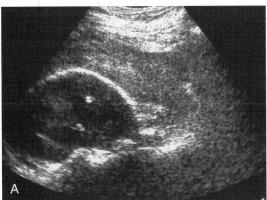

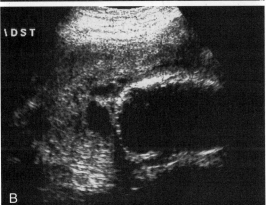

FIGURE 10-7 Aortic aneurysm in an unconscious, elderly patient seen in the emergency department. Longitudinal **(A)** and transverse **(B)** images show a dilated aorta. Transverse image also shows a large hematoma left of the umbilicus, which is worrisome for rupture.

also be explored for the presence of hemoperitoneum. Resolution of the disruption in the aortic wall may be impossible with sonography, but a periaortic hematoma may be identified, which would suggest rupture. Fluid in the gutters or a perinephric hematoma may also be identified.

AORTIC DISSECTION

Aortic dissection occurs with the rupture of the intima of the aorta, which separates from the media with a column of blood between the two layers. Causes of aortic dissection include hypertension, Marfan syndrome, and, less frequently, pregnancy and chest trauma. Dissection may also result from the degenerative changes that occur in the aorta with atherosclerotic disease or may result from a congenital defect or an iatrogenic event.

Based on the extent and location of the dissection, it can be characterized with the Stanford or DeBakey classification. The Stanford classification differentiates between dissections that involve the ascending aorta (type A) and dissections that do not involve the ascending aorta (type B). The DeBakey classification differentiates between dissections that involve the entire aorta (type I), dissections that involve only the ascending aorta (type II), and dissections that involve only the descending aorta (type III). The classifications are used in the determination of treatment and prognosis. Dissection of the ascending aorta has a much higher mortality rate than dissection of the descending aorta. Type B dissections may be treated conservatively when life-threatening complications are not present, whereas type A dissections are generally treated surgically.

The clinical presentation of dissection is usually acute onset of severe chest pain. Patients may also have neck or throat pain, pain in the abdomen or lower back, syncope, paresis, and dyspnea. If the patient history includes hypertension, aortic aneurysm, or Marfan syndrome, dissection should be strongly considered. Clinical examination may also reveal absent pulses in the legs.

Sonographic Findings

The sonographic technique used in the diagnosis of dissection varies depending on the location of the dissection. Transesophageal echocardiography (TEE) is the most common method of imaging for dissections of the ascending aorta. Transabdominal ultrasound is used for imaging dissections of the descending aorta, and CT and magnetic resonance imaging (MRI) may be used in evaluation of dissections of the ascending and descending aorta.

Dissection of the descending aorta may be diagnosed with identification of the intimal flap in the aorta (Fig. 10-8). Doppler can be used to document flow in the true lumen, and depending on whether the dissection is acute or chronic, flow may or may not be shown in the false

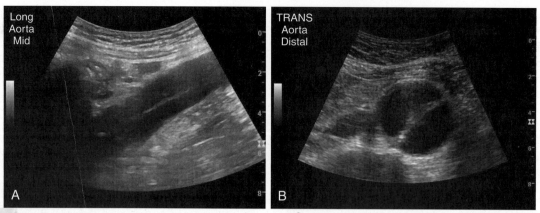

FIGURE 10-8 Dissection of abdominal aorta. Sagittal **(A)** and transverse **(B)** sonograms show intimal flap anteriorly separating true lumen from false lumen.

TABLE 10-1	Pathology of Aorta	
Pathology	**Symptoms**	**Sonographic Findings**
Aortic aneurysm	Pulsatile abdominal mass	Aortic AP diameter ≥3 cm, uniform or asymmetric dilation, with or without thrombus
Aortic rupture	Pulsatile abdominal mass, hypotension, abdominal pain, radiating pain	Aortic aneurysm, hemoperitoneum, periaortic hematoma
Aortic dissection	Severe chest pain, neck or throat pain, abdominal or back pain, syncope, paresis, dyspnea	Linear flap in aorta; flow may or may not be demonstrated on both sides of flap
Endoleak	Vary with type of leak	Blood flows into aneurysm sac; classified as one of four types

lumen located between the tunica intima and tunica media. Because rupture is a complication of dissection, the sonographic findings of aorta rupture should also be evaluated.

AORTIC ANEURYSM SCREENING

The U.S. Preventive Services Task Force released a statement summarizing recommendations for screening for AAA.[11-13] It stated that screening benefits patients who have a relatively high risk for dying from an aneurysm; major risk factors are age 65 years or older, male sex, and smoking at least 100 cigarettes in a lifetime. The guideline recommends one-time screening with sonography for AAA in men 65 to 75 years of age who have ever smoked. No recommendation was made for or against screening men 65 to 75 years of age who have never smoked, and it recommended against screening women. Men with a strong family history of AAA should be counseled about the risks and benefits of screening as they approach 65 years of age.[1,13]

Table 10-1 summarizes the pathology, symptoms, and sonographic findings of the aorta.

SUMMARY

Aortic aneurysm may be identified in patients with a pulsatile mass or as an incidental finding. Patients with a history of aneurysm and clinically significant symptoms should be considered at risk for dissection and rupture. Sonographic findings plus correlation with patient symptoms and clinical examination can aid with a speedy diagnosis in potentially life-threatening situations.

CLINICAL SCENARIO—DIAGNOSIS

The aorta is dilated, and thrombus is seen in the aneurysm. The hypotensive state and the fluid in the abdomen suggest aortic rupture. This diagnosis was confirmed at surgery, and the condition was successfully repaired. Incidentally, the large cystic structure anterior to the aorta was not the bladder, although it did provide an excellent window for visualization of the aneurysm. After the aneurysm was repaired, this mass was removed and was confirmed to be an ovarian cystadenoma.

CASE STUDIES FOR DISCUSSION

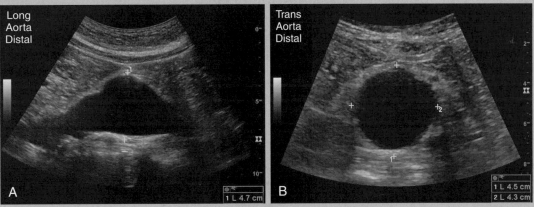

FIGURE 10-9 Longitudinal (A) and transverse (B) images of aorta with longitudinal AP diameter of 4.7 cm.

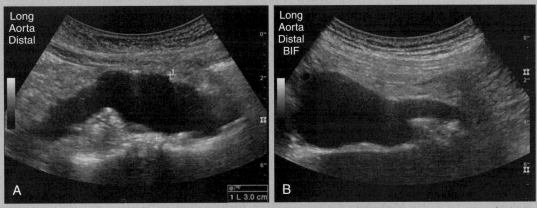

FIGURE 10-10 (A) and (B), Longitudinal images of distal aorta. Proximal left iliac artery is also identified (B).

1. A 63-year-old man is seen for evaluation of a possible renal mass seen on a radiograph. The sonogram reveals a right renal cyst. Incidentally noted are the findings in the aorta (Fig. 10-9). The aorta measured 4.7 cm in AP diameter. What is the most likely diagnosis of the findings in the aorta?

2. A 55-year-old man with a history of cigarette smoking undergoes sonography of the aorta because of a pulsatile mass over the area of the umbilicus on physical examination. The distal aorta is shown in Figure 10-10. What is the most likely diagnosis?

3. A 70-year-old man collapsed at a shopping mall and was transported via ambulance to the emergency department of the nearest hospital. The patient is hypotensive, is in shock, and has a pulsatile abdominal mass. A portable sonogram is requested immediately and reveals a dilated aorta that measures 8.5 cm in AP diameter (Fig. 10-11). What diagnosis do the clinical and sonographic findings suggest? How do the clinical findings contribute to the diagnosis?

4. A 60-year-old woman undergoes sonography of the aorta. She reports recent episodes of fainting and abdominal and back pain. She has a history of poorly controlled hypertension and an aortic aneurysm. An abdominal sonogram is performed to check the status of the aneurysm (Fig. 10-12). A new finding of linear echo is identified within the aorta, and color Doppler confirms flow on both sides of this flap. What is the most likely diagnosis? What symptoms, risk factors, and clinical presentation does she have to support the findings?

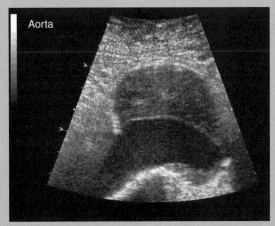

FIGURE 10-11 Longitudinal image of aorta with measurement of 8.5 cm in AP diameter.

5. A 75-year-old man is seen for follow-up of a known AAA. The sonogram reveals a dilated distal aorta that measures 3.9 cm in AP diameter. Mural thrombus is seen in the aneurysm (Fig. 10-13). No increase in size is noted from a sonogram performed 6 months previously. Considering the size of the aneurysm and the thrombus that is present, what is the recommended schedule of sonographic surveillance for this patient?

Continued

CASE STUDIES FOR DISCUSSION—cont'd

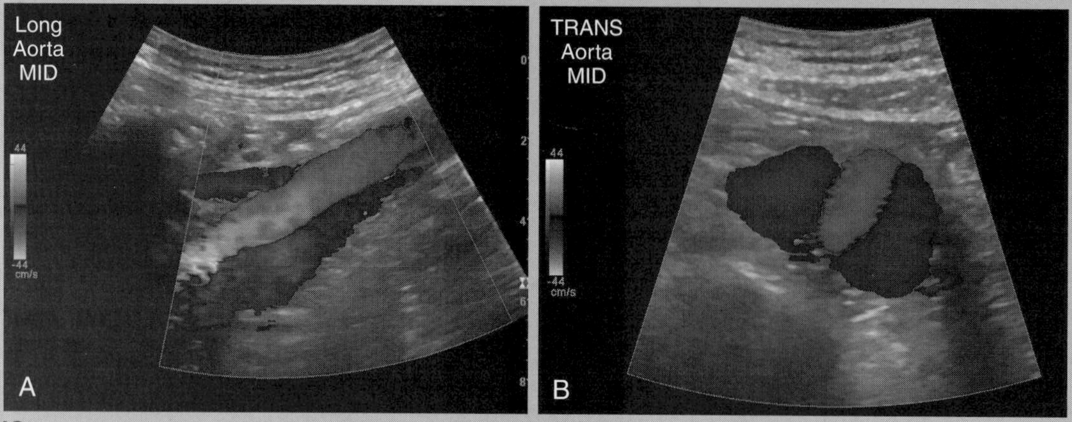

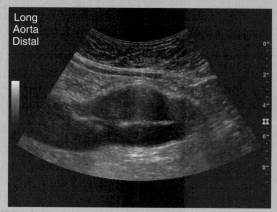

FIGURE 10-12 Longitudinal **(A)** and transverse **(B)** images of dilated aorta. Linear echo within vessel was documented with color flow on both sides.

FIGURE 10-13 Longitudinal image of aorta with mural thrombus.

STUDY QUESTIONS

1. Which of the following best describes the conventionally accepted definition of AAA?
   a. Focal dilation 1.5 times its normal diameter; an infrarenal diameter of 3 cm or larger
   b. Focal dilation 1.7 times its normal diameter in men and women
   c. Generalized dilation 3 times its normal diameter above the renal arteries
   d. Generalized dilation 1.7 times its normal diameter above the renal arteries

2. High blood pressure and current smoking increase the growth rate of aneurysms, and the resultant risk of rupture sharply increases with aneurysms of more than:
   a. 1.5 cm in diameter
   b. 3 cm in diameter
   c. 4.5 cm in diameter
   d. 6 cm in diameter

3. Repair of an AAA is indicated when the aneurysm becomes greater than ____ cm in diameter or grows more than ___ per year.
   a. 5.5 cm; 0.6 to 0.8 cm
   b. 4.5 cm; 0.6 to 0.8 cm
   c. 5.5 cm; 0.0 to 0.6 cm
   d. 4.5 cm; 0.0 to 0.6 cm

4. An endoleak occurs when blood is allowed to flow into the aneurysm sac after endograft placement. Based on the endoleak classifications, flow into the aneurysm owing to an inadequate seal between components of the device or a tear in the fabric of the graft would be given which of the following designations?
   a. Type 1
   b. Type 2
   c. Type 3
   d. Type 4

5. When performing a scan to rule out AAA, the abdominal aorta should be measured:
   a. AP in the transverse plane
   b. AP in the longitudinal plane
   c. Transverse at the level of the renal arteries
   d. Transverse at the level of the xiphoid process

6. The classic presentation of a ruptured AAA includes the triad of:
   a. Agitation, pulsatile abdominal mass, and low-grade fever
   b. Hypertension, referred shoulder pain, and abdominal mass
   c. Shortness of breath, epigastric pain, and abdominal mass
   d. Hypotension, abdominal or back pain, and pulsatile abdominal mass

7. Rupture of the intima of the aorta, which then separates from the media with a column of blood between the two layers, is the definition of:
   a. Dissection
   b. Endograft failure
   c. Aneurysm
   d. Thrombus
   e. Aneurysm rupture

8. The sonographic technique used in the diagnosis of dissection varies depending on the location of the dissection. Which section of the aorta may benefit from transabdominal sonography?
   a. Descending aorta
   b. Ascending aorta
   c. Aortic arch
   d. Ascending and descending aorta

9. The preferred method of evaluation and screening for AAA is:
   a. MRI
   b. CT angiography
   c. Sonography
   d. Radiograph
   e. Nuclear medicine positron emission tomography (PET) scan

10. Guidelines recommend a one-time screening with sonography for AAA in:
    a. Women who are hypertensive
    b. Men 65 to 75 years old who have ever smoked
    c. Men and women who have smoked more than 100 lifetime cigarettes
    d. Men and women 65 years old or older
    e. Men 65 to 75 years old who have persistent back pain

REFERENCES

1. Upchurch GR, Schaub TA: Abdominal aortic aneurysm, *Am Fam Physician* 73:1198–1204, 2006.
2. Anderson RN: Deaths: leading causes for 2000, *Natl Vital Stat Rep* 50:1–85, 2002.
3. Lederle FA, Johnson GR, Wilson SE, et al: Relationship of age, gender, race, and body size to infrarenal aortic diameter, *J Vasc Surg* 26:595–601, 1997.
4. Ebaugh JL, Garcia ND, Matsumura JS: Screening and surveillance for abdominal aortic aneurysms: who needs it and when, *Semin Vasc Surg* 14:193–199, 2001.
5. Kent KC, Zwolak RM, Jaff MR, et al: Screening for abdominal aortic aneurysm, *J Vasc Surg* 39:267–269, 2004.
6. Bromley PJ: A brief history of abdominal aortic endografting, *Appl Radiol* 30, 2001.

7. Pacanowski JP, Dieter RS, Stevens SL, et al: The Achilles heel of endovascular abdominal aortic aneurysm exclusion: a case report, *Wisc Med J* 101(7):57–58, 63, 2002.
8. Neumyer MM, Kidd J, Hodge M, et al: Sonographic evaluation of aortic endografts, *J Diag Med Sonogr* 27:55–64, 2011.
9. Brewster DC, Cronenwett JL, Hallett JW Jr, et al: Guidelines for the treatment of abdominal aortic aneurysms, *J Vasc Surg* 37:1106–1117, 2003.
10. Powell JT, Brown LC: The natural history of abdominal aortic aneurysms and their risk of rupture, *Acta Chir Belg* 101:11–16, 2001.
11. Wakefield TW, Whitehouse WM Jr, Wu SC, et al: Abdominal aortic aneurysm rupture, *Surgery* 91:586–596, 1982.
12. Dimick JB, Stanley JC, Axelrod DA, et al: Variation in death rate after abdominal aortic aneurysmectomy in the United States, *Ann Surg* 235:579–585, 2002.
13. U.S. Preventive Services Task Force: Screening for abdominal aortic aneurysm: recommendation statement, *Ann Intern Med* 142:198–202, 2005.

Suspect Appendicitis

Kristy Stohlmann, Kathryn Kuntz

CLINICAL SCENARIO

A mother brought her 8-year-old son to the emergency department after a 1-week episode of right lower quadrant (RLQ) pain, nausea, vomiting, and anorexia. During initial examination, the pediatrician found the boy to be lethargic and febrile with rebound tenderness in the RLQ (McBurney's sign). A blood test showed an elevated white blood cell (WBC) count of 13,000/mm³. A sonogram of the abdomen was ordered. Focusing on the appendix area, the sonogram revealed suspicious findings (Figs. 11-1 and 11-2). What is the mostly likely diagnosis of this boy's illness?

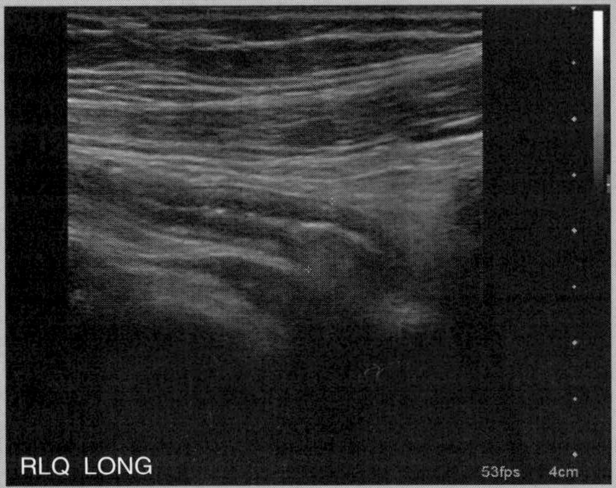

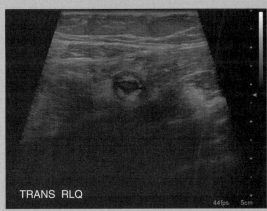

FIGURE 11-1 Longitudinal sonographic image of a noncompressible, blind-ended structure identified in the RLQ of an 8-year-old boy. Outer wall–to–outer wall AP measurement is 6.4 mm. The structure also contains echogenic material.

FIGURE 11-2 Transverse sonographic image of the same noncompressible RLQ structure in the 8-year-old boy shown in Figure 11-1.

OBJECTIVES

- Describe the epidemiology and causes of appendicitis.
- Describe the anatomy and pathophysiology of appendicitis.
- List the clinical presentation and sonographic findings of appendicitis.
- Describe the recommended method of imaging the appendix with sonography.

Sonography is an appropriate imaging method for the diagnosis of several types of gastrointestinal (GI) diseases, the most common of which is appendicitis. Appendicitis must be included in the differential diagnosis of patients of all ages with RLQ pain, nausea, and vomiting. Clinicians must presume the most likely cause of the symptoms and follow-up with diagnostic studies, such as sonography, to confirm or exclude the initial diagnosis.

Acute appendicitis is one of the most common diseases that necessitates emergency surgery and is the most common atraumatic surgical abdominal disorder in children 2 years old and older. Males and females have a lifetime appendicitis risk of 8.6% and 6.7%; the mortality rate in nonperforated appendicitis is less than 1%.[1] Early diagnosis of appendicitis is essential to prevent perforation, abscess formation, and postoperative complications. A delay in diagnosis often occurs with young, pregnant, or elderly patients, increasing the risk of perforation. The mortality rate can be 5% in these patients.[1,2] During the past 2 decades, sonography, along with nuclear medicine and computed tomography (CT), has been used in the diagnosis of appendicitis. Despite technologic advances, the diagnosis of appendicitis is still based primarily on patient history and physical examination.[1,2]

ANATOMY AND PHYSIOLOGY

The appendix is a long, thin diverticulum that arises from the inferior tip of the cecum (Fig. 11-3). Although the average length of the appendix is 3 inches, it can measure 9 inches. The appendix usually has an anterior intraperitoneal location that, when inflamed, may come in contact with the anterior parietal peritoneum and cause RLQ pain. The appendix may be "hidden" from the anterior peritoneum 30% of the time when in a pelvic, retroileal, or retrocecal position (Fig. 11-4).[3] The differing locations of the appendix can make sonographic imaging a challenge.

The shape of the appendix also differs depending on the patient's age. At birth, the appendix is funnel-shaped, which limits the chance for obstruction to occur. By age 2 years, the appendix assumes a more normal conic shape, which increases the chance for luminal obstruction (Figs. 11-5 and 11-6). Although the appendix itself is not necessary for survival, the lining of the appendix, composed of lymphatic tissue, is thought to play a specialized role in the immune system.

Epidemiology

Appendicitis usually results from an obstructing object, or obstructive disorder, within the appendix. The risk for an obstruction can be linked to diet or genetic predisposition. Generally, unhealthy diets, including decreased dietary fiber, along with increased refined carbohydrates (e.g., pure sugars and starches), can increase the incidence rate of appendicitis. A history of appendicitis in

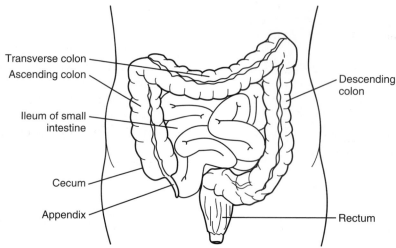

FIGURE 11-3 Diagram of the normal location of the appendix. The appendix lies at the inferior tip of the cecum near the junction of the terminal ileum of the small intestine and the proximal ascending colon.

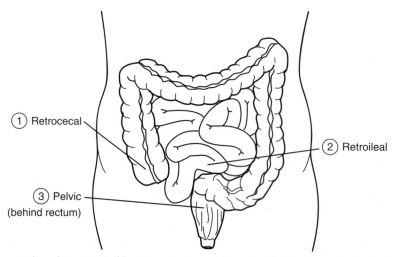

FIGURE 11-4 The appendix is sometimes in an atypical location. *1,* retrocecal location (behind cecum); *2,* retroileal location (behind ileum of small intestine); *3,* pelvic location (hidden behind uterus, rectum, or ovaries).

a first-degree relative is associated with a 3.5% to 10% relative risk. The strongest familial associations have been noted when children develop appendicitis at unusually young ages (birth to 6 years).[4]

Obstruction of the appendiceal lumen usually precedes appendicitis. This obstruction can be caused by several different diseases, including lymphoid follicle hyperplasia, fecalith (a hard, impacted mass of feces), foreign bodies, seeds, or parasites. An obstruction to the proximal lumen of the appendix inhibits the drainage of mucous secretions from the walls of the appendix, which eventually causes distention in the distal appendiceal lumen. This distention allows for bacterial invasion and edema to the wall of the appendix, and finally results in inflammation and pain.

Some cases of appendicitis have a different etiology. These less common cases begin with direct mucosal ulceration caused by a buildup of mucus within the appendix, sometimes called a mucocele, which leads to bacterial invasion and resultant appendicitis. Sonographically, a mucocele of the appendix is shown by a dilated, noncompressible appendix with an abnormal accumulation of debris (mucus) within the lumen. The appendiceal

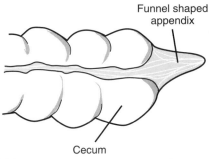

FIGURE 11-5 By age 2 years, the appendix assumes a more adult-like conic shape, increasing the chance for proximal luminal obstruction.

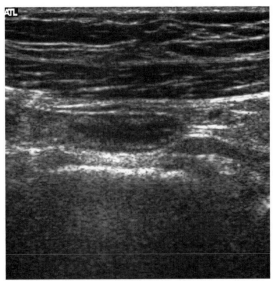

FIGURE 11-6 Longitudinal sonographic image of a normal conic-shaped appendix in a 9-year-old girl.

diameter can become very large, and the "onion sign" (sonographic layering of echogenic debris within a cystic mass) may be seen (see Table 11-1).

Regardless of the cause of appendicitis, the patient must seek immediate medical attention. If patients do not have symptoms, choose to ignore the symptoms, or cannot communicate their symptoms (e.g., infants and young children), rupture is a risk. Failure to receive medical attention within 36 hours is associated with an increased risk of rupture of the appendix, and the risk increases in ensuing 12-hour periods.[5]

A ruptured appendix places the patient at much greater risk for postsurgical complications. Rupture causes the bacteria-filled mucus to spill into the peritoneum and can lead to diffuse peritonitis, or abscess formation.[6] When the appendix has ruptured, sonographic visualization is much more difficult because the lumen is no longer distended, and the anatomy is distorted by surrounding inflammation and adjacent abscess (see Table 11-1).

Clinical Presentation

The first classic symptom of appendicitis is periumbilical pain, followed by nausea, RLQ pain, and subsequent vomiting with fever.[2] All of these symptoms are present in 50% of adult cases. Other adult cases and many pediatric cases may have more inconspicuous symptoms, such as irritability, lethargy, abdominal pain, anorexia, fever, or diarrhea, which make diagnosis more of a challenge. The most important clinical finding is RLQ pain with palpation. Physicians also use the quick release method to rule out appendicitis. The quick release is performed by applying pressure with the fingertips directly over the area of the appendix and then quickly letting go. With appendicitis, the patient usually has rebound tenderness (McBurney's sign) associated with peritoneal irritation. Although an elevated WBC count (>10,000/mm³) can be an indicator for appendicitis, the accuracy of this test alone is limited.

Vague abdominal pain that sometimes occurs with appendicitis may mimic several other GI diseases. It is important to obtain an accurate patient history to rule out other diseases, including gallbladder disease; acute pyelonephritis; urinary tract stone disease; infectious or inflammatory conditions of the cecum and ascending colon; and unusual diseases such as complicated ovarian cysts, cyst hemorrhage, and ovarian torsion.[3] A pelvic examination or pelvic sonography should be performed in women with suspicious RLQ pain because some painful gynecologic conditions can mimic appendicitis. A pregnancy test for all women of childbearing age is also recommended to rule out ectopic pregnancy.

Sonographic Findings. Graded compression sonography is a rapid, noninvasive, and inexpensive means of imaging a normal or inflamed appendix. When inflamed, the appendix does not compress. The technique requires no patient preparation, and scanning can be performed at the most tender site, which enables correlation of imaging findings with patient symptoms. A high-frequency linear array transducer ranging from 7 to 12 MHz is most commonly used. Before scanning, the patient is asked to point with one finger to the place of maximal pain. Graded compression uses gradual pressure, with the transducer moving in a cephalad-to-caudad fashion to displace the normal gas-containing bowel loops for visualization of the inflamed appendix. This technique also helps to identify the location of an abnormally positioned appendix.[6]

The graded compression technique used to image the appendix has been proven to be of considerable value in the diagnosis of acute appendicitis. Compression aids in relocating normal bowel loops and interfering air away from the site of interest. In more difficult cases, a technique called posterior manual compression can be used in addition to graded compression.[1,6] Posterior manual compression is performed by using both hands. The hand not holding the transducer is placed on the patient's back, and pressure is applied upward in an anterior direction. At the same time, pressure is applied on the abdomen by the transducer in the posterior direction. This technique helps visualize the appendix when it is located in a deep position.[6] Placing the patient in a left oblique lateral decubitus position may also be helpful in visualizing a retrocecal appendix.

If the patient is unable to point to a specific area of pain, the sonographer must locate the appendix. Real-time scanning is initiated in the transverse plane and directed toward the cecal tip and the origin of the appendix. Scanning begins laterally in the iliac fossa, at the level of the umbilicus. Gradual pressure (graded compression) is applied with the transducer to compress bowel loops and express all gas and fluid contents away from the site of interest. The ascending colon is first identified as a gas-filled peristaltic structure with the sonographic appearance of bowel (i.e., an inner echogenic ring surrounded by five concentric bowel wall layers) (Fig. 11-7). The ascending colon is scanned caudally to its termination at the cecum. With the transducer in the transverse plane, the cecum is scanned inferiorly to its tip. The normal cecum and terminal ileum are easily compressible with moderate pressure. The terminal ileum is identified as a compressible peristaltic bowel segment adjacent to the cecum. The examination is continued inferiorly with identification of the psoas and iliacus muscles and the external iliac artery and vein.

The examination is considered diagnostic when the psoas muscle and external iliac vessels are identified and when the cecum and terminal ileum can be adequately compressed by the transducer for evaluation of the retrocecal region. Because the appendix originates from the

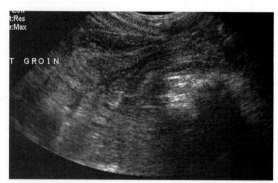

FIGURE 11-7 Sonographic image of ascending colon in a 4-year-old boy.

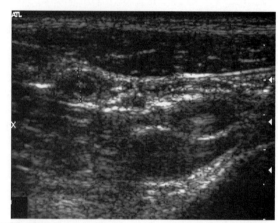

FIGURE 11-8 Transverse image of normal appendix in a 9-year-old boy. AP diameter is 4.1 mm (normal AP measurement <6 mm).

cecal tip but can vary in position, it is not always seen. It is most commonly directed medially or caudally but may be retrocecal or lateral to the cecum.

The appendix must be seen to rule out appendicitis. Tissue harmonic imaging has been shown to improve diagnostic resolution compared with conventional sonography, improving visualization of the normal appendix.[3] Visualization of a normal appendix during sonography is highly operator dependent and ranges from 0 to 82%.[3]

The normal appendix, when identified, appears as a tubular structure with a blind end that measures 6 mm or less in anteroposterior (AP) dimension from outer wall-to-outer wall (Figs. 11-8 to 11-10). The appendix should be scanned in both the longitudinal and the transverse planes, with several measurements obtained to reach the most accurate diagnosis. The area around the appendix should also be scanned to check for fluid collections and other GI or pelvic abnormalities.

APPENDICITIS

Sonographic findings in nonperforated appendicitis include a blind-ended tubular structure (Fig. 11-11) with a muscular wall thickness greater than 2 mm (Fig. 11-12), an appendiceal diameter (outer wall to outer

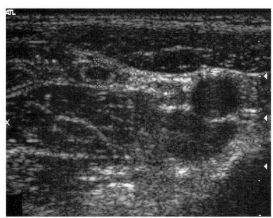

FIGURE 11-9 Normal transverse AP measurement in the same 9-year-old boy shown in Figure 11-8 demonstrating compression. With compression, the AP diameter is 3.5 mm. Compression of the appendix is not achievable in positive cases of appendicitis.

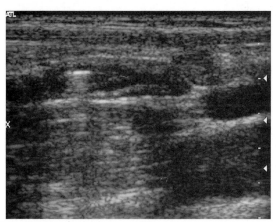

FIGURE 11-10 Longitudinal view of normal appendix in the same 9-year-old boy shown in Figures 11-8 and 11-9.

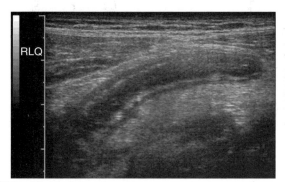

FIGURE 11-11 Blind-ended, tubular structure identified as an inflamed appendix in the RLQ.

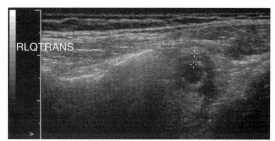

FIGURE 11-12 Transverse view of appendix wall with AP measurement of 2.5 mm (normal <2 mm).

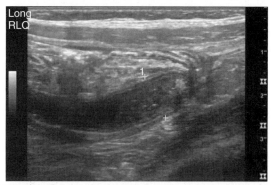

FIGURE 11-13 Longitudinal view of inflamed appendix with outer wall–to-–outer wall AP measurement of 1.1 cm (normal <6 mm).

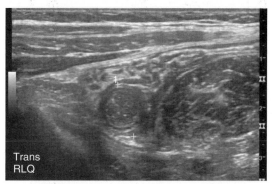

FIGURE 11-14 Transverse view of inflamed appendix with outer wall–to–outer wall AP measurement of 1.1 cm (normal <6 mm).

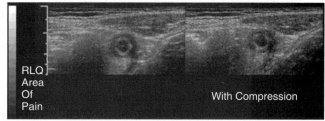

FIGURE 11-15 Transverse image of inflamed appendix that does not change with compression.

wall) greater than 6 mm (Figs. 11-13 and 11-14) that does not compress (Fig. 11-15), a nonperistaltic target sign (bull's-eye appearance) of abnormally thickened bowel wall layers when viewed in the short axis, and sometimes distention or obstruction of the appendiceal lumen accompanied by increased echogenicity (edema) surrounding the appendix (Fig. 11-16). Findings may also include an echogenic shadowing appendicolith (Fig. 11-17), pericecal or perivesical free fluid (Fig. 11-18), or increased color Doppler in the wall of the appendix, indicating increased appendiceal perfusion (Fig. 11-19).

The AP outer wall–to–outer wall measurement criterion for diagnosing appendicitis can vary between

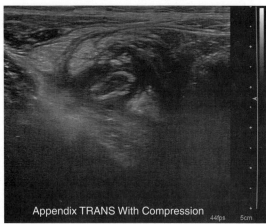

FIGURE 11-16 Transverse view of inflamed appendix with increased echogenicity in surrounding tissue representing edema.

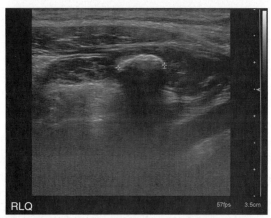

FIGURE 11-17 Longitudinal view of inflamed appendix with appendicolith. Acoustic shadowing is seen posterior to the appendicolith.

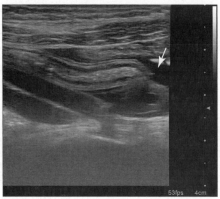

FIGURE 11-18 Free fluid near tip of inflamed appendix.

institutions. Some institutions use greater than 7 mm to prevent high rates of false-positive diagnoses of appendicitis. Care must be taken to diagnose or rule out appendicitis accurately by assessing the measurement criterion along with the other sonographic findings as well as the patient's clinical symptoms (see Table 11-1).

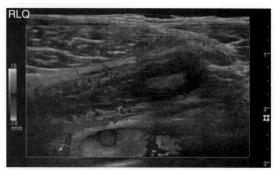

FIGURE 11-19 Longitudinal view shows increased color Doppler in the wall of appendix, indicating increased appendiceal perfusion.

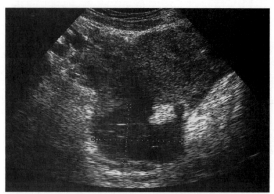

FIGURE 11-20 Abscess that developed following an appendectomy found in RLQ of a 22-year-old patient with a ruptured appendix. Abscesses generally appear as a vague hypoechoic or complex mass.

Sonographic findings with a perforated or ruptured appendix may include the target sign with inhomogeneous or missing layers in the wall and with inhomogeneous pericecal or perivesical mass without peristalsis or free fluid in the abdomen. Gangrenous appendicitis may be suggested when sonographic imaging shows a loss of the echogenic submucosal layer and absent color flow in that segment of the appendix. Periappendiceal abscesses may be found in cases of rupture either before or after appendectomy and generally appear as vague hypoechoic or complex masses (Fig. 11-20). Abscesses are usually successfully drained after appendectomy with a transrectal biopsy guide on an endocavitary transducer. Insertion of the transducer into the rectum allows for adequate visualization and drainage of the abscess with sonographic guidance.

A false-negative sonographic diagnosis is common when nonvisualization of the appendix occurs. Reasons for nonvisualization include superimposed air or feces, obesity, abdominal wall rigidity or pain, scanning of an uncooperative child, an abnormally large appendix, or atypical appendiceal location.[3,6] In these cases, a CT scan of the appendix may be ordered to confirm the diagnosis before surgery.

Table 11-1 summarizes the symptoms, sonographic findings, and laboratory values associated with appendicitis.

TABLE 11-1	Pathology of the Appendix	
Pathology	**Symptoms**	**Sonographic Findings**
Appendicitis—classic symptoms	Periumbilical pain, followed by nausea, RLQ pain, and subsequent vomiting with fever; rebound tenderness (positive McBurney's sign)	Primary findings: Noncompressible, nonperistaltic, blind-ended appendix with outer wall–to–outer wall AP measurement of >6 mm
		Other Findings*: Muscle wall AP measurement >2 mm; echogenic shadowing appendicolith; hyperemia with increase in color Doppler; inflamed, echogenic periappendiceal fat; pericecal or perivesical free fluid (ascites); complex mass representing an abscess
Appendicitis—other symptoms	Irritability, lethargy, abdominal pain, anorexia, or diarrhea*	
Rupture	Same as or indistinguishable from non-ruptured appendicitis.	Variable; distorted anatomy with or without distended appendiceal lumen; vague hypoechoic or complex periappendiceal mass; target sign with inhomogeneous or missing layers in wall; inhomogeneous pericecal or perivesical mass without peristalsis or free fluid in abdomen
Mucocele	Varies from asymptomatic to possible pain in the right lower abdominal quadrant, weight loss, nausea, vomiting, change in bowel habits, anemia, and hematochezia.	Dilated appendiceal lumen; cystic mass in expected region of appendix (with possible sonographic layering called the "onion sign"); possible internal echogenicity; lack of appendiceal wall thickening
Associated laboratory values for appendicitis		Elevated white blood cell count of >10,000/mm^3*

*May be present; accuracy of these findings alone is limited in the diagnosis of appendicitis.

SUMMARY

Suspected acute appendicitis is the most common condition requiring urgent abdominal surgery in pediatric patients.[2] Care must be taken to diagnose appendicitis properly because the symptoms may mimic other GI diseases. Confirmation of appendicitis by sonography requires skill on the part of the sonographer and interpreting physician. These skills should be acquired through education and experience. Although operator dependent, sonography has been an excellent tool for identifying the appendix for many years. A positive finding on sonographic examination speeds diagnosis and therapy in clinically doubtful cases and reduces the number of negative laparotomy cases. Because sonography has limitations in imaging of the GI tract, other methods such as CT scan may be needed to follow-up nondiagnostic or questionable findings.

CLINICAL SCENARIO—DIAGNOSIS

Before performing the sonogram, the patient was asked to point with one finger to the area of maximal pain. He pointed to the area of McBurney's point. The sonographer initiated scanning in that area and performed a complete abdominal and pelvis survey to rule out other pathologies. A noncompressible, blind-ended structure was found in the area of the appendix in the RLQ with an outer wall–to–outer wall AP measurement of 7 mm in longitudinal view and 6.7 mm in transverse view. The structure also contained echogenic material, which possibly represented small particles of an appendicolith. The sonologist diagnosed acute appendicitis. The patient was taken to surgery shortly after the sonogram, and pathologic specimens confirmed the diagnosis of acute appendicitis.

CASE STUDIES FOR DISCUSSION

1. A 5-year-old girl presents to the emergency department with RLQ pain, nausea, and vomiting. While questioning the mother, the physician finds out that the mother had an appendectomy as a child. Discuss the genetic association of familial appendicitis.
2. A 19-year-old woman presents to the emergency department 5 days after an appendectomy. She has been experiencing RLQ pain and fever for the past 3 days. On physical examination, she is tender along her entire right side. An endovaginal sonogram was performed and revealed a fluid-filled structure in the RLQ (Fig. 11-21). Taking her surgical history into consideration, what is the most likely diagnosis of this fluid-filled structure? What would the patient's treatment include?
3. A 42-year-old man presents to the emergency department after a motor vehicle accident. A series of radiographs was performed to rule out trauma. His blood test is negative for kidney or liver disease but shows an elevated WBC count (12,000/mm^3). The patient has a fever and is tender when the physician palpates the RLQ. On further examination, the patient admits he has been having RLQ pain for the past 5 days. The abdominal radiograph shows a calcification in the RLQ (Fig. 11-22). Discuss the differential diagnoses associated with this finding. What imaging test should be ordered next?
4. A 24-year-old woman presented to the emergency department with RLQ pain and fever. She was found to have RLQ tenderness on physical examination. Blood and urine tests were performed,

Continued

CASE STUDIES FOR DISCUSSION—cont'd

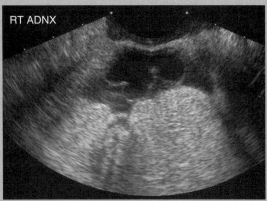

FIGURE 11-21 Fluid-filled structure identified in RLQ during an endovaginal sonogram of a 19-year-old woman with a history of appendectomy.

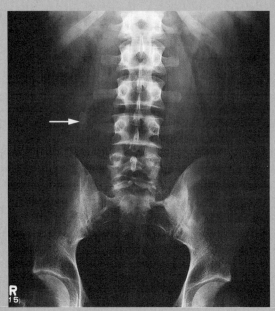

FIGURE 11-22 Abdominal radiograph of a 42-year-old patient following a motor vehicle accident shows calcification in RLQ. Calcification also is visible in RLQ (arrow).

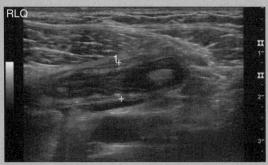

FIGURE 11-23 Longitudinal image of appendix in a 24-year-old pregnant woman with outer wall–to–outer wall AP measurement of 8 mm.

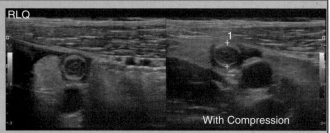

FIGURE 11-24 Transverse image of appendix with compression in the same 24-year-old pregnant woman shown in Figure 11-23 with outer wall–to–outer wall AP measurement of 6 mm.

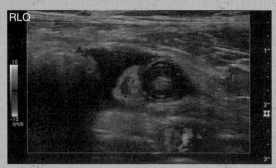

FIGURE 11-25 Transverse color Doppler image of appendix in the same 24-year-old pregnant woman shown in Figures 11-23 and 11-24.

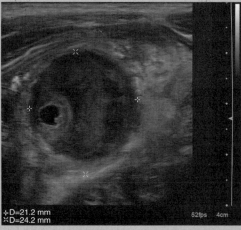

FIGURE 11-26 Transverse image of appendix in an 18-year-old man with a diameter of 21.2 mm × 24.2 mm.

and the results were positive for pregnancy. A pelvic sonogram showed a viable 13-week fetus. The sonographer also scanned the RLQ at the site of maximum tenderness. A blind-ended, tubular, distended, noncompressible, nonperistaltic structure with blood flow (color flow) measuring 8 mm × 6 mm was identified (Figs. 11-23 to 11-25). What is the most likely diagnosis of this mass?

5. An 18-year-old man presented to the emergency department with vague right-sided pain, vomiting, and nausea. An abdominal sonogram was ordered, focusing on the area of the appendix. Images showed an appendix measuring 21.2 mm × 24.2 mm (Fig. 11-26). What does the echogenic debris within the appendiceal lumen most likely represent? What other findings are seen in the image? What is the most likely diagnosis for this patient?

STUDY QUESTIONS

1. A _____ appendix must be identified to rule out appendicitis completely.
   a. Perforated
   b. Normal
   c. Pelvic
   d. Retroperitoneal

2. Sonographic imaging of the appendix includes using a technique called:
   a. Gradual compression
   b. Graduated compression
   c. Graded compression
   d. Grated compression

3. A linear transducer with a range of _____ MHz is used during sonographic evaluation of the appendix.
   a. 1 to 2
   b. 4 to 5
   c. 6 to 7
   d. 7 to 12

4. The appendix arises from the inferior tip of the _____, located near the junction of the terminal ileum of the small intestine, and the proximal ascending colon.
   a. Descending colon
   b. Transverse colon
   c. Sigmoid
   d. Cecum

5. Rebound tenderness in the RLQ found in patients with appendicitis is associated with:
   a. Peritoneal irritation
   b. Elevated WBC count
   c. Ascites
   d. Foreign bodies

6. The appendix can be "hidden" from the anterior peritoneum _____% of the time.
   a. 15
   b. 30
   c. 45
   d. 60

7. Rebound tenderness in the RLQ is called:
   a. Appendicolith
   b. McBurney's sign
   c. Pericecal sign
   d. Graduated sign

8. The risk of rupture increases significantly when appendicitis is not treated within _____ hours of the onset of symptoms.
   a. 36
   b. 24
   c. 12
   d. 2

9. An elevated _____ can be an indicator for appendicitis; however, the accuracy of this test alone is limited.
   a. Temperature
   b. Hematocrit
   c. WBC count
   d. Red blood cell count

10. Classic symptoms of appendicitis include periumbilical pain, followed by nausea, _____ pain, and subsequent vomiting with fever.
    a. LUQ
    b. LLQ
    c. RUQ
    d. RLQ

REFERENCES

1. Gaitini D, et al: Diagnosing acute appendicitis in adults: accuracy of color Doppler sonography and MDCT compared with surgery and clinical follow-up, *AJR Am J Roentgenol* 190:1300–1306, 2008.
2. Preeyacha P, et al: Sonography in the evaluation of acute appendicitis: are negative sonographic findings good enough, *J Ultrasound Med* 29:1749–1755, 2010.
3. Yabunaka K, et al: Sonographic appearance of the normal appendix in adults, *J Ultrasound Med* 26:37–43, 2007.
4. Rothrock SG, Pagane J: Acute appendicitis in children: emergency department diagnosis and management, *Ann Emerg Med* 36:39–51, 2000.
5. Bickell NA, Nina A, Aufses AH, et al: How time affects the risk of rupture in appendicitis, *J Am Coll Surg* 202:401–406, 2006.
6. Davie K, et al: Appendicitis in the deep pelvis, *J Diag Med Sonogr* 27:148–152, 2011.

Suspect Pyloric Stenosis or Other Gastrointestinal Findings

Holly Bostick

CLINICAL SCENARIO

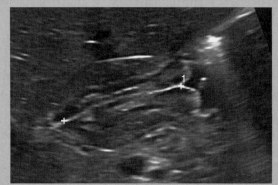

FIGURE 12-1 A 1-month-old infant with pyloric canal length of 2.6 cm.

A mother brought her 1-month-old twin girl to the emergency department because the infant had had projectile vomiting after every meal for the past 24 hours. The infant was also unusually irritable and would not stop fussing. During the pediatrician's initial examination, he felt a small 3 cm mass in the infant's right upper quadrant (RUQ), close to midline. The infant did not show signs of jaundice but was lethargic. The infant was immediately given intravenous fluids for dehydration, and a sonogram of the abdomen was ordered. The abdominal sonogram focused on the area of the pylorus (Figs. 12-1 to 12-3). What is the most likely diagnosis of this infant's illness?

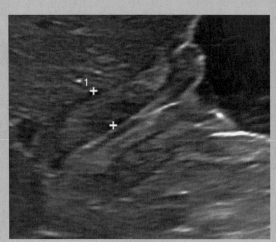

FIGURE 12-2 AP pyloric wall thickness of 6.3 mm.

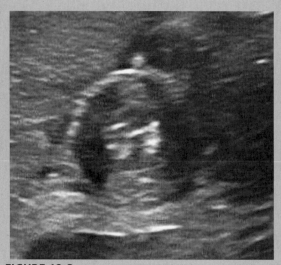

FIGURE 12-3 Transverse view of inflamed pyloric canal.

OBJECTIVES

- Describe the epidemiology, anatomy, and pathophysiology of infantile hypertrophic pyloric stenosis.
- Explain the clinical presentation, sonographic findings, and treatment of infantile hypertrophic pyloric stenosis.

- Describe the epidemiology, anatomy, and pathophysiology of intussusception.
- Describe the clinical presentation, sonographic findings, and treatment of intussusception.

Clinicians must consider patients presenting with symptoms including vomiting and pain to be at risk for various gastrointestinal (GI) diseases, including infantile hypertrophic pyloric stenosis (IHPS) and intussusception. Pyloric stenosis is common in infants, and sonography has become the preferred imaging method for evaluating and diagnosing this condition. Intussusception is often demonstrated with confidence via ultrasonography, avoiding the need for more invasive diagnostic imaging.

PYLORIC STENOSIS

Hypertrophic pyloric stenosis is a GI tract disorder common in infancy that can also occur in adults as the result of ulcer or fibrosis at the gastric outlet. The disorder causes projectile vomiting, weight loss, and fluid and electrolyte abnormalities. The problem can usually be diagnosed with clinical symptoms along with manual detection of an enlarged pylorus, described as an olive-sized lump to the right of the stomach. When diagnosis cannot be confirmed with clinical examination, imaging studies, including sonography and fluoroscopy, are appropriate.

Epidemiology

Infantile hypertrophic pyloric stenosis (IHPS) has a rate of occurrence of 3 per 1000 infants[1,2] and is four to five times more likely to occur in male infants than in female infants.[3] IHPS has been reported to have a familial predisposition, resulting in a higher incidence of occurrence in first-born white boys.[1,3,4] The symptoms usually begin within 3 to 6 weeks after birth; however, IHPS may infrequently occur in infants 1 week of age up to 5 months of age.[1] IHPS is thought to be an acquired condition with unknown cause, although various etiologic theories exist. The most notable of these theories is a possible association with oral administration of the medication erythromycin at an early age.[1,2,4]

Anatomy and Pathophysiology

Hypertrophic pyloric stenosis is the result of hypertrophy of the circular musculature that surrounds the pylorus, which causes constriction and obstruction of the gastric outlet. The pylorus is a tubular structure located on the right side of the stomach. It is the sphincter that connects the stomach with the duodenum of the small intestine. The most common position of the pylorus is about 3 cm to the right of the midsagittal axis at the level of the first lumbar vertebra (Fig. 12-4).

Clinical Presentation

Hypertrophic pyloric stenosis classically is seen with nonbilious projectile vomiting; if prolonged, vomiting could result in dehydration and metabolic alkalosis. Nonprojectile vomiting and jaundice may also occur. The hypertrophic pylorus can usually be palpated after a feeding and is described as an olive-shaped mass, about 2 cm in diameter, in the right side of the epigastrium, representing the constricted pyloric muscle. If this mass is felt, the diagnosis is confirmed; however, in many cases, the olive-shaped mass cannot be felt, so diagnostic sonography of the pylorus or fluoroscopic upper gastrointestinal (UGI) examination is required to rule out stenosis.

Sonographic Findings

Sonography is the imaging method of choice for IHPS because it is highly accurate and lacks the ionizing radiation associated with radiologic fluoroscopic procedures, such as UGI. With evaluation for IHPS, the role of any imaging method is first to identify the pyloric muscle, measure its length and anteroposterior (AP) wall thickness, and document passage of fluid from the stomach through the pylorus. Plain film radiographs or UGI contrast studies can be used; however, sonography is superior in direct visualization of the muscle hypertrophy and the pyloric channel length.

Hypertrophic pyloric stenosis can be viewed with real-time imaging of the pylorus muscle preferably 2 to 3 hours after the last meal. A high-frequency linear array probe ranging from 7 to 12 MHz is most commonly used; in older patients, a 3 to 7 MHz curvilinear probe may be necessary. Patients should undergo scanning in the right posterior oblique position (RPO) if possible. The RPO position helps with visualization of the pylorus with use of the fluid-filled stomach as a scanning window. The location of the pylorus can be identified with scanning in a transverse plane along the lesser curvature of the stomach through the left lobe of the liver just to the right of midline. The pylorus lies inferior and to the right of the antrum of the stomach. If the pylorus is not well visualized, the patient may drink some water for display of the gastric lumen. Gastric peristalsis can be seen in real time after the ingestion of approximately 60 to 120 mL of an electrolyte replacement fluid or water. The sonographer should remember to keep a towel handy because an infant is prone to vomiting after ingestion of the fluids. Absent peristalsis and lack of movement of fluid through the pylorus with a thickened AP muscle wall and increased pylorus channel length indicate stenosis. Measurements should be taken to document the size of the muscle. Although measurements may vary slightly between institutions, the most commonly accepted measurements for diagnosing pyloric stenosis include an AP muscle wall thickness of 3.0 mm or more (Figs. 12-5 and 12-6) with a pylorus length of 17 mm or more. A stenotic pyloric channel resembles the sonographic appearance of the cervix in pregnancy and is nicknamed the "cervix sign" (Figs. 12-7 and 12-8).

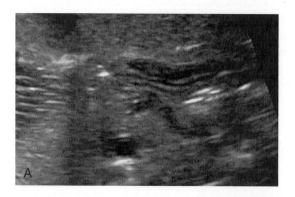

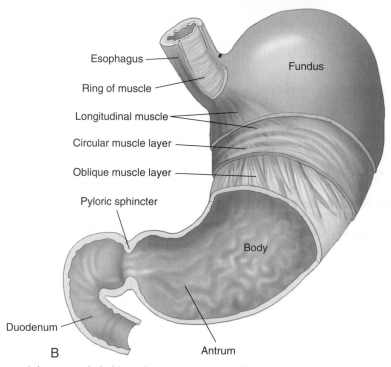

FIGURE 12-4 Diagram of pylorus. Pylorus muscle (sphincter) connects antrum of stomach with duodenum of small intestine. **(B),** Longitudinal image of normal pylorus.

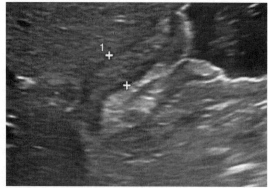

FIGURE 12-5 Longitudinal image of stenotic pylorus in a 4-week-old boy. AP wall thickness is 5.0 mm (normal wall thickness, <3.0 mm).

Hypertrophic pyloric stenosis can be dangerous if not diagnosed within several days of the onset of symptoms. Severe dehydration and biochemical disturbances, such as hypokalemic or hypochloremic metabolic alkalosis (Table 12-1), can occur when the condition is untreated.[2,3] Patients in whom the hypertrophied pylorus can be reliably palpated by an experienced clinician may not need sonographic evaluation. The use of sonography is best reserved for cases in which the clinical examination results are negative.

Treatment

When the diagnosis is made, the usual treatment for IHPS involves fluid replacement therapy followed by the Fredet-Ramstedt operation, or pyloromyotomy. This surgical procedure is performed with mild anesthesia and involves cutting the muscle fibers of the gastric outlet to widen the opening. Most patients successfully

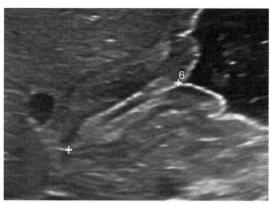

FIGURE 12-6 Longitudinal image of pyloric stenosis in a 4-week-old girl. Pyloric canal length is 1.8 cm (normal, <1.7 cm).

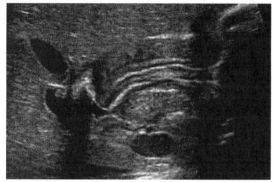

FIGURE 12-7 Longitudinal view of pyloric stenosis demonstrates the cervix sign. Canal length is 1.9 cm.

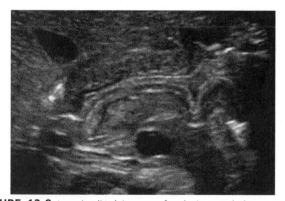

FIGURE 12-8 Longitudinal image of pyloric canal demonstrates the cervix sign. Canal length is 1.8 cm.

TABLE 12-1	Laboratory Findings of Gastrointestinal System
Pathology	**Laboratory Findings**
Pyloric stenosis	Hypochloremic metabolic alkalosis, hypokalemic metabolic alkalosis
Intussusception	Anemia, leukocytosis

recover from this procedure without recurrence of the stenosis.

INTUSSUSCEPTION

Intussusception is the acquired telescoping or invagination of a proximal portion of the intestine into a more distal portion, resulting in vascular compromise and subsequent bowel necrosis (Fig. 12-9). It is an emergent condition requiring prompt diagnosis; after IHPS, intussusception is the most common cause of intestinal obstruction in children. Peak occurrence is between 5 and 9 months of age, but the condition may occur in all age groups.[5,7] Intussusception is also common in patients with cystic fibrosis, a disease that causes the exocrine glands to produce abnormally thick secretions of mucus that result in chronic cough, frequent foul-smelling stools, and persistent upper respiratory infections. Although various imaging tools, including abdominal radiographs, computed tomography (CT), and enema, may be used to diagnose intussusception, abdominal sonography has increased in popularity and reliability when diagnosing the condition. In experienced hands, sonographic evaluation reaches a sensitivity of 98% to 100% and specificity of 88% to 100%.[5,8]

Epidemiology

Intussuception has been reported to occur in approximately 56/100,000 children per year in the United States, with a 3:2 male predominance ratio.[5,7] Although intussusception is most common in infants 5 to 9 months of age, children with cystic fibrosis may also have intussusception because of meconium ileus, an obstruction of the small bowel by viscid stool in the terminal ileum. A seasonal incidence has also been noted, with peaks in the spring, summer, and middle of winter. These periods correspond to peaks in the occurrence of seasonal gastroenteritis and upper respiratory tract infections.

Anatomy and Pathophysiology

Intussusception may involve segments of the small intestine, colon, or terminal ileum and is described as a prolapse of one segment of bowel into the lumen of another segment. It can be ileoileal, colocolic, ileoileocolic, or, most commonly, ileocolic (Fig. 12-10). A specific lead point, which draws the proximal intestine and its mesentery inward, propagating it distally through peristalsis, is identified in only 5% of cases and is most commonly seen in ileoileal intussusception. Lead points are more commonly found in older children and nearly always in adults. A lead point is any intestinal disorder that can cause an intussusception. Meckel's diverticulum (an anomalous sac of embryologic origin protruding from the wall of the ileum usually 30 to 90 cm from the ileocecal sphincter) is the most common lead point, followed by polyps, and then tumors such as lymphoma. The

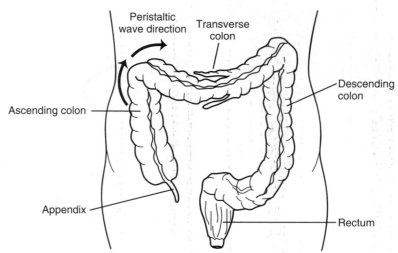

FIGURE 12-9 Diagram of colocolic intussusception. Proximal transverse colon is undergoing peristalsis into distal transverse colon.

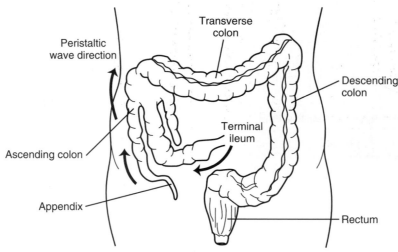

FIGURE 12-10 Diagram of ileocolic intussusception (most common type) in ascending colon. Distal ileum of small intestine is being drawn by peristalsis into proximal ascending colon.

cause of intussusception in patients without a lead point is mostly unknown; however, infantile cases are more common in fat and healthy infants than in thin, undernourished infants.

Clinical Presentation

The most common triad of clinical symptoms in patients with intussusception includes crampy abdominal pain, vomiting, and bloody stools. Patients may also have lethargy, fever, diarrhea, abdominal distention, irritability, or RUQ mass. A rectal examination, with testing for occult blood or mucus, is an important part of the evaluation and frequently has positive results. Laboratory testing may also reveal dehydration, anemia, or leukocytosis (see Table 12-1). The peristaltic nature of the intestine may cause abdominal pain to occur in spasms. Careful palpation during physical examination reveals an ill-defined or sausage-shaped mass in the RUQ in 85% of patients.

Sonographic Findings

The patient should undergo scanning in the supine position. A complete survey of the upper abdomen should always be performed, followed by an examination of the lower abdomen, with focus on the bowel with a 5 to 7 MHz linear or curved array transducer. The classic sonographic appearance of intussusception includes the "doughnut," or target, sign and the "pseudokidney," or "sandwich," sign. A doughnut sign, a hypoechoic rim of homogeneous thickness and contour with a central hyperechoic core, is seen in a transverse view of intussusception (Fig. 12-11). A hyperechoic tubular center is seen longitudinally covered by a hypoechoic ring 3 to 5 cm in diameter, resembling a pseudokidney (Fig. 12-12). Free peritoneal fluid or ascites is a common finding with uncomplicated intussusception. Color Doppler can be used to help determine whether the involved bowel should be reduced (cured with retrograde fluid pressure) or surgically resected. Absent blood flow in the bowel

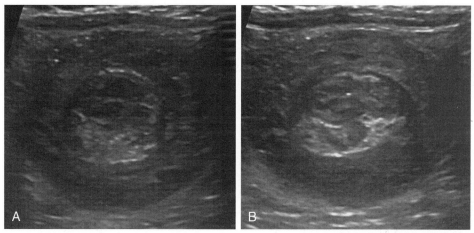

FIGURE 12-11 (A) Transverse view (doughnut sign) of ileocolic intussusception in an 8-year-old boy. **(B)** Image of intussusception showing the target sign.

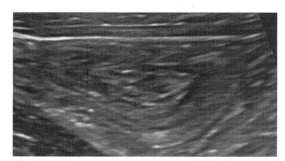

FIGURE 12-12 Longitudinal view of ileocolic intussusception resembling a pseudokidney.

walls means that the bowel has probably necrosed and needs surgical resection. If adequate color flow is seen to all areas of the telescoping bowel, the chances are better for a reduction (Fig. 12-13).

Diagnostic fluoroscopic enema studies have remained the imaging method of choice for intussusception for both diagnosis and therapy in patients with stable conditions. However, in recent years, increasing numbers of radiologists are relying on sonography for diagnosis or exclusion of intussusception. The quality of the study and its interpretation are operator dependent, although sonographic diagnosis in positive cases has shown an accuracy rate of 100%. Sonography is best used as a diagnostic tool of exclusion in patients with low suspicion of intussusception.

Treatment

Air and liquid enemas are routinely relied on in the treatment of intussusception because they are associated with decreased risk of perforation, more limited radiation exposure, and greater efficiency of reduction. However, air, as opposed to liquid enemas, is being used with a higher prevalence (Figs. 12-14 and 12-15).[5,8] In instances in which the enema fails to reduce the intussusception, reduction may be attempted a second or third time; or if the patient's condition is unstable, surgery can provide

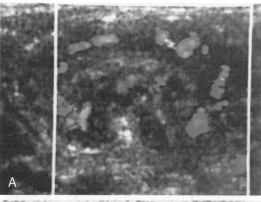

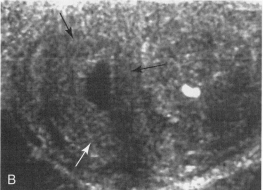

FIGURE 12-13 (A) Color Doppler demonstrates substantial blood flow within the wall of the intussusceptum. Hydrostatic reduction was successful in this patient with no further complications. **(B)** In another patient, power Doppler shows very little flow within the wall of the intussusception. At surgery, the bowel was necrotic.

a mode for manual reduction. Patients in whom a lead point is suspected or diagnosed are not candidates for radiologic enema reduction and would undergo surgery directly. Without treatment, the patient may have complications, such as bowel obstruction, perforation, peritonitis, and vascular compromise, which could lead to edema or gangrene of the bowel.

Table 12-2 summarizes the symptoms and sonographic findings in positive cases of GI disease.

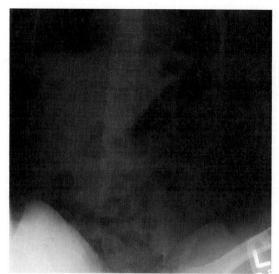

FIGURE 12-14 Preliminary barium enema scout radiograph of a 2-year-old girl. Mass effect is seen outlined by air in right side of abdomen. The mass was found to be intussusception at hepatic flexure, which was successfully reduced during barium enema examination (see Fig. 12-15).

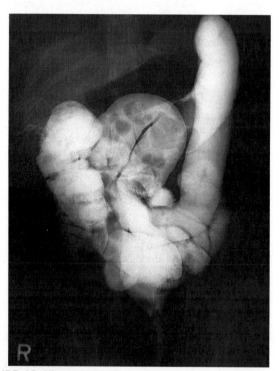

FIGURE 12-15 Postreduction radiograph of the same 2-year-old girl shown in Figure 12-14.

TABLE 12-2	Pathology of Gastrointestinal System	
Pathology	**Symptoms**	**Sonographic Findings**
Pyloric stenosis	Projectile vomiting, weight loss, dehydration, RUQ mass	AP muscle wall, >3.0 mm; pyloric channel length, >17 mm
Intussusception	Abdominal pain, vomiting, bloody stool, lethargy, fever, diarrhea, abdominal distention, RUQ mass	Doughnut or target sign (transverse), pseudokidney or sandwich sign, ascites

SUMMARY

The confirmation of GI diseases such as IHPS and intussusception by sonography requires skill on the part of the sonographer and radiologist. These skills can easily be acquired through education and experience. Sonography has limitations in imaging of the GI tract, and other methods such as fluoroscopic radiography or CT scan may be needed to follow-up nondiagnostic or questionable sonographic findings.

ACKNOWLEDGMENT

The author acknowledges the sonographers of Florida Hospital Orlando, in particular, Robyn Aguilar and Aimee Vargas, for assisting in the acquisition of images. The author also acknowledges Dr. Gregory Logsdon; Dr. Logsdon provided multiple image possibilities and taught the author extensively about pediatric imaging.

CLINICAL SCENARIO—DIAGNOSIS

The abdominal sonogram was performed by the sonographer while the pediatric surgeon and pediatric radiologist observed. Although the infant had eaten 4 hours previously, the stomach was still full of fluid. No additional fluid was needed for the diagnosis. The radiology report indicated that the pyloric muscle was thickened. Single-wall thickness was measured at 6.3 mm, with a channel length of 2.6 cm. These findings were compatible with IHPS. Surgery was scheduled and performed the same afternoon.

CASE STUDIES FOR DISCUSSION

1. A 19-day-old boy born at term presents weighing 10.5 lb with projectile vomiting. Initially suspecting that the infant has the flu, the physician does not order any diagnostic imaging. The infant presents again 3 days later with failure to thrive, weighing close to 6 lb and with severe dehydration and an electrolyte imbalance. Additionally, the infant has decreased urine output as a result of the initial stages of renal failure. Fluoroscopic UGI imaging is ordered and reveals the findings shown in Figure 12-16. A subsequent sonogram is also ordered (Fig. 12-17). These findings are consistent with what diagnosis?

2. A 6-week-old first-born boy is seen by the pediatrician; his mother reports the infant has had multiple episodes of vomiting for the past 2 days. She indicates to the pediatrician that the infant is bottle-fed and that she recently switched the infant's brand of

formula to reduce gastric upset. The infant is also noted to have a slight fever of 100.6° F and has become increasingly irritable. With a familial history of IHPS, the physician decides to err on the side of caution and orders a sonogram of the abdomen to rule out any abnormalities. Extra imaging time is spent over the area of the pylorus, and the sonographer documents the findings in Figure 12-18.

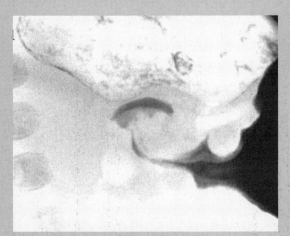

FIGURE 12-16   UGI image of IHPS.

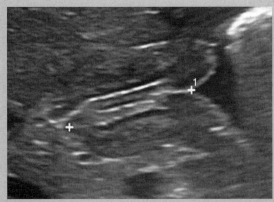

FIGURE 12-17   Longitudinal image of pylorus muscle. Channel length measures 1.7 cm.

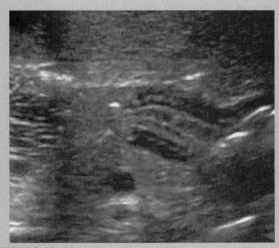

FIGURE 12-18   Longitudinal image shows pyloric channel.

Additionally, fluid is seen freely passing through the pyloric channel. What is the most likely diagnosis?

3. A normally healthy 8-year-old girl presents to the emergency department with diffuse abdominal pain for several hours. The physician notes that her abdomen appears slightly distended and that she has a mild fever. With trepidation, she mentions to the physician that she had a slightly bloody stool earlier that day. Palpation of the patient's abdomen reveals an RUQ mass. The physician orders a sonogram of the abdomen, which reveals the findings in Figure 12-19. What is the most likely diagnosis?

4. A healthy 7 lb girl is born at 39 weeks' gestation. The infant appears slightly jaundiced 2 weeks after birth, and the pediatrician requests that serum bilirubin levels be obtained. Bilirubin levels are determined to be elevated. Levels continue to increase despite phototherapy treatment, and the infant becomes lethargic. Additionally, the infant is losing weight and vomiting, and the physician palpates a 3 cm movable mass in the infant's epigastric region. Sonographic imaging of the abdomen focuses on the area of the pylorus. What sonographic finding is demonstrated in Figure 12-20?

5. An 8-month-old boy is seen by the pediatrician for a history of vomiting for 2 days. The physician found nothing of significance during the examination, and the infant was sent home. The parents returned to the pediatrician with the infant because of continued emesis. They were also concerned at a small amount of blood found in the infant's stool. The physician requests abdominal x-rays, which demonstrated a questionable mass in the right lower quadrant. What is the most likely diagnosis?

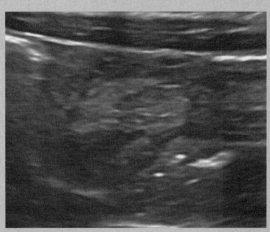

FIGURE 12-19   Transverse image of RUQ in an 8-year-old girl.

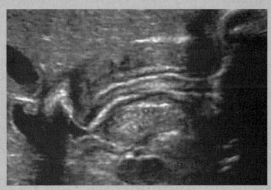

FIGURE 12-20   Longitudinal image of enlarged pyloric channel.

STUDY QUESTIONS

1. All but which of the following might occur with IHPS?
   a. Dehydration
   b. Metabolic alkalosis
   c. Projectile vomiting
   d. Weight gain

2. A 4-week-old girl with projectile vomiting for 2 days is seen. She is jaundiced, and the physician is able to palpate an olive-shaped mass in the RUQ on physical examination. What is the most likely diagnosis?
   a. Intussusception
   b. Pyloric stenosis
   c. Reflux
   d. Ulcer

3. The most common clinical symptoms demonstrated in patients with intussusception include all but which of the following?
   a. Abdominal pain
   b. Bloody stool
   c. Dehydration
   d. Vomiting

4. All but which of the following must be evaluated when using ultrasonography to image the pylorus?
   a. Channel length
   b. Muscle thickness
   c. Gastric peristalsis
   d. Duodenum

5. An 8-month-old boy with a history of new-onset irritability presents with lethargy, abdominal distention, and fever. A moderate amount of blood is found to be present in the infant's stool. What is the most likely diagnosis?
   a. Gastric upset
   b. Intussusception
   c. Peritonitis
   d. Pyloric stenosis

6. The classic sonographic appearance of intussusception includes all but which of the following?
   a. Cervix
   b. Doughnut
   c. Pseudokidney
   d. Sandwich

7. A 46-year-old man presents with a history of stomach ulcers, electrolyte imbalance, and persistent vomiting. What is the most likely diagnosis?
   a. Bowel perforation
   b. Cholecystitis
   c. Intussusception
   d. Pyloric stenosis

8. An 8-year-old girl with a history of cystic fibrosis is seen with nonspecific abdominal pain and diarrhea. Sonographic evaluation of the patient's abdomen reveals a mass in the RUQ similar in appearance to a kidney. What is the most likely diagnosis?
   a. Abdominal abscess
   b. Diverticulitis
   c. Intussusception
   d. Pyloric stenosis

9. What is the imaging method of choice for diagnosing IHPS?
   a. CT
   b. Nuclear medicine
   c. Sonography
   d. UGI

10. The diagnosis of IHPS can be determined with confidence via sonography when which of the following diagnostic criteria are demonstrated?
    a. >3.0 mm muscle wall, >17 mm channel length
    b. <3.5 mm muscle wall, <15 mm channel length
    c. <3.0 mm muscle wall, <17 mm channel length
    d. >3.5 mm muscle wall, >15 mm channel length

REFERENCES

1. Walker K: Sonographic evaluation of hypertrophic pyloric stenosis, *J Diag Med Sonogr* 26:209–211, 2010.
2. Glatstein M, Carbell G, Boddu SK, et al: The changing clinical presentation of hypertrophic pyloric stenosis: the experience of a large, tertiary care pediatric hospital, *Clin Pediatr* 50:192–195, 2011.
3. Piroutek MJ, Brown L, Thorp AW: Bilious vomiting does not rule out infantile hypertrophic pyloric stenosis, *Clin Pediatr (Phila)* 51:214–218, 2012.
4. Reed A, Michael K: Hypertrophic pyloric stenosis, *J Diag Med Sonogr* 26:157–160, 2010.
5. Pineda C, Hardasmalani M: Pediatric intussusception: a case series and literature review, *Internet J Pediatr Neonatol* 11:13, 2009.
6. DeGoff W, Anderson JE, Chen T: Back pain as the only presenting symptom of intussusception: a case report, *Clin Pediatr (Phila)* 49:43–44, 2010.
7. Kaiser A, Applegate K, Ladd A: Current success in the treatment of intussusception in children, *Surgery* 142:469–476, 2007.
8. Lehnert T, Sorge I, Till H, et al: Intussusception in children—clinical presentation, diagnosis and management, *Int J Colorectal Dis* 24:1187–1192, 2009.

PART II

Gynecology

Abnormal Uterine Bleeding

Diane J. Youngs

CLINICAL SCENARIO

A 46-year-old multiparous woman sees her physician because of concerns about abnormal menses. Her last normal menstrual period occurred several months ago; however, 3 weeks before her visit, she experienced a heavy menstrual period that lasted 7 days. Physical examination findings are unremarkable and include a normal-size, nontender uterus. The sonographer notes a normal endometrium, a globular appearance to the uterus, and a diffusely heterogeneous myometrium (Fig. 13-1). Discuss two differential diagnoses for the sonographic appearance and an additional imaging modality that can aid in the diagnosis.

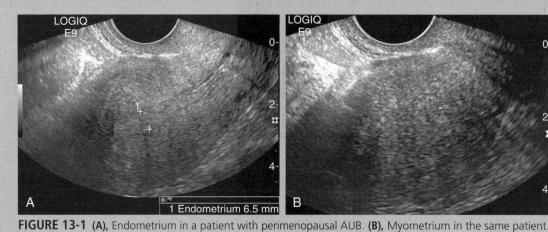

FIGURE 13-1 (A), Endometrium in a patient with perimenopausal AUB. **(B),** Myometrium in the same patient.

OBJECTIVES

- List the most common conditions associated with abnormal uterine bleeding in nonpregnant patients.
- Differentiate the sonographic appearances of pathologies involving the myometrium and endometrium.
- Describe appropriate imaging studies available for evaluation of abnormal uterine bleeding.
- Discuss treatment options for the most common causes of abnormal uterine bleeding.

Abnormal uterine bleeding (AUB) is a common problem for which pelvic sonography is indicated. Patients may see a health care provider because of infrequent menses, prolonged and heavy menses (menorrhagia), intermenstrual bleeding or spotting, postcoital spotting, or irregular and heavy menses (menometrorrhagia). Many possible diagnoses are considered in the evaluation of AUB. AUB may arise from structural causes, such as a lesion within the uterus or endometrium, or from a reproductive tract abnormality. AUB that is not caused by a structural problem is usually endocrine in nature and is called dysfunctional uterine bleeding (DUB). Causes of AUB are listed in Box 13-1.

Multiple treatment options exist for patients with AUB; the choice of treatment is guided by the patient's symptoms, the impact of the symptoms on her quality of life, expectations of treatment, and whether the patient wishes to maintain fertility. Current treatments include hysterectomy, myomectomy, uterine artery embolization, magnetic resonance imaging (MRI)–guided focused ultrasound treatment, medical treatment based on hormone therapy (e.g., progestin or gonadotropin-releasing

BOX 13-1	Causes of Abnormal Uterine Bleeding in Nonpregnant Patients

Reproductive
Cervicitis (cervical infection)
Carcinoma (cervical or endometrial)
Endometrial infection
Hyperplasia
Iatrogenic (e.g., contraceptives, hormone replacement medications, some psychotropic medications)
Leiomyoma
Lost or misplaced IUD
Ovarian or fallopian tube malignancy (uncommon)
Pelvic inflammatory disease
Polyps (cervical or endometrial)
Retained products of conception
Trauma (iatrogenic, sexual intercourse, sexual assault)

Systemic
Cirrhosis
Leukemia
Thrombocytopenia
Uremia
von Willebrand's disease

Endocrinologic
Anorexia
Anovulation (postmenopausal atrophy, polycystic ovary syndrome, significant stress)
Hyperprolactinemia
Hypothyroidism
Polycystic ovary syndrome
Prolongation of corpus luteum cyst*

*Controversial.

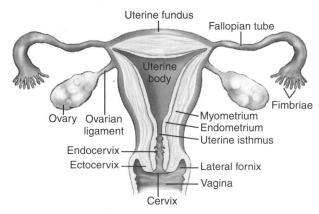

FIGURE 13-2 Uterine divisions include vagina, cervix, body, and fundus. Uterine layers include serosa, myometrium, and endometrium.

hormone agonists), and endometrial ablation for women who are finished with childbearing. The initial step in evaluating a woman with AUB is a pelvic examination, and if pathology is suspected, a pelvic sonogram should be obtained.

Pelvic sonography plays an important role in the diagnosis of uterine abnormalities in nonpregnant patients. The extended field of view provided by transabdominal pelvic sonography gives a global overview of the pelvis and is more likely to include large uterine masses such as fibroids. Transvaginal sonography provides the level of detail necessary to evaluate the endometrium and myometrium further for possible causes of AUB. Sonographic evaluation is useful in detecting anatomic causes of AUB, such as fibroids, adenomyosis, endometrial carcinoma, endometrial hyperplasia, endometrial polyps, and retained products of conception in a postpartum patient. Clinicians find pelvic sonography useful for development of a coherent treatment plan.

NORMAL UTERINE ANATOMY

The normal uterus is a pear-shaped organ located in the midpelvis, posterior to the urinary bladder and anterior to the rectum. The uterine divisions include the cervix, body, and fundus. The entrance to each fallopian tube, called the cornu (pl. cornua), is located in the uterine fundus. Uterine tissue consists of three layers: serosa, myometrium, and endometrium. The serosal layer (perimetrium) is the thin outer layer surrounding the uterus, the myometrium is the thick middle muscular layer, and the endometrium is the functional inner lining of the uterus (Fig. 13-2). The endometrium consists of a basal and a functional layer. The functional layer responds to hormonal stimulation throughout the menstrual cycle and is the layer that sheds during menses.

The uterine artery enters the uterus around the level of the isthmus, giving rise to the arcuate arteries, which lie in between the outer and intermediate layers of the myometrium. The arcuate arteries branch to radial arteries, extending through the intermediate myometrial layer and into the inner layer. The radial arteries branch to spiral arteries, which enter the endometrium and supply the functional layer.

UTERINE PHYSIOLOGY

The uterus is the reproductive organ responsible for growth, maintenance, and delivery of the fetus. The secretory endometrium provides embryonic nourishment during early pregnancy, whereas the myometrium provides the muscular contractions necessary for delivery. Estrogen and progesterone are the hormones responsible for preparing the endometrium for pregnancy. During menses, lack of hormonal stimulation causes atrophy of the spiral arteries, and the functional layer of the endometrium sloughs and bleeds. Soon after menses, the proliferative phase of rebuilding and growth of endometrial tissue takes place under the influence of estrogen. After ovulation, under the influence of progesterone, the secretory phase of the uterus begins by stimulating glandular changes. These secretory changes cause the endometrial glands and stroma to produce glycogen-rich secretions capable of supporting an early embryo. If no pregnancy occurs, the corpus luteum of the ovary regresses, and the lack of hormones causes menses again. After menopause, the ovaries no longer function, and the endometrium undergoes atrophy.

NORMAL SONOGRAPHIC APPEARANCE

The normal sonographic appearance of the uterus depends on age, menstrual status, and parity. Uterine size varies throughout a woman's life, depending on hormonal stimulation, pregnancy, and anatomic disorders. After menarche but before childbirth, the uterus measures approximately 8 cm long, 5 cm wide, and 4 cm thick. Parity generally increases uterine size by about 1 cm in all dimensions. After menopause, the uterus decreases in size. By age 65 years, uterine size ranges from 3.5 to 6.5 cm in length and 1 to 2 cm in diameter.[1] The length and anteroposterior (AP) diameter of the uterus are obtained in the longitudinal midline view by measuring from the top of the uterine fundus to the external cervical os (Fig. 13-3).

The sonographic appearance of the normal endometrium depends on the menstrual phase or status of the patient and should be homogeneous in appearance and of appropriate thickness for the woman's menstrual status (Table 13-1). An AP measurement of the double layer endometrial thickness should be obtained while in the longitudinal scanning plane, with placement of the calipers at the outer edges of each echogenic basal layer (Fig. 13-4, A). When intercavitary fluid is present, the endometrial layers should be measured separately, with the sum of the two measurements representing endometrial thickness (Fig. 13-4, B). For menstrual age women, normal double layer endometrial thickness is 4 to 14 mm,

with maximum thickness occurring during the secretory phase. Endometrial pathology is very unlikely in a postmenopausal woman if endometrial thickness is less than 5 mm.[2] Postmenopausal women taking hormone replacement therapy can experience a slightly thickened endometrium during the estrogen cycle (up to 8 mm) and should undergo repeat scanning during the progesterone cycle.

The functional layer of the endometrium demonstrates changes in sonographic appearance throughout the menstrual cycle. During menses, the endometrium is thin and appears as a hyperechoic line (Fig. 13-5, A). As the proliferative phase progresses and ovulation approaches, a triple line appearance is created by the opposite hyperechoic basal layers, hypoechoic functional layer, and hyperechoic endometrial cavity (Fig. 13-5, B). The secretory phase results in a thickened endometrium hyperechoic to the myometrium (Fig. 13-5, C). The inner layer of myometrium adjacent to the basal layer of the endometrium appears as a hypoechoic rim and is sometimes referred to as the junctional zone or subendometrial halo (Fig. 13-6); this should not be included in endometrial measurements.

The normal myometrium has a homogeneous echotexture, and the sonographer should assess for focal masses, diffuse heterogeneity, distortions in uterine contour, and size. The uterine veins are larger than the arteries and can be identified sonographically as focal anechoic areas around the periphery of the uterus (Fig. 13-7). In older women, atherosclerotic changes within the arcuate arteries of the uterus may be seen as hyperechoic, shadowing foci around the periphery of the uterus (Fig. 13-8).

Although there are many causes of AUB in a nonpregnant patient, sonographic assessment for endometrial and myometrial abnormalities is important because they are a common cause of AUB. Endometrial abnormalities may appear sonographically as a thickened endometrium, a focal mass, or a heterogeneous endometrium. Some common endometrial abnormalities that are discussed in this chapter include endometrial hyperplasia, endometrial carcinoma, polyps, changes caused by tamoxifen therapy, and retained products of conception. The most common cause of postmenopausal bleeding is endometrial atrophy, which appears sonographically as an endometrium less than 4 mm in thickness. Common myometrial abnormalities resulting in AUB include leiomyomas and adenomyosis. Myometrial abnormalities may affect the sonographic appearance of the uterus in the following ways: diffuse heterogeneity, focal

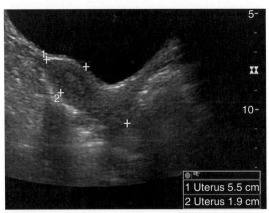

1 Uterus 5.5 cm
2 Uterus 1.9 cm

FIGURE 13-3 Transabdominal longitudinal midline image demonstrating caliper placement for uterine length and AP measurement of the uterine body.

TABLE 13-1	Normal Endometrial Thickness (mm)		
Early Proliferative Phase	**Periovulatory (Late Proliferative) Phase**	**Secretory Phase**	**Postmenopausal (No HRT)**
4-8	6-10	7-14	1-4

HRT, Hormone replacement therapy.
From Salem S: Gynecologic ultrasound. In: Rumack C, Wilson S, Charboneau J, et al, editors: *Diagnostic ultrasound,* vol 1, ed 4, Philadelphia, 2011, Mosby:547-612.

hypoechoic or hyperechoic masses, distortion of the uterine contour, or overall uterine enlargement.

MYOMETRIAL ABNORMALITIES

Leiomyoma

Leiomyomas, also called myomas or fibroids, are benign smooth muscle tumors that develop within the myometrium, but they may intrude into any of the uterine layers (Fig. 13-9). Uterine fibroids represent the most common pelvic tumor and are a leading cause of hysterectomy.

Less commonly, fibroids can develop within the vagina, cervix, broad ligament, or fallopian tubes or on the omentum (so-called parasitic fibroids). They are more common in African American women than in women of other ethnicities.[3] Fibroids range in size from 1 mm to more than 20 cm. Many women have multiple fibroids of varying sizes. Fibroids are known to grow in response to estrogen stimulation and tend to stabilize or regress during menopause.

Fibroids are myometrial in origin, and they can be surrounded by myometrium, intrude into the endometrium, or come in contact with the serosal layer (Fig. 13-10).

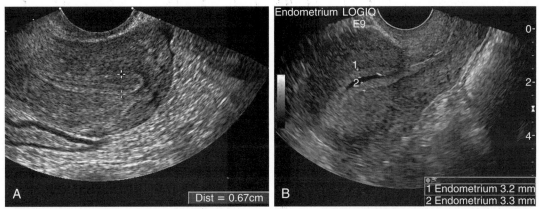

FIGURE 13-4 **(A),** Longitudinal midline image demonstrating caliper placement for endometrial thickness measurements. Caliper placement includes hyperechoic basal layers. **(B),** Measurement of each layer is required in cases of endometrial layers separated by intercavitary fluid.

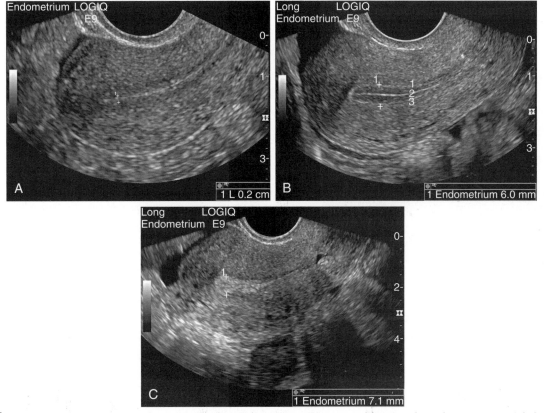

FIGURE 13-5 **(A),** Early proliferative phase demonstrates thin endometrium. **(B),** Late proliferative phase demonstrates triple line appearance of endometrium. **(C),** Secretory phase demonstrates thicker, hyperechoic appearance.

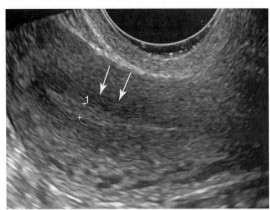

FIGURE 13-6 Hypoechoic area adjacent to hyperechoic endometrium represents the inner myometrial layer known as the junctional zone *(arrows)* and should not be included in endometrial measurements.

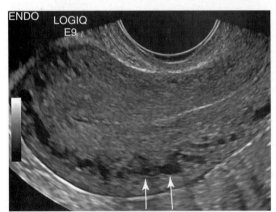

FIGURE 13-7 Anechoic spaces *(arrows)* around the periphery of the uterus are normal uterine veins and should not be mistaken for an abnormality.

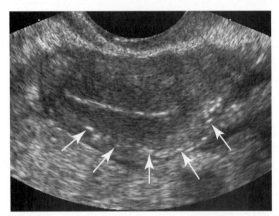

FIGURE 13-8 Arterial calcifications *(arrows)* within myometrium.

Fibroids surrounded predominantly by myometrium are the most common and are referred to as intramural fibroids. Fibroids that project into the endometrium are referred to as submucosal fibroids. Subserosal fibroids are in contact with the serosal layer and distort the uterine contour. In some cases, subserosal fibroids grow off of a stalk into the adnexal regions seemingly separate from the uterus; these are referred to as pedunculated

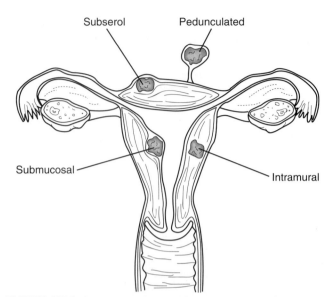

FIGURE 13-9 Illustration of cut uterus showing classification and location of fibroids.

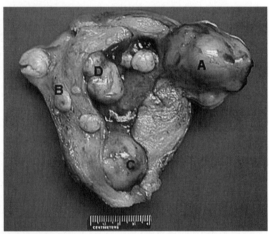

FIGURE 13-10 Cut pathology specimen shows multiple fibroids including subserosal **(A)**, intramural **(B)**, and submucosal **(C** and **D)**. *(Courtesy Michael Radi, MD, Department of Pathology, Florida Hospital, Orlando.)*

fibroids. Generally, only submucosal or large intramural fibroids cause AUB. Pedunculated fibroids are remote from the endometrium and myometrium and typically do not cause menorrhagia. The exact cause of menorrhagia with fibroids is unknown, but fibroid-associated changes in uterine vasculature, contractility, and endometrial surface area may contribute to the problem.[4] Fibroids can undergo degeneration, which may cause pain.

Clinicians may suspect uterine fibroids based on patient history or physical examination. Pelvic sonography may be performed to assess the location and size of the fibroids, which can assist in development of a treatment plan. Some gynecologists obtain a sonogram before surgery to help determine the best surgical procedure plan for the patient. A patient who undergoes removal of fibroids (myomectomy) may need a combined approach in which the gynecologist removes large subserosal fibroids via an abdominal incision and removes submucosal fibroids with placement of an operative hysteroscope into the endometrial cavity. Treatment is not always necessary because many women with uterine fibroids are asymptomatic. Clinicians base treatment plans on the size and location of the fibroid, patient symptoms, and patient wishes regarding whether or not to undergo surgery.

Medical therapy for uterine fibroids includes birth control pills to reduce menstrual blood loss or short-term use of progestin to treat menorrhagia. Progestin-releasing intrauterine devices (IUDs) are also an option. A more recent treatment for uterine fibroids is uterine artery embolization. For this procedure, a catheter is introduced into the femoral artery and into the uterine artery. Microspheres injected through the catheter undergo embolization and block perfusion of the distal branches of the uterine artery that supply the fibroid, which results in necrosis and shrinkage of the fibroid. MRI-guided focused ultrasound therapy is another recent treatment for fibroids. This treatment involves using focused converging ultrasound beams to generate heat at a focal point causing necrosis of tissue. MRI is used for accurate targeting of the focal point and for monitoring tissue temperatures.[4]

Sonographic Findings. Fibroids visualized with sonography may cause obvious distortion of the uterine contour, generalized enlargement of the uterus, an altered echotexture, hypoechoic or hyperechoic focal masses, calcifications with shadowing, or heterogeneous masses with cystic areas (usually within degenerating fibroids). Fibroids are usually multiple. Documentation should include the size, location, and appearance of each fibroid. If it is not possible or practical to document each of the multiple fibroids, measurement and localization of the largest fibroid helps assess growth or regression on subsequent sonographic examinations. The fibrous nature of fibroids causes attenuation of the sound beam, and decreasing transducer frequency to increase penetration may be necessary to image large, dense fibroids.

Submucosal fibroids focally distort the endometrium, creating an area of increased or decreased echogenicity within the endometrium, which may be difficult to differentiate from endometrial polyps. Sonohysterography, the infusion of saline as a contrast agent into the uterine cavity, may help differentiate fibroids from polyps. Generally, submucosal fibroids tend to appear hypoechoic to the secretory endometrium, have a broad base of attachment, and display sonographic evidence of attenuation (Fig. 13-11). Intramural fibroids are relatively easy to visualize when they are hypoechoic and well encapsulated within the myometrium (Fig. 13-12).

However, visualization of multiple fibroids can be challenging, and this is particularly true when large fibroids distort the myometrium or when calcified fibroids cast shadows (Fig. 13-13). Subserosal fibroids can distort the uterine contour (Fig. 13-14), and pedunculated fibroids

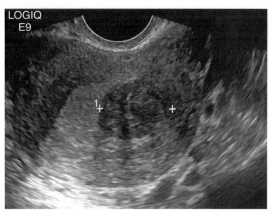

FIGURE 13-11 Submucosal fibroid (calipers) appears as a hypoechoic mass within the endometrium on this transverse image.

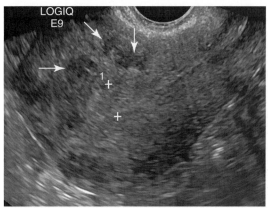

FIGURE 13-12 Focal hypoechoic masses within the myometrium represent intramural fibroids (arrows).

can extend laterally, possibly mimicking an adnexal mass or a bicornuate uterus (Fig. 13-15). Differentiation of a pedunculated fibroid from a solid ovarian mass is possible if the ipsilateral ovary is demonstrated separate from the fibroid. Fibroids may undergo degeneration, in which the central portion loses its blood supply and becomes necrotic. Other sonographic findings associated with uterine fibroids include diffuse enlargement and diffuse heterogeneity of the uterus. However, these findings are nonspecific and are also associated with another uterine pathologic condition called adenomyosis.

Adenomyosis

Adenomyosis is a common gynecologic condition in which glands and stroma from the basal layer of the endometrium penetrate into the myometrium causing distortion of the myometrium from smooth muscle hyperplasia. Because the glands arise from the basal layer, they do not have the typical response to hormonal stimulation that endometrial tissues from the functional layer do. The most definitive method for diagnosis of adenomyosis is a pathologic specimen of the myometrium obtained at hysterectomy; this condition is found in 70% of hysterectomy specimens (Fig. 13-16).[5]

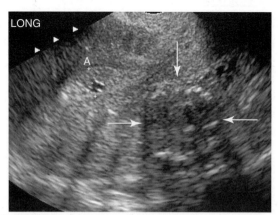

FIGURE 13-13 Calcified fibroid demonstrating shadowing *(arrows)*.

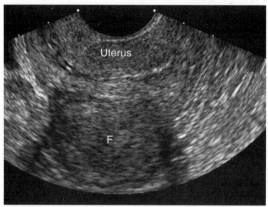

FIGURE 13-14 Distortion of the uterine contour caused by a sub-serosal fibroid *(F)*.

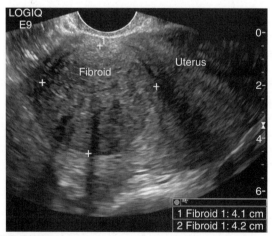

FIGURE 13-15 Pedunculated fibroid extending into right adnexa from the uterine body.

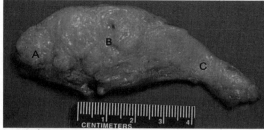

FIGURE 13-16 Cut pathology specimen of uterus shows fundal adenoma **(A)** and extensive adenomyosis within myometrium **(B)**. **(C)**, Cervix. *(Courtesy Michael Radi, MD, Department of Pathology, Florida Hospital, Orlando.)*

Symptoms of adenomyosis include painful menstruation (dysmenorrhea) and AUB; these symptoms are associated with numerous other common gynecologic conditions. Attribution of a patient's symptoms to adenomyosis may be difficult because fibroids, hyperplasia, endometriosis, and other gynecologic conditions may coexist. The mechanism with which adenomyosis causes or contributes to AUB is unknown. Treatment options other than hysterectomy are limited and include gonadotropin-releasing hormone agonist therapy, endometrial ablation or resection, narcotic analgesics, and oral contraceptives.[5]

Sonographic Findings. Adenomyosis can be classified as either diffuse or focal. Diffuse adenomyosis, in which endometrial glands and stroma are diffusely incorporated into the myometrium, is more common and can result in ill-defined myometrial heterogenicity and uterine enlargement. The presence of adenomyosis may result in hyperplasia and hypertrophy of the myometrium surrounding the heterotopic endometrial tissue, causing hypoechoic striations demonstrated as refraction artifacts (Fig. 13-17, *A*), myometrial cysts (Fig. 13-17, *B*), heterogeneous areas, thickened posterior uterine wall, diffuse vascularity, and a globular uterine configuration.[6] Sonographic imaging of diffuse adenomyosis may be difficult, particularly if the uterus is markedly enlarged or fibroids are present. The focal form of adenomyosis results in a less typical appearance and is characterized by focal masses called adenomyomas (Fig. 13-17, *C*).

Besides myometrial alterations, sonographic evaluation of the junctional zone can contribute to the diagnosis of adenomyosis. Transvaginal sonography may demonstrate poor definition of the endometrial and junctional zone caused by endometrial tissue extending from the basal layer. However, subjective evaluation of a poorly defined junctional zone has a low sensitivity value. More recent studies have shown that sonographic three-dimensional coronal images of the uterus allow improved evaluation of the thickness and regularity of the junctional zone.[6] The ability of MRI to image heterotopic endometrial tissue as small foci of increased signal intensity in the junctional zone is also subjective, although comparing minimum and maximum focal junctional zone thickness can provide objective criteria.[6]

ENDOMETRIAL ABNORMALITIES

Endometrial Hyperplasia

Endometrial hyperplasia is an abnormal proliferation (growth) of the endometrium in response to excess or unopposed estrogen. Patients taking estrogen-only

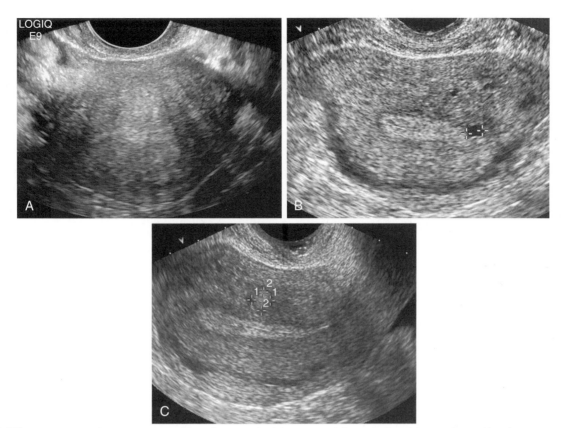

FIGURE 13-17 (A), Myometrial striations caused by adenomyosis. **(B),** Myometrial cyst (calipers) in a patient with adenomyosis. **(C),** Adenomyoma indicated by calipers.

hormone replacement medications or women with chronic anovulation are at risk for endometrial hyperplasia. An anovulatory patient does not always produce a corpus luteum cyst, so the endometrium does not receive adequate progesterone stimulation. The unopposed estrogen causes continual endometrial proliferation potentially leading to abnormal growth (Fig. 13-18). Pathologists and gynecologists use specific terminology to categorize endometrial hyperplasia as without cellular atypia or with cellular atypia (atypical hyperplasia), depending on the appearance of the endometrial glands and whether or not cellular abnormalities (atypia) are visible microscopically. Each category can also be subdivided into simple (cystic) or complex (adenomatous). Sonography cannot be used to distinguish between the different classifications of endometrial hyperplasia. However, this information is important clinically because 25% of atypical hyperplasia progresses to carcinoma.[1]

The treatment of endometrial hyperplasia depends on the degree of atypia and the age and health of the patient. In some cases, hormonal therapy with progestin is effective for treatment of endometrial hyperplasia, and hysterectomy may be indicated for older patients finished with childbearing or patients with significant atypia.

Sonographic Findings. Sonographically, the endometrium is diffusely thickened (Fig. 13-19), although asymmetric or focal thickening may be present. Besides endometrial thickening, some forms of hyperplasia

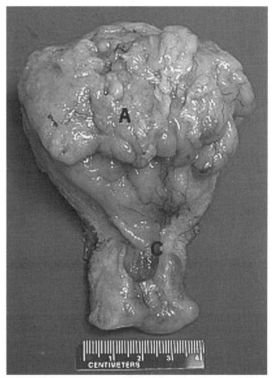

FIGURE 13-18 Cut hysterectomy specimen shows endometrial hyperplasia at fundal portion of specimen **(A)**. *C,* Cervix. *(Courtesy Michael Radi, MD, Department of Pathology, Florida Hospital, Orlando.)*

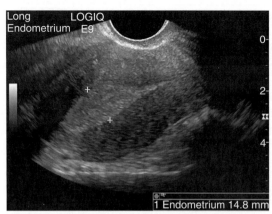

FIGURE 13-19 Sagittal view of uterus shows a thickened endometrium in a patient with endometrial hyperplasia.

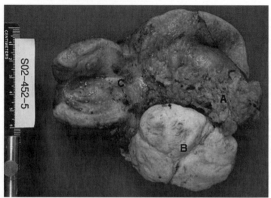

FIGURE 13-20 Cut hysterectomy specimen shows endometrial carcinoma **(A)** and associated leiomyoma **(B)**. Distinguishing hyperplasia from carcinoma with visualization is often difficult. **(C)**, Cervix. *(Courtesy Michael Radi, MD, Department of Pathology, Florida Hospital, Orlando.)*

can cause cystic changes within the endometrium. For women with AUB, endometrial hyperplasia or endometrial carcinoma must be considered as the possible etiology. Because both conditions have similar symptoms, risk factors, and sonographic appearance, biopsy is necessary for diagnosis.

Endometrial Adenocarcinoma

Endometrial adenocarcinoma is the most common gynecologic cancer, affecting almost 1 in every 50 women, with most cases diagnosed in postmenopausal women. The most common clinical presentation is postmenopausal bleeding; however, only 10% of women with postmenopausal bleeding have endometrial carcinoma.[1] Risk factors for endometrial carcinoma include unopposed estrogen stimulation, obesity, nulliparity, diabetes, hypertension, tamoxifen therapy for breast cancer, chronic anovulation, and the presence of atypical endometrial hyperplasia.[1] Endometrial carcinoma is highly curable because it is usually confined to the uterus at clinical presentation. A pelvic sonogram may be performed when patients have AUB, particularly when heavy and prolonged or frequent bleeding (menorrhagia or menometrorrhagia) or postmenopausal bleeding is present. When endometrial carcinoma is present, some patients have an enlarged uterus, but most patients have normal physical examination findings. Although the most accurate method for diagnosis of endometrial carcinoma is an endometrial biopsy or a hysterectomy specimen (Fig. 13-20), many patients with AUB undergo pelvic sonography before a biopsy or as part of a triage system to determine the need for a biopsy.

The treatment for endometrial carcinoma depends on the age and health of the patient, the histologic characteristics of the tumor, and the degree of spread. Cancers limited to the endometrium or inner uterus without metastases have cure rates in the 90% range. Generally, endometrial carcinoma limited to the uterus may be treatable with hysterectomy. Carcinoma that has spread

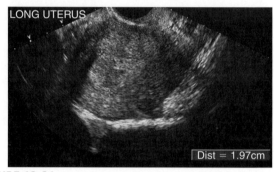

FIGURE 13-21 Endometrial cancer with thickened endometrium.

to adjacent or distant organs may require hysterectomy, chemotherapy, or radiation therapy.

Sonographic Findings. Only a biopsy can be used to differentiate between endometrial hyperplasia and carcinoma, but useful information may be obtained from a sonographic examination that may point to or help exclude either of these diagnoses. The sonographic findings associated with endometrial carcinoma include abnormally thickened endometrium (Fig. 13-21), heterogeneous echotexture, hematometra, and an enlarged uterus. The presence of trapped blood in the uterine cavity (hematometra) in a postmenopausal patient with a thickened endometrium is worrisome for endometrial carcinoma (Fig. 13-22). The thickened endometrium may be irregular and even masslike in appearance and may demonstrate invasion into the myometrium. Because uterine enlargement and hematometra are findings associated with endometrial carcinoma in advanced stages, evaluation of the endometrium is more specific for determination of the potential for or the exclusion of this condition.

An abnormally thickened endometrium on sonography along with the patient's menstrual status and symptoms may be the first clue to endometrial carcinoma. Postmenopausal patients with AUB and an endometrial thickness greater than 4 mm are at greater risk for endometrial carcinoma and should undergo a biopsy. An endometrium that is clearly visualized in its entirety, is

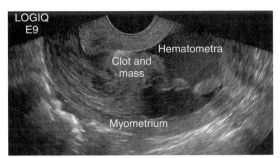

FIGURE 13-22 Advanced endometrial cancer resulting in trapped blood within the uterine cavity (hematometra).

regular in appearance, and is thinner than 5 mm presents a very low risk for endometrial carcinoma or other serious endometrial disease, and patients with these measurements may forgo further invasive procedures.[2]

Endometrial Polyps

Endometrial polyps are benign focal overgrowths of endometrial glands and stroma. Their size is variable; some measure 1 mm, and others fill the entire endometrial cavity and extend into the cervix or vagina. Endometrial polyps are soft, fleshy, tan or red growths attached to the endometrium by a narrow pedunculated stalk, or, less commonly, a broad base of attachment may be present. Pedunculated polyps can prolapse from the cervix and are difficult to remove with endometrial curettage (dilatation and curettage) because they tend to move away from the curette. Polyps are most prevalent in perimenopausal and postmenopausal women, and most polyps are asymptomatic. Polyps can cause coital spotting, intermenstrual bleeding, menorrhagia, and menometrorrhagia.

Endometrial polyps contain blood vessels, stroma, and endometrial glands that can respond to hormonal stimuli. Less commonly, endometrial polyps may harbor foci of endometrial hyperplasia or carcinoma. Gynecologists treat endometrial polyps with hysteroscopic endometrial polypectomy because uterine curettage can miss endometrial polyps. With hysteroscopy, gynecologists can directly visualize the polyp, its base, and the entire endometrial cavity, allowing removal of the polyp (Fig. 13-23; see Color Plate 9). Pathologists can examine the excised polyps for hyperplasia or malignant disease.
Sonographic Findings. Sonographic findings depend on the echogenicity of the surrounding endometrium. During the secretory phase, a polyp is typically isoechoic to the surrounding endometrium causing the appearance of either focal or global endometrial thickening (Fig. 13-24). Polyps are well defined when outlined by saline instilled during sonohysterography (Fig. 13-25) or by the hypoechoic functional layer during the proliferative phase (Fig. 13-26). Additional sonographic findings associated with polyps include cystic spaces within the polyp (Fig. 13-27) and evidence of a vascular feeding vessel on color Doppler imaging (Fig. 13-28; see Color Plate 10).

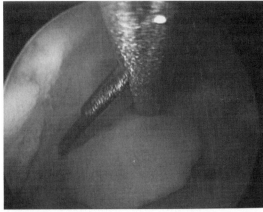

FIGURE 13-23 Gynecologist removing endometrial polyp during hysterectomy.

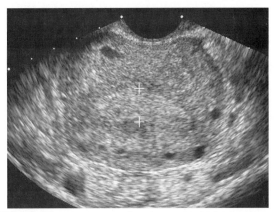

FIGURE 13-24 Appearance of endometrial thickening caused by isoechoic polyp in a secretory endometrium.

Tamoxifen

Tamoxifen is a drug administered to women with breast cancer to block estrogenic effects on breast tissue. Although tamoxifen acts as an estrogen antagonist in the breast, it has an opposite effect in the uterus by acting as an estrogen agonist. This agonistic effect of tamoxifen can stimulate cell growth and proliferation in endometrial tissue, enhancing the risk of endometrial abnormalities including carcinoma, hyperplasia, and polyps.[7]
Sonographic Findings. The sonographic findings of endometrium exposed to tamoxifen are related to the resultant pathology, with endometrial thickening a common finding. Tamoxifen exposure also causes cystic changes in the endometrium and in the area of the junctional zone (Fig. 13-29) representing adenomyosis-like changes.

Retained Products of Conception

After delivery of an infant or after an abortion, some of the gestational contents may remain within the uterine cavity and cause bleeding or infection. The retained products of conception (RPOC) typically consist of placental tissue, which can persist for months and result in AUB.

Sonographic Findings. The uterus immediately postpartum is enlarged and typically returns to normal size and shape within 6 to 8 weeks after delivery. Besides an enlarged uterus, immediate postpartum findings may include residual fluid and echogenic material representing hemorrhage within the endometrial cavity. When the clinical indication is to rule out RPOC, the sonographer should evaluate the endometrial cavity for a focal echogenic mass and assess endometrial thickness. Studies indicate that with an endometrial thickness less than 10 mm, RPOC is unlikely; however, RPOC is likely if an echogenic mass with vascularity is present.[1] An echogenic mass without vascularity may represent either RPOC (Fig. 13-30) or blood clots.

SONOHYSTEROGRAPHY

Sonohysterography is transvaginal sonography enhanced with infusion of sterile saline solution to provide a contrasting backdrop for localizing solid lesions projecting into the uterine cavity. Similar to hysterosalpingography,

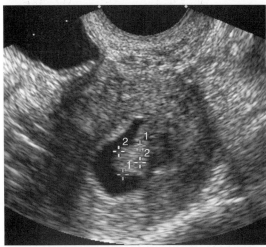

FIGURE 13-25 Polyp outlined by saline from hysterosonography.

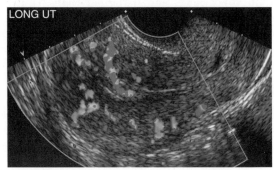

FIGURE 13-28 Endometrial polyp demonstrating a vascular feeding stalk.

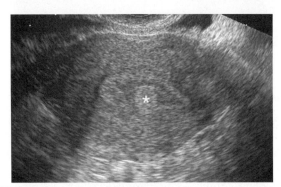

FIGURE 13-26 Hyperechoic polyp *(asterisk)* in a proliferative endometrium.

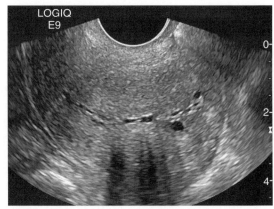

FIGURE 13-29 Endometrial changes caused by tamoxifen.

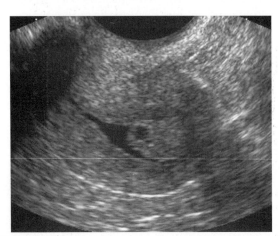

FIGURE 13-27 Polyp outlined by saline, demonstrating small cystic area.

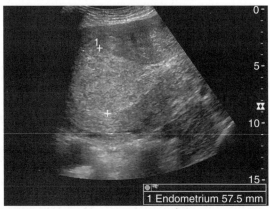

FIGURE 13-30 Retained products of conception in a postpartum patient.

sonohysterography allows visualization of the endometrial cavity; however, instead of having a static image, it allows the operator to image the endometrium, uterus, and adnexa in real time.

Imaging technique involves insertion of a sterile catheter into the uterine cavity. With the catheter in place, transvaginal scanning is performed while sterile saline is slowly injected through the catheter. The entire endometrial cavity is systematically evaluated, endometrial measurements are taken, and representative images of normal and abnormal anatomy are documented.

Sonohysterography is a well-tolerated procedure; however, there are some contraindications. This procedure should not be performed in women who are or could be pregnant or women with acute pelvic inflammatory disease. Premenopausal women with regular cycles should have the procedure performed during the early proliferative phase to avoid disrupting an early pregnancy. Postmenopausal women can have the examination performed at any time unless there is known endometrial cancer. Box 13-2 lists current indications and relative contraindications for sonohysterography.

Sonohysterography is an accurate technique for diagnosis of endometrial polyps and submucosal fibroids, particularly compared with traditional transvaginal sonography. Because the anterior and posterior uterine walls compress the endometrium, identifying endometrial masses may be difficult with conventional transvaginal sonography. Infusion of saline solution removes the compression and allows visualization of endometrial abnormalities that may be present. Figure 13-31 demonstrates the use of sonohysterography to outline endometrial abnormalities.

Table 13-2 summarizes pathology, symptoms, and sonographic findings of the anatomic causes of AUB.

BOX 13-2 Indications and Contraindications for Sonohysterography

Indications
Evaluation of AUB
Detection of endometrial polyps
Detection of submucosal fibroids
Diagnosis of intrauterine adhesions
Diagnosis of residual placental tissue
Evaluation of patients with recurrent pregnancy loss
Evaluation of infertility patients

Contraindications
Known or suspected intrauterine pregnancy
Unstable uterine hemorrhage
Acute salpingitis (pelvic inflammatory disease)
Known endometrial carcinoma

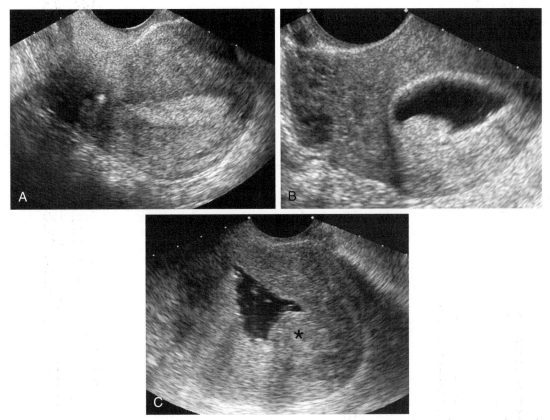

FIGURE 13-31 (A), Standard transvaginal sonography demonstrates thickened endometrium. **(B),** Sonohysterography in the same patient outlines polyp, which caused the endometrium to appear thickened. **(C),** Submucosal fibroid *(asterisk)* outlined by saline.

TABLE 13-2   **Anatomic Causes of Abnormal Uterine Bleeding**

Pathology	Symptoms	Sonographic Findings
Adenomyosis	May be asymptomatic or cause uterine tenderness, dysmenorrhea, menorrhagia, uterine enlargement	Diffuse uterine enlargement, ill-defined myometrial heterogeneity, myometrial striations, thickened posterior uterine wall, loss of distinct junctional zone, myometrial cysts, focal myometrial masses; minimal distortion of endometrial or serosal contour
Endometrial atrophy	Postmenopausal bleeding	Thin endometrium measuring <5 mm
Endometrial carcinoma	AUB, postmenopausal bleeding	Thickened endometrium (>4 mm in postmenopausal patient), may be uniformly echogenic or heterogeneous; cystic changes may be present; fluid with or without echoes may be present within uterine cavity
Endometrial hyperplasia	AUB most commonly in perimenopausal and postmenopausal women	Diffusely thickened, echogenic endometrium with or without small cystic spaces (more commonly without)
Endometrial polyps	May be asymptomatic or may cause intermenstrual bleeding or menometrorrhagia	Focal or diffuse endometrial thickening with or without small cystic areas; vascularity within feeding vessel may be seen on color Doppler
Leiomyomas	Uterine enlargement, pelvic pain, pelvic pressure, AUB	Uterine or endometrial contour irregularity, heterogeneous echotexture, generalized uterine enlargement, focal hypoechoic or hyperechoic masses with or without cystic spaces and calcifications
Retained products of conception	Postpartum bleeding or pain	Thickened endometrium (>10 mm) with endometrial mass
Tamoxifen	Drug administered to women with breast cancer	Similar to findings associated with carcinoma, hyperplasia, and polyps; cystic changes within polyps and in subendometrial area are common

SUMMARY

AUB is a common gynecologic problem that is often an indication for pelvic sonography. Sonographers are able to provide clinicians with valuable information that directly affects treatment plans. In the case of postmenopausal bleeding, the results of a pelvic sonogram may prevent the patient from undergoing unnecessary invasive surgery.

CLINICAL SCENARIO—DIAGNOSIS

A 46-year-old perimenopausal patient has experienced an episode of menorrhagia. Sonographic evaluation reveals a normal endometrium, a globular uterine appearance, and a heterogeneous myometrium. The striations evident in the images are typical of adenomyosis; however, the uterine shape and heterogeneity can also be attributed to fibroids. MRI can provide further evaluation of the junctional zone to evaluate for adenomyosis.

CASE STUDIES FOR DISCUSSION

1. A 65-year-old nulliparous woman with postmenopausal bleeding is evaluated by her physician. She is not receiving hormone replacement therapy. A pelvic sonogram is ordered. The adnexae appear normal; however, the sonographer notes an abnormality on the longitudinal midline image of the uterus (Fig. 13-32). List

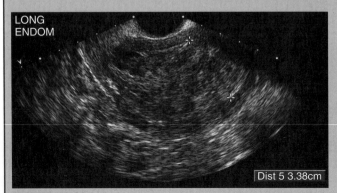

FIGURE 13-32 Longitudinal midline view of the uterus in a postmenopausal patient with bleeding.

at least two differential diagnoses for this finding. Which imaging study can help differentiate the anatomic cause for the finding? Discuss how these imaging findings might influence further diagnostic procedures.

2. A 35-year-old multiparous woman is referred for a pelvic sonogram because of menorrhagia. The endometrial and myometrial findings are demonstrated in Figure 13-33. What is the most likely diagnosis?

3. A 59-year-old woman with new-onset postmenopausal spotting is seen. A pelvic sonogram is ordered, and the sonographer notes no masses in the myometrium or adnexal regions. The endometrium measures 0.14 cm, and the appearance is as shown in Figure 13-34. What is the most likely diagnosis?

4. A 37-year-old woman undergoes a pelvic sonogram for AUB. The endometrium appears abnormally thick, so a sonohysterogram is performed. The findings are demonstrated in Figure 13-35. What is the most likely diagnosis?

5. A 42-year-old woman undergoes a pelvic sonogram because of pelvic fullness and menorrhagia. The sonographic findings are shown in Figure 13-36. What is the most likely diagnosis?

CASE STUDIES FOR DISCUSSION—cont'd

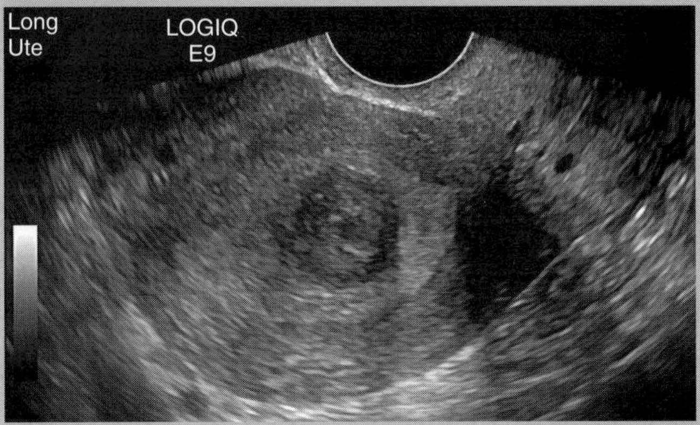

FIGURE 13-33 Longitudinal midline view of the uterus in a 35-year-old patient with menorrhagia.

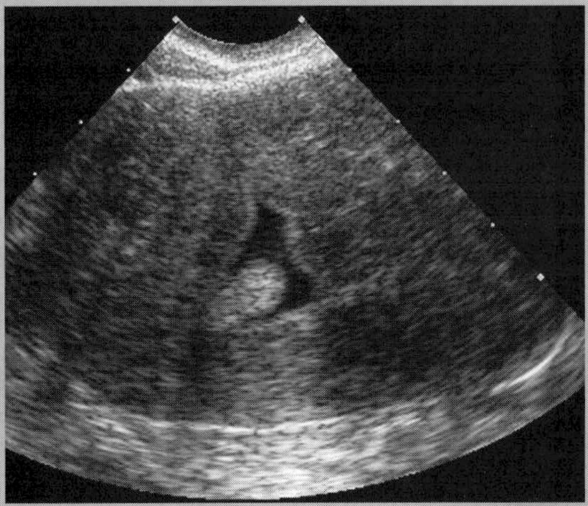

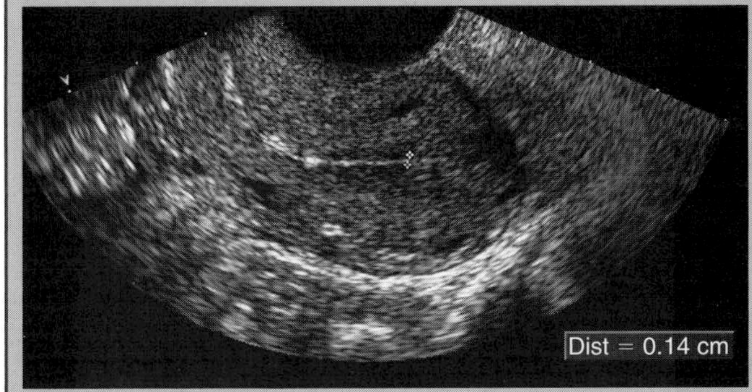

FIGURE 13-34 Longitudinal midline view of the uterus in a post-menopausal patient with bleeding.

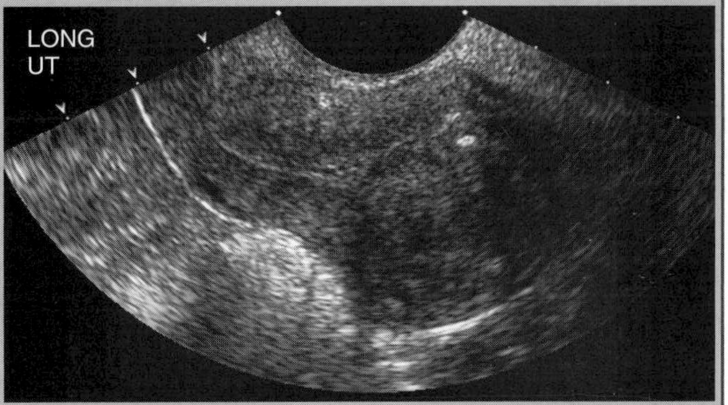

FIGURE 13-35 Sonohysterogram image of the uterus in a 37-year-old patient with AUB.

FIGURE 13-36 Longitudinal view of the uterus in a 42-year-old patient with pelvic fullness and menorrhagia.

STUDY QUESTIONS

1. A 50-year-old woman with AUB undergoes a pelvic sonogram. Transvaginal sonography reveals a thickened endometrium with a single vascular feeding vessel apparent on color Doppler imaging. What is the most likely diagnosis?
   a. Adenomyosis
   b. Submucosal fibroid
   c. Endometrial polyp
   d. Intramural fibroid

2. A 48-year-old woman undergoes a pelvic sonogram because of AUB. The uterus has a homogeneous echotexture, and the endometrial thickness is 1.7 cm. Sonohysterography reveals diffuse endometrial thickening with no intraluminal masses. What is the most likely diagnosis?
   a. Endometrial hyperplasia
   b. Submucosal fibroid
   c. Endometrial polyp
   d. Adenomyosis

3. A 30-year-old woman 2 months postpartum with AUB undergoes transvaginal sonography. The examination reveals a normal-size uterus, a 12 cm thick endometrium, and an echogenic mass within the uterine cavity. Serum β human chorionic gonadotropin testing is negative. What is the most likely cause of AUB?
   a. Endometrial hyperplasia
   b. Ectopic pregnancy
   c. Endometrial carcinoma
   d. RPOC

4. A 42-year-old woman with a history of breast cancer undergoes a pelvic sonogram, which demonstrates cystic changes within the endometrium. Which of the following is the most likely cause of the endometrial appearance?
   a. Submucosal fibroid
   b. Tamoxifen changes
   c. Adenomyosis
   d. Intramural fibroid

5. A 30-year-old woman with menorrhagia undergoes a pelvic sonogram that reveals a hypoechoic mass distorting the endometrium. This mass attenuates the sound beam, it has a broad base, and the endometrium courses over it. What is the most likely diagnosis?
a. Tamoxifen changes
b. Endometrial polyps
c. Submucosal fibroid
d. Endometrial hyperplasia

6. A 45-year-old woman with intermenstrual spotting undergoes transvaginal sonography. Endometrial thickness is 20 mm, and saline introduced during hysterosonography outlines a focal mass isoechoic to the endometrium. What is the most likely diagnosis?
a. Submucosal fibroid
b. Intramural fibroid
c. Adenomyosis
d. Endometrial polyp

7. A 25-year-old woman with menorrhagia undergoes a pelvic sonogram, which demonstrates multiple intramural and subserosal fibroids, with the largest measuring 8 cm. The physician presents several treatment options. The patient wishes to maintain fertility. Which of the following is *not* a treatment option likely to be offered?
a. Myomectomy
b. Endometrial ablation
c. Uterine artery ablation
d. Progestin-releasing IUD

8. A 75-year-old woman with postmenopausal bleeding undergoes pelvic sonography, which reveals a 1.5 cm endometrium. What is the most likely diagnosis?
a. Endometrial carcinoma
b. Subserosal fibroids
c. Submucosal fibroids
d. Adenomyosis

9. An adnexal mass is palpated in a 34-year-old woman with pelvic pressure. Pelvic sonography reveals a 4 cm solid adnexal mass with a normal-appearing ovary adjacent to the mass. What is the most likely diagnosis?
a. Submucosal fibroid
b. Pedunculated fibroid
c. Intramural fibroid
d. Uterine cancer

10. A 50-year-old woman experiencing AUB undergoes pelvic sonography. The uterine body is globular and slightly heterogeneous in appearance, several myometrial cysts are identified, and the endometrial-myometrial junction is not clearly delineated. What is the most likely diagnosis?
a. Endometrial polyps
b. Endometrial hyperplasia
c. Adenomyosis
d. Pedunculated fibroids

REFERENCES

1. Salem S: Gynecologic ultrasound. In Rumack C, Wilson S, Charboneau J, et al: *Diagnostic ultrasound*, vol 1, ed 4, Philadelphia, 2011, Mosby, pp 547–612.
2. Van den Bosch T, Van Schoubroeck D, Vergote E, et al: A thin and regular endometrium on ultrasound is very unlikely in patients with endometrial malignancy, *Ultrasound Obstet Gynecol* 29:674–679, 2007.
3. Day B, Dunson D, Hill M, et al: High cumulative incidence of uterine leiomyoma in black and white women: ultrasound evidence, *Am J Obstet Gynecol* 188:100–107, 2003.
4. Van Voorhis B: A 41-year-old woman with menorrhagia, anemia, and fibroids: review of treatment of uterine fibroids, *JAMA* 301:82–89, 2009.
5. Poder L: Ultrasound evaluation of the uterus. In Callen P, editor: *Ultrasonography in obstetrics and gynecology*, ed 5, Philadelphia, 2008, Saunders, pp 919–941.
6. Exacoustos C, Brienza L, Di Giovanni A, et al: Adenomyosis: three-dimensional sonographic findings of the junctional zone and correlation with histology, *Ultrasound Obstet Gynecol* 37:471–479, 2011.
7. Ignatov T, Eggemann H, Semczuk A, et al: Role of GPR30 in endometrial pathology after tamoxifen for breast cancer, *Am J Obstet Gynecol* 203: 595.e9-595.e16, 2010.

14

Localize Intrauterine Device

Susanna Ovel

CLINICAL SCENARIO

A 30-year-old woman undergoes a pelvic sonogram. A nonhormonal intrauterine device (IUD) was inserted 2 months ago. She complains of pelvic cramping and intermittent vaginal spotting. Her gynecologist attempted to remove the device, but the strings broke and are no longer visible. A coronal three-dimensional (3D) rendering of the uterus demonstrates a homogeneous uterus with an echogenic structure in the endometrial cavity (Fig. 14-1). No adnexal or ovarian abnormalities were noted. Is an IUD visible on this sonogram? If so, where is it most likely located? Does this image reveal an additional uterine anomaly?

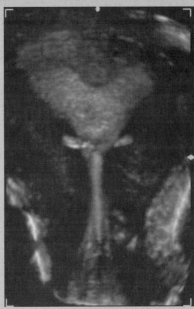

FIGURE 14-1 3D image of uterus. *(Courtesy Ted Whitten.)*

OBJECTIVES

- Describe the sonographic appearance of properly positioned intrauterine devices (IUDs).
- Describe the sonographic appearance of abnormally positioned IUDs.

- Differentiate the sonographic characteristics of IUDs in association with complicating factors, including infection, perforation, and intrauterine and ectopic pregnancy.
- Identify gynecologic symptoms associated with IUD use.
- List the factors associated with lost IUDs.

An intrauterine device (IUD) is a flexible contraceptive device inserted through the vaginal canal into the endometrium. It is typically T-shaped, made of plastic, wrapped in copper, and may or may not contain hormones. Plastic strings tied to the end of the IUD generally suspend through the cervix into the superior portion of the vaginal canal. When the IUD has been properly inserted, the device expands from its temporarily constricted state (used for insertion through the endocervical canal) and lies in the midline of the endometrial cavity. The top bars of the "T" unfold after insertion to lie across the fundal portion of the endometrial cavity, and the stem lies vertically (Fig. 14-2). The IUD strings (usually two) are attached to the bottom of the stem and pass through the endocervical canal into the upper portion of the vagina, where they typically coil causing no symptoms. When the patient or clinician cannot locate the strings, a sonogram is ordered to localize the IUD. Missing strings might indicate the IUD has been expelled, the strings have fallen off, the strings have retracted into the uterus, malposition of the IUD, or perforation of the IUD into the myometrium or peritoneal cavity. Other indications for sonographic evaluation of an IUD include pelvic pain following insertion, abnormal bleeding, and a positive pregnancy test with a known IUD.[1]

The most common IUDs currently used in the United States include ParaGard and Mirena. These are small, safe, and highly effective contraceptive devices. ParaGard is a nonhormonal T-shaped plastic device wrapped in copper. Copper has a stimulating effect on the uterus, thickening the cervical mucus and producing a fluid that is toxic to sperm. This type of IUD is preferred but may cause menometrorrhagia and pelvic cramping. Copper-wrapped IUDs are approved for 10 years of continuous use before removal is necessary. Mirena is a T-shaped plastic device that releases low amounts of progestin. This type of IUD stimulates the endometrial glands to shrink and atrophy, reduces sperm survival, and inhibits embryo implantation. The hormones may prevent or decrease menstrual bleeding and cramping.[2] This type of levonorgestrel-releasing device requires removal every 5 years. Discontinued IUDs include the serpentine-shaped Lippes Loop (Fig. 14-3), Copper 7 (shaped like a 7), Saf-T Coil (coil-shaped), and Dalkon Shield.[3]

NORMAL SONOGRAPHIC APPEARANCE OF AN INTRAUTERINE DEVICE

Sonographic appearance varies depending on the type of IUD. All types of IUDs should be located in the midline portion of the endometrial cavity. The ParaGard IUD demonstrates two parallel hyperechoic linear echoes with intense posterior acoustic shadowing. The two echogenic parallel structures (entrance-exit reflections) represent the anterior and posterior surfaces of the IUD. The intense attenuation of the sound beam is caused by the copper wire (Fig. 14-4, *A*). The Mirena IUD demonstrates a hypoechoic or mildly echogenic stem with thin echogenic "T-arms" (Fig. 14-4, *B*). 3D imaging in the coronal plane displays the IUD in its entirety, which is advantageous when evaluating location. The strings are the consistency of fine fishing line and are occasionally visualized sonographically (Fig. 14-5).

INTRAUTERINE DEVICE COMPLICATIONS

Complications associated with IUDs are rare but may develop into a serious medical condition. Abnormal or ectopic locations of IUDs include migration from the superior fundal portion to the inferior portion of the endometrium or vaginal canal, myometrial penetration, and perforation into the peritoneal cavity. Additional complications include pelvic inflammatory disease, ectopic pregnancy, and a coexisting intrauterine pregnancy.

Expulsion of Intrauterine Device

Expulsion of the IUD generally occurs within the first year, most commonly during the first few months after insertion. Expulsion is more likely to occur when inserted soon after childbirth or in women with a history of

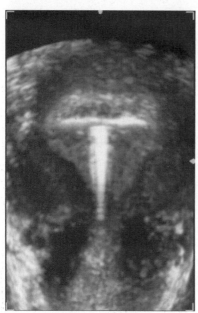

FIGURE 14-2 3D coronal image of properly placed copper wire IUD. *(Courtesy Ted Whitten.)*

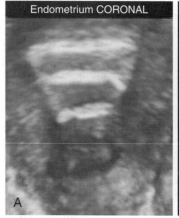
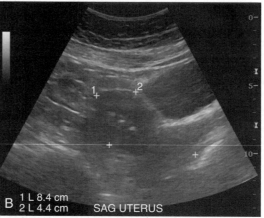

FIGURE 14-3 (A), Coronal 3D rendering of Lippes Loop IUD. **(B),** Sagittal view shows Lippes Loop IUD that appears as multiple echogenic dots in the sagittal plane. *(Courtesy Radiological Associates of Sacramento.)*

previous expulsion, nulliparity, or severe menorrhagia.[4] Clinically, women can be asymptomatic or complain of cramping, vaginal discharge, intermenstrual or postcoital bleeding or spotting, and dyspareunia.[5]

Sonographic Findings. When expulsion of an IUD has occurred, there is absence of the IUD within the endometrial cavity. Thickness and echo pattern of the endometrium vary according to the endometrial phase of the menstrual cycle. When the IUD is not visualized sonographically, a plain film radiograph of the abdomen and pelvis should be obtained to rule out perforation into the peritoneal cavity.

Migration

An IUD is abnormally located if it is inferiorly located within the endometrial cavity or if any part extends past the confines of the cavity into the uterus or cervix. An inferior location of the IUD may be a result of migration or improper insertion of the device, and patients may experience pain or be asymptomatic. An IUD in this location decreases the contraceptive effectiveness and is at risk for being expelled.[6] If the IUD is embedded in the myometrium, operative hysteroscopy may be required for removal.

Sonographic Findings. An IUD that has migrated appears as a hyperechoic linear structure within the lower uterine segment, cervix, or vaginal canal with mild or intense attenuation of the sound beam posterior to the device (Fig. 14-6).

Myometrial Penetration

Extension or penetration of the IUD through the basal layer of the endometrium into the uterine myometrium may occur. Generally, the "T" portion of the IUD extends partially or completely through the lateral and fundal portions of the endometrial layers embedding into the myometrium of the uterus.[7] Women may be asymptomatic or experience pelvic pain or irregular bleeding. According to one study, patients presenting for 3D

sonography with pain or irregular bleeding are at higher risk of having an abnormally located IUD compared with patients with a normally positioned IUD.[1]

Sonographic Findings. Myometrial penetration of an IUD results in an eccentric position of the IUD within the endometrial cavity or myometrium (Fig. 14-7). The linear hyperechoic "arms" of the IUD breach the basal layer of endometrium and extend into the myometrium. 3D imaging in the coronal plane has greatly improved sonographic detail of IUDs by enhancing visualization of

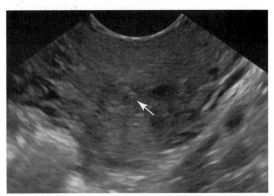

FIGURE 14-5 Transvaginal coronal sonogram of uterine cervix shows strings from IUD *(arrow). (Courtesy Sharon Ballestero.)*

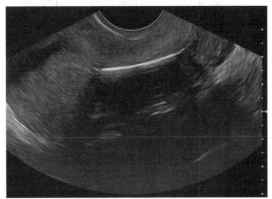

FIGURE 14-6 Sagittal sonogram of improperly placed IUD. *(Courtesy Ted Whitten.)*

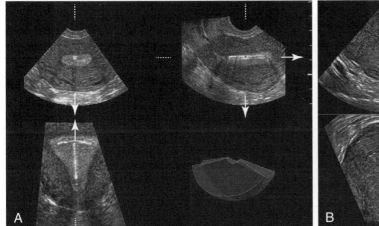
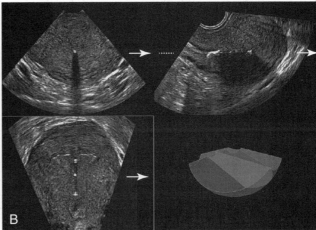

FIGURE 14-4 Multiplane images of ParaGard **(A)** and Mirena **(B)** IUDs.

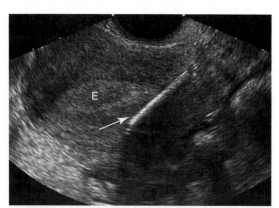

FIGURE 14-7 Transvaginal sonogram of perforated IUD. There is extension into posterior myometrium *(arrow)*.

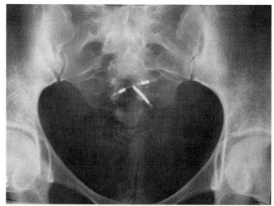

FIGURE 14-8 Radiograph of pelvis shows T-shaped IUD.

the shape and location of the device within the endometrial cavity.[3]

Perforation

Perforation is rare occurring in approximately 1 per 1000 insertions.[8] Perforation almost always occurs during insertion and is associated with an inexperienced clinician, retroverted uterus, and congenital uterine anomalies. Pelvic pain is the principal clinical finding. Complications include damage and scarring of the surrounding organs and pelvic infection.[9]

Sonographic Findings. If an IUD has perforated to the extent that it is no longer within the endometrial cavity, the endometrial cavity is clearly delineated separately from the location of the IUD. The IUD may be visible in the myometrium, the cervix, or the pelvic or abdominal cavity. It is possible that no IUD is seen at all, suggesting expulsion or perforation into the peritoneum. A radiograph should be obtained whenever the IUD cannot be visualized sonographically because IUDs are radiopaque and show up on radiographic images (Fig. 14-8).

Infection

Bacteria may enter the endometrial cavity as the IUD is inserted through the vaginal canal. A woman's risk for infection is strongly related to previous history of a sexually transmitted disease and insertion technique.[10] Although rare, pelvic infection can develop into a serious condition affecting the uterus, fallopian tubes, adnexa, and peritoneum resulting in endomyometritis, pyosalpinx, and tuboovarian abscess. Most infections are treated with antibiotics, but additional therapy may be needed in some instances.

Sonographic Findings. In cases of endomyometritis, the endometrium may appear thick and irregular, and the uterus may appear enlarged and inhomogeneous. A hypervascular endometrium and myometrium may be evident with color Doppler imaging (Fig. 14-9, *A*; see Color Plate 11) As the infection progresses into the

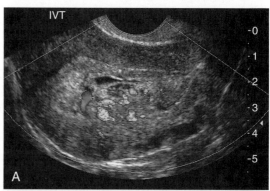

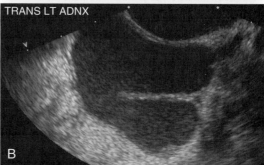

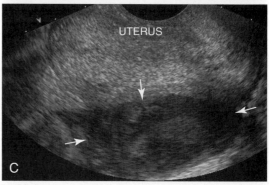

FIGURE 14-9 Sonographic examples of infection. **(A)**, Transvaginal sagittal image of hypervascular uterus with thick endometrium. **(B)**, Transvaginal image of dilated fallopian tube with echogenic debris. **(C)**, Transvaginal sagittal image of uterus with large complex mass *(arrows)* adjacent and separate from the uterus.

fallopian tubes, sonographic findings may include a complex irregular tubular structure in the adnexal region (Fig. 14-9, *B*). In cases of tuboovarian abscess, the resultant pelvic mass appears complex and multilocular with ill-defined wall margins and breakdown of normal adnexal anatomy (Fig. 14-9, *C*). The IUD is typically noted in its usual endometrial location.

Pregnancy with an Intrauterine Device

The risk of pregnancy with an IUD in place is highest in the first year after IUD insertion.[5] Pregnancy in the presence of an IUD is associated with several complications; the most noted complication is ectopic pregnancy.[11] Spontaneous abortion with an IUD that remains in situ is 40% to 50%, a rate twice as high as that of the general obstetric population. Other complications include chorioamnionitis, premature rupture of membranes, preterm labor, septic abortion, and maternal death.[12]

When a pregnancy occurs with an IUD in place, the World Health Organization and U.S. Food and Drug Administration recommend that if the IUD is seen and the strings are visible, the device should be removed by pulling the strings.[13] In recent years, with the increased availability of 3D imaging, sonography has been helpful in the removal of IUDs with strings that are not visible with excellent fetal and maternal results.[6] As stated earlier, 3D imaging in the coronal plane increases detail and accuracy in the location of an IUD.

Intrauterine Pregnancy

In the event of a coexisting intrauterine pregnancy, removal of the IUD early in pregnancy reduces the risk of spontaneous abortion or preterm labor. IUD removal reduces the risk for adverse obstetric outcomes but does not eliminate it.[6]
Sonographic Findings. When an intrauterine pregnancy coexists with an IUD, the echogenic IUD is commonly found displaced to the inner surface of the myometrium, outside of the amniotic sac, and may be in any orientation (Fig. 14-10).

Ectopic Pregnancy

Using an IUD does not increase a woman's risk for ectopic pregnancy. Although rare, a pregnancy that occurs with an IUD is more likely to be an ectopic pregnancy

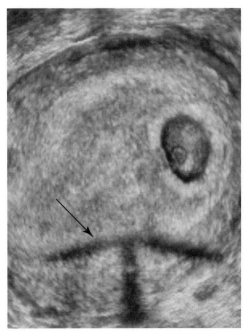

FIGURE 14-10 First-trimester pregnancy at 6 weeks showing gestational sac with a yolk sac. Note the shape of an IUD *(arrow)* located below the level of the gestational sac. This is actually the shadow of the IUD, which is located in a different plane. Such a shadow is an artifact, which is reconstructed in a plane different from the location of the IUD itself.

compared with the general population, and the risk is slightly greater with hormone-releasing IUDs.[11] Most ectopic pregnancies are located in the ampulla segment of the fallopian tube. Treatment of an ectopic pregnancy may include medical therapy (methotrexate) or surgical intervention. Clinical findings of ectopic pregnancy include abnormal rise in β human chorionic gonadotropin levels, pelvic pain, bleeding, palpable pelvic mass, and hypotension when the tube has ruptured.
Sonographic Findings. Sonographic evaluation of the uterus with an IUD coexisting with an ectopic gestation demonstrates the IUD within the endometrial cavity, no evidence of an intrauterine pregnancy, and possibly a centrally located endometrial fluid collection. A complex mass may be present in the adnexal region separate from the ovary. An extrauterine gestation with or without an embryo may be visualized, but this is generally a less common finding. Fluid in the posterior cul-de-sac may be anechoic or contain echoes representing hemorrhage.

Table 14-1 summarizes the symptoms and pathologic findings of the complications of IUDs.

TABLE 14-1	Intrauterine Device Complications	
Complication	**Symptoms**	**Sonographic Finding**
Expulsion	Asymptomatic	Normal-appearing uterus, no evidence of IUD
Migration	Asymptomatic	Abnormal low placement of IUD in endometrial cavity
Myometrial penetration	Pelvic pain	Eccentric position, hyperechoic "arms" breach the endometrial-myometrial junction
Perforation	Pelvic or abdominal pain	IUD not visualized within uterus
Infection	Pelvic pain, fever, leukocytosis	Thick and hypervascular endometrium, dilated fallopian tubes
Tuboovarian abscess	Pelvic pain, fever, leukocytosis, purulent discharge	Complex adnexal mass, inability to distinguish adnexal structures
Ectopic pregnancy	Positive pregnancy test, pelvic pain, vaginal bleeding, slowly rising β hCG values	No evidence of intrauterine pregnancy, complex adnexal mass, echogenic cul-de-sac fluid

hCG, Human chorionic gonadotropin.

SUMMARY

The use of an IUD for contraception is prevalent, and sonography is commonly used to determine the proper placement, location, and orientation of the device. Sonography can be used to evaluate the nature of concurrent complications, such as migration, myometrial penetration, perforation, infection, and intrauterine and extrauterine pregnancies. IUDs currently available in the United States are small, safe, and highly effective contraceptive devices. Use of an IUD does not protect women from sexually transmitted diseases or prevent physiologic ovarian changes.

Evaluation of IUD placement and associated complications has greatly improved with the use of 3D sonography. This technique enables imaging of both the arms and the stem of the entire IUD simultaneously, allowing for faster and more accurate localization.

CLINICAL SCENARIO—DIAGNOSIS

The fact that the IUD strings were initially visible suggests that the IUD is in the uterus and not abdominally located. The sonogram demonstrates a small separation between the superior portion of the endometrial cavity. The contour of the uterine fundus appears smooth and regular. The endometrial cavities appear to be separated by a small amount of myometrial tissue. The most likely diagnosis is uterus subseptus.

CASE STUDIES FOR DISCUSSION

1. A 28-year-old woman with a last menstrual period of approximately 1 week prior and an IUD insertion 6 months ago undergoes a sonogram. The songraphic findings are shown in Figure 14-11. What is the most likely diagnosis?
2. A 25-year-old asymptomatic woman is seen for pelvic sonogram for a "lost" IUD string. The sonogram reveals the findings in Figure 14-12. What is the likely diagnosis for this patient?
3. A 35-year-old woman with a palpable IUD string undergoes a pelvic sonogram. She complains of vaginal spotting, and a laboratory

test is positive for pregnancy. The sonographic findings are demonstrated in Figure 14-13. What is the most likely diagnosis?
4. A 32-year-old woman undergoes a pelvic sonogram 1 month after insertion of an IUD. She complains of pelvic pain and cramping. The sonographic findings are shown in Figure 14-14. What is the most likely diagnosis?

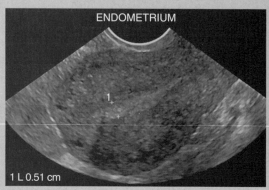

FIGURE 14-11 Transvaginal sagittal sonogram of uterus. *(Courtesy Radiological Associates of Sacramento.)*

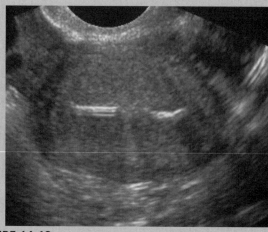

FIGURE 14-12 Transvaginal coronal sonogram of uterine fundus.

CASE STUDIES FOR DISCUSSION—cont'd

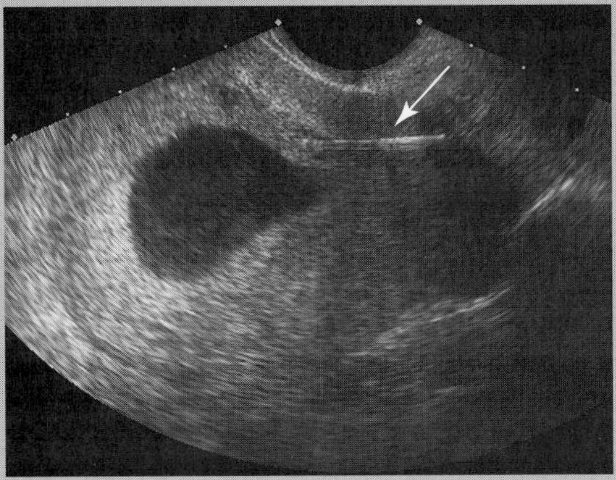

FIGURE 14-13 Transvaginal sonogram of early intrauterine pregnancy.

5. A 40-year-old woman had an IUD inserted 2 months ago and is experiencing pelvic pain, especially when seated. She is referred for a pelvic sonogram. The sonographic findings are shown in Fig. 14-15. What is the most likely diagnosis?

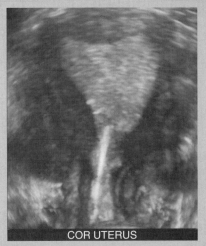

COR UTERUS

FIGURE 14-14 Coronal 3D rendering of uterus

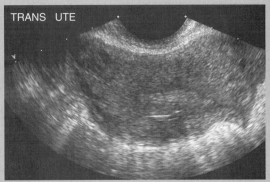

TRANS UTE

FIGURE 14-15 Transvaginal coronal sonogram of uterus.

STUDY QUESTIONS

1. A 27-year-old woman complaining of severe pelvic pain undergoes a pelvic sonogram. The patient has a history of IUD insertion after her most recent pregnancy. The IUD is eccentrically located with the right T-arm extending lateral to the endometrium. What is the most likely diagnosis?
   a. Ectopic pregnancy
   b. Myometrial penetration
   c. Tuboovarian abscess
   d. Peritoneal perforation
   e. Migration of the IUD

2. The sonographic appearance of a copper wire IUD includes which of the following?
   a. Hypoechoic stem with mild posterior shadowing
   b. Highly echogenic stem with mild posterior shadowing
   c. Hypoechoic stem with intense posterior shadowing
   d. Highly echogenic stem with intense posterior enhancement
   e. Highly echogenic stem with intense posterior shadowing

3. A patient presents with a history of severe pelvic pain, fever, and purulent discharge. A pelvic sonogram demonstrates a properly placed IUD and a complex adnexal mass. The ovary cannot be identified within or adjacent to the adnexal mass. What is the most likely diagnosis?
   a. Ectopic pregnancy
   b. IUD perforation
   c. Endomyometritis
   d. Myometrial penetration
   e. Tuboovarian abscess

4. A patient who is scheduled for a pelvic sonogram states that she currently has a Mirena IUD in place. What is the shape of this IUD?
   a. Circle
   b. T
   c. 7
   d. Serpiginous
   e. Triangle

5. A patient with an IUD in place has a positive pregnancy test. A sonogram reveals a 7-week, viable gestation within the uterus. The IUD is identified in the lower uterine segment; however, the strings are not visible to the obstetrician. Leaving the IUD in situ during the pregnancy increases the risk for which one of the following complications?
   a. Birth defects
   b. Amniotic band syndrome
   c. Incompetent cervix
   d. Preterm labor
   e. Uterine rupture

6. A patient with a positive serum pregnancy test and an IUD in place is seen for sonographic examination. The sonogram reveals an IUD within the uterine cavity with no evidence of an intrauterine gestation. A complex adnexal mass separate from the ovary is identified, and a moderate amount of hypoechoic fluid is noted in the cul-de-sac and right upper quadrant. The patient's last menstrual period was 7 weeks prior. What is the most likely diagnosis for this patient?
   a. Ectopic pregnancy
   b. Spontaneous abortion
   c. Endomyometritis
   d. Tuboovarian abscess
   e. Early intrauterine pregnancy

7. A 27-year-old woman with a history of IUD insertion 6 months prior is seen now because the IUD strings are missing. Her last menstrual period was 3 weeks ago. The pelvic sonogram reveals a normal-appearing uterus without evidence of an IUD. A radiograph demonstrates an IUD within the pelvis. What is the most likely explanation regarding the IUD?
   a. Unrecognized IUD expulsion
   b. Perforation of IUD into the peritoneal cavity
   c. A normally placed hormone-releasing IUD
   d. Blood clots within the endometrium preventing recognition of the IUD
   e. A normally placed copper wire IUD

8. A 35-year-old woman with pelvic pain undergoes a pelvic sonogram. She has had an IUD for the past 3 years without complication. The sonogram reveals a normal-appearing uterus with an IUD located in the lower uterine segment. This is consistent with which of the following?
   a. IUD migration
   b. Ectopic pregnancy
   c. Myometrial penetration
   d. A normally positioned IUD
   e. Peritoneal perforation

9. A 23-year-old woman undergoes a pelvic sonogram for missing IUD strings. Her last menstrual period was 6 months prior, and a recent pregnancy test was negative. An IUD with a hypoechoic stem and hyperechoic arms is identified in the endometrial cavity. Based on the patient's history and sonographic findings, what type of IUD is imaged?
   a. Mirena
   b. Copper 7
   c. ParaGard
   d. Lippes Loop
   e. Dalkon Shield

10. A 40-year-old woman presents for a pelvic sonogram because of abnormal menses. The sonogram reveals a Copper 7 IUD, which has been in place for 12 years. What is the most likely course of treatment for this patient?
   a. Assess for toxic shock syndrome because the IUD has been in place too long
   b. IUD removal and antibiotic treatment because older IUDs cause infections
   c. Leave the IUD in place because it is not causing problems
   d. IUD removal because copper IUDs lose effectiveness after 10 years
   e. Replace the Copper 7 IUD with a Lippes Loop IUD

REFERENCES

1. Benacerraf B, Shipp T, Bromley B: Three-dimensional ultrasound detection of abnormally located intrauterine contraceptive devices which are a source of pelvic pain and abnormal bleeding, *Ultrasound Obstet Gynecol* 34:110–115, 2009.
2. Fraser I: Non-contraceptive health benefits of intrauterine hormonal systems, *Contraception* 82:396–403, 2010.
3. Peri N, Graham D, Levine D: Imaging of intrauterine contraceptive devices, *J Ultrasound Med* 26:1389–1401, 2007.
4. Muller L, Ramos L, Martins-Costa S, et al: Transvaginal ultrasonographic assessment of the expulsion rate of intrauterine devices inserted in the immediate postpartum period: a pilot study, *Contraception* 72:192–195, 2005.
5. Grimes D: Intrauterine devices (IUDs). In Hatcher R, Trussel J, Stewart F, et al: *Contraceptive technology*, ed 18, New York, 2004, Ardent Media, pp 495–530.
6. Moschos E, Twickler D: Intrauterine devices in early pregnancy: findings on ultrasound and clinical outcomes, *Am J Obstet Gynecol* 204:427, 2011. e1-427.e6.
7. Naftalin J, Jurkoovi D: The endometrial-myometrial junction: a fresh look at a crossing, *Ultrasound Obstet Gynecol* 34:1–11, 2009.
8. Harrison-Woolrych M, Aston J, Coulter D: Uterine perforation on intrauterine device insertion: is the incidence higher than previously reported? *Contraception* 67:53–57, 2003.
9. Vasquez P, Schreber C: The missing IUD, *Contraception* 82:126, 2010.
10. Mohllajee A, Curtis K, Peterson H: Does insertion and use of an intrauterine device increase the risk of pelvic inflammatory disease among women with sexually transmitted infection? A systematic review, *Contraception* 73:145–153, 2006.
11. Furlong L: Ectopic pregnancy risk when contraception fails: a review, *J Reprod Med* 47:881, 2002.
12. Ganer H, Levy A, Ohel I, et al: Pregnancy outcome in women with an intrauterine contraceptive device, *Am J Obstet Gynecol* 201:381, 2009. e1-381.e5.
13. American College of Obstetricians and Gynecologists: Intrauterine device. ACOG practice bulletin no. 59, January 2005.

15

Pelvic Inflammatory Disease

Winslow (Ted) Whitten

CLINICAL SCENARIO

A 21-year-old woman presents to the emergency department with lower abdominal pain and fever. The patient states that the abdominal pain has become increasingly severe since her period finished 3 days ago. She has been using an over-the-counter treatment for what she thought was a vaginal infection that somewhat improved her symptoms of itching and burning. Physical examination reveals abdominal guarding and rebound tenderness. Manual pelvic examination elicits such severe pain that a thorough examination of the pelvic organs cannot be completed. Laboratory test results show elevated white blood cell (WBC) counts and a negative human chorionic gonadotropin level. The patient also denies pregnancy.

A sonogram of the pelvis is ordered. Transabdominal scanning shows bilateral complex masses, fluid in the cul-de-sac, and ovarian enlargement (Fig. 15-1). Thickening of the endometrium is also noted. Endovaginal scanning is attempted, although only a limited amount of information is gained, because the patient experiences severe pain during the procedure. What is the possible diagnosis?

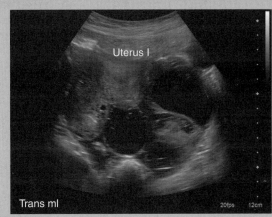

FIGURE 15-1 Transverse scan of the uterus shows bilateral adnexal masses, pyosalpinx, and thickened endometrium.

OBJECTIVES

- List and describe the etiology and risk factors associated with pelvic inflammatory disease (PID).
- Describe the progression of PID, and identify the specific sequelae of PID.
- Describe the sonographic appearances of PID, including endometritis, salpingitis, pyosalpinx, hydrosalpinx, and tuboovarian abscess.
- Identify Doppler findings associated with PID.
- Identify pertinent laboratory values and related diagnostic studies associated with PID.

Pelvic inflammatory disease (PID) is a type of sexually transmitted disease, although bilateral infection may be associated with the use of an intrauterine device (IUD).[1] Less commonly, unilateral PID may result from direct extension of primary lower abdominal or pelvic abscesses or complications following abortion or childbirth. The diagnosis of PID is usually made clinically through the assessment of patient history and symptoms, pelvic examination, urine test, and culture of vaginal secretions.[2] Early and vigorous antibiotic treatment is needed to stop the progression of the disease and prevent the development of infertility.

Chlamydia is more common than gonorrhea as a source of infection, but numerous aerobic and anaerobic organisms may also be present. In many cases, the symptoms of chlamydia and gonorrhea are mild or nonexistent in both female and male patients; however, men are more likely to seek treatment when symptoms are present.

Normally, the endocervical mucous plug provides a barrier against the ascension of both normal vaginal flora and pathogens. Chlamydia and gonorrhea can damage the endocervical canal and allow an easier ascent of these infectious bacteria into the uterus.[3] It also has been noted that other factors may allow for easier spread of disease. Bacteria can gain easier access through the cervical canal shortly after menstruation, when the mucous plug is normally expelled. Easier access also can occur with cervical ectopy, which is the extension of endocervical columnar epithelium beyond the cervix. Cervical ectopy also is more common in teenagers, who represent the age group with the highest incidence of PID.[3]

Risk factors for PID include female gender, age younger than 35 years, sexual activity (two or more partners), and use of an IUD. The risk of recurrent infection is high, and the consequences of PID include chronic pelvic pain from adhesions, peritonitis, ectopic pregnancy, maternal death from ectopic pregnancy, and infertility (risk increases with each occurrence of PID). Early and appropriate treatment is usually with two antibiotics to cover the possibility of multiple organisms; the patient's partners also must be treated. Symptoms may abate without the infection being cured, which can lead to the patient not completing the course of medication.

Because PID is readily diagnosed with assessment of the patient's symptoms and signs, sonography of the pelvis may not provide additional diagnostic information because the anatomy often appears normal. However, pelvic sonography is frequently performed because of physical findings such as fever, severe pain with manipulation of the cervix or adnexal areas, presence of purulent vaginal discharge, abdominal or rebound tenderness, and possible elevated WBC count and erythrocyte sedimentation rate (ESR). Sonography shows the presence and extent of endometritis, salpingitis, pyosalpinx, hydrosalpinx, and tuboovarian abscess (TOA). Occasionally, the only sonographic feature of PID is a loss of definition of the posterior uterine border.

Both transabdominal and endovaginal scanning techniques are recommended for evaluation of the presence and extent of PID. With transabdominal scanning, the entire pelvis can be evaluated and large structures and masses can be delineated. With endovaginal scanning, high-resolution evaluation of the uterus and endometrial cavity, fallopian tubes, ovaries, cul-de-sac, and adnexal areas can be performed. However, the patient's condition (i.e., pelvic pain) may make full distention of the urinary bladder or insertion and manipulation of the endovaginal transducer impossible. The sonographer must be aware of these possibilities and should tailor the examination to decrease pain for the patient and increase information gained. Gentle and slow scanning motions are imperative, and a thorough explanation of the procedure may help to increase patient compliance.

The symptoms of acute PID include fever (low or high), shaking chills, abdominal pain (mild, moderate, or severe), nausea, vomiting, vaginal discharge, and irregular vaginal bleeding. Signs of acute PID include abdominal guarding, rebound tenderness, increased pain with cervical or adnexal manipulation, dyspareunia, leukocytosis, elevated ESR, paralytic ileus, and shock from peritonitis.[4] Symptoms of chronic PID are persistent pelvic or lower abdominal pain, irregular menses, and possibly infertility. Chronic PID often results in

a hydrosalpinx and may include presence of an adnexal mass without fever.[3] Peritoneal inclusion cysts also may be seen in women with a history of PID, endometriosis, or prior pelvic surgery or trauma.[5] These cysts are created by the trapping of fluid arriving from the ovary by adhesions that are created by an inflammatory process.[5]

Related diagnostic studies include the following:

- Urine test, cultures of vaginal secretions or discharge, culdocentesis, laparoscopy, and computed tomography (CT) and magnetic resonance imaging (MRI)
- Endometrial biopsy and histology showing evidence of endometritis—these are the most specific studies for diagnosis of PID[2]
- Transvaginal sonography or MRI showing thickened, fluid-filled tubes with or without free pelvic or tubo-ovarian complex or Doppler studies suggesting pelvic infection (tubal hyperemia)
- Laparoscopy showing abnormalities consistent with PID

SONOGRAPHIC FINDINGS

Fallopian Tubes

The fallopian tubes are contained within the broad ligament and are not appreciated with sonography unless surrounded by ascites or involved in a disease process, such as salpingitis, pyosalpinx, or hydrosalpinx. Fallopian tubes are best shown with radiographic salpingography, which involves pressure injection of radiopaque contrast material through the tubes.

Salpingitis

Salpingitis is an infection of the fallopian tubes that may be acute, subacute, or chronic. The sonographic appearance of acute salpingitis includes nodular thickening of the walls of the fallopian tubes with diverticula. Hyperemia is also present and can be shown with color Doppler imaging. Anechoic or echogenic (pus-containing) fluid may be seen in the posterior cul-de-sac (pouch of Douglas), as may uterine enlargement with endometrial fluid or thickening (endometritis). Subacute salpingitis indicates that infectious changes have occurred without significant clinical signs and symptoms.

Chronic salpingitis is related to recurrent bouts of PID and may result in significant tubal scarring and the presence of hydrosalpinx (Fig. 15-2). The patient may have pain during intercourse or bowel movements (from adhesions involving the bowel and peritoneal surface) and during menses. Tubal scarring may be seen sonographically as several cystic structures extending from the uterus to the adnexa; this is sometimes referred to as the "chain of lakes" or "string of pearls" sonographic appearance (Fig. 15-3). Infertility and ectopic pregnancy may result from the tubal scarring.

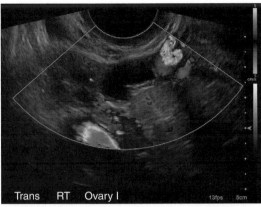

FIGURE 15-2 Hydrosalpinx. No flow is seen in the anechoic tubular structure; blood flow is seen in vessels around the structure.

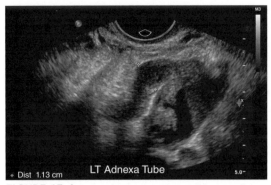

FIGURE 15-4 Left salpingitis and possible pyosalpinx.

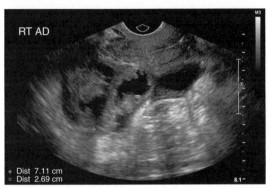

FIGURE 15-3 Right hydrosalpinx showing the "chain of lakes" or "string of pearls" sonographic appearance.

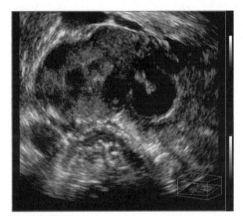

FIGURE 15-5 Hydrosalpinx using 3D technology.

Pyosalpinx

Pyosalpinx is a progression of PID in which the fallopian tubes become swollen with purulent exudates (Fig. 15-4). The sonographic appearance of pyosalpinx is consistent with visualization of thick-walled tubular or serpiginous structures surrounding the ovaries. The interstitial portion of the tube is tapered at the cornu of the uterus. The tube also may be described as sausage-shaped. Echogenic material or debris related to the presence of pus may be seen within the fallopian tubes. In addition, blurring of the normal tissue planes in the pelvis can occur, making delineation of the organs and structures difficult.

Endovaginal scanning can differentiate pyosalpinx from other pelvic masses by showing the tubular nature of the tube. Pyosalpinx also can be differentiated from fluid-filled bowel with visualization of peristalsis in the bowel. Color Doppler imaging shows increased flow in the pelvic structures.

Hydrosalpinx

Hydrosalpinx is a consequence of PID in which the fallopian tube or tubes become closed at the fimbriae, and the pus within a pyosalpinx gradually liquefies, leaving serous fluid. In addition, the walls of the tubes become thinner, and the tubes may dilate to twice the normal

diameter. The patient may be asymptomatic or may have colicky pain. Hydrosalpinx may be present for a significant length of time before diagnosis of infertility from blockage of the fallopian tubes.

Sonographically, the fallopian tubes appear as anechoic thin-walled structures with a multicystic or fusiform mass effect (Fig. 15-5). Color Doppler is useful to differentiate hydrosalpinx from bowel or prominent pelvic veins. The sonographer should take care to show the pathway of the tube and the ovary. Three-dimensional (3D) endovaginal sonography has increased the ability of imaging abnormal fallopian tubes, which may be tortuous and be positioned in a plane that is not easily accessible by standard two-dimensional sonography. In the regular two-dimensional image, multiple cystic areas are seen medial to the right ovary (Fig. 15-6). In the 3D image, a tortuous, fluid-filled tube is easily identified (see Fig. 15-5).

Tuboovarian Abscess

TOA results from pus leaking from an infected fallopian tube (pyosalpinx) and may occur from communication with the ovary. TOA is a result of a serious pelvic infection and is generally seen in the later stages of PID. Small abscesses develop but still respond to the antibiotic treatment. Large abscesses may necessitate surgical removal

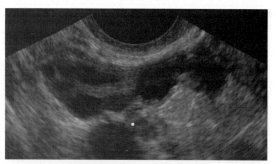

FIGURE 15-6 Hydrosalpinx.

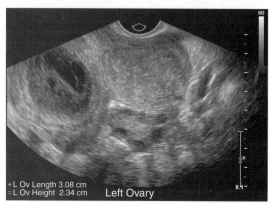

FIGURE 15-7 Left pyosalpinx and abscess.

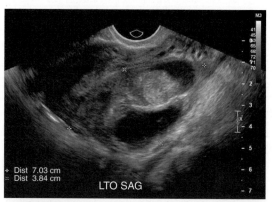

FIGURE 15-8 Longitudinal image of left TOA.

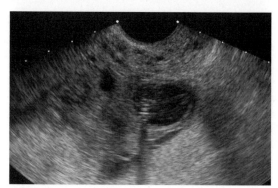

FIGURE 15-9 TOA containing a small amount of air or gas.

or drainage with transrectal or transvaginal guidance (Fig. 15-7).[6] A surgical emergency can occur with massive perforation by a pelvic abscess during which the patient has a rapid progression of severe abdominal pain, nausea, vomiting, peritonitis, shock from peritonitis, and endotoxemia.[6]

Sonographically, TOA appears as a thick-walled, complex hypoechoic mass with fluid in the cul-de-sac and adnexa (Fig. 15-8). TOA may be bilateral or unilateral and can be found in the adnexa or in the posterior cul-de-sac. Other sonographic appearances include a mass with septations, irregular margins, and fluid-debris levels. Serial sonographic examinations can follow the response of the TOA to antibiotic therapy or can provide guidance during a drainage procedure. If untreated, TOA may progress to peritonitis. The presence of air or gas within the abscess (Fig. 15-9) may make sonographic detection and delineation of the disease process difficult unless the examination correlates with clinical findings.

In pelvic abscess with peritonitis, the patient has a high fever and a significantly elevated WBC count associated with severe lower abdominal pain, nausea, and vomiting. Diffuse spread of purulent fluid into the surrounding pelvic cavity is seen. Fitz-Hugh–Curtis syndrome, which involves right upper quadrant pain, may develop in 10% of patients.[3] Sonographically, free fluid may be noted in the cul-de-sac and the hepatorenal space (Morison's pouch), with an indistinct appearance of the pelvic organs secondary to tissue edema and abscesses.

Endometritis

Of patients with endometritis, inflammation of the endometrium, 50% to 80% are asymptomatic. The most common symptoms are vaginal discharge, urethral burning, pelvic pain, and elevated WBC and ESR. Endometritis may result from cesarean section birth, IUD perforation, retained products of conception, or contamination with gonorrhea or chlamydia. Endometritis is not always related to PID but may be the first manifestation of PID.

Sonographic appearances of endometritis include normal uterus in approximately 75% of cases, uterine enlargement, widened or thickened echogenic endometrium, air in the endometrium (from gas-forming infection), fluid in endometrial cavity, or hypoechoic halo around the endometrium. The ovaries may be enlarged and indistinct because of inflammation. Endometritis may progress to myometritis, parametritis, pelvic abscess, or peritonitis.

Table 15-1 summarizes the pathology, symptoms, and sonographic findings of PID.

SUMMARY

Sonographic examination of the female pelvis is performed to determine the extent of PID and to demonstrate the sequelae of the disease process. Sonography can follow the course of PID, enabling the physician to treat the disease successfully. Guidance for drainage procedures in the case of TOA or pelvic abscess can be provided with ultrasound imaging. Because of the severe pain often experienced with PID, a pelvic sonogram can be a challenging examination to perform. Sonographic appearances must be correlated with clinical and laboratory findings to provide a definitive sonographic diagnosis.

CLINICAL SCENARIO—DIAGNOSIS

Although the sonogram was limited in quality because of the inability of the patient to cooperate fully for the examination, a diagnosis of PID with bilateral TOA was made. The patient was treated with antibiotics, and follow-up sonograms revealed resolution of PID and bilateral TOA. Additional follow-up was recommended to determine whether the PID affected her fertility status.

TABLE 15-1 Pelvic Inflammatory Disease

Pathology	Symptoms	Sonographic Findings
Endometritis	Often asymptomatic; vaginal discharge, urethral burning, pelvic pain; patient history of cesarean section, IUD perforation, retained POC; STD	Normal uterus; uterine enlargement, thickened endometrium, air or fluid in endometrial cavity, hypoechoic halo around endometrium, ovarian enlargement with indistinct borders
Salpingitis	Subacute: no clinical symptoms	
	Acute: fever, chills, abdominal pain, nausea, vomiting, vaginal discharge, irregular vaginal bleeding, abdominal guarding, rebound tenderness, pain with manipulation of cervix, ectopic pregnancy	Subacute/acute: nodular thickening of fallopian tube walls with diverticula, hyperemia, anechoic or echogenic fluid in cul-de-sac, uterine enlargement, endometrial fluid or thickening
	Chronic: dyspareunia, painful bowel movements, infertility, ectopic pregnancy	Chronic: hydrosalpinx, cystic structures extending from uterus to adnexa
Pyosalpinx	Fever, chills, abdominal pain, nausea, vomiting, vaginal discharge, irregular vaginal bleeding, abdominal guarding, rebound tenderness, pain with manipulation of cervix	Swollen, thick-walled fallopian. tubes; echogenic debris within tubes; blurring of normal tissue planes
Hydrosalpinx	Asymptomatic or colicky pain	Dilated, thin-walled fallopian tubes filled with fluid
TOA	High fever, elevated WBC count, severe lower abdominal pain, nausea and vomiting, RUQ pain, peritonitis	Variable appearance; unilateral or bilateral thick-walled, complex hypoechoic mass in adnexa or cul-de-sac; mass with septations, irregular margins, fluid-debris levels; air within mass; free fluid in cul-de-sac and Morison's pouch; blurring of normal tissue planes

POC, Products of conception; *RUQ,* right upper quadrant; *STD,* sexually transmitted disease.

CASE STUDIES FOR DISCUSSION

1. A 20-year-old woman presents to the emergency department for the second time in 1 week complaining of severe pelvic pain. She was given a diagnosis of PID during the previous visit and prescribed a course of antibiotics. The patient states that she saw slight improvement after 3 or 4 days, but now the pain has become unbearable. Pelvic sonography is ordered to evaluate the pelvic organs as well as check for a potential abscess. On the transabdominal sonogram, there is enlargement of both ovaries, and a complex cystic mass is identified posterior to the uterus. The patient was premedicated with pain medication, and a limited endovaginal examination was performed, which confirmed the presence of a complex fluid collection posterior to the uterus (Fig. 15-10). The patient was subsequently admitted, administered intravenous antibiotics, and referred to a gynecologist. What is the most probable diagnosis?

2. A 29-year-old married woman presents to the emergency department for lower abdominal pain, cramping, and dysuria that has

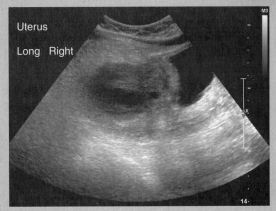

FIGURE 15-10 Abscess located posterior to the uterus and toward the right adnexa.

Continued

CASE STUDIES FOR DISCUSSION—cont'd

been present for 4 or 5 days. She states that she has had a low-grade fever "off and on" for a couple of days. During the pelvic examination, the physician notices a small amount of foul-smelling cervical discharge. Initial laboratory work shows an elevated WBC count and elevated ESR. Qualitative human chorionic gonadotropin is negative. On pelvic sonography, the endometrium appears mildly prominent, and the left adnexa appears prominent and complex. Endovaginal sonography was of limited value because of patient pain but was able to show hyperemia within the endometrium. It was also noted that the left ovary appeared separate from the adnexal mass (see Fig. 15-7). What is the most probable diagnosis?

3. A 27-year-old woman is seen in the emergency department for severe pelvic pain. She states that she has had pelvic discomfort since having an IUD placed by her gynecologist 2 weeks ago, but the pain has progressed over the 2 weeks and is now severe. A physical examination is limited by the patient's pain, and a pelvic sonogram is ordered. Transabdominal pelvic sonography is performed and shows an IUD centrally located within the endometrial canal. Transvaginal sonography is limited by patient pain but with the use of 3D technology clearly shows a normally placed IUD (Fig. 15-11). The uterus also appears slightly prominent with a thickened endometrium (Fig. 15-12). On transabdominal sonography, the ovarian volumes appear slightly prominent, and color Doppler shows some hyperemia. What is the most probable diagnosis?

4. Pelvic sonography is ordered for a 32-year-old woman who presents to her physician's office with mild, chronic pain in the right pelvis. The patient describes dyspareunia and occasional pain with bowel movements. She denies any nausea, vomiting, or fever. Laboratory test results reveal a negative qualitative human chorionic gonadotropin, normal blood work, and normal urinalysis. Transabdominal pelvic sonography shows a cystic area adjacent to the right ovary but no other abnormal findings. Transvaginal sonography is performed to evaluate the cystic structure better and shows a completely anechoic cystic area adjacent to but separate from the right ovary. The uterus and left ovary appear normal. What is the most probable diagnosis?

5. A 23-year-old woman is seen in the emergency department for pelvic pain. The patient's history and physical examination are limited by poor patient cooperation with obtaining accurate information. She is homeless with a history of polysubstance abuse; she was in her usual state of health up until 1 week ago when she developed severe pelvic pain and a foul-smelling vaginal discharge. On physical examination, there is lower abdominal guarding; the pelvic examination is limited by severe pelvic pain, but a foul-smelling discharge is noted. Laboratory test results reveal a negative qualitative human chorionic gonadotropin and an elevated WBC count. Pelvic sonography is ordered. Transabdominal examination shows a right complex-appearing adnexal mass, thickened endometrium, and free fluid in the cul-de-sac. The right adnexal mass and the uterus appear to have increased blood flow (Fig. 15-13). Limited endovaginal sonography was performed, owing to the patient's pain, but no additional information was obtained. What is the most probable diagnosis?

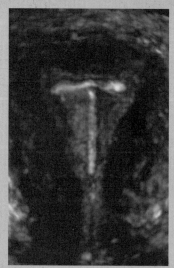

FIGURE 15-11 3D image of a properly positioned IUD.

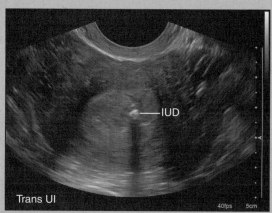

FIGURE 15-12 Transverse image of a thickened endometrium containing an IUD.

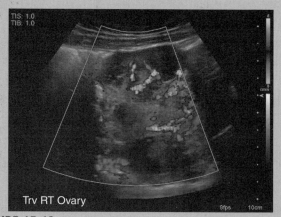

FIGURE 15-13 Color Doppler image of TOA showing increased blood flow (hyperemia).

STUDY QUESTIONS

1. An 18-year-old female college student presents to the emergency department with pelvic pain. Initial laboratory work shows an elevated WBC count, elevated ESR, negative human chorionic gonadotropin, and normal urinalysis. During a pelvic examination, the patient experiences severe pain with any manipulation of the cervix. Sonography of the pelvis was ordered for suspected PID. On transabdominal sonogram, the uterus and ovaries appear normal with no free fluid seen. The patient refused endovaginal sonography because of the pain. What is the likely diagnosis?
   a. Ruptured ovarian cyst
   b. PID is still likely, even with a normal transabdominal sonogram
   c. Acute pyosalpinx
   d. PID is not likely because the uterus and ovaries appear normal

2. A 28-year-old woman presents to the emergency department with increasing abdominal and pelvic pain. The patient states that she has been treated twice within the last year for PID, but she has not felt like this during the previous episodes. She thinks she may have a pelvic infection again, but she is also having pain in her right upper quadrant that is more severe when she coughs or moves. Sonography of the gallbladder appears normal. What is the likely diagnosis?
   a. Hepatitis
   b. Kidney stones
   c. Fitz-Hugh–Curtis syndrome
   d. Gallbladder disease

3. A 19-year-old woman is seen in her obstetrician's office 1 week after cesarean section. The cesarean section was urgent in nature and was performed at 27 weeks, 3 days gestational age for ruptured membranes, breech presentation, and extended period of fetal heart rate decelerations. The patient states that she has had increasing uterine tenderness over the last few days, which now is severe. She also says that she has had very minimal bleeding but a foul-smelling discharge and fever. The patient has no history of pelvic infections in the past. What is the most likely diagnosis?
   a. Hydrosalpinx
   b. Endometritis
   c. Normal postoperative changes
   d. PID

4. A pelvic sonogram is performed on a 33-year-old woman with pelvic pain. She describes the pain as a constant dull ache that seems to increase when standing. Transabdominal sonography shows an enlarged, fibroid uterus, normal ovaries, and bilateral cystic areas that appear to be tubular. What should the sonographer do next?
   a. Use color Doppler to see if the tubular structures are prominent veins
   b. Have the physician order laboratory work to see if she has PID
   c. Perform an endovaginal sonogram to evaluate the fibroid better
   d. Nothing because there is enough information

5. A 32-year-old woman is seen by her gynecologist in the office for pelvic pain. She describes the pain as chronic that comes and goes. On pelvic examination, there is fullness in the right adnexa. The patient has no history of PID or IUD use but has had previous surgery for an ovarian cyst. Endovaginal sonography shows a completely anechoic structure near the right ovary, but the uterus and ovaries appear normal. What is the most likely diagnosis?
   a. Corpus luteum cyst
   b. Ectopic pregnancy
   c. Endometriosis
   d. Peritoneal inclusion cyst

6. A mother brings her 15-year-old daughter to her pediatrician's office for increasing pelvic pain over the last few days. The mother is concerned that the daughter may have an ovarian cyst. While obtaining the patient's history, the patient seems hesitant to answer questions and seems elusive but does state that she had her appendix removed when she was 10 years old. After the pediatrician asks the mother to step out for a few minutes, the daughter states that she has been sexually active with a guy she met online a few months ago. A urine test is negative for pregnancy, but the patient's temperature is 100.7° F. What is the likely diagnosis?
   a. Hydrosalpinx
   b. Endometriosis
   c. Chronic PID
   d. Acute PID

7. A 28-year-old woman is seen in the emergency department for pelvic pain that has increased over the last 4 to 5 days. She states that she had an IUD placed by a physician in a clinic approximately 2 weeks ago and has had "problems" since then. While obtaining the patient's history, the patient says that she has had PID in the past but has not had any problems lately. On pelvic examination, the patient experiences severe pain with any movement of the cervix. Laboratory work shows an elevated WBC count and elevated ESR. What is the diagnosis?
   a. Adhesions from prior infections
   b. PID from an IUD placement
   c. Hydrosalpinx
   d. Endometriosis

8. A 26-year-old white woman presents to the emergency department with acute left lower quadrant and flank pain. The patient reports the pain was better when she laid still and worse with movement or sitting. She claims no sexual activity for the last few months. Initial laboratory work shows a WBC count of 20,550/μL with a shift to the left, and urinalysis is negative for red blood cells. A CT scan shows no evidence of a kidney stone but reveals bilateral cystic masses in the pelvis. Sonography shows a 4-cm right ovarian cyst and a left adnexal tubular structure with internal echoes and hyperemia. What is the most likely diagnosis?
   a. Endometriosis
   b. Ovarian torsion
   c. Appendicitis
   d. Acute left pyosalpinx

9. Pelvic sonography is requested for a 45-year-old, postmenopausal woman who has a history of chronic right pelvic discomfort. The patient states that she has a history of endometriosis but denies a history of PID. Sonography shows an anechoic tubular structure between the uterus and right ovary, but there are no signs of hyperemia. What is the most likely diagnosis?
   a. Ovarian torsion
   b. Right hydrosalpinx
   c. Ectopic pregnancy
   d. Right pyosalpinx

10. A 38-year-old woman presents to the emergency department complaining of intermittent right adnexal pain for the last 2 weeks. The pain became severe the night before following intercourse, but symptoms have slightly improved today. The patient states that she has a history of endometriosis. The pelvic examination reveals mild right adnexal tenderness. The right ovary appears normal on pelvic sonography, but a moderate amount of adjacent fluid with internal echoes is identified. Neither color nor spectral Doppler was performed. The report states suspicion of a right TOA, but the laboratory test results are normal. What is the most likely diagnosis?
   a. Ruptured endometrioma
   b. Acute right pyosalpinx
   c. Chronic right hydrosalpinx
   d. Right TOA

REFERENCES

1. Peri N, Graham D, Levine D: Imaging of intrauterine contraceptive device, *J Ultrasound Med* 26:1389–1401, 2007.
2. Jaiyeoba O, Soper DE: A practical approach to the diagnosis of pelvic inflammatory disease, *Infect Dis Obstet Gynecol* 2011: 753037, 2011.
3. Horrow MM: Ultrasound of pelvic inflammatory disease, *Ultrasound Q* 20:171–179, 2004.
4. Allison SO, Lev-Toaff AS: Acute pelvic pain: what we have learned from the ER, *Ultrasound Q* 26:211–218, 2010.
5. Guerriero S, Ajossa S, Mais V, et al: Role of transvaginal sonography in the diagnosis of peritoneal inclusion cysts, *J Ultrasound Med* 23:1193–1200, 2004.
6. Sudakoff GS, Lundeen SJ, Otterson MF: Transrectal and transvaginal sonographic intervention of infected pelvic fluid collections: a complete approach, *Ultrasound Q* 21:175–185, 2005.

Infertility

Daniel Breitkopf

An 18-year-old woman is seen for pelvic sonography with 1 week of severe pelvic pain and spotting. She is nauseated but not vomiting. A pregnancy test is ordered and is positive. The sonographic examination reveals the findings in Figures 16-1 and 16-2. What is the most likely diagnosis for this patient?

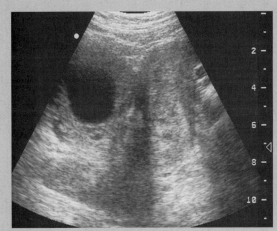

FIGURE 16-2 Two horns are identified. The horn on the right has a gestational sac.

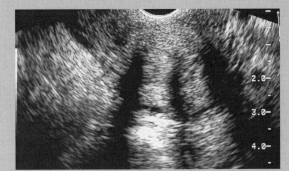

FIGURE 16-1 Transverse image demonstrating two cervices.

OBJECTIVES

- List and describe the ovarian factors that can lead to infertility.
- Differentiate the sonographic appearances of ovarian causes of infertility.
- Describe the normal embryologic development of the uterus.

- Identify various congenital uterine anomalies.
- Describe the sonographic features that differentiate the types of congenital uterine anomalies.
- Discuss the role of sonography in evaluating the ovaries and endometrium during assisted reproductive technology procedures.

Pelvic sonography may be used in the identification of various causes of infertility. Many abnormalities may be found incidentally because the patient is asymptomatic. Clinical examinations and correlative imaging procedures may assist in a definitive diagnosis so that treatment, surgery, or pregnancy options can be explored.

This chapter discusses factors linked with infertility that may be identified sonographically. The most common ovarian factors linked with infertility are explored, and differentiations of congenital uterine anomalies are discussed. Tubal factors associated with infertility are discussed in Chapter 15.

ENDOMETRIOSIS

Endometriosis is the result of functioning endometrial tissue being located outside the uterus. The condition is hormonally stimulated during the reproductive years and can affect 25% to 35% of infertile women.[1,2] Besides infertility, symptoms of endometriosis include pelvic pain, dyspareunia, abnormal uterine bleeding, and dysmenorrhea; however, some patients may be asymptomatic. Endometriosis can be localized or diffuse. The ovaries are the most common place for endometriosis to occur, although endometrial implants may be located anywhere in the body. Endometriosis can be treated medically, with

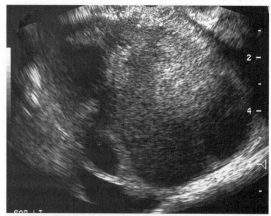

FIGURE 16-3 Transvaginal image of endometrioma.

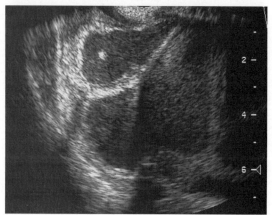

FIGURE 16-4 Endometrioma.

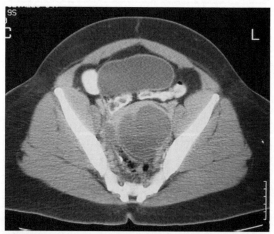

FIGURE 16-5 Computed tomography scan of endometrioma.

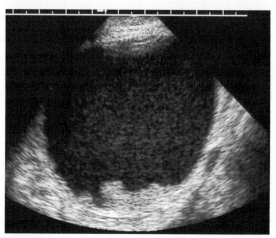

FIGURE 16-6 Transvaginal image of left ovarian endometrioma with internal debris.

hormones or hormone suppression therapy, or surgically, depending on the extent of disease and the desired outcome. The purpose of treatment may be to decrease or alleviate symptoms of pain associated with endometriosis or to improve the chances of pregnancy with removal of endometrial implants that may be impeding ovulation or obstructing fallopian tubes. Surgery is the better option if endometriosis is moderate to severe, although recurrence of the disease is possible. Patients who no longer desire fertility may elect hysterectomy and bilateral salpingo-oophorectomy to decrease symptoms of the disease.

Sonographic Findings

The localized form of endometriosis, endometrioma, appears as a mass involving the ovary and is also known as a chocolate cyst. The classic sonographic appearance is a well-defined, thin-walled mass containing low-level, internal echoes with through transmission. Endometriomas can be unilocular or multilocular and are frequently multiple in number. Other sonographic appearances include masses with thick walls, internal septations, or fluid/debris levels in the dependent portion of the lesion (Figs. 16-3 to 16-8). Endometriomas are most easily characterized transvaginally with better definition of the

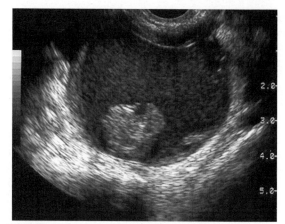

FIGURE 16-7 Endometrioma with complex appearance.

degree of internal echoes compared with transabdominal scanning. Endometrioma is also discussed in Chapter 17.

The diffuse form of endometriosis is more difficult to evaluate because the implants of diffuse endometriosis are usually too small to be seen. Endometriosis may be suggested when the tissue planes between the pelvic

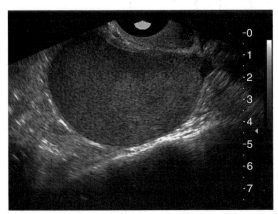

FIGURE 16-8 Endometrioma completely filled with internal echoes.

structures blend indistinctly as the result of adhesions. When the focal form is not visualized, sonographic examination is usually nondiagnostic.

POLYCYSTIC OVARIAN SYNDROME

Polycystic ovarian syndrome (PCOS) is an endocrine disorder that produces anovulation and results in infertility. Women with PCOS often have high levels of androgen hormones and may be resistant to the effect of insulin. Among women with PCOS, 80% are obese and are at risk for development of diabetes.[3,4]

PCOS is a cause for infertility in approximately 6% of women of reproductive age. Clinical symptoms include infertility, early pregnancy loss, hirsutism, acne, and amenorrhea; however, some patients with PCOS have no symptoms. The diagnosis is generally made with evaluation of the clinical presentation and hormone levels; sonographic criteria also are helpful in confirming the condition (Box 16-1). In addition, patients with PCOS may incur the risks associated with unopposed estrogen and may be monitored for endometrial carcinoma and breast cancer.

Sonographic Findings

Sonographic examination of PCOS may reveal bilateral ovaries that contain multiple small follicles. The follicles are usually located in the periphery of the ovary and are 0.5 to 0.9 cm in size. The follicles produce a sonographic appearance of a "string of pearls" (Figs. 16-9 and 16-10). The ovaries also have an increase in stromal echogenicity (Fig. 16-11). The size of the ovaries may be normal or enlarged. Sonographic criteria for diagnosis of PCOS include presence of 12 or more follicles measuring 2 to 9 mm or increased ovarian volume greater than 10 mL.[3,4]

CONGENITAL UTERINE ANOMALIES

Congenital uterine anomalies can be a contributing factor in infertility and adverse pregnancy outcomes. The uterus and fallopian tubes develop from paired müllerian

BOX 16-1	2003 Rotterdam Consensus Diagnostic Criteria for Polycystic Ovarian Syndrome

Two of three of the following are required for the diagnosis of PCOS:
1. Oligoovulation or anovulation
2. Clinical or biochemical signs of hyperandrogenism
3. Polycystic ovaries: ≥12 follicles measuring ≤9 mm, ovarian volume >10 mL, or both

From Rotterdam ESHRE/ASRM-Sponsored PCOS Consensus Workshop Group: Revised 2003 consensus on diagnostic criteria and long-term health risks related to polycystic ovary syndrome, *Fertil Steril* 81:19-25, 2004.

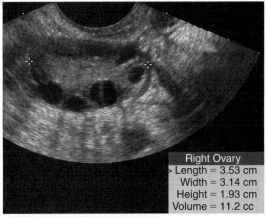

Right Ovary
Length = 3.53 cm
Width = 3.14 cm
Height = 1.93 cm
Volume = 11.2 cc

FIGURE 16-9 Polycystic ovary with a volume of 11.2 mL.

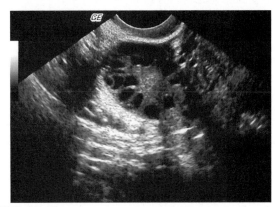

FIGURE 16-10 Transvaginal image of polycystic ovary showing "string of pearls."

ducts that fuse, and then the uterine septum formed from the fusion is reabsorbed. Development of the uterus occurs between 7 and 12 weeks of gestation.[5] Anomalies that occur may be caused by failure of development of one or both of the müllerian ducts (uterine agenesis, unicornuate uterus), failure of fusion of the müllerian ducts (uterus didelphys, bicornuate uterus), or failure of the sagittal septum to reabsorb (Fig. 16-12). Septate uteri are associated with infertility, miscarriage, preterm birth, and fetal malpresentation (e.g., breech). Unicornuate, bicornuate, and didelphic uteri are associated with preterm birth and fetal malpresentation.[6]

The development of the uterus is closely associated with the development of the excretory system. When a uterine anomaly is identified, the kidneys should also be evaluated for the presence of congenital anomalies, such as unilateral renal agenesis or renal ectopia.

Sonographic identification and differentiation of uterine anomalies can be difficult because imaging the uterus in the coronal plane best shows the uterine cavity and the shape of the fundus. Careful transducer angulation may attain this view, but when available, three-dimensional ultrasound imaging can be used to acquire this plane. Identification of the endometrium is also easier when patients undergo imaging in the secretory phase of the menstrual cycle when the endometrium is thick and echogenic. Three-dimensional multiplanar imaging is useful for evaluating the uterine fundal contour, which is helpful in differentiating between septate and bicornuate uteri as noted subsequently.

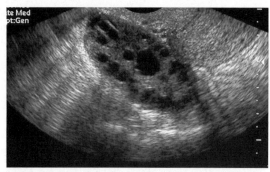

FIGURE 16-11 Ovary with increased echogenicity containing multiple, tiny follicles.

Uterus Didelphys

Uterus didelphys is a rare, complete duplication of the uterus, cervix, and vagina that results from the complete failure of the müllerian ducts to fuse together. Both uteri may be similar in size, or one may be smaller than the other. The vaginal duplication may result in one smaller vagina (hemivagina) opening within the other vagina, so this anomaly may not be identified on external visual inspection. The condition can be associated with unilateral hematocolpos. The symptoms associated with uterus didelphys when the hemivagina is obstructed include dysmenorrhea beginning shortly after menarche, progressive pelvic pain after menses, and a unilateral pelvic mass.

Sonographic Findings.   The sonographic appearance of uterus didelphys is of two separate endometrial echo complexes. A deep fundal notch is present, separated widely with a full complement of myometrium (Figs. 16-13 to 16-16). Two cervices and vaginas should be visualized. The initial impression of uterus didelphys may suggest a normal uterus with an adjacent pelvic mass, especially if the uteri are asymmetric. This appearance is related to an obstructed hemivagina causing hematocolpos or hematometracolpos.

Bicornuate Uterus

Bicornuate uterus is a duplication of the uterus entering one cervix or two cervices, with only one vagina. This results from partial fusion of the müllerian ducts during embryologic development. Bicornis bicollis describes the duplication of both cervix and uterus. Bicornis unicollis describes the duplication of the uterus without

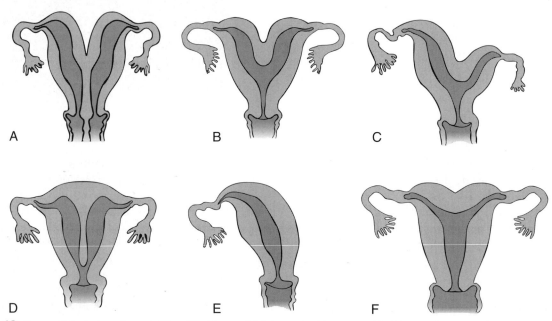

FIGURE 16-12 Congenital uterine abnormalities. **(A),** Uterus didelphys—double uterus. **(B),** Bicornuate uterus. **(C),** Bicornuate uterus with rudimentary left horn. **(D),** Septate uterus. **(E),** Unicornuate uterus. **(F),** Arcuate uterus.

duplication of the cervix; the cervix fuses normally, and the fundus fails to fuse. Fertility problems can occur when one of the cornua does not communicate and is rudimentary.

Sonographic Findings. Sonographic examination of a bicornuate uterus shows a deep fundal notch. The endometrial echoes appear as two different complexes widely separated; this gives the same appearance as uterus didelphys in the fundal region (Figs. 16-17 to 16-21). Bicornuate uterus and uterus didelphys can be differentiated with the identification of duplication of the vaginal canal, which is evident in uterus didelphys.

Septate Uterus

Septate uterus is the most common congenital uterine abnormality. It is the result of a failure in reabsorption of the median septum. Fusion of the müllerian ducts occurs. This process leaves the uterine cavity completely separated by a thin septum known as uterus septus or a partially reabsorbed septum known as uterus subseptus.

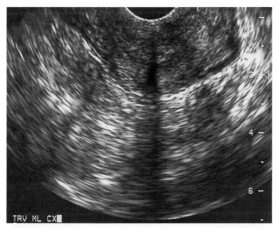

FIGURE 16-13 Transverse image showing two cervices.

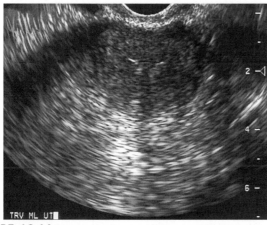

FIGURE 16-14 Transverse image of lower uterine segment with uterus didelphys.

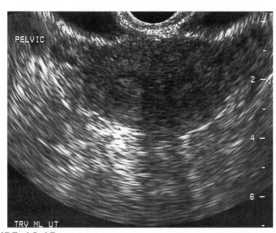

FIGURE 16-15 Transverse image at level of uterine corpus that shows uterus didelphys.

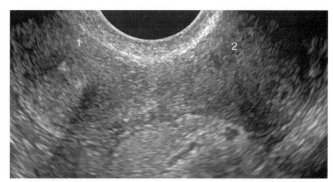

FIGURE 16-16 Two fundal horns shown in uterus didelphys.

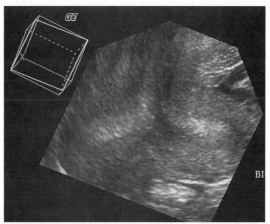

FIGURE 16-17 Three-dimensional image of bicornuate uterus. *(Courtesy GE Medical Systems.)*

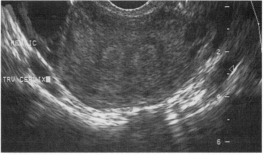

FIGURE 16-18 Transverse image of cervical region in a patient with uterus bicornis bicollis.

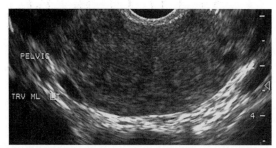

FIGURE 16-19 Transverse image of bicornuate uterus at level of uterine corpus.

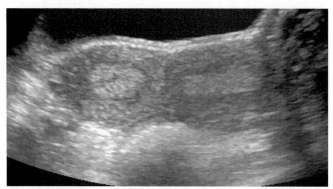

FIGURE 16-20 Transverse image shows bicornuate uterus near fundal region. Note widely separated endometria.

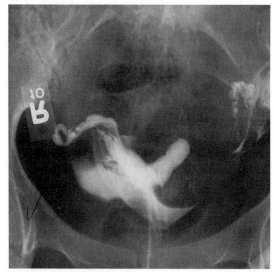

FIGURE 16-21 Hysterosalpingogram shows bicornuate uterus.

The presence of the anomaly leads to fertility problems; however, when the condition is identified, treatment is available. Patients with this defect can have the septum removed via hysteroscopy. Use of three-dimensional pelvic ultrasound or magnetic resonance imaging to determine whether the abnormality is actually a septate uterus is very important.

Sonographic Findings. The sonographic appearance of a septate uterus shows a convex, flat, or minimally indented fundal contour.[7] Two endometrial echoes

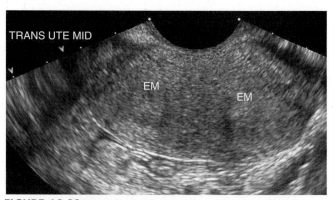

FIGURE 16-22 Transverse transvaginal image of fundus in a septate uterus.

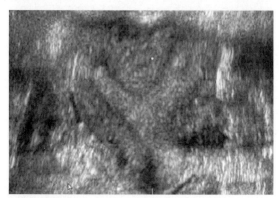

FIGURE 16-23 Three-dimensional image of septate uterus.

appear close together because they are separated only by a thin septum, which is best demonstrated with three-dimensional imaging (Figs. 16-22 and 16-23).

Arcuate Uterus

Arcuate uterus is the mildest congenital uterine anomaly. It represents a minor lack of fusion of the fundal region that results in a slight depression in that area. The endometrium is fairly normal, which is why this anomaly is considered a normal variant. The clinical significance of an arcuate uterus is a matter of debate. Some studies do not support an increase in the incidence of adverse reproductive outcomes for women with an arcuate uterus.[8]

Sonographic Findings. Arcuate uterus is difficult to diagnose sonographically. The uterus appears normal with a subtle fundal indentation, and the uterine cavity is slightly concave (Fig. 16-24).

Table 16-1 summarizes the sonographic findings of uterine anomalies.

SONOGRAPHIC MONITORING OF ASSISTED REPRODUCTIVE TECHNOLOGY CYCLES

Sonography plays a key role in the evaluation and management of infertility treatment. Depending on

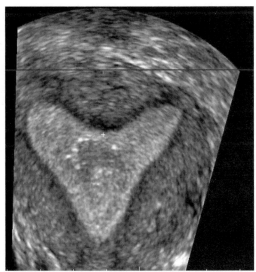

FIGURE 16-24 Three-dimensional image of arcuate uterus with slight indentation of the endometrium.

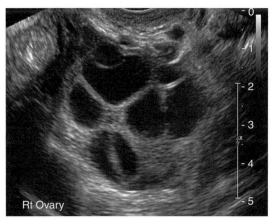

FIGURE 16-25 Image of the ovary after stimulation with gonadotropins.

TABLE 16-1	Congenital Uterine Anomalies	
Uterine Anomalies	**Development**	**Sonographic Findings**
Uterine didelphys	Complete failure of müllerian ducts to fuse	Two separate endometrial echoes, two cervices, and two vaginas
Bicornuate uterus	Müllerian ducts only partially fused	Two separate endometrial echoes, one or two cervices, and one vagina
Septate uterus	Müllerian ducts fuse with failure of reabsorption of median septum	Two close endometrial echoes
Arcuate uterus	Only minor lack of fusion of uterus in fundal region	One normal endometrial echo with slight fundal indentation

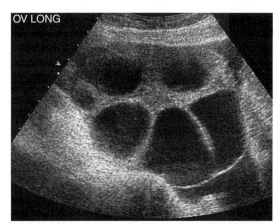

FIGURE 16-26 Hyperstimulated ovary with large theca lutein cysts.

the specific cause for infertility, treatment may include ovarian stimulation to induce ovulation, intrauterine insemination, or in vitro fertilization (IVF). Stimulation of the ovaries is often monitored with serum estradiol levels and transvaginal sonography to determine follicle size and number. This information is used to help decide when to induce ovulation or harvest the oocytes in the case of an IVF cycle.

During IVF, the ovaries are stimulated to produce multiple follicles with gonadotropin medications, usually comprising follicle-stimulating hormone. The ovaries are monitored for follicle size and number during stimulation by transvaginal sonography (Fig. 16-25). When the follicles reach maturity (17 to 18 mm in diameter), the oocytes are harvested using a transvaginally guided needle aspiration procedure. Fertilization occurs in the laboratory, and the embryos are transferred to the uterus via a transcervically placed catheter under transabdominal ultrasound guidance.

Ovarian Hyperstimulation Syndrome

Ovarian hyperstimulation syndrome is a serious complication that can result from stimulation of the ovaries for induction of ovulation. The ovaries massively enlarge with multiple luteinized follicles, called theca lutein cysts (Fig. 16-26), caused by excessive human chorionic gonadotropin levels. Ascites and pleural effusions may develop and lead to hypovolemia, hypotension, and impaired renal function. Patients may become critically ill and need care in an intensive care unit. The disease is usually self-limited, and withdrawal of the stimulation medications and supportive care allow for resolution.

SUMMARY

Pelvic sonography combined with an accurate patient history and physical examination plays a vital role in the diagnosis of possible causes of infertility and other symptoms. Three-dimensional ultrasound scanning techniques may improve the accuracy of diagnosis of congenital uterine anomalies by allowing easier access to the coronal plane of the uterus for better visualization of the contour of the fundal region. When abnormalities are confirmed, surgical and medical treatment options may be available to increase the chances for successful pregnancy.

CLINICAL SCENARIO—DIAGNOSIS

The sonographic findings are consistent with duplication of the cervix and uterus. Additional conversation with the patient reveals that she had a hemivagina, which would be consistent with uterus didelphys. A gestational sac is revealed in the right horn without evidence of a live embryo or yolk sac, consistent with her last menstrual period, which was 9 weeks prior. Quantitative pregnancy tests confirm a failed pregnancy.

CASE STUDIES FOR DISCUSSION

1. A 14-year-old girl presents with acute pain in her left lower abdomen following menses. Her periods began 6 months ago. She recently became sexually active. Transvaginal sonography (transverse plane image shown) demonstrates a normal uterus with a mass on the left side of the pelvis (Fig. 16-27). The left ovary is noted to be separate from the mass. What is the most likely cause for her pain?

2. A 33-year-old woman presents with a history of three first-trimester miscarriages. She and her husband are frustrated with the recurrent pregnancy losses and are seeking answers as to the potential cause. Pelvic sonography was performed as part of the evaluation and a coronal image was obtained using three-dimensional multiplanar rendering (Fig. 16-28). The fundal contour is normal. What is the most likely diagnosis?

3. A 23-year-old woman presented with a history of 3 years of increasingly painful periods. She also noted worsening pain with intercourse. She has never been pregnant despite several years of unprotected intercourse with her husband. She was sent for sonography after her gynecologist palpated a mass to the right of her uterus. The image of the mass is shown in Figure 16-29. What is the most likely cause for the mass and her symptoms?

4. A 28-year-old woman has irregular menstrual periods and excessive hair growth on her chin and lip. She has had irregular periods since age 12 when she started menstruating. She is overweight and has never conceived despite unprotected intercourse for 1 year. Her physician orders a pelvic sonogram; the right ovarian findings are shown in Figure 16-30. The left ovary has a similar appearance. What is the most likely cause for the abnormal appearance of the ovaries?

5. A 27-year-old woman has a history of two pregnancies complicated by breech deliveries. At her last delivery by cesarean section, the physician told her that the uterus appeared abnormal. She is 3 months postpartum and is sent for a sonogram. The uterine findings are shown in Figure 16-31. Which uterine anomaly is present in this patient?

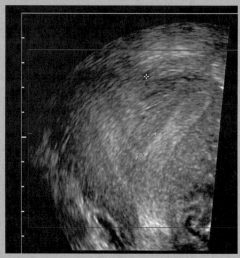

FIGURE 16-28 Uterus visualized with three-dimensional sonography in the true coronal plane.

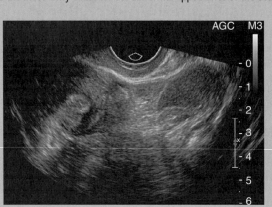

FIGURE 16-27 Transverse image of the uterus and left pelvic mass that is separate from the ovary.

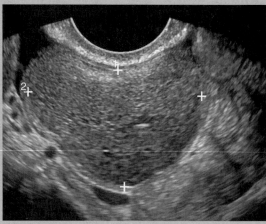

FIGURE 16-29 Transvaginal image of right adnexal mass.

CASE STUDIES FOR DISCUSSION—cont'd

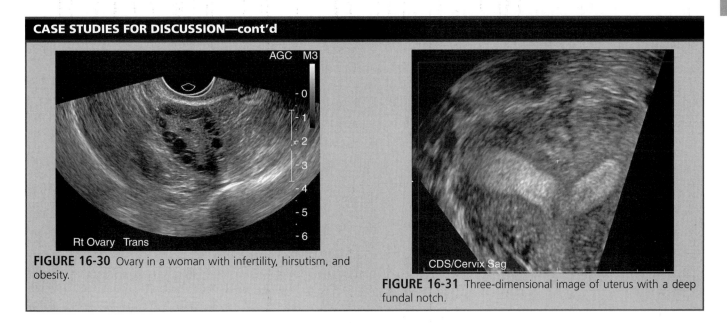

FIGURE 16-30 Ovary in a woman with infertility, hirsutism, and obesity.

FIGURE 16-31 Three-dimensional image of uterus with a deep fundal notch.

STUDY QUESTIONS

1. A 31-year-old woman with irregular menses and infertility presents for pelvic sonography. The ovaries have eight follicles measuring 3 to 6 mm in diameter. The most likely reason for this sonographic finding is:
   a. Ectopic pregnancy
   b. Endometriosis
   c. PCOS
   d. Pelvic inflammatory disease

2. A 13-year-old girl started menses 6 months ago and has cyclic pain on the left side during menses. On the sonogram, an endometrial echo is present in addition to a thick-walled oblong mass attached to the uterus on the left side. What is the most likely diagnosis?
   a. Uterus didelphys
   b. Septate uterus
   c. Endometrioma
   d. Bicornuate uterus

3. A 26-year-old woman has abnormal hair growth on her chin and elevated serum testosterone levels. Her last menses were 2 years ago. Her urine pregnancy test was negative. On transvaginal sonography, both ovaries are enlarged, measuring greater than 15 mL in volume. What is the most likely cause for her symptoms and sonographic findings?
   a. Endometriosis
   b. Pelvic inflammatory disease
   c. Uterus didelphys
   d. PCOS

4. A 22-year-old woman with irregular menses presents for a transvaginal sonogram. The right ovary contains 15 follicles in the periphery measuring 3 to 6 mm in diameter. The left ovary and the uterus appear normal. The sonographic findings are compatible with:
   a. Endometriosis
   b. Ectopic pregnancy
   c. PCOS
   d. Rudimentary uterine horn

5. For evaluation of infertility, three-dimensional ultrasound of the pelvis has the most utility for the diagnosis of:
   a. Endometriosis
   b. Septate uteri
   c. PCOS
   d. Rudimentary uterine horn

6. A 27-year-old woman with recurrent miscarriages presents for a pelvic sonogram. Sonography reveals a subtle fundal indentation on the uterus with a slightly concave uterine cavity. These findings are associated with which uterine anomaly?
   a. Arcuate uterus
   b. Septate uterus
   c. Bicornuate uterus
   d. Uterus didelphys

7. A 37-year-old woman is undergoing IVF. After receiving gonadotropins, her physician orders a transvaginal sonogram. The purpose for this sonogram is to:
   a. Measure follicle size
   b. Ascertain uterine version
   c. Calculate ovarian volume
   d. Guide embryo transfer

8. Which uterine anomaly is always characterized by two cervices and two vaginas?
   a. Bicornuate uterus
   b. Uterus didelphys
   c. Septate uterus
   d. Arcuate uterus

9. A 30-year-old woman with pelvic pain and dyspareunia presents for a pelvic sonogram. Sonography demonstrates a thin-walled cystic mass with low-level internal echoes and through transmission in the left adnexa. The right ovary and uterus appear normal. What is the most likely diagnosis?
   a. Hydrosalpinx
   b. Rudimentary uterine horn
   c. Follicular ovarian cyst
   d. Endometrioma

10. A 28-year-old woman with dysmenorrhea since age 14 comes in for a pelvic sonogram. A right ovarian cyst is seen with thick walls and a fluid/debris level. This same mass was seen sonographically 3 months ago. It is tender on imaging with the vaginal probe. What is the most likely diagnosis?
   a. Follicular cyst
   b. Hemorrhagic corpus luteum
   c. Endometrioma
   d. Hydrosalpinx

REFERENCES

1. Falcone T, Lebovic D: Clinical management of endometriosis, *Obstet Gynecol* 118:691–705, 2011.
2. American College of Obstetricians and Gynecologists: Management of endometriosis. ACOG Practice Bulletin No. 114, *Obstet Gynecol* 116:223–236, 2010.
3. American College of Obstetricians and Gynecologists: Polycystic ovary syndrome. ACOG Practice Bulletin No. 108, *Obstet Gynecol* 114:936–949, 2009.
4. Rotterdam ESHRE/ASRM-Sponsored PCOS Consensus Workshop Group: Revised 2003 consensus on diagnostic criteria and long-term health risks related to polycystic ovary syndrome, *Fertil Steril* 81:19–25, 2004.
5. Olpin J, Heilbrun M: Imaging of Müllerian duct anomalies, *Clin Obstet Gynecol* 52:40–56, 2009.
6. Chan Y, Jayaprakasan K, Tan A, et al: Reproductive outcomes in women with congenital uterine anomalies: a systematic review, *Ultrasound Obstet Gynecol* 38:371–382, 2011.
7. Homer H, Li T, Cooke I: The septate uterus: a review of management and reproductive outcome, *Fertil Steril* 73:1–14, 2000.
8. Mucowski S, Herndon C, Rosen M: The arcuate uterine anomaly: a critical appraisal of its diagnostic and clinical relevance, *Obstet Gynecol Surv* 65:449–454, 2010.

17

Ovarian Mass

Diane J. Youngs, Douglas L. Brown

CLINICAL SCENARIO

A 21-year-old woman who is 10 weeks pregnant presents to the emergency department with acute pelvic pain. The physician palpates a pelvic mass adjacent to the uterus and orders a pelvic sonogram. Transabdominal sonography of the uterus reveals a viable 10-week gestation with no evidence of subchorionic hemorrhage. Gray-scale, pulsed, and color Doppler imaging of the adnexa reveal the findings in Figure 17-1 (see Color Plate 12). What is the most likely diagnosis for these findings?

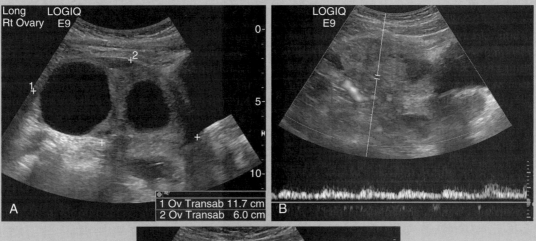

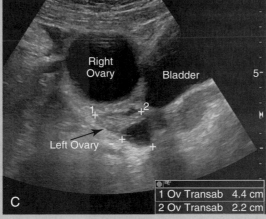

FIGURE 17-1 (A), Longitudinal sonogram of right ovary measuring 11.7 cm × 6.0 cm. **(B),** Doppler imaging of right ovary. **(C),** Longitudinal view of left ovary *(arrow)* measuring 4.4 cm × 2.2 cm.

OBJECTIVES

- Describe normal ovarian anatomy and function.
- Describe the sonographic features of benign ovarian masses.
- Describe the sonographic features of malignant ovarian masses.
- Identify factors useful in differentiation of ovarian masses.

Pelvic sonography plays an important role in the detection and evaluation of ovarian masses. Although many ovarian masses are found incidentally, indications that may prompt a sonographic evaluation to assess for an ovarian mass include pelvic pain, pelvic fullness, palpable mass, or a family history of ovarian or breast cancer.

Ovarian cancer usually produces nonspecific symptoms. In more than 70% of patients, malignant ovarian disease is diagnosed during the later stages, which significantly reduces the survival rate.[1] Although early detection may improve survival, reliable ovarian cancer screening for the general population has not yet been developed. The most widely used serum tumor marker for epithelial ovarian cancer is cancer antigen 125 (CA 125). If a woman's serum concentration of CA 125 is elevated, transvaginal sonography may be performed to assess for an ovarian mass. Only 50% to 60% of women with stage 1 epithelial ovarian cancer have elevated serum levels, and other benign conditions can elevate serum concentrations of CA 125 as well.[2] The resultant low sensitivity and specificity limit the value of this test in detecting ovarian cancer. A combination of CA 125 testing with transvaginal sonography is sometimes performed as a screening method in women at high risk of having ovarian cancer.[2]

Despite the poor prognosis in most patients diagnosed with ovarian cancer, the lack of complete understanding of the pathogenesis of ovarian cancer, the increasingly recognized occurrence of interval cancers (cancers detected within a year after a negative screening test), and the high proportion of ovarian masses that are benign all make screening difficult. Multicenter trials are ongoing, and the results of these trials should provide useful information to determine whether screening is beneficial. Screening is not recommended for the general population at the present time.[3] Women with a higher risk because of family history or known *BRCA1* or *BRCA2* (breast cancer gene) mutations may request sonographic screening, but even in these women, no benefit from screening has yet been shown.[3]

A variety of ovarian masses are examined in this chapter, including benign and malignant masses. Specific sonographic features of the mass can usually help determine the most likely diagnosis or significantly narrow the list of likely diagnoses, and this helps in determining treatment options. Although only pathology after surgical removal can determine the diagnosis with certainty, a sonographic diagnosis of an ovarian mass can often be strongly suggested based on morphologic features, Doppler findings, clinical signs and symptoms, and the age of the patient. To understand better how all of these factors contribute to a differential diagnosis, it is helpful to review ovarian anatomy and physiology and key sonographic observations to be made when evaluating ovarian masses.

NORMAL OVARIAN ANATOMY AND PHYSIOLOGY

Anatomy

The ovaries are almond-shaped intraperitoneal endocrine organs that are composed of cortical and medullary tissue covered by epithelium. The ovarian cortex is the site of follicular development, and the medulla is the vascular core of the ovary. The ovary is supplied with blood from two sources: the ovarian artery arising from the aorta and the ovarian branch of the uterine artery.

Although the ovaries are attached to the uterus by the ovarian ligament and to the infundibulum of the fallopian tube and pelvic side wall by the suspensory ligament, the ovaries are relatively mobile organs that typically reside in the adnexa anterior to the internal iliac vessels and medial to the external iliac vessels. Ovarian size varies with a woman's menstrual status and age; mean ovarian volume is approximately 3.0 cm^3 in premenarchal girls, 10 cm^3 in menarchal women, and 6.0 cm^3 in postmenopausal women.[4]

Ovarian follicles contain the oogonia, and the appearance of these follicles depends on the stage of their development. Multiple follicles begin maturation, but ultimately a single follicle called a dominant or graafian follicle matures until it reaches a size of 2.0 to 2.5 cm before ovulation causes it to rupture. After ovulation, the collapsed follicle transforms into a corpus luteum.

Physiology

Follicular development is influenced by follicle-stimulating hormone (FSH) and luteinizing hormone (LH), which are gonadotropins produced by the pituitary gland. FSH stimulates follicular development within the ovaries. As the follicle matures, it secretes estrogen, which stimulates endometrial growth and proliferation. Around day 14 of the menstrual cycle, increased levels of estrogen provide a negative feedback mechanism to the pituitary gland causing it to stop secreting FSH and begin production of LH. The follicular phase of the ovarian cycle refers to the events leading to ovulation.

Around day 14 of the menstrual cycle, a surge of LH stimulates ovulation. Continued LH production promotes development and maintenance of the corpus luteum, which promotes and maintains a secretory endometrium. The corpus luteum secretes estrogen and progesterone, which stimulate glandular changes within the endometrium necessary for supporting an early pregnancy. If pregnancy does not occur within approximately 9 days, LH production ceases, and the corpus luteum regresses into a structure known as the corpus albicans. Persistence of the corpus luteum may delay menstruation or cause abnormal bleeding from continued progesterone production. The postovulatory period is known as the luteal phase.

Normal Sonographic Appearance

The ovaries are homogeneous in texture, with an echogenicity similar to that of the uterus and hypoechoic to surrounding bowel (Fig. 17-2). Anechoic follicles may be seen in the ovarian periphery, and the vascular medulla may appear echogenic compared with the cortex. The dominant follicle typically reaches 2.0 to 2.5 cm in size; however, it can reach 2.8 cm. Simple cysts seen within the ovary that measure less than 3.0 cm are assumed to be ovarian follicles.

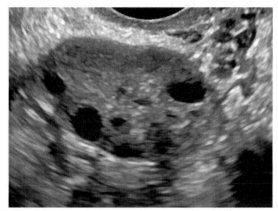

FIGURE 17-2 Normal menarchal ovary containing several small follicles.

The corpus luteum forms from the ruptured dominant follicle, and luteinization is made possible by the development of numerous capillaries and a rich blood supply. Hemorrhage into the corpus luteum is very common, resulting in a hemorrhagic corpus luteum. The corpus luteum remains intact until about week 12 of a pregnancy or until day 23 of the menstrual cycle if pregnancy does not occur. The sonographic appearance of a corpus luteum is variable, but the corpus luteum is often irregular in shape with a thick wall that may be crenulated (Fig. 17-3, A and B). The corpus luteum is often highly vascular with abundant flow evident on color Doppler imaging (Fig. 17-3, C; see Color Plate 13). It is a normal structure and should not be misinterpreted as pathology.

After menopause, the ovaries atrophy and are frequently devoid of follicles, which make them difficult to identify. Postmenopausal women may occasionally have small cysts or residual follicles; generally, a simple cyst less than 1 cm can be ignored in postmenopausal women.[5]

KEY SONOGRAPHIC OBSERVATIONS

When an adnexal mass is discovered during sonographic evaluation, the location, echotexture, size of the mass, and any associated findings such as ascites should be documented. Determining whether a mass is cystic, solid, or complex (a nonspecific term generally used to denote

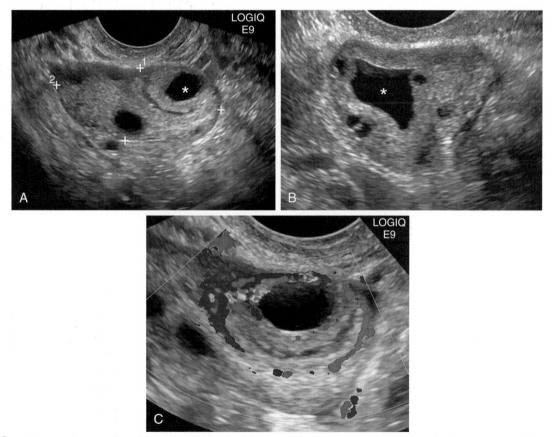

FIGURE 17-3 (A), Corpus luteum *(asterisk)* with thick walls. **(B),** Corpus luteum *(asterisk)* with crenulated appearance. **(C),** Color Doppler image demonstrating flow around highly vascular corpus luteum.

a combination of cystic and solid components) requires observation of the following: acoustic enhancement or attenuation, the presence of internal echoes by optimized gain and frequency, loculation, thickness and regularity of any septations, and whether solid components represent tissue versus blood or debris, which can be determined by applying color or power Doppler imaging. One also needs to consider nonovarian causes for findings such as tuboovarian abscess, pyosalpinx or hydrosalpinx (see Chapter 15), ectopic pregnancy (see Chapter 21), or pedunculated fibroid (see Chapter 13).

Besides the sonographic findings, the patient's age, menstrual status, symptoms, and family history need to be considered. Women in their reproductive years are much more likely to present with benign ovarian pathology, whereas postmenopausal women and women of reproductive age with a family history of ovarian or breast cancer are at higher risk for malignant ovarian pathology. Most ovarian masses found sonographically are benign. A complex-appearing ovarian mass in a woman during her reproductive years usually represents a hemorrhagic physiologic cyst, whereas a solid adnexal mass is more likely to be a pedunculated fibroid than a malignant ovarian tumor. However, a complex-appearing ovarian mass in a postmenopausal woman is more worrisome for ovarian malignancy. Many appearances can result in a complex adnexal mass, and it is important to identify specific sonographic features that the physician can use to make a likely diagnosis.

Many benign ovarian masses do not demonstrate sonographic evidence of vascularity in the internal components by Doppler imaging. Color Doppler imaging demonstrates peripheral flow around a simple cyst, a hemorrhagic cyst, an endometrioma, or cystic teratoma, but vascularity is not evident within the internal components. When the solid-appearing components of an ovarian mass demonstrate vascularity on color Doppler imaging, a benign or malignant neoplastic process must be considered. Table 17-1

TABLE 17-1	Benign and Malignant Characteristics of Ovarian Masses	
Benign Characteristics	**Malignant Characteristics**
Purely cystic	Complex with thick septations
Findings consistent with hemorrhagic cyst, endometrioma, or cystic teratoma	Complex with mural nodules or other solid areas not typical of a dermoid
No internal flow by Doppler imaging	Ascites (more than normal small amount often seen in premenopausal women)
Complex mass is thin walled, has thin septations, no papillary projections or other solid areas	Solid components of mass demonstrate vascularity on color Doppler imaging
Benign solid masses tend to demonstrate mild to no vascularity	

presents sonographic characteristics associated with benign and malignant ovarian masses.

The sonographic appearance of adnexal masses can occasionally be confusing. Hemorrhage can make a cystic mass appear complex or solid, whereas a solid mass may produce attenuation that obscures the borders of the mass. There are well-established findings associated with ovarian masses that make it possible to offer a differential diagnosis based on the patient's clinical history and the sonographic appearance of the mass. For indeterminant masses, other imaging modalities such as magnetic resonance imaging (MRI) may be used.

FUNCTIONAL OR PHYSIOLOGIC OVARIAN CYSTS

If an ovarian follicle or corpus luteum fails to regress, it can continue to fill with fluid and result in a functional or physiologic cyst. The term "functional cyst" means that the cyst is ovarian in origin and responds to cyclic hormonal changes. The functional ovarian cysts discussed in this chapter are follicular cysts and hemorrhagic cysts. Theca lutein cysts are functional cysts related to human chorionic gonadotropin exposure and are discussed in Chapter 16.

Follicular Cyst

Follicular cysts are one of the most common causes of ovarian enlargement in young women. They occur when a dominant follicle fails either to ovulate or to regress. Anechoic cystic spaces within the ovary are assumed to be follicles and are referred to as a "cyst" only when they measure greater than 3.0 cm. The walls of follicular cysts are smooth and thin. Follicular cysts typically range in size from 3.0 to 8.0 cm but may attain larger diameters. They are usually asymptomatic but may produce dull adnexal pressure and pain. In most cases, these cysts eventually rupture or are resorbed. In premenopausal women who are or become asymptomatic, follow-up sonography is generally suggested if the cyst is larger than 5.0 cm.[5] Although the ovaries cease to function during menopause, it is not unusual to identify ovarian cysts in a postmenopausal patient. MRI or surgical evaluation is generally recommended only if an ovarian cyst measures more than 7.0 cm in premenopausal and postmenopausal patients.[5]

Sonographic Findings. Follicular cysts most commonly appear as anechoic, thin-walled unilocular structures demonstrating acoustic enhancement (i.e., as simple cysts). Occasionally, these cysts may contain diffuse, low-level echoes that reflect bleeding into the cyst. Ovarian tissue can be seen around the periphery of the cyst (Fig. 17-4). If follow-up sonography is performed on a symptomatic patient, most follicular cysts resolve within about 2 months.

Hemorrhagic Cyst

Hemorrhage into a follicular cyst or excess hemorrhage into a corpus luteum may result in a hemorrhagic ovarian cyst. Most hemorrhagic cysts resolve within 8 weeks. However, as with follicular cysts, asymptomatic women with cysts less than 5.0 cm probably do not need routine sonographic follow-up.[5]

Sonographic Findings. Hemorrhage within the cyst creates predictable patterns described as the "fishnet" or reticular pattern (Fig. 17-5, A) or retracting clot (Fig.

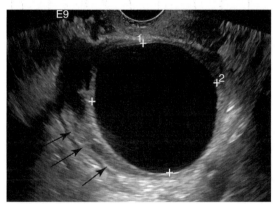

FIGURE 17-4 Follicular cyst 4.0 cm in size, with a thin rim of ovarian tissue *(arrows)* surrounding the cyst.

17-5, B). Hemorrhagic cysts may also demonstrate internal echoes with a fluid/fluid level (Fig. 17-5, C). Sometimes a hemorrhagic cyst has a predominantly solid appearance, but color Doppler sonography demonstrates no blood flow within the cyst and may show a highly vascular rim around the periphery of the cyst (Fig. 17-6; see Color Plate 14).

NONFUNCTIONAL CYSTS

Nonfunctional cysts generally refer to cysts that do not respond to cyclic hormonal stimulation. These include cysts of ovarian origin, such as endometriomas, and cysts not of ovarian origin, such as paraovarian cysts and peritoneal inclusion cysts.

Paraovarian Cyst

Paraovarian cysts originate from the wolffian structures located in the broad ligament. They occur in women of all ages but are most often found in menstruating women. They are benign and typically asymptomatic, but larger cysts may cause symptoms. Paraovarian cysts vary in size, with larger cysts at an increased risk for the same complications as other cysts, such as torsion, hemorrhage, or rupture.

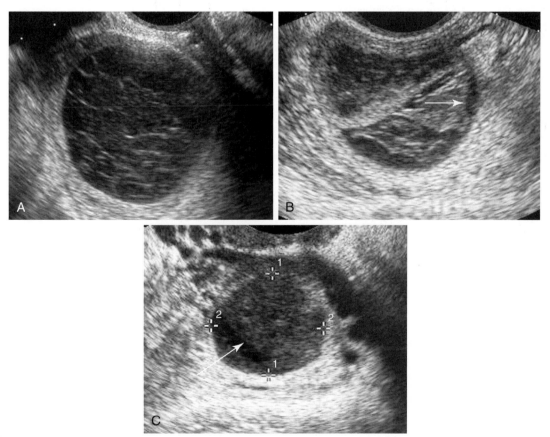

FIGURE 17-5 Patterns of hemorrhage typically seen within a hemorrhagic cyst. **(A)**, Reticular pattern. **(B)**, Retracting clot *(arrow)*. **(C)**, Hemorrhagic cyst demonstrating low-level echoes and fluid/fluid level *(arrow)*.

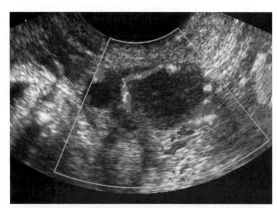

FIGURE 17-6 Hemorrhagic cyst with peripheral flow shown on color Doppler imaging.

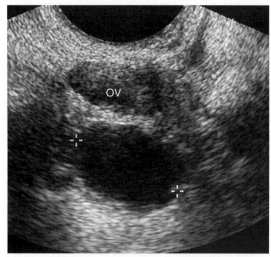

FIGURE 17-7 Paraovarian cyst (calipers) shown adjacent to ovary.

Sonographic Findings.

Most paraovarian cysts appear as a small, simple cyst separate from the ovary (Fig. 17-7). If the cyst is close to the ovary, it may be difficult to differentiate it from a follicular cyst. Application of gentle hand or transducer pressure may help separate the cystic structure from the ovary. Because there is no rim of ovarian tissue, large paraovarian cysts may resemble the urinary bladder. Differentiation from the bladder can be made by having the patient void. Because paraovarian cysts do not respond to the hormone cycle, follow-up examination is likely to demonstrate little or no change in size and appearance.

Peritoneal Inclusion Cyst

Patients who have experienced abdominal surgery, trauma, pelvic inflammatory disease, or endometriosis may develop peritoneal adhesions. Peritoneal inclusion cysts result when adhesions surround an ovary, and the follicular fluid that normally escapes into the peritoneum accumulates within the confines of the surrounding adhesions. Pain and a pelvic mass are the most common clinical presentations. Treatment is usually conservative,

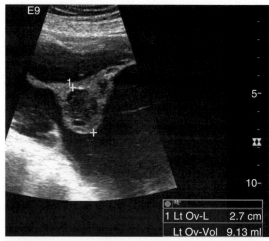

FIGURE 17-8 Peritoneal inclusion cyst. Multiloculated fluid collection surrounds ovary (calipers).

with fluid aspiration or administration of oral contraceptives to limit ovarian activity.

Sonographic Findings.

Peritoneal inclusion cysts appear as a multiloculated cystic mass either adjacent to or surrounding an ovary (Fig. 17-8). The ovary may be in the center of the septations and fluid or peripherally located. The fluid is usually anechoic, but echoes may be evident if hemorrhage or protein is present.

Endometrioma

Another ovarian mass commonly encountered in women during the reproductive years is endometrioma. A localized form of endometriosis results when endometrial tissue implants on an ovary creating one or multiple walled-off collections of blood, known as an endometrioma or chocolate cyst. The etiology of the disorder is unclear, but it is thought to relate to migration of endometrial tissue from the uterus or to primary ectopic development of endometrial tissue outside the uterus. The most common form of endometriosis is diffuse, with minute implants of endometrial tissue throughout the pelvic region, including the fallopian tubes, broad ligaments, and cul-de-sac. Because the ectopic endometrial tissue responds to varying levels of estrogen and progesterone during the menstrual cycle, the endometrial implants also undergo cyclic bleeding. Repetitive bleeding, inflammation, and resultant scarring can cause cyclic pain and infertility.

Endometriomas are virtually always benign with malignant transformation occurring in only a few, usually older women with large cysts. If an endometrioma ruptures or undergoes torsion, the patient experiences pain, and emergency surgery may be performed.

Sonographic Findings.

Endometriomas are generally well-defined unilocular or multilocular cystic masses that contain diffuse low-level echoes caused by the blood (Fig. 17-9, *A* and *B*). Small, punctate, hyperechoic foci are sometimes apparent in the wall of the mass. An

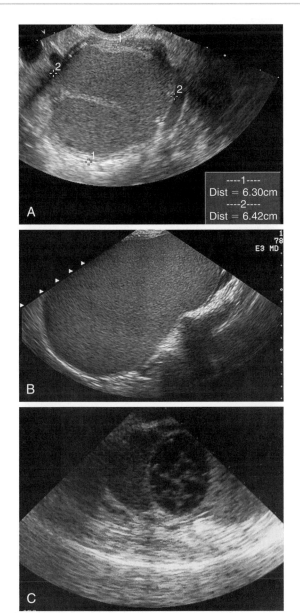

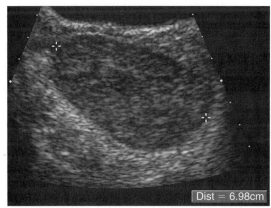

FIGURE 17-10 Right ovarian torsion resulting in enlarged ovary measuring 7.0 cm in length compared with the left ovary, which measured 2.0 cm.

FIGURE 17-9 (A) and **(B)**, Endometriomas containing low-level echoes. **(C)**, Endometrioma resembling hemorrhagic cyst

endometrioma typically does not demonstrate internal vascularity, which helps differentiate it from a neoplasm. When an endometrioma is unilocular, it may resemble a hemorrhagic ovarian cyst (Fig. 17-9, C). Follow-up sonograms of an endometrioma usually demonstrate persistence, whereas follow-up of a hemorrhagic cyst typically demonstrates resolution. A few endometriomas may contain a small, solid-appearing area; such masses are problematic because the solid area raises concern for a neoplasm, yet these are usually benign endometriomas.

OVARIAN TORSION

Ovarian torsion is a significant condition that often requires prompt surgical intervention. Ovarian torsion occurs when the ovary twists on its pedicle resulting in impaired blood flow to and from the ovary. The lack of

venous drainage can cause the ovary to enlarge, whereas compromised arterial perfusion can cause the ovary to infarct and necrose. Torsion usually occurs in childhood and during the reproductive years and is associated with mobile adnexa or a preexisting ovarian cyst or mass. Clinically, there is severe pain, nausea, and vomiting; a palpable mass may also be present.

Sonographic Findings

The sonographic appearance of a torsed ovary is variable but ovarian enlargement is always present (Fig. 17-10). The ovary may contain a cyst or other ovarian mass. Free fluid in the cul-de-sac is a common but nonspecific finding. Depending on the degree of torsion, color and spectral Doppler findings can range from absent to diminished arterial flow within the ovary; it is important to recognize that the presence of arterial flow does not exclude ovarian torsion. Venous flow is typically compromised before arterial flow, which may contribute to ovarian enlargement. Arterial flow, with absent venous flow in the ovary, is a fairly common sonographic appearance for ovarian torsion. Spectral Doppler is needed to determine arterial versus venous flow. Torsion may still be present in an enlarged ovary even with arterial and venous flow because Doppler findings likely vary with the degree of torsion, and there may be intermittent detorsion. Another finding associated with ovarian torsion is the coiled appearance of the twisted vessels at the pedicle, known as the "whirlpool" sign. [6] Depending on the degree of torsion, flow may or may not be detected in the twisted vessels by Doppler imaging.

OVARIAN NEOPLASMS

Ovarian tumors, or neoplasms, represent a small but significant subset of ovarian masses discovered sonographically in premenopausal and postmenopausal women. Ovarian neoplasms can be benign or malignant; postmenopausal women have a threefold increased risk of having a malignant ovarian neoplasm compared with premenopausal women.[7] Ovarian neoplasms are classified by the type of ovarian tissue from which they arise: germ cell, epithelial, and sex cord–stromal tumors. The two most common types of ovarian neoplasms are germ cell tumors, specifically benign cystic teratoma, and surface epithelial neoplasms, such as serous cystadenoma. Germ cell tumors are most commonly found in young women, whereas epithelial tumors are more common in women in their fourth and fifth decades. Metastatic ovarian disease is a fourth source of ovarian neoplasms.

Sonography has been accepted as the diagnostic modality of choice for noninvasive assessment of ovarian tumors. Sonographic assessment includes pattern recognition, assessment of morphologic gray-scale and Doppler features, clinical signs and symptoms, and consideration of age and menopausal status.

GERM CELL NEOPLASMS

Germ cell neoplasms are the most frequent ovarian neoplasm among women younger than 50 years of age; benign cystic teratomas are the most common type of germ cell tumor.[4] Malignant ovarian germ cell tumors are rare and are classified into several subgroups: dysgerminomas, endodermal sinus tumors, yolk sac tumors, immature teratomas, choriocarcinomas, and embryonal carcinomas. Benign cystic teratomas and malignant dysgerminomas are discussed in this chapter.

Benign Cystic Teratoma

Benign cystic teratomas, which are also referred to as cystic teratomas, dermoids, or dermoid cysts, are composed of a combination of the three germ cell layers: ectoderm (dermoid), mesoderm, and endoderm, with ectoderm being the most common component. Germ cells form teeth, bone, skin, fingernails, hair, fat, and sebum; a cystic teratoma commonly contains sebum with varying amounts of fat, hair, teeth, and bone fragments.

Patients with cystic teratomas are commonly asymptomatic, although larger masses may cause abdominal swelling or pain. Cystic teratomas are also prone to torsion or rupture. Malignant transformation has been reported in approximately 2% of cases.[4] These masses may be bilateral. Cystic teratomas are often surgically removed to prevent torsion or rupture, and these lesions are excised without removal of the involved ovary whenever possible. Because of the typically slow growth rate of these tumors, surgery can sometimes be delayed until patients have completed their childbearing.

Sonographic Findings. The internal components of benign cystic teratomas demonstrate variable but often unique sonographic features described as the "tip-of-the-iceberg" sign, fat/fluid level, dermoid plug, or dermoid mesh. When the echogenic tissue contained within a cystic teratoma obscures the entire back wall of the mass

because of attenuation, it is referred to as the "tip-of-the-iceberg" sign (Fig. 17-11, A). Sebum and fat can liquefy at body temperature, and as the liquids separate, a fat/fluid level may be apparent (Fig. 17-11, B). When hair is mixed with sebum, a hyperechoic dermoid plug becomes evident, sometimes with acoustic shadowing behind it (Fig. 17-11, C). Hair within serous fluid within the cyst creates hyperechoic lines and dots, often referred to as a dermoid mesh appearance (Fig. 17-11, D). Less commonly, a tooth or small bone fragment within the cyst or dermoid plug creates an intensely hyperechoic area with a strong acoustic shadow. Because of the hyperechoic interfaces and acoustic shadowing, cystic teratomas may blend in with the surrounding bowel. Color Doppler evaluation may demonstrate flow only in the periphery of the mass because the internal components consist of avascular fat and hair.

Malignant Dysgerminoma

Ovarian dysgerminomas are malignant tumors; they constitute only 1% to 2% of all malignant ovarian tumors and occur predominantly in 20- to 30-year-old women. Invasive malignant ovarian tumors discovered during pregnancy are typically dysgerminomas.[8] These neoplasms may be detected incidentally or in patients with abdominal enlargement because of a palpable mass. Occasionally, pain or menstrual abnormalities are present. When discovered during the early stages, ovarian dysgerminomas have a good prognosis with a 95% 5-year survival rate.[9]

Sonographic Findings. The most characteristic sonographic findings of an ovarian dysgerminoma include a solid, smoothly lobulated mass with well-defined borders and a heterogeneous internal echotexture (Fig. 17-12). Color or power Doppler imaging may demonstrate a highly vascularized mass with tortuous vessels and irregular branching.[9]

EPITHELIAL OVARIAN NEOPLASMS

Ovarian neoplasms of epithelial origin are the most common ovarian tumor among women 50 years or older and account for most malignant ovarian neoplasms.[4] The most common types of epithelial neoplasms include serous and mucinous cystadenoma or cystadenocarcinoma, borderline ovarian tumors, and endometrioid tumors. Other epithelial ovarian neoplasms include clear cell tumors and Brenner or transitional cell tumors.

Serous Cystadenoma and Cystadenocarcinoma

Serous tumors are the most common type of epithelial neoplasm, with approximately 50% to 70% of them being benign. The benign form is known as a serous cystadenoma, and it occurs most frequently in women

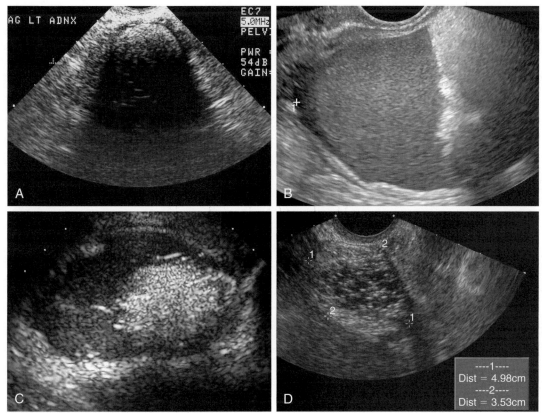

FIGURE 17-11 Findings associated with benign cystic teratomas. **(A)**, Strongly attenuating tissues in dermoid plug obscure back wall of mass, producing characteristic "tip-of-the-iceberg" sign. **(B)**, Fat/fluid level as evidenced by varying echogenicity of fat and fluid. **(C)**, Dermoid plug with shadowing. **(D)**, Dermoid mesh created by hair within mass.

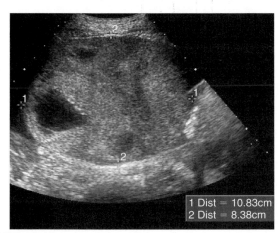

FIGURE 17-12 Malignant dysgerminoma demonstrating predominantly solid appearance.

40 to 50 years old.[4] The malignant form, serous cystadenocarcinoma, occurs predominantly in perimenopausal and postmenopausal women. Serous cystadenocarcinomas account for about 50% of all malignant ovarian neoplasms. Approximately 20% of benign serous tumors and 50% of malignant serous tumors are bilateral.[4] These tumors are lined with mesothelial, ciliated, and secretory cells, which cause the tumor to fill with serous fluid. The size can vary greatly; however, these tumors can become quite large causing abdominal or pelvic fullness.

As discussed earlier, ovarian malignancies produce few distinct symptoms, although malignant epithelial tumors can produce elevated levels of CA 125. Monitoring CA 125 levels during and after treatment can help determine if a cystadenocarcinoma is in remission. The treatment for benign and malignant serous tumors is surgical excision with chemotherapy if the tumor is malignant.

Sonographic Findings. Serous cystadenomas typically appear sonographically as a simple cyst, although they may also have thin septations or papillary projections or both in the cyst cavity (Fig. 17-13). Serous cystadenocarcinomas tend to exhibit internal papillary projections, sometimes with thick septations producing multiple locules. The presence of a cystic mass that contains a solid area with detectable flow by Doppler imaging is the most predictive sonographic feature for malignancy (Fig. 17-14; see Color Plate 15). Detectable flow in septations and solid areas may still occur in benign masses but should raise concern for a malignant neoplasm. Cystadenomas and cystadenocarcinomas vary in size and can be quite large.

Mucinous Cystadenoma and Cystadenocarcinoma

Mucinous tumors are less common than serous tumors, and most mucinous neoplasms are benign

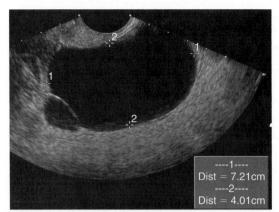

FIGURE 17-13 Serous cystadenoma with single septation.

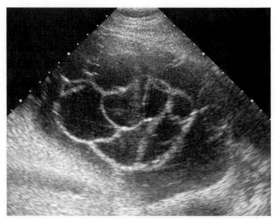

FIGURE 17-15 Mucinous cystadenoma containing multiple septations.

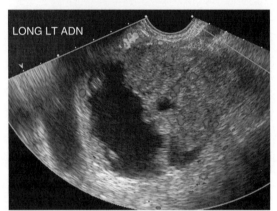

FIGURE 17-14 Serous cystadenocarcinoma measuring 9.0 cm, demonstrating a solid component with internal vascularity evident on color Doppler imaging.

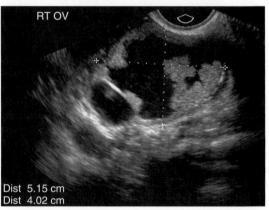

FIGURE 17-16 Borderline ovarian tumor with septations and papillary projections. These features are indistinguishable from cystadenocarcinoma.

cystadenomas. Younger women are more likely to present with the benign form, whereas older women are at higher risk for mucinous cystadenocarcinomas. Mucinous tumors are less frequently bilateral than serous tumors and may become quite large, measuring 30 cm. The internal contents consist of a thick mucinous material. Rupture of the tumor capsule may cause spillage of the gelatinous contents into the abdomen resulting in a condition called pseudomyxoma peritonei. Serum CA 125 testing is insensitive to this type of tumor, and clinical signs and symptoms are nonspecific ranging from abdominal fullness to gastric problems. Mucinous ovarian neoplasms are treated with surgery, sometimes combined with radiation therapy or chemotherapy.

Sonographic Findings. Mucinous tumors tend to appear sonographically as multiloculated cystic masses containing low-level echoes (Fig. 17-15). Internal septations tend to be thicker and papillary projections less common than in the serous variety; however, the sonographic findings of serous and mucinous neoplasms overlap enough to make differentiation between the two difficult. Pseudomyxoma peritonei may resemble ascites, and the fluid filling much of the pelvis and abdomen may contain multiple septations.

Borderline Tumors or Tumors of Low Malignant Potential

An intermediate group of epithelial tumors, most commonly serous or mucinous, demonstrates histologic features of malignancy but no invasive characteristics. The histologic categorization has been termed "borderline" or "low malignant potential" tumors. Borderline tumors tend to occur in younger women than cystadenocarcinomas and have a much better prognosis.[10]

Sonographic Findings. Slight differences have been reported for borderline tumors compared with frankly malignant or benign tumors, but the appearances overlap enough that it is usually difficult to make a specific diagnosis of borderline tumors by sonography.[10] Mural nodules may be seen in borderline tumors (Fig. 17-16). Normal ovarian tissue may be seen adjacent to the lesion, which suggests that it is not invasive, but this finding can also occur with benign neoplasms.

Endometrioid Tumor

Endometrioid tumors occur most frequently in women in their 50s and 60s and may be associated with endometrial adenocarcinoma and endometriosis. About 80% of endometrioid tumors are malignant, they account for 20% to 25% of all ovarian malignant tumors, and they rank as the second most common malignant epithelial tumor.[4] Although most are malignant, endometrioid tumors have a better prognosis than either serous or mucinous cystadenocarcinomas, probably because of diagnosis at an earlier stage.[4]

Sonographic Findings. Endometrioid tumors usually appear sonographically as a cystic mass that contains solid areas. Endometrioid (and clear cell) carcinomas tend to have more solid components within them compared with serous or mucinous carcinomas. Of these tumors, 25% to 30% are bilateral.[4]

Brenner Tumors

Brenner tumors, also known as transitional cell tumors, are almost always benign. These dense fibrous tumors are usually less than 2 cm in diameter and rarely exceed 10 cm. Brenner tumors are occasionally associated with an ipsilateral cystic neoplasm, such as a cystadenoma or cystic teratoma. Most patients are asymptomatic, and the tumors are discovered incidentally.

Sonographic Findings. Most Brenner tumors appear as a unilateral solid mass that measures less than 1 to 2 cm in diameter. These solid masses are typically hypoechoic and may have posterior attenuation of the sound beam. Calcifications may be present. Cystic areas are uncommon but may occur as the result of a coexisting cystic neoplasm. Brenner tumors may be difficult to differentiate sonographically from other solid pelvic masses, including ovarian fibromas, thecomas, and pedunculated subserosal uterine leiomyomas.

SEX CORD–STROMAL TUMORS

Sex cord–stromal neoplasms arise from the sex cords of the embryonic gonad and from the ovarian stroma. These tumors are less common than germ cell and epithelial ovarian neoplasms and tend to produce predominantly solid masses that are hormonally active. The most common tumors in this category include granulosa cell tumor, Sertoli-Leydig cell tumor (androblastoma), fibroma, and thecoma.

Granulosa Cell Tumor

Granulosa cell tumors are considered low-grade malignant tumors and often secrete estrogen. They occur predominantly in postmenopausal women but can occur in patients younger than 30 years and in children. Excess estrogen production can cause endometrial carcinoma in 10% to 15% of patients.[11] Excess estrogen in children can result in precocious puberty or premature breast development.

Sonographic Findings. Granulosa cell tumors have a variable sonographic appearance, ranging from a solid mass (more common in smaller tumors) resembling a fibroid to a complex, multiloculated cystic mass (more common in large tumors). Because of the estrogen production, uterine evaluation may reveal a thickened endometrium.

Sertoli-Leydig Cell Tumor

Sertoli-Leydig cell tumors, or androblastomas, are rare ovarian neoplasms occurring predominantly in menstruating women. These tumors may be hormonally active, producing the androgen testosterone, which results in virilization in about 30% of patients.[4] Occasionally, these tumors produce estrogen. Malignancy occurs in 10% to 20% of Sertoli-Leydig cell neoplasms.

Sonographic Findings. Sertoli-Leydig cell tumors usually appear as unilateral solid hypoechoic masses. They may be small and difficult to identify.

Fibroma and Thecoma

Fibromas and thecomas are similar benign neoplasms both arising from the ovarian stroma. They may occur individually, but sometimes there are histologic components of both, and such tumors are termed fibrothecomas. Fibromas occur most often in perimenopausal and postmenopausal women. Fibromas consist of fibrous tissue, are not usually hormonally active, and tend to be asymptomatic. Thecomas contain a variable combination of thecal and fibrous tissue. Thecomas, in contrast to fibromas, may show clinical signs of estrogen production. Occasionally, a benign solid ovarian mass, of which fibroma is the most common, causes Meigs' syndrome, a condition characterized by the presence of ascites and a pleural effusion.

Sonographic Findings. Fibromas and thecomas comprise dense, fibrous tissue that usually appears as a hypoechoic solid mass (Fig. 17-17). The tissue may appear homogeneous or heterogeneous. In some cases, there is marked attenuation of sound by the hypoechoic mass.

METASTATIC OVARIAN TUMORS

The most common tumors to metastasize to the ovary are tumors of the breast and of the gastrointestinal tract. The term "Krukenberg tumor" is sometimes erroneously used as synonymous with any metastatic tumor to the ovary but is actually best reserved for tumors containing mucin-secreting signet ring cells, which usually arise from the gastrointestinal tract. Endometrial carcinoma can metastasize to the ovaries, and differentiation from endometrioid tumors is difficult. Lymphoma may also involve the ovaries.

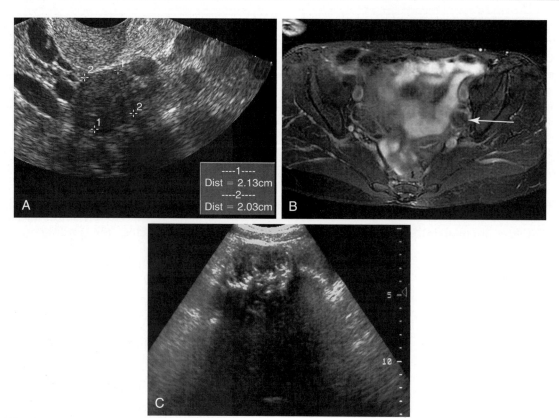

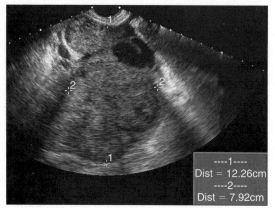

FIGURE 17-17 **(A)**, Sonographic image of fibroma consisting of dense, solid, fibrous tissue. **(B)**, Axial T2-weighted MRI of the same fibroma, demonstrating low signal mass in left ovary *(arrow)*. **(C)**, Thecoma appears as a heterogeneous solid mass with acoustic shadowing. The appearance is similar to that of a fibroma.

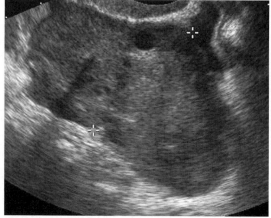

FIGURE 17-18 Solid ovarian mass representing metastatic neoplasm. Metastatic ovarian neoplasms tend to be bilateral.

FIGURE 17-19 Solid ovarian mass representing metastatic neoplasm resulting from lymphoma.

Sonographic Findings

Metastatic ovarian neoplasms are usually bilateral solid masses (Fig. 17-18), but they can also appear as complex, large, predominantly cystic masses. Complex cystic masses may occur secondary to colon cancer. Ascites may also be present. Ovaries affected by lymphoma appear as a solid hypoechoic mass (Fig. 17-19).

Table 17-2 lists differential diagnoses based on the sonographic appearance of an ovarian mass.

TABLE 17-2	Differential Diagnosis for Ovarian Masses Based on Sonographic Appearance			
Completely Cystic/Unilocular	**Cystic with Echoes (Unilocular or Multilocular)**	**Cystic with Septations**	**Complex (Cystic and Solid Components)**	**Solid**
Ovarian follicle	Hemorrhagic cyst	Peritoneal inclusion cyst*	Cystic teratoma (color Doppler imaging does not demonstrate flow within mass)	Pedunculated fibroid*
Paraovarian cyst*	Endometrioma	Serous or mucinous cystadenoma	Serous or mucinous cystadenoma	Ovarian torsion
Serous cystadenoma	Cystic teratoma	Theca lutein cysts	Serous or mucinous cystadenocarcinoma	Fibroma or thecoma
	Serous or mucinous cystadenoma		Granulosa cell tumor	Brenner tumor
			Dysgerminoma	Sertoli-Leydig cell tumor
				Metastatic tumors
				Dysgerminoma
				Granulosa cell tumor

*Nonovarian masses that can mimic ovarian masses.

SUMMARY

Sonographic characterization of ovarian masses provides information valuable in differentiation of benign and malignant masses. Most adnexal masses are benign and can be correctly categorized by sonography. Knowledge of the typical sonographic features of benign and malignant masses, combined with patient history and clinical presentation, can suggest a diagnosis and assist the clinician with patient management decisions.

CLINICAL SCENARIO—DIAGNOSIS

The sonographic appearance of the enlarged right ovary is suggestive of ovarian torsion. The clinical symptoms and presence of arterial flow suggest possible intermittent episodes of torsion and detorsion. The patient underwent a right oophorectomy/salpingectomy, which removed the corpus luteum, necessitating progesterone suppositories. Follow-up visits indicated mother and baby were doing well.

CASE STUDIES FOR DISCUSSION

1. A 20-year-old woman is seen for an annual pelvic examination, and the physician palpates an adnexal mass. The patient denies pelvic pain or abnormal bleeding. Serum pregnancy testing is negative. Sonographic evaluation demonstrates an ovarian mass (Fig. 17-20, A). Computed tomography (CT) scan demonstrates fat within the mass (Fig. 17-20, B). What is the most likely diagnosis?
2. A 68-year-old woman is referred for pelvic sonography to follow-up a known adnexal cystic mass (Fig. 17-21). This mass has been stable in size for the last 2 years. What is the most likely diagnosis?
3. Pelvic sonography in a 24-year-old woman experiencing cyclic pain reveals a right adnexal mass (Fig. 17-22). Follow-up examination in 5 weeks demonstrates no change in appearance or size. What is the most likely diagnosis?
4. A 43-year-old woman with breast cancer and a history of tamoxifen therapy is referred for a pelvic sonogram to rule out endometrial pathology and metastatic ovarian disease. Sonography reveals a normal-appearing uterus. However, a mass is noted in the right adnexa (Fig. 17-23). Follow-up pelvic sonography in 5 weeks demonstrates resolution of the mass. What is the most likely diagnosis?
5. A 60-year-old woman with an elevated CA 125 level is referred for a pelvic sonogram. A mass is noted in the right adnexa (Fig. 17-24; see Color Plate 16). What is the most likely diagnosis?

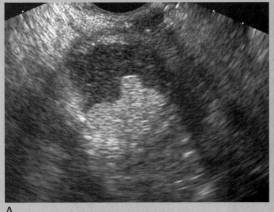
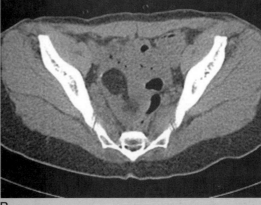

A   B

FIGURE 17-20 **(A)**, Sonographic image of adnexal mass in an asymptomatic 20-year-old patient. **(B)**, CT image demonstrates fat within mass.

Continued

CASE STUDIES FOR DISCUSSION—cont'd

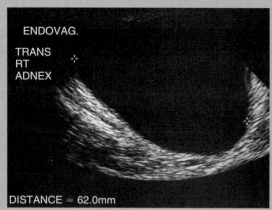

FIGURE 17-21 Adnexal mass in a postmenopausal patient. Mass has remained stable in size and appearance for 2 years.

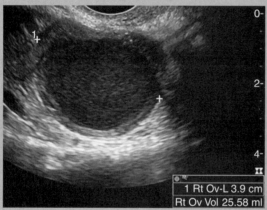

FIGURE 17-22 Adnexal mass in a 24-year-old patient. Follow-up sonogram demonstrates no change.

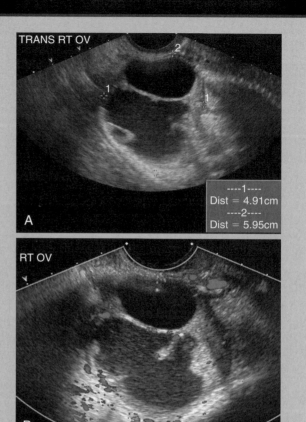

FIGURE 17-24 Adnexal mass in a 60-year-old patient with increased CA 125.

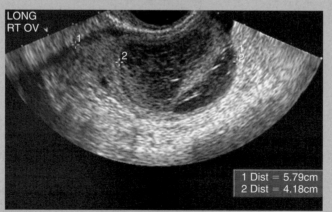

FIGURE 17-23 Adnexal mass in a 43-year-old patient with a history of breast cancer. Follow-up sonogram demonstrates resolution of the mass.

STUDY QUESTIONS

1. A 25-year-old woman is referred for a pelvic sonogram because of left lower quadrant pain. A pregnancy test is negative. The sonogram reveals a 2.0 cm unilocular, simple cyst adjacent to the left ovary. Which of the following statements is true regarding this finding?
   a. This is most likely an ectopic pregnancy and should be handled on an emergent basis.
   b. The findings are most consistent with a cystic teratoma, and surgical removal should be advised.
   c. The findings are consistent with a corpus luteum.
   d. This most likely represents a paraovarian cyst, and no treatment is necessary.

2. A 75-year-old woman undergoes a pelvic sonogram because of increasing abdominal girth and complaints of feeling exhausted. Sonographic evaluation demonstrates a 20 cm, complex, predominantly cystic mass occupying her pelvis and abdomen. Multiple papillary projections and septations are evident within the mass, which demonstrate vascularity on color Doppler imaging. What is the most likely diagnosis?
   a. Pelvic abscess
   b. Cystadenocarcinoma
   c. Metastatic tumor
   d. Hemorrhagic corpus luteum

3. A 45-year-old woman with mild pelvic discomfort undergoes a sonographic examination, and a 3.0 cm hypoechoic solid ovarian mass is discovered. The images also demonstrate ascites and marked attenuation posterior to the mass. Which of the following is the most likely diagnosis?
   a. Fibroma with Meigs' syndrome
   b. Cystadenocarcinoma with ascites
   c. Cystic teratoma with free fluid
   d. Ovarian torsion with free fluid

4. A pediatric patient with elevated estrogen levels is referred for a pelvic sonogram after receiving a diagnosis of precocious puberty. A solid mass is discovered in the left adnexa, with no evidence of a normal left ovary. What is the most likely diagnosis?
   a. Ovarian torsion
   b. Cystic teratoma
   c. Endometrioma
   d. Granulosa cell tumor

5. A 55-year-old woman with stomach cancer is referred for a pelvic sonogram because of pelvic discomfort. The sonogram reveals bilateral solid ovarian masses. This finding is most consistent with which of the following?
   a. Fibromas
   b. Endometriomas
   c. Metastatic tumors
   d. Cystadenocarcinoma

6. A 19-year-old woman was referred for a pelvic sonogram because of a palpable right adnexal mass and no other symptoms. The sonographer was unable to identify a normal right ovary but noticed a discrete area with hyperechoic dots and lines, including a rounded echogenic area that produced a shadow. At first, the area was thought to be bowel, but on observation, there was no peristalsis. These findings are most consistent with which type of ovarian mass?
   a. Hemorrhagic corpus luteum
   b. Follicular cyst
   c. Mucinous cystadenoma
   d. Cystic teratoma

7. A 45-year-old woman with menorrhagia undergoes a pelvic sonogram that reveals a multiloculated cystic mass adjacent to the right ovary. The patient's medical history includes prior pelvic surgery for endometriosis 15 years ago. The patient denies any right lower quadrant pain. Which of the following is the most likely diagnosis?
   a. Cystadenocarcinoma
   b. Peritoneal inclusion cyst
   c. Paraovarian cyst
   d. Cystic teratoma

8. The sonographic images of a unilateral ovarian mass in a 25-year-old woman with menstrual irregularities demonstrate a well-defined, 5.0 cm homogeneous unilocular mass containing low-level internal echoes and posterior acoustic enhancement. These findings are most consistent with which ovarian pathology?
   a. Thecoma
   b. Fibroma
   c. Endometrioma
   d. Cystic teratoma

9. A 45-year-old woman undergoes a pelvic sonogram because of a family history of ovarian cancer. Her CA 125 levels are not elevated, and she is not experiencing any unusual symptoms other than weight gain. Sonography reveals a 15 cm, predominantly cystic mass with multiple septations, several papillary projections, and low-level echoes within the mass. Color Doppler imaging reveals vascularity within the solid components. Given the patient's history and sonographic findings, which of the following is the most likely diagnosis?
   a. Dysgerminoma
   b. Metastatic tumor

c. Peritoneal inclusion cyst

d. Mucinous cystadenocarcinoma

10. A 29-year-old woman with left lower quadrant pain is referred for a pelvic sonogram to rule out ovarian torsion. The images demonstrate a 4.0 cm left ovarian mass containing a reticular pattern of echoes with posterior enhancement and peripheral ovarian flow by color Doppler imaging. A follow-up sonogram performed 2 months later demonstrates a normal left ovary and a 2.5 cm dominant follicle on the right ovary. By the time of the follow-up sonogram, the patient was asymptomatic. Which of the following is the most likely diagnosis for the first examination?

a. Hemorrhagic ovarian cyst

b. Endometrioma with rupture

c. Intermittent ovarian torsion

d. Cystic teratoma with rupture

REFERENCES

1. Valentin L, Callen P: Ultrasound evaluation of the adnexa (ovary and Fallopian tubes). In Callen P, editor: *Ultrasonography in obstetrics and gynecology*, ed 5, Philadelphia, 2008, Saunders, pp 968–985.

2. Moore R, MacLaughlan S, Bast R Jr: Current state of biomarker development for clinical application in epithelial ovarian cancer, *Gynecol Oncol* 116:240–245, 2010.

3. Brown D, Andreotti R, Lee S, et al: ACR appropriateness criteria ovarian cancer screening, *Ultrasound Q* 26:219–223, 2010.

4. Salem S: Gynecologic ultrasound. In Rumack C, Wilson S, Charboneau J, Levine D, editors: ed 4, *Diagnostic ultrasound*, vol. 1, Philadelphia, 2011, Mosby, pp 547–612.

5. Levine D, Brown D, Andreotti R, et al: Management of asymptomatic ovarian and other adnexal cysts imaged at US: Society of Radiologists in Ultrasound Consensus Conference Statement, *Radiology* 256:943–954, 2010.

6. Valsy E, Esh-Broder E, Cohen SM, et al: Added value of the gray-scale whirlpool sign in the diagnosis of adnexal torsion, *Ultrasound Obstet Gynecol* 36:630–634, 2010.

7. Howlader N, Noone A, Krapcho M, et al: SEER Cancer Statistics Review, 1975-2008. Bethesda, MD, National Cancer Institute, 2011.

8. Pectasides D, Pectasides E, Kasanos D: Germ cell tumors of the ovary, *Cancer Treat Rev* 34:427–441, 2008.

9. Guerriero S, Testa D, Timmerman D, et al: Imaging of gynecological disease: clinical and ultrasound characteristics of ovarian dysgerminoma, *Ultrasound Obstet Gynecol* 37:596–602, 2011.

10. Exacoustos C, Romanini ME, Rinaldo D, et al: Preoperative sonographic features of borderline ovarian tumors, *Ultrasound Obstet Gynecol* 25:50–59, 2005.

11. Van Holsbeke C, Domali E, Holland T, et al: Imaging of gynecological disease (3) clinical and ultrasound characteristics of granulosa cell tumors of the ovary, *Ultrasound Obstet Gynecol* 31:450–456, 2008.

PART III

Obstetrics

Uncertain Last Menstrual Period

Jill Trotter

A 19-year-old woman is seen for prenatal care after a positive home pregnancy test. The patient has a history of irregular menstrual periods; she cannot remember the date of her last normal period. A sonogram is performed, and the various fetal measurements obtained during the examination are listed on the obstetrics report form (Fig. 18-1).

Are all of the biometric measurements consistent with each other? Are there any measurements that are abnormal or worrisome? Should a follow-up sonographic evaluation be recommended? If so, what specific observations should be made?

AUA	17w5d					
		GA	**Range**	**Author**	**Percent**	**Author**
BPD	3.88 cm	17w6d	(+/−1w2d)	Hadlock	74%	Hadlock
HC	14.39 cm	17w5d	(+/−1w2d)	Hadlock	59%	Hadlock
AC	11.55 cm	17w3d	(+/−1w5d)	Hadlock	50%	Hadlock
FL	2.44 cm	17w3d	(+/−1w3d)	Hadlock	48%	Hadlock
Heart Rate	156 bpm					

— **Advanced OB** —

AUA	17w5d					
Lat Vent	0.78 cm					
Cerebellum	1.80 cm	18w6d	(17w4d-20w1d)	Chitty		
Cist Mag	0.35 cm					
Nuch Fold	3.34 mm					
Humerus	2.70 cm	18w4d	(15w6d-21w3d)	Jeanty	91%	Jeanty

FIGURE 18-1 Obstetrics report form for a patient with an uncertain LMP. *OB*, obstetrics; *AUA*, actual ultrasound age; *GA*, gestational age; *BPD*, biparietal diameter; *HC*, head circumference; *AC*, abdominal circumference; *FL*, femur length; *LMP*, last menstrual period.

OBJECTIVES

- Describe the purpose of biometric measurements during the first trimester of pregnancy for estimation of gestational age.
- Demonstrate appropriate techniques used for accurate first-trimester biometric measurements.
- Describe the purpose of biometric measurements during the second and third trimesters of pregnancy for estimation of gestational age.
- Demonstrate appropriate techniques used for accurate second-trimester and third-trimester biometric measurements.

- Describe additional measurements that may be performed throughout pregnancy for confirmation of gestational age.
- Describe additional measurements that may be performed for diagnostic purposes during specific gestational age ranges.
- Identify the technical limitations of delayed biometric imaging in cases of uncertain last menstrual period.

For more than four decades, sonography has engraved a mark in the estimation of gestational age. Diagnostic sonography plays a role in the management of a pregnant patient whose history leaves the clinician with the task of estimating a due date on the basis of an uncertain last menstrual period (LMP). Advances in equipment and techniques have made sonographic determination of gestational age possible even earlier in the pregnancy than previously. The acceptance of routine transvaginal imaging in the first trimester has been one of the biggest advances. The gestational sac diameter may be measured before the embryo is seen, but the first-trimester crown-rump length (CRL) continues to be the most accurate sonographic predictor for gestational age. Early second-trimester biometry can also be of predictive value when obtained and interpreted accurately. A patient who does not seek prenatal care until the late third trimester creates the most difficult clinical scenario. This increased difficulty is the result of biologic variations in fetal size later in the pregnancy, which decrease the accuracy of biometry performed for the first time at this advanced gestational age. At any stage in the pregnancy, precise technique must be used to estimate gestational age accurately with sonographic measurements.

FIRST-TRIMESTER BIOMETRY

Before the advent of pregnancy testing and sonography, the LMP was the most identifiable reference point for the beginning of the pregnancy. With advances in prenatal testing, pregnancy is now known to have a duration of approximately 280 days from the first day of the LMP, also referred to as 9 calendar or 10 lunar months. This is also known as Nägele's rule. In clinical practice, the term "gestational age" is often used interchangeably with "menstrual age," which dates a pregnancy based on a woman's LMP. In this chapter, gestational age references are based on LMP. The knowledge of an accurate gestational age is needed to manage the pregnancy optimally; to reduce the risks of preterm and postterm deliveries; and to coordinate elective procedures, such as biochemical screening evaluation, chorionic villus sampling, and amniocentesis, and delivery method, such as a repeat cesarean section or pregnancy induction. Because many women who potentially become pregnant in any given month may have variable cycle lengths, bleeding in early pregnancy, or inaccurate accounts of menstrual dates, estimation of a due date can be a clinical challenge. Patients who seek prenatal care during the first or second trimester of pregnancy without a strong knowledge of LMP or normal cycle lengths may undergo a sonographic examination to estimate gestational age with biometric measurements of the structures of pregnancy or the fetus. Among the measurements that may be obtained for dating purposes during the first trimester using sonographic techniques are the gestational sac diameter and the CRL. First-trimester measurements are considered to

| BOX 18-1 | First-Trimester Measurements |

Biometry
Gestational sac (mean sac diameter)
Crown-rump length

Additional Measurements
Yolk sac (2-6 mm)
Nuchal translucency (<3 mm between 11 and 14 weeks)

be reliable indicators because pathologic states and fetal abnormalities have the least impact on fetal size during this time, and biologic variation is at a minimum during the first few weeks of pregnancy (Box 18-1).

Gestational Sac

The appearance of an anechoic fluid collection surrounded by an echogenic ring in the fundal region of the endometrial cavity is the first sonographic evidence of an intrauterine pregnancy (Fig. 18-2, *A*). This echogenic ring is a vital structure of a normal pregnancy because it represents the chorion and decidua capsularis. Absence of the echogenic ring should prompt suspicion of a pseudogestational sac associated with ectopic pregnancy and may warrant clinical correlation with beta-hCG levels. As the pregnancy progresses and displacement of the endometrial echo occurs, a second outer echogenic ring may be seen that represents the remainder of the endometrial lining, known as the decidua parietalis or decidua vera. The appearance of these two echogenic rings has become known as the double decidual sac sign and may be seen between 4 to 6 weeks of gestational age. The space between the two decidual rings is the unoccupied endometrial cavity, which becomes obliterated as the pregnancy progresses.

With two scan planes, a measurement made in each of the three dimensions of the gestational sac can be used to calculate a mean sac diameter (MSD). These sac measurements should be made at the interface between the echogenic border and the fluid (Fig. 18-2, *B*). The introduction of transvaginal ultrasound techniques has allowed visualization of this normal progression of early pregnancy. With high-frequency transvaginal technique, a pregnancy dating only 4 weeks and 1 or 2 days from the LMP may be visualized as a 2- to 3-mm fluid collection within the uterus. The MSD should correlate closely with suspected gestational age, and any significant variance or suspicion of pregnancy loss should be closely correlated with beta-hCG levels. The MSD is not a true fetal parameter, but its correlation to the estimated gestational age and growth rate may prove to be valuable in the prediction of spontaneous abortion. Normal first-trimester gestational sac growth rate should be approximately 1 mm per day. During this time of rapid embryologic change, a repeat examination may be performed within a few days to show the progression of the pregnancy and confirm it

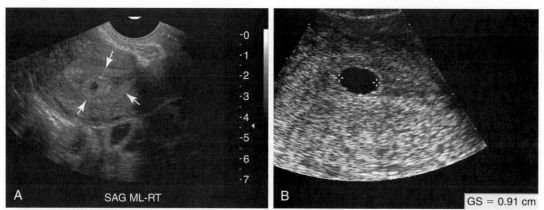

FIGURE 18-2 (A), Well-defined anechoic collection surrounded by echogenic decidualized endometrium *(arrows)*. **(B)**, Correct caliper placement is shown at fluid interface with the echogenic borders.

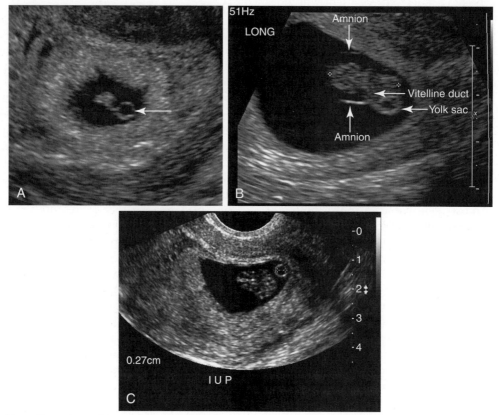

FIGURE 18-3 (A), The yolk sac *(arrow)* is seen as a round anechoic structure within the gestational sac. **(B)**, The yolk sac and embryo can be seen separated by the echogenic amnion but connected by the vitelline duct. **(C)**, Correct caliper placement is shown for measurement of the yolk sac.

as normal or abnormal. Evidence of a developing intrauterine pregnancy should be seen transvaginally with a serum beta-hCG level greater than 1000 to 2000 mIU/mL using the International Reference Preparation (IRP) standard.

Yolk Sac

The sonographically visualized yolk sac is more accurately called the secondary yolk sac. Most sonographers and sonologists loosely use the term "yolk sac" in discussion of this structure in pregnancy when visualized.

The sonographic presence of the yolk sac in an early gestational sac may be considered a predictor of a normally progressing pregnancy before visualization of the embryo. With transvaginal technique, a gestational sac measuring 8 mm or more should demonstrate a yolk sac, which is consistent with a 5 to 5.5-week gestation. The secondary yolk sac appears as a round anechoic structure with an echogenic rim (Fig. 18-3, *A*). This yolk sac supplies nutrition for the developing embryo through the vitelline duct (Fig. 18-3, *B*). The size of the yolk sac is most often measured to be 2 to 6 mm throughout the first trimester, and an abnormally small or large

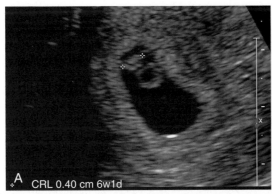
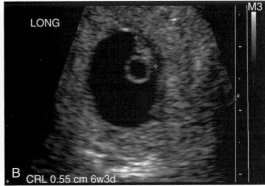

A   CRL 0.40 cm 6w1d

B   CRL 0.55 cm 6w3d

FIGURE 18-4 (A) and **(B)**, Tiny embryo (between calipers) of an early pregnancy is adjacent to the yolk sac. Its disklike appearance becomes more evident as pregnancy progresses between weeks 5 and 7. The embryo should be measured in its longest axis, excluding the yolk sac. Cardiac activity should be evident when the embryo measures 5 mm.

measurement may be indicative of pending loss or fetal abnormality. The yolk sac diameter should be measured with placement of calipers along the inner borders of the echogenic ring (Fig. 18-3, C). The yolk sac is also often used to assist in locating the developing embryo. After the yolk sac is located, close evaluation of adjacent structures often identifies the embryonic disk, recognized with the flicker of cardiac activity.

Crown-Rump Length

After the gestational sac has formed and a yolk sac has developed, the next structure of pregnancy visualized with sonography is the embryo. The embryonic period is considered to be week 6 through week 10 of the pregnancy. In the earliest stage of the embryonic period, the yolk sac may be used as a landmark for locating the very early embryo and possible cardiac activity. Initially, the embryo is found adjacent to the yolk sac and appears on the sonographic image as a flat, disklike structure (Fig. 18-4). Faint flickering of this structure, which represents early cardiac activity, may be seen on real-time sonography at 5.5 weeks or when the CRL measures 5 mm. The normal embryonic heart rate range is 120 to 180 beats per minute. If the embryonic heart rate is 100 beats per minute or less, it should be compared with the maternal heart rate to ensure that maternal uterine vessels are not being sampled and inaccurately represented as embryonic cardiac activity (Fig. 18-5).

With transvaginal technique, the embryo should be visualized in a gestational sac that measures 25 mm. Evaluation of the embryo must include multiple scan planes to obtain the longest axis for accurate gestational dating. A measurement of the longest axis, excluding the yolk sac, provides accurate information for estimation of gestational age. This measurement may be difficult because of the small size of the embryo early in the pregnancy. By approximately 8 weeks' gestational age, the embryo begins to assume a C-shaped appearance, the cystic rhombencephalon can be seen in the posterior embryonic head (Fig. 18-6, A), and limb buds may

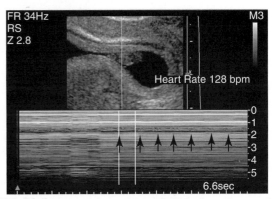

Heart Rate 128 bpm

6.6sec

FIGURE 18-5 Early embryo shows flicker of cardiac motion as demonstrated in this M-mode tracing *(arrows)*. Embryonic heart rate should be between 120 and 180 beats per minute.

be apparent (Fig. 18-6, *B*). At around 11 to 12 weeks, the distinction between the head and torso of the fetus is more easily recognized (Fig. 18-7). An accurate CRL is obtained by placement of the calipers at the top of the fetal head (crown) to the bottom of the torso (rump). Care must be taken not to include the yolk sac or fetal extremities within this measurement. Inclusion of these structures undermines the accuracy of gestational age. Care should also be taken to avoid CRL measurements on an embryo or fetus that is flexed.

Nuchal Translucency

The final measurement that may be performed during a sonographic examination in the first trimester is not a measurement for gestational age estimation but rather a secondary measurement and early screening tool for possible fetal aneuploidy. The nuchal translucency (NT) refers to the normal subcutaneous translucent space along the back of the fetal neck. The thickness of this space has been the source of numerous studies. A thickened NT is associated with fetal aneuploidy, most specifically trisomy 21 (Down syndrome). Increased NT thickness is also associated with genetic syndromes, structural anomalies, and adverse outcome.[1] Techniques

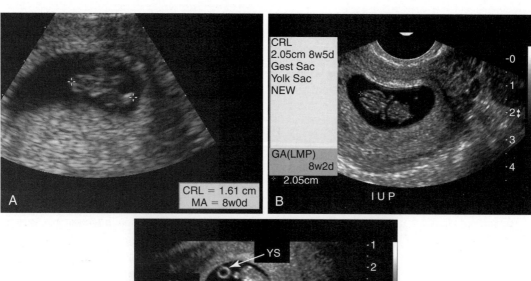

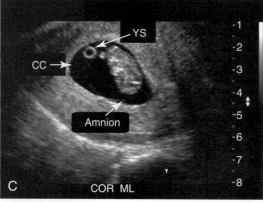

FIGURE 18-6 (A), Normal cystic rhombencephalon *(arrow)* in the hindbrain of an 8-week embryo. **(B),** Limb buds may be seen in an 8-week embryo *(arrows).* **(C),** Surrounding structures include thin amnion, yolk sac *(YS),* and chorionic cavity *(CC).*

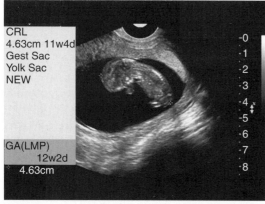

FIGURE 18-7 By 11 weeks, it is easier to distinguish the fetal head and torso; however, obtaining a CRL at this stage can be challenging because of fetal flexion.

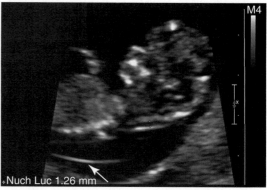

FIGURE 18-8 Caliper placement for measurement of the nuchal translucency in the first trimester. Care should be taken not to confuse the amnion *(arrow)* as the similar-appearing nuchal translucency *(between calipers).*

for measurement of the NT require accuracy and precision in the sonographic view, caliper placement, and gestational age at the time of imaging. To assess NT thickness, the true sagittal plane of the embryo must be acquired. The appropriate technique for measurement of the NT involves placement of the calipers at the fetal skin and the posterior aspect of the nuchal membrane (Fig. 18-8). This technique must be performed with precision because spaces of this small size can be misinterpreted as abnormal with even the slightest variation. The amnion is often found along the posterior edge of the fetus. With the fetus in the supine position, the amniotic

cavity behind the fetus may be confused as the NT and measured as abnormally thickened. Sonographer training and experience in this technique are important to prevent inaccurate measurements that may create false-positive results.

Studies performed to determine the validity of the thickened NT and a cutoff value for this thickening have generated a narrow window of time for evaluation of the NT to be a predictor for fetal chromosomal abnormality. Before the NT measurement is used, gestational age must be assessed with the CRL. The NT may be evaluated with a CRL of no less than 45 mm and no more than 84 mm, which corresponds to a gestational age of 11+0 and 13+6 weeks. Reporting of the nuchal translucency should not be considered if the CRL suggests gestational age outside of this range. The NT is considered to be thickened if it measures 3 mm or more during this gestational time frame. The risk for adverse outcome increases as nuchal translucency increases.

An additional limitation in the validity of NT evaluation is the potentially normal resolution of the thickening, which has been recognized even in cases of fetal aneuploidy. Resolution of an abnormal measurement earlier in the pregnancy does not rule out an abnormality. Close clinical correlation and patient counseling should be performed in cases of an abnormally thickened NT. The significance of NT thickening and sonographic measurement techniques are also discussed in Chapter 24.

SECOND- AND THIRD-TRIMESTER BIOMETRY

After the first 12 weeks of pregnancy, the pregnancy enters the second of three trimesters. The early portion of the second trimester can still yield an accurate gestational age using multiple biometric measurements. Performance of one long-axis measurement of the fetus is no longer acceptable or possible in this trimester, and multiple anatomic structures must be evaluated and measured.

Through approximately 20 weeks, the primary biometric parameters of biparietal diameter (BPD), head circumference (HC), abdominal circumference (AC), and femur length (FL) have minimal biologic variation unless a pathologic condition is present, and estimation of gestational age with these measurements is still accurate with the appropriate technique. With identification of sonographic landmarks of fetal anatomy, these measurements may be obtained with consistency and accuracy. In the case of suspected pathology, biometric measurements should be interpreted using only the unaffected anatomy and may be supplemented with secondary biometric parameters (Box 18-2). After midterm, or 20 gestational weeks, the fetus enters the growth stage of pregnancy, and considering that all newborns are not the same size, the estimation of gestational age is more challenging. Measurements performed in the late second and third trimesters are more accurate for estimation of gestational size rather than age. For this reason, gestational age is more easily determined with fetal biometry in the first half of pregnancy. All subsequent examinations performed in the pregnancy should be based on the earliest examination for gestational age and interval growth.

Primary Biometric Parameters

Biparietal Diameter. As the patient enters the second trimester of pregnancy, the fetal cranium and intracranial structures become more evident and permit sonographic measurements to be performed with a high level

Primary Parameters
Biparietal diameter (BPD)
Head circumference (HC)
Abdominal circumference (AC)
Femur length (FL)

Secondary Parameters
Occipitofrontal diameter (OFD)
Transcerebellar diameter (1 mm per week between weeks 15 and 25)
Binocular distance

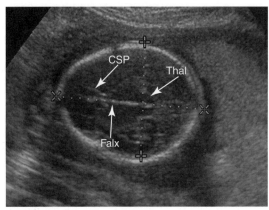

FIGURE 18-9 Location for BPD is shown with the visualized thalamus *(thal)* and cavum septum pellucidum *(CSP)*. Caliper placement is shown from outer edge to inner edge of the cranium perpendicular to cerebral falx *(Falx)*. OFD is demonstrated by the caliper line over the cerebral falx. By using BPD and OFD, HC and cephalic index can also be calculated.

of accuracy. The BPD is considered to be one of the best predictors for gestational age, second only to the CRL performed in the first trimester. The BPD is a biometric measurement performed in the transaxial view of the fetal head just above the level of the ears. For this measurement to provide valuable information, it must be performed with an image of the fetal head at a plane that allows visualization of certain intracranial sonographic landmarks.

The BPD measurement should be performed from the lateral aspect of the fetal head, with the sound beam perpendicular to the interhemispheric fissure, also known as the cerebral falx. The diamond-shaped, hypoechoic thalamus should be seen near the center of the cranium. This view should not demonstrate the orbital rims anteriorly or the cerebellum posteriorly. The BPD should be calculated at the widest point of the fetal head at this level. Calipers should be placed on the outer edge of the near-field cranium and the inner edge of the far-field cranium (Fig. 18-9).

The BPD can be an excellent predictor for gestational age, especially in the early second trimester, but it is not without limitations for accuracy. Among these limitations are the lack of sonographer knowledge and precision, fetal head molding, and biologic variation in the third trimester. The outer-to-inner measurement, described previously, is the most common technique used, but it must be performed correctly to be valuable. Fetal head shape may influence the accuracy of the BPD. This occurs more commonly in cases of oligohydramnios or other sources of fetal crowding. In any circumstance, fetal head shape (cephalic index [CI]) should be evaluated when the BPD is in an unexpected range. An abnormally widened BPD may be a result of a rounded fetal head, also known as brachycephaly. An abnormally shortened BPD may be a result of a flattened fetal head, also known as dolichocephaly. With any fetal head shape, the third trimester creates more biologic variation in fetal head size than any other time in the pregnancy. This variation prevents accurate estimation of gestational age during the later stages of pregnancy.

Head Circumference. The HC provides the interpreting physician with an additional cranial measurement for gestational age assessment. The HC may be calculated with the BPD and the occipitofrontal diameter (OFD) by using the formula $(D1 + D2) \times 1.57$ (see Fig. 18-9). With advances in technology and ultrasound equipment, the HC is now most often performed within the scanner as an ellipse measurement. This measurement should be performed using the same transverse image of the fetal head as the BPD. The ellipse tracing should be placed along the outer border of the fetal cranium and should not include the soft tissues of the fetal scalp (Fig. 18-10). HC is helpful in cases of abnormal fetal head shape because it is least influenced by shape.

Abdominal Circumference. Gestational age may also be determined with measurement of the AC of the fetus. This biometric measurement is used in estimation of gestational age but is better used for estimation of fetal size or weight. The AC should be obtained with the true transverse plane of the fetal abdomen at the level of the umbilical vein junction with the left portal vein. This image should show the fetal stomach along with a hockey stick–shaped appearance of the portal sinus anteriorly in the fetal abdomen (Fig. 18-11). The accuracy of the angle through the fetal abdomen may be confirmed with the appearance of the three ossification centers of the fetal spine seen in a true transverse axis. The fetal kidneys should not be seen along this level of the transverse fetal abdomen, and inclusion of the kidneys undermines the accuracy of the measurement for estimation of gestational age.

Once the correct landmarks are visualized and an image is acquired, the AC may be obtained with the ellipse tracing around the edge of the skin surface on the fetal abdomen (see Fig. 18-11). If the ellipse measurement is unavailable on the equipment, abdomen diameters may be obtained perpendicular to one another in the anteroposterior (AP) and transverse dimensions of the fetal abdomen. Calculation of the AC may be performed with these two diameters.

The AC measurement has limitations for assessment of gestational age. Fetal crowding can alter the fetal abdomen shape and its size. The same conditions that may cause fetal head molding, such as oligohydramnios and advanced gestational age, may influence fetal AC. Sonographer recognition of these conditions may prevent false interpretation of gestational age. The fetal abdomen also has a large variation during the third trimester because of biologic influences. Fetal AC is influenced more by fetal size than fetal age, especially in the third trimester. Gestational age assessment should not rely heavily on the AC, particularly in the third trimester.

Femur Length. Fetal FL is second to the BPD in accuracy for prediction of gestational age in the second trimester. The FL has little biologic variation in the second trimester and is least affected by surrounding structures. To obtain FL, the sonographer should follow the transverse plane of the fetal torso from the level of the AC to the pelvic region. While scanning inferiorly to the iliac wings, the fetal lower extremities can be visualized. The long axis of the femur should be easy to locate because of its limited range of motion. Once the femur is identified, a pivoting motion or rotation of the transducer should allow demonstration of its longest axis. The femur closest to the transducer should be used in estimation of gestational age and imaged perpendicular to the beam's axis. Complete fetal anatomic surveys should include

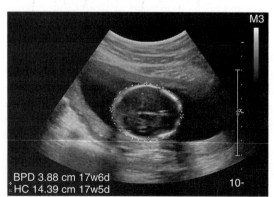

FIGURE 18-10 BPD and HC are acquired at the same location. Ellipse calipers are demonstrated around the fetal cranium for calculation of HC.

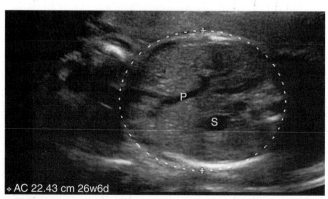

FIGURE 18-11 AC is shown with an ellipse at the level of the fetal stomach (S) and portal sinus (P).

visualization of both femurs for the presence of ossification and gross symmetry.

The FL should be measured in the long axis to include only the diaphysis, or shaft, of the femur (Fig. 18-12). The cartilaginous portion of the femoral head should not be included in the measurement, and the distal femoral epiphysis, seen after approximately 32 weeks, should not be included. If gestational age is completely unknown, visualization of the distal femoral epiphysis has been described to estimate a gestational age of 32 weeks or more. An accurate measurement of the FL can be a valuable predictor of gestational age until the late third trimester. Limitations to this assessment exist, such as biologic influences that may become more evident near term or in cases of suspected skeletal dysplasia. Care should be taken to recognize these limitations to prevent inaccurate assessment of gestational age.

Secondary Biometric Parameters

Occipitofrontal Diameter. The occipitofrontal diameter (OFD) is a secondary biometric measurement that may be used along with the BPD to determine the fetal head shape and size. The OFD is performed at the same transverse image as the BPD, with calipers placed directly on the fetal cranium measuring along the interhemispheric fissure (see Fig. 18-9). A comparison of the BPD and OFD measurements will generate the cephalic index (CI) with the following formula:

$$CI = BPD/OFD \times 100$$

A cephalic index of 76 to 84 is considered to be within the normal range, indicating normal fetal head shape. A cephalic index of more than 84 indicates a brachycephalic shape, and a cephalic index of less than 76 indicates a dolichocephalic shape.

Transcerebellar Diameter. The posterior fossa region of the fetal head should be evaluated for evidence of pathology, and the transcerebellar diameter (TCD) may be used as a secondary biometric measurement to assess gestational age. The cerebellum can be visualized by angling the transducer inferiorly in the posterior skull from the plane of the BPD. This angulation allows visualization of the cerebellum, cerebral peduncles, and thalamus from posterior to anterior in the fetal cranium. The cerebellum can be identified as two hypoechoic circular structures with echogenic borders, also known as the cerebellar hemispheres, on both sides of the midline. The hemispheres are adjacent to a brightly echogenic wedge between them. This echogenic wedge represents the vermis. Other structures included in the posterior fossa view include the cisterna magna and nuchal fold (Fig.18-13, A).

The TCD may be measured with placement of the calipers on the most lateral borders of the cerebellar hemispheres (Fig. 18-13, B). This measurement in millimeters is considered to correlate directly with gestational age between weeks 15 and 25. The TCD is not considered to be the most accurate of head measurements, but in cases of fetal head molding, it may assist in calculation of gestational age. Correlation with the TCD and gestational age can also assist in the diagnosis of cerebellar hypoplasia.

Binocular Distance. At any time during a pregnancy, the fetal head may be found in an extremely low position within the maternal pelvis. This position may make an accurate BPD technically impossible, even after patient manipulation. If the BPD is unobtainable,

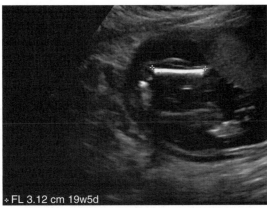

FIGURE 18-12 Diaphysis of the femur is visualized perpendicular to the beam with proper caliper placement demonstrated.

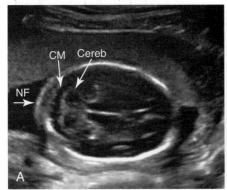
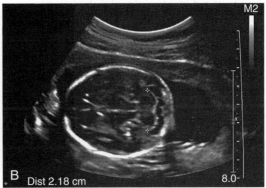

FIGURE 18-13 (A), Posterior fossa structures in a second-trimester fetus include nuchal fold *(NF)*, cisterna magna *(CM)*, and cerebellum *(Cereb)*. **(B),** Proper caliper placement for transcerebellar diameter.

the binocular distance may be performed as a secondary parameter in calculation of gestational age. Although this is not the method of choice for dating the pregnancy, a measurement from the lateral borders of the fetal orbits in the transverse plane may provide an acceptable substitute. The measurement across the distance of both orbital rims is called the binocular distance. Calipers should be placed at the most lateral border of the orbits. Additional measurements may be performed between each orbital rim and between the medial borders of the orbits. The comparison of these measurements with the binocular distance may assist in diagnosis of facial abnormalities, such as hypotelorism and hypertelorism.

Miscellaneous Fetal Measurements of the Second and Third Trimesters

Cisterna Magna. The cisterna magna is found in the posterior fossa immediately posterior to the cerebellum. It appears on sonographic images as an anechoic space between the cerebellum and the posterior cranium (Fig. 18-14). The AP thickness of the cisterna magna is not considered to correlate with gestational age, but if abnormal in size, it is found to be an early indication of fetal pathologic conditions. The cisterna magna should measure 1 cm or less in its AP dimension. An abnormally large cisterna magna has been identified and associated with fetal abnormalities such as ventriculomegaly, cerebellar hypoplasia, and Dandy-Walker malformation. Absence or obliteration of the cisterna magna is a finding associated with fetal spinal dysraphism.

Nuchal Fold. The nuchal fold measurement is a second-trimester sonographic observation used to identify fetuses at risk for trisomy 21. The nuchal fold is the skin at the posterior edge of the fetal cranium. A

measurement of this skin thickness may be taken at the same image plane as the TCD. Calipers must be placed at the midline along the outer edge of the cranium and the outer edge of the fetal skin surface (see Fig. 18-14). Studies have indicated that a nuchal fold thickness of 5 to 6 mm or more between weeks 18 and 24 is associated with trisomy 21.[2] For the nuchal fold thickness to be used as a marker for trisomy 21, care must be taken that fetal head flexion or extension does not influence the measurement. The interpretation of this measurement should be used only in the early second trimester.

Thoracic Circumference. The circumference of the fetal thorax is used for diagnosis of potentially lethal fetal abnormalities rather than for gestational dating purposes. The normal fetus has a thoracic circumference slightly smaller in size than the abdomen circumference. The comparison of these two circumferences may provide valuable information regarding possible pathology, especially skeletal dysplasias. An abnormally small thoracic to AC ratio ($< 0.94 \pm 0.05$) may assist in the assessment for risk of pulmonary hypoplasia.[3] The thoracic circumference should be performed in the transverse plane of the fetal chest at the level of the four-chamber fetal heart. On this same image, the heart circumference may be compared with the thoracic circumference. The normal heart circumference is approximately one third of the thoracic circumference.

Long Bones. In addition to the femur, all other long bones of the extremities may be measured to assist in management of the pregnancy. These measurements may include the humerus, radius, ulna, tibia, or fibula. Charts for each bone measurement have been derived. Gestational age determination itself does not rely on the measurement of these other bones, but identification of pathologic conditions may be possible with comparison of all of these measurements. Visualization of these bones to complete a survey of fetal anatomy should become routine for the sonographer. Sonographer knowledge of the anatomy is important because this evaluation may be more complex and challenging if measurements are needed. In the lower extremities, the smaller fibula is found along the lateral aspect of the lower leg. In the upper extremities, the smaller radius is found along the lateral edge of the forearm and closest to the thumb side of the wrist. An organized technique must be used to identify the bones, given the wide range of motion associated with them. Box 18-3 includes a review of miscellaneous measurements.

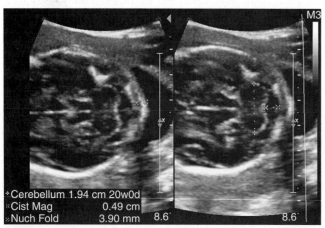

FIGURE 18-14 Proper caliper placement for the measurement of nuchal fold thickness is demonstrated in the image on the left. The image on the right demonstrates transcerebellar and cisterna magna measurements. All three posterior fossa view measurements are within normal limits for a 20-week fetus.

BOX 18-3	Miscellaneous Measurements

Cisterna magna (<1 cm)
Nuchal fold (<5-6 mm between weeks 15 and 19)
Thoracic circumference to abdominal circumference ratio (0.94)
Long bones

SUMMARY

Accurate sonographic measurements are essential for the management of pregnancies with a certain or uncertain LMP. Sonography can be of significant value for assessment of gestational age because of the variability of the female reproductive cycle length. Sonographers must have a thorough knowledge of pregnancy development and embryonic and fetal anatomy as well as an expertise in fetal sonography to provide accurate biometric measurements. Although limitations exist in the prediction of gestational age because of biologic variations or the presence of pathologic conditions, an accurate estimation can be made with strong certainty during the first half of the pregnancy using sonographic biometry. Manufacturers of sonography equipment have incorporated computerized calculation packages that report a composite gestational age using primary biometric parameters. Sonographers and sonologists should recognize the importance of evaluating each biometric parameter individually for avoidance of misinterpretation of gestational age with asymmetric growth. The use of secondary biometric parameters and additional anatomic measurements may assist in determination of a more accurate estimation of gestational age.

The accurate interpretation of sonographic findings can be of significant value in management of a pregnancy with an uncertain LMP. Subsequent sonographic examinations during the pregnancy may be performed to assess and chart fetal growth. The accuracy of fetal biometry is greatest earlier in the pregnancy. All subsequent examinations performed in the pregnancy should be based on the earliest examination for gestational age and interval growth.

CLINICAL SCENARIO—DIAGNOSIS

The primary biometric parameters all are consistent with an adjusted ultrasound age of 17 weeks 5 days. Secondary parameters (transcerebellar diameter, humerus length) are within acceptable deviation standards for this date range and are of no cause for concern. Ventricular diameter, cisterna magna diameter, and nuchal fold thickness are also within normal limits. A follow-up examination is unnecessary based on the findings listed on this report.

CASE STUDIES FOR DISCUSSION

1. A 20-year-old woman is seen for sonographic evaluation of the pelvis because of complaints of right lower quadrant pain. She states that her periods are irregular, but she thinks her last menstrual period was 2 months ago. The sonogram reveals a 4-mm fluid collection surrounded by an echogenic ring within an endometrial layer of the uterus. Adnexal findings include a corpus luteum, and no additional adnexal masses or cul-de-sac fluid is noted. What is the most likely diagnosis?

2. A 24-year-old woman with a positive home pregnancy test is referred for a sonogram to date the pregnancy. The patient states that her last menstrual period was 10 weeks prior. The sonogram demonstrates a gestational sac with a mean sac diameter consistent with 6 weeks' gestation and a living embryo with a crown rump length consistent with 6.5 weeks. What gestational age should be assigned to this pregnancy?

3. A 30-year-old woman with a recent positive pregnancy test is seen for a sonogram because of bleeding. According to her last menstrual period, she should be about 8 weeks pregnant. Transvaginal sonography reveals an intrauterine 30 mm gestational sac containing a yolk sac but no embryo. What is the prognosis for this pregnancy?

4. A sonogram of a 12-week fetus demonstrates a 3.1 mm nuchal translucency measurement. A follow-up scan shows resolution of the thickening. Is this pregnancy at risk for poor outcome? What should be the next step?

5. A fetal sonogram demonstrates BPD, HC, FL, and AC measurements consistent with 20 weeks of gestation. Follow-up sonographic measurements 10 weeks later are consistent with 28 weeks. Should the due date be changed based on the most recent examination? Why or why not?

STUDY QUESTIONS

1. The cystic space within the embryonic head visualized at approximately 8 weeks' gestational age is the developing:
   a. Nuchal fold
   b. Nuchal translucency
   c. Cerebellum
   d. Rhombencephalon

2. Evidence of a developing intrauterine pregnancy should be recognized endovaginally with a serum beta-hCG (IRP) of:
   a. 100 to 200 mIU/mL
   b. 200 to 400 mIU/mL
   c. 500 to 1000 mIU/mL
   d. 1000 to 2000 mIU/mL

3. In the early first trimester of pregnancy, the gestational sac is expected to grow at a rate of:
   a. 1 mm/day
   b. 10 mm/day
   c. 5 mm/day
   d. 1 cm/week

4. The absence of the thick echogenic rim surrounding the early gestational sac within the endometrial cavity is suspicious for:
   a. Pseudogestational sac of ectopic pregnancy
   b. Missed abortion
   c. Molar pregnancy
   d. Partial molar pregnancy

5. In the development of a normal intrauterine pregnancy, the yolk sac should be demonstrated transvaginally in a gestational sac with what minimum measurement?
   a. 1 to 2 mm
   b. 5 mm
   c. 8 mm
   d. 12 mm

6. The occipitofrontal diameter may be measured in the second or third trimester of pregnancy. This measurement in conjunction with BPD is best used to:
   a. Assess for frontal bossing associated with skeletal anomalies
   b. Determine fetal head shape (CI)
   c. Assess fetal risk for Down syndrome
   d. Determine the risks of complicated vaginal delivery

7. The nuchal translucency thickness used for genetic screening in the first trimester of pregnancy must be obtained in the:
   a. Coronal plane
   b. Transverse plane
   c. Sagittal plane
   d. Plane that demonstrates it most easily depending on embryonic position

8. The fetal thoracic circumference should be closely evaluated and compared with the abdominal circumference in the event of a suspected:
   a. Skeletal dysplasia
   b. Abdominal wall defect
   c. Chromosomal abnormality
   d. Growth-restricted fetus

9. A secondary yolk sac measuring greater than what measurement is considered to be abnormal and suspicious for abnormal pregnancy development?
   a. 2 cm
   b. 2 mm
   c. 5 mm
   d. 6 mm

10. The sonographic measurement of what fetal biometric parameter is least influenced by shape?
    a. AC
    b. HC
    c. OFD
    d. BPD

REFERENCES

1. Nicolaides K: Screening for fetal aneuploidies at 11 to 13 weeks, *Prenat Diagn* 31:7–15, 2011.
2. Yeo L, Vintzileos A: The second trimester genetic sonogram. In Callen P, editor: *Ultrasonography in obstetrics and gynecology*, ed 5, Philadelphia, 2008, Saunders, pp 968–985.
3. Goncalves L, Kusanovic J, Gotsch F, et al: The fetal musculoskeletal system. In Callen P, editor: *Ultrasonography in obstetrics and gynecology*, ed 5, Philadelphia, 2008, Saunders, pp 968–985.

Size Greater than Dates

Terry J. DuBose

CLINICAL SCENARIO

A pregnant woman presents to the sonographic laboratory for dating with an unknown last menstrual period (LMP). A wide range of multiple fetal ages was found to be approximately 6 weeks between the relatively smallest and largest parameters. The largest parameter was the femur length estimated at 40 weeks, the smallest was the head circumference (HC) estimated near 34 weeks, and the mean of four parameter ages was 36 weeks, 2 days. The HC-to-abdominal circumference (AC) ratio was 89%, which would indicate a relatively large abdomen. Normal HC-to-AC ratio at 36 weeks is between 87% (large AC) and 109% (small AC).[1] An AC of 340.4 mm at 36 weeks average of the parameter's ages is near the 95th percentile and HC at 32 weeks would be well above the 95th percentile.[2] On a superficial look, one might consider this fetus to have an AC large for dates or fat when compared only with the HC; however, the femur length estimate of age was at term (40 weeks).

OBJECTIVES

- Define terms associated with excessive fetal growth.
- Differentiate between large for gestational age and macrosomia.
- Identify the common causes of large-for-gestational-age pregnancies.
- Describe the sonographic appearance of macrosomia.
- List risk factors associated with macrosomia.
- Describe the management of and interventions for suspected macrosomia.
- Assess the relative size and age of multiple fetal parameters.

Obstetric sonographic examinations are frequently requested because the patient's size is greater than the size expected for gestational age (size greater than dates) if the LMP is unknown or incorrect. The size expected for gestational age is based on the patient's LMP and the physical examination that may include a fundal height measurement. The fundal height measurement is performed with external palpation of the uterus and measurement of the distance from the symphysis pubis to the uterine fundus. The fundal height roughly correlates in centimeters with the gestational age in weeks. This measurement is not highly accurate and may not always be a reflection of excessive fetal growth and can be affected by multiple factors, including the technique of the clinician, maternal weight, fetal position, increase in amniotic fluid, and size of the placenta. In addition, size greater than dates may be suspected when the patient has had a significant weight gain. The uterus may also present large for dates when leiomyomas are present or when ovarian masses mimic an enlarged uterus or hamper the ability to measure the uterus accurately. This chapter explores the possible results and outcomes when a patient is seen for an obstetric sonogram for size greater than dates.

EXCESSIVE FETAL GROWTH

Excessive fetal growth is typically divided into two categories with fetal weight in the determination. Large for gestational age (LGA) is a term suggested when the estimated fetal weight is greater than the 90th percentile for gestational age. Chapter 20 discusses the term small for gestational age, which is suggested when the estimated fetal weight is less than the 10th percentile for gestational age. Macrosomia is determined when the estimated fetal weight is greater than or equal to 4500 g. Appropriate fetal growth is clinically significant and a direct indicator of fetal well-being. Identification of fetuses that are not growing appropriately is important because as fetal growth discrepancy becomes progressively greater, whether from macrosomia or growth restriction, the risk of perinatal morbidity and mortality is significantly increased.

Estimation of Fetal Weight

The estimation of fetal weight is simply that—an estimation. Multiple variables contribute to fetal weight discrepancies. The very nature of the process for determination of fetal weight involves much variability in that sonographic measurements of the fetal head, abdomen, and femur bones, regardless of the degree of care and accuracy by the sonographer, are assigned a weight approximation on the basis of previous research data. Even the best sonographic determination of fetal weight has been estimated to be 10% discrepant of the actual weight. This potential discrepancy percentage would not appreciably affect a fetus of average size with regard to the determination of fetal weight. However, in cases of LGA, it can result in a significant discrepancy of several hundred grams. One study showed that for a confidence level of 90% that a newborn would actually weigh more than 4000 g, one must estimate the sonographic fetal weight at 4750 g.

The most reliable formula used to determine the estimated fetal weight incorporates several fetal parameters, including biparietal diameter, HC, AC, and femur length. The accuracy of this determination is associated with limitations and ranges of discrepancy. Patients and their families need to be properly educated with regard to the degree of accuracy in the estimation of fetal weight with sonographic examination.

Calculation Software. Most current sonographic instruments provide the sonographer with the ability to record a multitude of obstetric measurements and perform calculations during the examination. Because of the various regression models available, it is important to know which is being used to obtain consistency within the laboratory. With regard to diversity, it is also important to understand the obstetric population with which one is working and to make appropriate adjustments to the regression models when necessary.

Pregnancy Dating. Crucial information used in the proper dating of a pregnancy includes an accurate LMP date and the performance of an early baseline sonogram for later comparison. However, in about 20% to 40% of all pregnancies, the correct menstrual age is uncertain because of unknown or unclear LMP dates. Accurate assessment of the fundal height of the uterus during physical examination in cases of maternal obesity may be extremely difficult. In addition, pregnancy dating and the determination of estimated fetal weight involve the following basic assumptions:

- Menstrual cycles last 28 days.
- Women ovulate 14 days into their menstrual cycles.
- Fertilization occurs within 24 hours of ovulation.
- Implantation occurs within 2 days of fertilization.
- Pregnancies last 280 days (menstrual dating).
- Newborns weigh 7.5 lb at delivery.
- Fetal growth is constant.

These assumptions are averages calculated over time and across multiple populations. Just one of these assumptions may have a significant impact on the calculation of pregnancy dating. Taken together, a much wider potential range of error exists. A common source of LMP errors is due to implantation bleeding or spotting, which is mistaken for the LMP. This implantation bleeding often occurs 2 to 3 weeks after the normal LMP and leads to an estimated gestational age that is less than the true age, resulting in sonographic estimates that appear larger than dates. For these reasons, an early baseline sonographic examination is the most reliable indicator of fetal age that may be referenced throughout the duration of the pregnancy.

Macrosomia

The term macrosomia is defined as an abnormally large size of the body. The term refers to the entire fetus, neonate, or newborn. Fetal macrosomia complicates more than 10% of all pregnancies in the United States. With respect to delivery, any fetus that is too large for the maternal pelvis through which it must pass is macrosomic. The most straightforward approach to the sonographic determination of macrosomia is to use the estimated fetal weight.

Risk Factors. The major risk factor for macrosomia is gestational diabetes, which accounts for 40% of all cases. The prevalence rate of macrosomia is 25% to 42% among diabetic mothers versus 8% to 10% among nondiabetic mothers. Despite the higher frequency in diabetic mothers, nondiabetic mothers account for 60% of macrosomic cases because of their majority compared with the smaller number of diabetic mothers. Macrosomia is associated with enlargement of the placenta (Fig. 19-1; see Color Plate 17). A placental thickness obtained at a right angle to its long axis that measures greater than 3 cm before 20 weeks' gestation or greater than 5 cm before 40 weeks' gestation is considered abnormal.

Time of delivery is an important factor to consider. One study showed an increased incidence of macrosomia

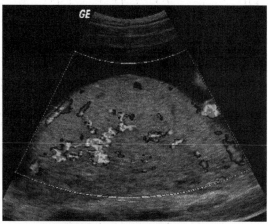

FIGURE 19-1 Enlarged placenta.

from 1.7% at 36 weeks' gestation to 21% at 42 weeks' gestation. Chronic and progressing macrosomia is in direct proportion to an elevated risk of associated conditions, and women who have previously delivered a macrosomic infant are at an increased risk in future pregnancies. Primary perinatal complications include shoulder dystocia, soft tissue trauma, humeral and clavicular fractures, brachial plexus injury, facial palsies, meconium aspiration, prolonged labor, and asphyxial injuries. Shoulder dystocia (Fig. 19-2) occurs when the arm of the fetus prevents or complicates delivery and may result in serious traumatic injury. Because many of these injuries are unpredictable events, available evidence suggests that planned interventions on the basis of estimates of fetal weight may not significantly reduce the incidence of shoulder dystocia and the adverse outcomes attributable to fetal macrosomia. However, because evidence strongly suggests an increased risk of prenatal complications for pregnancies with fetuses weighing greater than 4500 g, the option for cesarean delivery should be considered with fetal macrosomia in diabetic patients with small pelvic structures and in any pregnancy where macrosomia is a concern.

The sonographic fetal AC measurement has been determined to be helpful in identification of potential macrosomic infants. One study reported a less than 1% incidence rate of infant birth weights greater than 4500 g with AC measured less than 35 cm. The incidence rate significantly increased to 37% in cases where the AC was greater or equal to 38 cm. Macrosomic infants of diabetic mothers usually have organomegaly, especially a disproportional enlargement of the heart, liver, adrenals, and adipose tissue.

Hydrops fetalis is also associated with macrosomia and may manifest sonographically with one or more of the following: increased placental thickness, increased thickness of scalp or body wall greater than 5 mm (Figs. 19-3 and 19-4), hepatosplenomegaly, pleural and pericardial effusions, ascites, and structural fetal anomalies.

Prenatally diagnosed syndromes associated with macrosomia include Beckwith-Wiedemann, Marshall-Smith, Ruvalcaba-Myhre, Sotos', and Weaver's syndromes. Other risk factors for macrosomia include prolonged gestation and maternal obesity. Fetal infections can lead to visceromegaly and an enlarged AC. Pregnancies that extend beyond the normal term length tend to fall eventually under the macrosomic category simply because of continued growth before delivery.

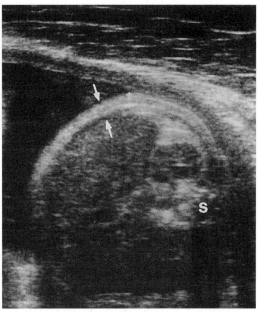

FIGURE 19-3 Increased subcutaneous fat *(arrows)* of body wall thickness. *S,* Spine.

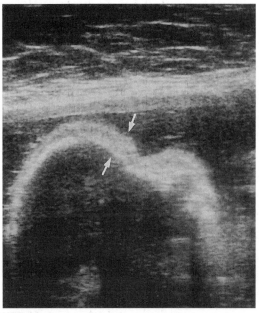

FIGURE 19-4 Increased subcutaneous fat *(arrows)* on scalp.

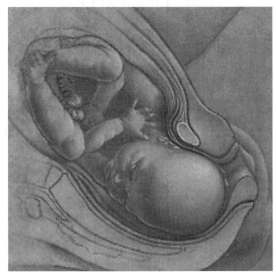

FIGURE 19-2 Fetal position leads to potential shoulder dystocia at delivery.

INCREASED FUNDAL HEIGHT

Other factors contribute to a patient with size greater than dates. A patient with a multiple gestation (Fig. 19-5) may present with an increased fundal height on clinical examination, and the cause for the increased size is easily clarified with sonographic examination. Complications of multiple gestations may contribute significantly to a size discrepancy. Conjoined twins (Fig. 19-6) are a potentially lethal complication that may be identified when a sonographic evaluation is performed because of increased fundal height. Twin-to-twin transfusion syndrome is a serious condition in monozygotic twins where fetal size discrepancy is shown. Because of arteriovenous shunting of blood within a shared placenta, the recipient twin sonographically displays an increase (while the donor twin shows a decrease) in size and amniotic fluid.

Another complication of pregnancy that may manifest with a size-date discrepancy is gestational trophoblastic disease, also known as molar pregnancy. Patients also frequently have hyperemesis. The most common form, the benign hydatidiform mole (Fig. 19-7), appears sonographically as an inhomogeneous or complex mass within the uterus with or without the presence of a fetus. Gestational trophoblastic disease is discussed in detail in Chapter 21.

Polyhydramnios may contribute to an increased fundal height with singleton pregnancies as well. Frequently, a subjective assessment by an experienced sonographer raises suspicion of polyhydramnios when noting that the fetus looks like a "small fish in a big fishbowl." Two primary methods used to quantify the amount of amniotic fluid have been defined and are useful for the less experienced sonographer and for following patients over time.[3] The single pocket assessment can be performed with identification of the largest vertical pocket of amniotic fluid and measurement of the anteroposterior depth. Polyhydramnios is indicated when the pocket exceeds 8 cm (Fig. 19-8), and oligohydramnios is indicated when the pocket is less than 2 cm. At the present time, the amniotic fluid index (AFI) is more often used to assess amniotic fluid. The method involves dividing the maternal uterus into four quadrants and adding the anterior-to-posterior measurements of the amniotic fluid in each of

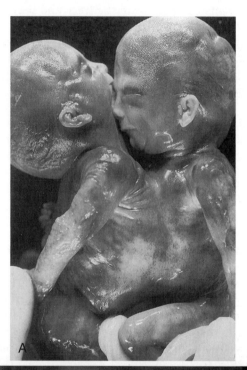
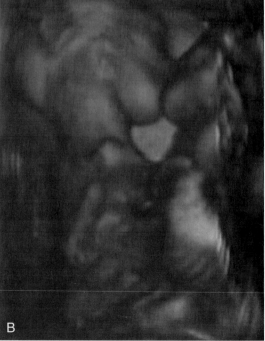

FIGURE 19-6 (A), Thoracoomphalopagus conjoined twins, gross specimen. **(B),** Thoracoomphalopagus conjoined twins, three-dimensional sonography.

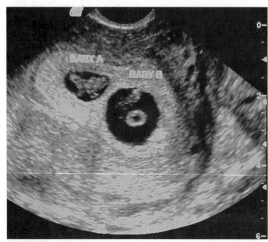

FIGURE 19-5 Increased uterine size was noted clinically in 7-week, 1-day twin gestation.

the quadrants. The AFI total is normally 10 to 13 ± 5 cm. The normal range for the AFI is usually 5 to 20 cm. These measurements are not absolute limits of normal but simply guidelines. Increasing AFI correlates linearly with increasing birth weight. One study reported more than double the risk of a macrosomic infant birth with an AFI greater than 15 and a risk of more than six times with an AFI greater than 18. Although several studies have been conducted in recent years to identify a more accurate assessment of the upper and lower limits of normal amniotic fluid levels to define clinically significant polyhydramnios, less than exact correlations have been the result. It continues to be a nonspecific finding but one that warrants further investigation because more than 100 fetal anomalies are associated with this condition, including diabetes (Fig. 19-9).

Genetic constitution, including familial physical traits such as parental stature, needs to be considered in cases of suggested macrosomia. Larger parents are more likely to produce larger than average-sized infants, whereas smaller parents tend to have smaller than average-sized infants.

In addition, a history of size greater than dates may not relate to the pregnancy. Leiomyomas (fibroids) are benign uterine tumors that can be significant in size, contributing to an increased fundal height (Fig. 19-10). They can also increase in size during pregnancy. Leiomyomas typically appear as well-defined masses of variable echogenicity within the myometrium. Sonographic evaluation of a patient with an increased fundal height may also reveal ovarian enlargement, which may be from an ovarian cyst or neoplasm such as a benign cystic teratoma or cystadenoma. The sonographic appearance of a cyst should be anechoic and thin-walled and exhibit enhancement. Teratomas and cystadenomas (Fig. 19-11) often have a complex appearance, although a teratoma often has a characteristic shadowing from the presence of calcifications.

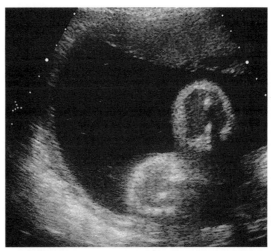

FIGURE 19-9 Polyhydramnios noted in a patient was the result of diabetes.

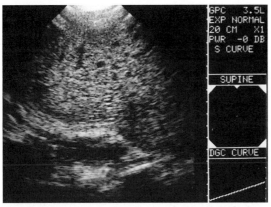

FIGURE 19-7 Patient was seen for sonography because of size greater than dates. Sonogram reveals molar pregnancy.

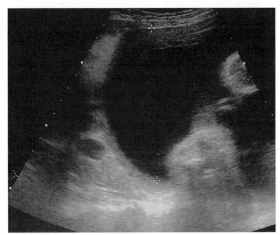

FIGURE 19-8 Patient with polyhydramnios has single pocket measurement of more than 10 cm.

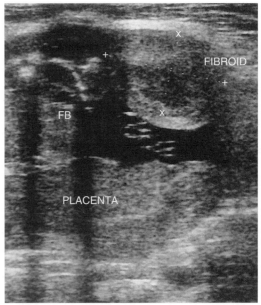

FIGURE 19-10 Fibroid identified in image was a contributing factor in a patient having increased fundal height.

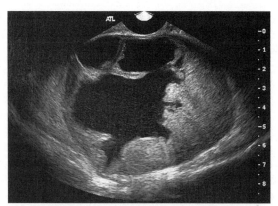

FIGURE 19-11 Mucinous cystadenoma.

TABLE 19-1	Causes for Size Greater than Dates
Diagnosis	**Findings**
LGA	Fetal weight >90th percentile
Macrosomia	Fetal weight ≥4500 g
Implantation bleeding	Underestimation of normal LMP and gestational age by 2-3 weeks
Enlarged abdomen	Large AC, which may be due to fetal infection and visceromegaly
Hydrops fetalis	Fluid in two body cavities (ascites, pericardial effusion, pleural effusion) or skin edema plus fluid in one body cavity; also associated with placentomegaly, hepatosplenomegaly, structural anomalies
Multiple gestation	More than one fetus, one or more placentas
Molar pregnancy	Heterogeneous mass within uterine cavity, no fetus; associated with large, bilateral, multilocular ovarian cysts
Polyhydramnios	Single pocket, >8 cm; AFI, >18 cm
Leiomyomas	Well-defined lesions of variable echogenicity

SUMMARY

The cause (Table 19-1) for size greater than dates can be evaluated with diagnostic medical sonography. However, sonography continues to have limitations based on myriad variables relative to the complexity of pregnancy and fetal development. Although sonographic estimations of fetal weight have shown poor accuracy in the prediction of macrosomia, use of a combination of specific maternal and fetal characteristics has shown the ability to estimate birth weight more accurately. Some significant predictors of term birth weight are gestational age, parity, fetal gender, maternal height, maternal weight, and third-trimester rate of maternal weight gain. In addition, three-dimensional sonography and magnetic resonance imaging are expected to generate estimates of fetal weight that are more accurate than the estimates for two-dimensional sonography or clinical estimates. Sonography continues to be used in the determination of fetal weight and can be useful in evaluation of the anatomic structures of the fetus and mother to identify other possible causes for a size greater than dates presentation.

CLINICAL SCENARIO—DIAGNOSIS

On closer examination, it was found that both the liver and the spleen were enlarged. The liver measured 96.0 mm in length and the spleen measured 84.8 mm in length, indicating visceromegaly (Fig. 19-12). The large abdominal organs, with the relatively small HC, led to a tentative diagnosis of a fetal infection. Subsequent assays found the fetus did have a TORCH (*t*oxoplasmosis, *o*ther [congenital syphilis, viruses] *r*ubella, *c*ytomegalovirus, *h*erpes simplex virus) infection. This case illustrates the complexity of the assessment of fetal parameters. It is important to look at the big picture and not focus on one or two fetal parameters.

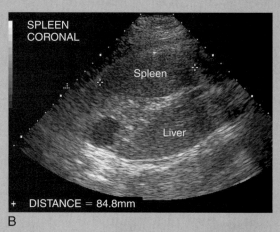

MEAN (mm)	MA		
BPD 79.5	31W6D(±22D)	HC/AC	0.89(0.92-1.11)
HC 304.5	33W6D(±21D)	CI	75.1(70-86)
AC 340.4	38W0D(±21D)		
FL 78.6	40W1D(±22D)		

AFI= 256mm

EFW = 3139 ± 383g

CLINICAL	ULTRASOUND
LMP=UNKNOWN	ACUSON
MA =UNKNOWN	MA=36W2D(±16D)
EDD=UNKNOWN	EDD=28-APR-98

A

SPLEEN CORONAL

Spleen

Liver

+ DISTANCE = 84.8mm

B

FIGURE 19-12 (A), Sonographic fetal parameters size and age calculations. **(B)**, Sonogram showing enlarged liver and spleen.

CASE STUDIES FOR DISCUSSION

1. During a dating obstetric sonographic study (Fig.19-13), the fetal abdomen appears to be large compared with the thorax. The arms and legs appear to be short. The head appears to be a normal size, but the skull and other bones appear to be hypoechogenic. What is the most likely diagnosis?

2. A sonographer is asked to be an expert witness in an obstetric medicolegal case in which the mother had gestational diabetes. During the difficult delivery, there was dystocia, with neurologic damage to the left arm and shoulder. The neonate was found to be at the 95th percentile for weight, and the length was normal. Which sonographic images would be the most important to study and why?

3. A woman is referred for sonographic dating of pregnancy. The LMP, 12 weeks before the sonogram, is reported to be lighter than normal. Four fetal parameters are measured with an estimated gestational age of 15 LMP weeks. What are the possible explanations for the 3-week difference in the reported LMP and the sonographic gestational age?

4. A 25-year-old woman is seen for obstetric sonography at 24 weeks' gestation by LMP for increased fundal height. The sonogram reveals the finding in Figure 19-14 in addition to absence of the fetal calvaria and brain. What is the cause of the size-date discrepancy?

5. A woman is referred for sonographic examination at 35 weeks by LMP because of increased fundal height. Figure 19-15, *A*, shows a coronal plane of the fetal abdomen. Figure 19-15, *B*, shows the measurements taken during the sonogram. What is the most likely diagnosis?

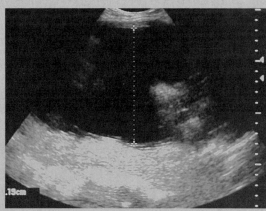

FIGURE 19-14 An 11.2-cm, single pocket measurement of amniotic fluid is identified in a 24-week gestation.

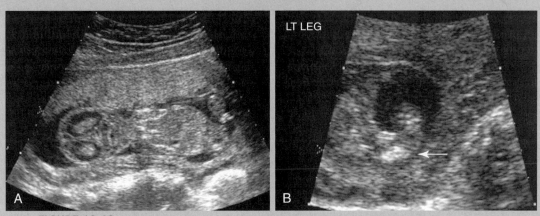

FIGURE 19-13 **(A)**, Coronal plane of fetal head and trunk. **(B)**, Left fetal leg with femur *(arrow)*.

Continued

CASE STUDIES FOR DISCUSSION—cont'd

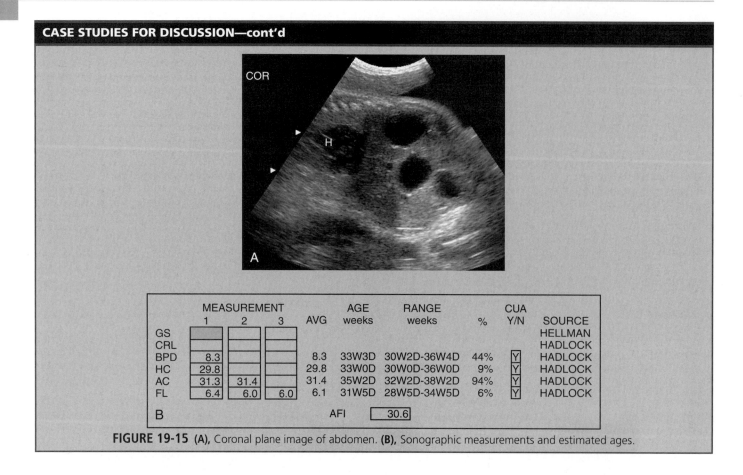

	MEASUREMENT				AGE	RANGE		CUA	
	1	2	3	AVG	weeks	weeks	%	Y/N	SOURCE
GS									HELLMAN
CRL									HADLOCK
BPD	8.3			8.3	33W3D	30W2D-36W4D	44%	Y	HADLOCK
HC	29.8			29.8	33W0D	30W0D-36W0D	9%	Y	HADLOCK
AC	31.3	31.4		31.4	35W2D	32W2D-38W2D	94%	Y	HADLOCK
FL	6.4	6.0	6.0	6.1	31W5D	28W5D-34W5D	6%	Y	HADLOCK
B				AFI	30.6				

FIGURE 19-15 (A), Coronal plane image of abdomen. **(B),** Sonographic measurements and estimated ages.

STUDY QUESTIONS

1. A woman is referred to the sonography laboratory for gestational dating. Reported LMP was 10 weeks earlier than the current examination date and lighter than normal. The average age of multiple fetal parameters was 13 weeks, and all parameter ages were within 1 week of that age. What is the most likely explanation of the fetal age discrepancy?
   a. The fetus is growing too fast, the mother should be checked for diabetes, and the fetus should be remeasured in 4 to 6 weeks.
   b. The reported LMP was most likely implantation breakthrough bleeding, and the true LMP was 13 weeks earlier.
   c. The fetal measurements were incorrect.
   d. The fetal age should be adjusted to the age estimated by the 10-week LMP.

2. A routine obstetric sonogram was performed in a patient with a reported LMP of 20 weeks. The estimated age by femur length was 19 weeks, and the AC was calculated to 22 weeks; liver and spleen were normal. The HC indicated a gestational age of 20 weeks. What is the most likely explanation of this age assessment?
   a. The fetus is most likely a dwarf.
   b. The fetus is normal with slightly short femurs and a fat abdomen.

   c. The AC was probably measured incorrectly.
   d. The fetus is likely a dwarf with microcephaly.

3. A 29-year-old woman is seen for an obstetric sonogram for an increased fundal height at 27 weeks' gestation by LMP. The sonographic examination reveals two fetuses sharing a single placenta. Fetus A measures 28 weeks and shows mild polyhydramnios. Fetus B measures 25 weeks and shows moderate oligohydramnios. What is the most likely diagnosis?
   a. Normal twin pregnancy
   b. Marshall-Smith syndrome
   c. Trophoblastic disease
   d. Twin-to-twin transfusion syndrome

4. A 21-year-old woman is seen for an obstetric examination with an indication of large for gestational age at 28 weeks by first-trimester sonography. The sonogram shows a fetus measuring 28 weeks. The AFI is 25 cm. What is the most likely diagnosis?
   a. Oligohydramnios
   b. Polyhydramnios
   c. Macrosomia
   d. Hydrops fetalis

5. A 29-year-old woman presents for obstetric sonography at 35 weeks' gestation. She has a history of gestational diabetes in two prior pregnancies.

Sonograms at 11 weeks and 23 weeks have confirmed gestational age and have been otherwise unremarkable. The current examination reveals an average sonographic age of 38 weeks, 4 days. The placenta appears generous in size, measuring 6.2 cm. What is the most likely diagnosis?
a. Inaccurate LMP date
b. Hydrops
c. Microsomia
d. Poor nutrition
e. Macrosomia

6. A 22-year-old woman is seen for an obstetric sonogram at 16 weeks' gestation by LMP for increased uterine size and absent heart tones. The sonogram shows a large heterogeneous mass within the uterus. No identifiable fetus or amniotic fluid can be detected. What is the most likely diagnosis?
a. Fetal demise
b. Hydatidiform mole
c. Hydropic placenta
d. Ruvalcaba-Myhre syndrome

7. A 25-year-old woman is referred for sonographic dating, with unknown LMP, no prior studies, and a fundal height measuring approximately 35 weeks. The average of four fetal parameters measured calculate to 32 weeks. AFI measures 17 cm. What is the most likely diagnosis?
a. The fetus is most likely normal, with mild polyhydramnios.
b. The fetus has intrauterine growth restriction and needs to be followed.
c. The fetus is most likely abnormal, with mild polyhydramnios.
d. The fetus needs to be remeasured to correlate the growth pattern.

8. A 24-year-old woman with a history of reduced fetal movement presents for an obstetric sonogram. There is no indication of bleeding, pain, or other complications. Based on previous unremarkable sonography in the first trimester, the pregnancy should currently measure 37 weeks' gestation. The patient is 5 feet, 11 inches in height, and the father is 6 feet, 7 inches in height. The average age by sonography is 40 weeks' gestational age. The remainder of the examination is unremarkable. What is the most likely diagnosis?
a. Abnormally increased growth
b. Hydrops fetalis
c. Normal growth from tall parents
d. High suspicion for anomaly

9. A 30-year-old woman with a gestational age by LMP of 30 weeks is referred for gestational dating and fetal assessment. The sonogram showed the fetal age by HC and femur length to be 31 weeks, and the AC measured to 35 weeks. The liver, kidneys, and other viscera appeared large, and the fetal face showed macroglossia. What is the most likely diagnosis?
a. Beckwith-Wiedemann syndrome
b. Marshall-Smith syndrome
c. Sotos' syndrome
d. Turner's syndrome

10. A 35-year-old woman presents for sonographic dating and is found to have a fetus with severe abnormalities. Findings included scalp edema, generalized skin edema, ascites, plural effusion, and a large cystic structure at the occipital area. What is a likely diagnosis?
a. Beckwith-Wiedemann syndrome
b. Marshall-Smith syndrome
c. Sotos' syndrome
d. Turner's syndrome

REFERENCES

1. DuBose T: *Fetal sonography*, Philadelphia, 1996, Saunders.
2. Jeanty P: Fetal biometry. In Fleischer AC, Manning FA, Jeanty P, et al: *Sonography in obstetrics and gynecology*, ed 6, New York, 2001, McGraw-Hill, p 155.
3. Magann EF, Sandlin AT, Ounpraseuth ST: Amniotic fluid volume dynamics and clinical correlation, *J Ultrasound Med* 30:1573–1585, 2011.

Size Less than Dates

Jennie Durant, Diane Youngs

CLINICAL SCENARIO

A 39-year-old woman, gravida 1, para 0, is seen at the high-risk obstetric clinic for a sonogram of the fetus. She is a professional in a high-stress career who works 70 to 80 hours a week. On her last prenatal visit, the uterine fundal height measured 30 cm and lagged behind the gestational age of 33 weeks, 4 days. She had a prior sonographic examination at 16 weeks that confirmed the gestational age was consistent with her last menstrual period. The prior sonogram also failed to reveal any obvious fetal congenital anomalies, and a genetic amniocentesis showed normal fetal chromosomes. Her medical history is significant for type 1 diabetes mellitus since age 12 years; her condition is well controlled with an insulin pump. During her pregnancy, blood pressures have been normal and she has always had a trace of proteinuria.

The current sonogram reveals a single viable fetus in the vertex presentation. Fetal biometry shows an average ultrasound age of 31 weeks, 5 days, and an amniotic fluid index (AFI) of 6.7 cm. The estimated fetal weight is at the 8th percentile for gestational age. The placenta is posterior-fundal and unremarkable. Clinically, her blood pressure is 149/100 mm Hg, and her urine dipstick test reveals significant protein. She also has a severe headache. What are the possible explanations for these findings?

OBJECTIVES

- Discuss the clinical scenarios associated with a pregnancy size less than dates.
- Describe the sonographic appearance and technique for a diagnosis of oligohydramnios.
- Describe the sonographic appearance of common fetal renal diseases associated with size less than dates.
- Describe clinical conditions, basic physiology, and sonographic findings to understand and make a diagnosis of intrauterine growth restriction.
- Discuss the role of sonography in the diagnosis of premature rupture of membranes.

Measurement of the uterine fundal height during every prenatal visit after 20 weeks of gestation is an integral part of obstetric care. It is a simple, safe, inexpensive, and reasonably accurate method to screen for fetal growth and amniotic fluid volume abnormalities, although it is less accurate in identifying small-for-gestational-age (SGA) fetuses. Longitudinal studies have shown that symphysis-to-fundus measurements correctly identify less than 35% of SGA fetuses.[1] The standard of care is to order or perform an obstetric sonogram when the uterine fundal height is in discordance with the estimated gestational age.

When evaluating a woman considered to have a pregnancy size less than dates, obtaining a medical history, vital signs, social and family history, and recent symptoms is warranted. Some patients may have decreased fetal movement, which would suggest the finding of oligohydramnios. Others may be found to have recently elevated blood pressure or a history of vascular disease, such as pregestational diabetes mellitus or systemic lupus erythematosus. Family history may reveal prior cases of neonates with renal abnormalities or a tendency for small infants. Evaluation of social habits, such as work, nutrition, and use of alcohol or recreational drugs, can be useful. Generally, a carefully performed obstetric sonogram together with pertinent clinical data is more likely to yield an accurate diagnosis.

OLIGOHYDRAMNIOS

Oligohydramnios is a significant decrease in the normal volume of amniotic fluid. Amniotic fluid volume (AFV) results from a balance between what enters and exits from the amniotic cavity. From 20 weeks of gestation to term, the amniotic fluid is mostly made up of fetal urination and respiratory secretions, and fluid is resorbed via fetal swallowing. Alteration of these dynamics can have a significant impact on the pregnancy. The functions of amniotic fluid are numerous, including preventing fetal injury, regulating temperature, providing mobility for practicing breathing, swallowing exercises, fighting infection, discouraging contractions, and maintaining cervical length and consistency. A decrease in AFV is directly correlated with perinatal mortality and many serious morbidities.[2]

Oligohydramnios or anhydramnios (absence of amniotic fluid) can result from amniotic fluid loss from premature rupture of membranes (PROM) (Fig. 20-1) or can be a result of decreased fetal urinary production or excretion. Decreased urine output is associated with fetal renal anomalies in which both kidneys are dysplastic and with severe intrauterine growth restriction (IUGR) when perfusion to the kidneys is reduced. Decreased excretion is associated with urinary outlet obstruction. Ruptured membranes may be suggested with the finding of decreased amniotic fluid on sonography and a fetus that is of an appropriate size without structural anomalies. Fetal anomalies, medication or drug use by the mother (nonsteroidal antiinflammatory drugs, angiotensin-converting enzyme inhibitors, cocaine), maternal medical disease, placental insufficiency, and chromosome alterations all can explain a finding of oligohydramnios. Chronic oligohydramnios, with or without fetal abnormalities, may cause pulmonary hypoplasia, abnormal chest wall compliance, contractures, and infection.[2]

Sonographic Findings

Although the most accurate methods to determine total AFV are direct measurement during hysterotomy or dye-dilution techniques, sonographic estimation is the only practical method. Sonographic methods include qualitative assessment (subjective) and quantitative assessment (objective). Most clinicians use some form of objective measurement to estimate the AFV, such as the maximum vertical pocket (MVP) or AFI.

MVP involves a survey of the entire amniotic cavity and measurement of the largest vertical pocket of amniotic fluid, free of umbilical cord or fetal parts. The criteria for oligohydramnios vary, but a deepest pocket of less than 2 cm is most widely accepted.[3]

AFI is calculated by adding the largest vertical pocket of fluid measured from each of the four quadrants of the uterus. Measurement of pockets of fluid should be void of umbilical cord or any fetal parts. AFI should be measured with the patient supine and can be obtained in the transverse or sagittal plane orientating the transducer perpendicular to the floor. To divide the uterus into four quadrants, the midsagittal line is used as the vertical landmark, and an imaginary line halfway between the symphysis pubis and the fundus of the uterus is used as the horizontal landmark. Using excessive transducer pressure can cause an inaccurate AFI assessment. It is important to use color Doppler imaging while obtaining an AFI measurement (Fig. 20-2; see Color Plate 18) because this eliminates the inaccuracy of measuring the umbilical cord instead of the amniotic fluid, especially on patients who are difficult to scan. AFI of less than 5 cm is the generally accepted criterion used to diagnose oligohydramnios, and AFI between 5.1 cm and 18 cm is considered normal.[3]

The ability of the described sonographic methods to detect normal AFV is high; however, abnormal AFV detection is poor, especially for oligohydramnios.

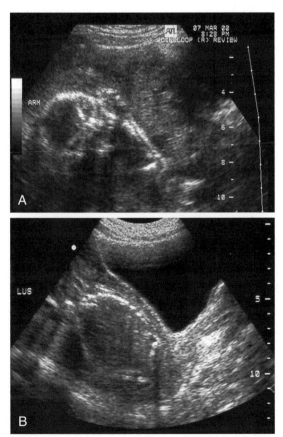

FIGURE 20-1 Severe oligohydramnios in a fetus at gestational age 20 weeks, 3 days. Note lack of fluid around fetal head **(A)** and abdomen **(B)**. The fetus is in breech position. A single pocket of amniotic fluid measuring 0.9 cm is identified. This patient had reported abdominal pain and leaking fluid.

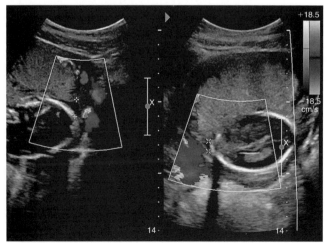

FIGURE 20-2 Oligohydramnios is noted in a pregnancy at gestational age 19 weeks. Only 1.9 cm of fluid is noted around the fetus. Color Doppler imaging helps identify the umbilical cord.

Studies have compared AFI and MVP, and results indicate that AFI overestimates and MVP underestimates fluid volumes.[3,4]

When the diagnosis of oligohydramnios is made, detailed sonographic examination of the fetus should follow; however, evaluation of other anatomic structures may be limited because of the lack of an acoustic window. Sonographic evaluation determines if the kidneys are present and functioning, and fetal biometry and Doppler assessment can evaluate for IUGR. When major anomalies are not present, onset, duration, and severity of amniotic fluid loss are important cofactors, but the gestational age at delivery remains the overriding issue.[2]

FETAL RENAL ANOMALIES

Renal Agenesis

Renal agenesis is the congenital absence of one or both kidneys from the complete lack of formation. The incidence rate of renal agenesis is 1 in 3000 births and 1 in 240 stillbirths.[5,6] It is 2.5 times more common in male fetuses than in female fetuses. Bilateral absence of the kidneys is more common in twins than in singletons. An increased incidence is not seen with advanced maternal age or maternal medical disease.

Renal agenesis is a developmental anomaly that occurs at 4 to 6 weeks of embryonic life. Three main embryologic events are necessary for normal formation of the kidneys. Failure of one of the steps in renal formation (the development of the metanephros) results in complete absence of the kidney. Because of the absence of fetal urination, oligohydramnios develops in a woman with a fetus with bilateral renal agenesis, which may be clinically identified as size less than dates. In unilateral renal agenesis, one of the kidneys does not develop, and the contralateral fetal kidney undergoes compensatory hypertrophy. This hypertrophy occurs prenatally. Because renal function exists in the presence of unilateral renal agenesis, the AFV is usually within normal limits.

Sonographic Findings. The sonographic criteria for the diagnosis of bilateral renal agenesis are (1) presence of severe oligohydramnios or anhydramnios after 14 to 16 weeks of gestation and (2) failure to visualize the fetal kidneys and the urinary bladder (Fig. 20-3, *A*; see Color Plate 19). After 26 to 28 weeks of gestation, preterm premature rupture of membranes (PPROM) or placental dysfunction may be the cause for the low or absent AFV.

First-trimester diagnosis of renal agenesis is rare because AFV is often not reduced at that point in gestation because its volume is primarily from the placenta. The fetal kidneys may be visualized from 10 weeks of gestation with

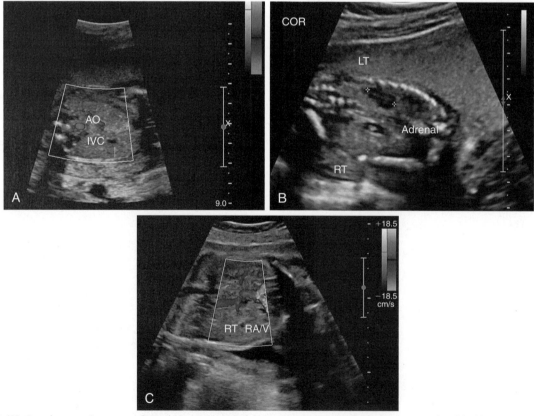

FIGURE 20-3 (A), Renal agenesis was confirmed in this breech fetus with severe oligohydramnios. Neither bladder nor renal arteries were identified. **(B),** Renal agenesis in a 29-week fetus shows enlarged adrenal glands *(calipers)* occupying renal spaces. Oligohydramnios and an absent bladder confirmed the diagnosis. **(C),** Normal renal arteries are apparent. Color Doppler maps out renal arteries bilaterally in a growth-restricted fetus with oligohydramnios, confirming the presence of kidneys that are poorly visualized.

transvaginal sonography. In contrast to the fetal adrenals, which are relatively hypoechogenic, the fetal kidneys appear as bilateral echogenic masses with a similar density to that of the fetal lungs. The fetal adrenal glands have served as a source of false-negative diagnoses in cases of renal agenesis. They may appear enlarged and be confused for fetal kidneys. However, adrenal hypertrophy has been found not to occur, and the false-negative diagnosis of renal agenesis is related to a change in the normal adrenal shape and not to any enlargement of the fetal adrenal gland. In the absence of a fetal kidney, the adrenal gland, which is no longer in its transverse lie draped over the superior pole of the kidney, now is primarily in a longitudinal lie (Fig. 20-3, *B*). This position gives it an enlarged appearance within the renal fossa.

Difficulty may arise in identifying the fetal kidneys in the presence of oligohydramnios. Color or power Doppler imaging is recommended as an adjunct in the diagnosis of bilateral renal agenesis. With correct Doppler settings, color Doppler imaging can aid in identifying the renal arteries (Fig. 20-3, *C*; see Color Plate 20), and renal agenesis is strongly suspected when the renal arteries are not identified.

Autosomal Recessive Polycystic Kidney Disease

Autosomal recessive polycystic kidney disease (ARPKD) occurs in approximately 1 in 20,000 births.[7] This type of polycystic kidney disease is caused by mutations in the *PKHD1* gene and is characterized by nonobstructive dilations of the collecting ducts in the kidneys and hepatic fibrosis.[8] Severe cases can result in perinatal death when pulmonary hypoplasia is caused by long-standing oligohydramnios. Both kidney and liver disease are progressive in most patients, requiring kidney transplantation before the age of 20 years or treatment of early-onset severe hypertension, esophageal varices, and recurrent cholangitis, or both transplantation and treatment of the aforementioned complications.[8] Fetal liver changes may not be evident sonographically; however, 30% of patients with ARPKD present perinatally with enlarged kidneys.[8] DNA previously collected from the first fetus affected with ARPKD is invaluable to facilitate early prenatal diagnosis in subsequent pregnancies.

Sonographic Findings. Typical in utero presentation of ARPKD is the finding of enlarged, echogenic kidneys with loss of corticomedullary differentiation, along with oligohydramnios (Fig. 20-4). The echogenicity of the renal parenchyma is thought to be the result of numerous, closely spaced small cysts that cannot be detected sonographically. Increased echogenicity has been identified by 12 to 16 weeks of gestation. An accurate diagnosis of ARPKD may be difficult early in pregnancy because the size of the fetal kidneys may still be normal. Evidence of renal enlargement and marked echogenicity is usually present by 24 weeks of gestation. Occasionally,

the diagnosis cannot be made until the third trimester or after birth. Oligohydramnios is associated with renal dysfunction, and marked oligohydramnios is a common finding. A detailed family history, together with sonographic evaluation of the parents' kidneys, is helpful in obtaining the correct diagnosis because both ARPKD and autosomal dominant polycystic kidney disease can manifest with oligohydramnios.

Multicystic Dysplastic Kidneys

Dysplastic kidneys can be of any size, ranging from small kidneys (with or without cysts) to large kidneys distended from multiple large cysts up to 9 cm in diameter. Multicystic dysplastic kidneys (MCDK) occur when parenchymal dysplasia causes renal cysts; this condition is not known to be inheritable.[7] The incidence rate of unilateral dysplasia is 1 in 3000 to 5000 births. It occurs with less frequency in the bilateral form, with an incidence of 1 in 10,000.[9] Prenatal diagnosis of unilateral dysplastic kidneys is variable. Bilateral MCDK is more likely to be diagnosed earlier in the pregnancy because of the associated finding of oligohydramnios.

A strong association exists between MCDK and obstruction. Multicystic kidneys are usually attached to atretic ureters. A detailed examination of the fetus should be performed to identify contralateral renal anomalies (Fig. 20-5, *A*) or associated extrarenal anomalies, including heart, spine, extremities, face, and umbilical cord. Genetic counseling and karyotyping should be offered to rule out chromosomal abnormalities.

Sonographic Findings. The classic presentation of MCDK is a multiloculated abdominal mass consisting of multiple, thin-walled cysts that do not appear to connect. The cysts are distributed randomly, the kidney is enlarged with an irregular outline, and no renal pelvis is usually identified (Fig. 20-5, *B*). Parenchymal tissue between the cysts is usually echogenic because of the enhancement from the surrounding cysts.

In the unilateral form, oligohydramnios is uncommon. In the bilateral form, oligohydramnios or anhydramnios

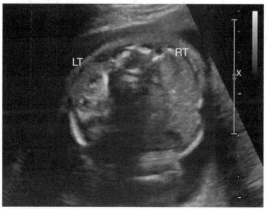

FIGURE 20-4 Enlarged echogenic kidneys are noted bilaterally. Oligohydramnios is also identified in association with ARPKD.

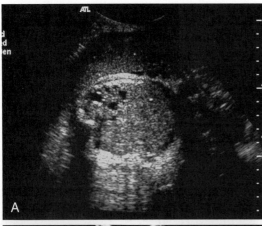

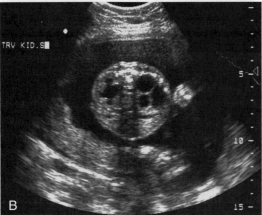

FIGURE 20-5 **(A)**, Unilateral cystic dysplasia was noted in association with contralateral renal agenesis. Note absence of amniotic fluid surrounding the fetus. **(B)**, Unilateral MCDK is identified in a fetus with contralateral UPJ obstruction. There is a normal amount of amniotic fluid.

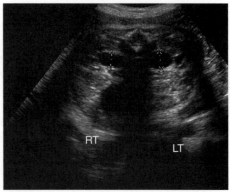

FIGURE 20-6 Transverse image of a fetal abdomen with bilateral pyelectasis (calipers).

Hydronephrosis

Hydronephrosis is a dilation of the renal collecting system. It may be accompanied by dilation of the ureters with or without dilation of the bladder, depending on the level of obstruction. The severity of hydronephrosis can be defined as mild, moderate, or severe. Mild hydronephrosis is described as dilation of the renal pelvis. Moderate hydronephrosis is described as dilation of the renal pelvis and calyces. Severe hydronephrosis is described as gross dilation of the collecting system with a decrease in the renal cortical tissue. Mild pyelectasis, when identified with other findings, has been

is present, and the bladder is not visualized. Bilateral, severe MCDK may be difficult to distinguish from renal agenesis because the dysplastic kidneys commonly decrease in size as pregnancy progresses. Color Doppler imaging can be useful in the diagnosis of MCDK because the renal artery is always small or absent, and the Doppler waveform, when identified, is markedly abnormal with high resistance. Renal cystic diseases are also discussed in Chapter 9.

associated with Down syndrome.[10] Oligohydramnios may accompany hydronephrosis when the obstruction is severe, bilateral, or associated with a serious contralateral anomaly. The most common congenital obstructive genitourinary anomalies include ureteropelvic junction (UPJ) obstruction, ureterovesical junction (UVJ) obstruction, and posterior urethral valves (PUV). The purpose of the sonographic examination includes the identification of the renal obstructive disorder and the level of obstruction because this affects the treatment options and the prognosis for the fetus.

Ureteropelvic Junction Obstruction. UPJ obstruction is the most common cause of congenital hydronephrosis. This condition may occur secondary to arrested or hypoplastic development of the junction of the renal pelvis and the proximal ureter. UPJ obstruction is bilateral in 30% of cases, but when unilateral, it may be accompanied by a contralateral anomaly, including MCDK, renal agenesis, or duplication. Extrarenal anomalies have also been associated with UPJ obstruction, including cardiovascular and central nervous system anomalies.[11]

Sonographic Findings. UPJ obstruction can be diagnosed when the renal pelvis is dilated (Fig. 20-6). The anteroposterior (AP) diameter on a transverse scan should measure less than 7 mm for mild dilation, 7 to 15 mm for moderate dilation, and more than 15 mm for marked dilation.[7] One study concluded that an AP diameter of 11 mm or more is a reliable indicator of neonatal nephrouropathy requiring surgery.[12] With UPJ obstruction, there is absence of ureteral dilation, and the bladder appears normal. When UPJ obstruction is isolated, the amniotic fluid should also be within normal limits.

Ureterovesical Junction Obstruction. UVJ obstruction describes an obstruction at the junction of the distal ureter and bladder and is usually accompanied by duplication of the ureters. The ureter inserting into the upper pole is typically obstructed because that ureter inserts ectopically. An ectopic ureter may insert into various places, including the superior bladder, the urethra, or the vagina. A ureterocele in the bladder, resulting in a dilated upper pole of the kidney, is often contiguous with a dilated ureter.

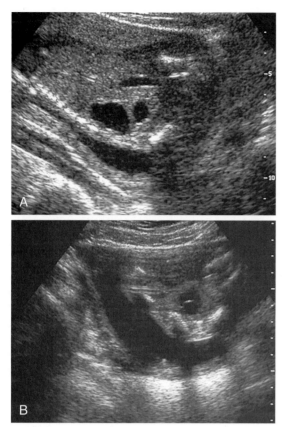

FIGURE 20-7 (A), Dilated right renal pelvis was identified in addition to dilated ureter in a fetus, confirming the diagnosis of UVJ obstruction. **(B)**, Ectopic ureterocele was also noted in fetal bladder.

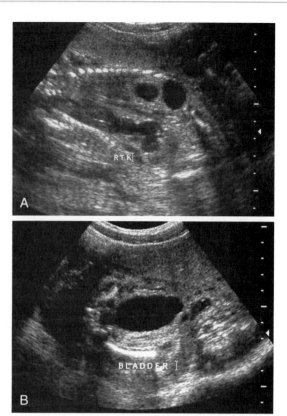

FIGURE 20-8 (A), Bilateral severe hydronephrosis is identified in a male fetus with PUV. **(B)**, Keyhole bladder appearance can be seen. Note lack of amniotic fluid surrounding the fetus.

Sonographic Findings. The diagnosis of UVJ obstruction can be made when hydronephrosis is identified with an accompanying hydroureter (Fig. 20-7, *A*). The identification of the dilated ureter helps to differentiate between UPJ obstruction (in which the ureter is not distended) and UVJ obstruction. The bladder should appear normal in size. An ectopic ureterocele (Fig. 20-7, *B*) may be identified, although in utero identification of the ureterocele may be difficult because of its small size.

Posterior Urethral Valves. PUV is the most common cause of bladder outlet obstruction resulting from the development of abnormal valves in the posterior urethra. The anomaly is accompanied by an enlarged bladder, bilateral hydronephrosis, and hydroureters. It occurs only in male fetuses and may be accompanied by prune-belly syndrome. The female equivalent that has similar findings occurs with urethral atresia. It is important to identify the sex of the fetus to diagnose the pathologic condition correctly. When PUV is identified early in pregnancy, patients may be offered prenatal vesicoamniotic shunting to decompress the bladder and kidneys and provide a pathway for fluid from the fetus into the amniotic cavity. If successful, this shunt also aids in fetal lung development and reduces fetal growth restriction anomalies.

Sonographic Findings. The sonographic appearance of PUV may vary. The fetal bladder may be grossly dilated, and the dilated proximal urethra may create a "keyhole" appearance (Fig. 20-8). The distended bladder may have significant bladder wall thickening, or spontaneous bladder decompression can occur with accompanying urinary ascites. Bilateral hydronephrosis and hydroureters may also be identified in the fetus. Severe oligohydramnios may be present, depending on the gestational age.

INTRAUTERINE GROWTH RESTRICTION

IUGR refers to a fetus that has not reached growth potential because of genetic or environmental factors; the fetus is most likely SGA. SGA is generally defined as a birth weight or fetal weight less than the 10th percentile at any given gestational age; however, constitutional factors, such as the gender of the infant; race, parity, and body mass index of the mother; and environmental factors, can affect the distribution of normal birth weight in any population. These factors must be considered when evaluating fetal growth for a mother referred for size less than dates. Generally, standards for fetal growth have been incorporated with ultrasound equipment computer software, and different programs exist that can be applied to various geographic locations. SGA describes fetuses with weight less than the 10th percentile without reference to the cause. It is important to attempt to distinguish SGA from IUGR by close monitoring because

IUGR is associated with stillbirth, neonatal death, and perinatal morbidity.[13]

IUGR has traditionally been subdivided into two growth restriction patterns: symmetric and asymmetric. In the symmetric form, both the fetal head and the abdomen are proportionately decreased. Historically, symmetric IUGR has been associated with intrinsic insults, such as chromosomal alterations or fetal infections; however, an extrinsic insult that occurs early in gestation may cause symmetric IUGR. In the asymmetric form, a greater decrease in abdominal size is seen, and asymmetric IUGR has been associated with extrinsic insults such as placental insufficiency. Mixed patterns of fetal growth restriction are also possible, limiting even further the clinical utility of separating IUGR into two distinct patterns. It is now recognized that the timing of the pathologic insult is more important than the actual nature of the underlying pathologic process. Approximately 20% to 30% of all cases of IUGR are symmetric, with the remaining 70% to 80% asymmetric.

The causes of IUGR are many and have been divided into three categories according to fetal, placental, and maternal factors. The most common fetal factors associated with IUGR include chromosomal abnormalities, fetal infections (e.g., toxoplasmosis, cytomegalovirus), multiple pregnancies, and fetal malformations. Placental factors include tumors and placental or umbilical cord accidents or abnormalities, such as a velamentous or marginal cord insertion.

Maternal Diseases Associated with Intrauterine Growth Restriction

Although many maternal factors may contribute to a growth-restricted fetus, not all of them involve maternal medical disease. Factors such as race, height and weight, older age, and nutritional factors such as low prepregnancy weight and poor weight gain may negatively affect fetal growth. A poor obstetric history, including previous stillbirth, preterm birth, or IUGR, has been associated with an elevated risk for a growth-restricted infant with the next pregnancy. Environmental factors such as cigarette smoking, substance abuse, use of certain medications, and high altitude may also negatively affect the rate of fetal growth. Generally, maternal diseases that compromise oxygen availability or cause endothelial vascular damage are associated with fetal growth restriction. Maternal diseases associated with IUGR include hypertension, renal disease, insulin-dependent diabetes mellitus, systemic lupus erythematosus, sickle cell anemia, severe lung disease, and cyanotic heart disease.

Preeclampsia is characterized by the new onset of hypertension and proteinuria after 20 weeks of gestation. Risk factors for preeclampsia include a history of preeclampsia, first pregnancy, family history, multiple gestation, obesity, preexisting hypertension, renal disease, collagen vascular disease, advanced age, prolonged interval between pregnancies, and a change of partners between pregnancies.[14] Preeclampsia itself or superimposed on chronic vascular conditions may cause fetal growth failure, especially when the onset is early.[15] The finding of IUGR in the context of preeclampsia makes that condition severe and is considered an indication for delivery.

Sonographic Findings. Sonography is the method of choice for diagnosis and evaluation of fetuses with possible IUGR. The finding of a significant discrepancy in some or all of the fetal biometric parameters compared with measurements expected (based on gestational age) is consistent with the diagnosis of fetal growth restriction. Biometric parameters commonly measured include the biparietal diameter, head circumference, abdominal circumference, and femur length. Various formulas are used to calculate an estimated fetal weight. Sonographic prediction of fetal weight is not accurate, which is why the evaluation and management of fetuses suspected to have IUGR is based on serial sonographic examinations.

Symmetric IUGR is characterized by measurements of the fetal head, abdomen, and femur that all are below the expected values for a given gestational age. In asymmetric fetal growth restriction, the abdominal circumference is smaller than expected, but fetal head and femur measurements are appropriate for gestational age. However, the sonographic differentiation of these two patterns of IUGR does not provide an etiology.

When the diagnosis of IUGR is made, a careful anatomic survey of the fetus should be performed. Oligohydramnios is a common component of IUGR when placental function is insufficient. Normal or increased AFV in the context of IUGR should prompt the search for fetal congenital anomalies and lead the clinician to suspect the presence of a chromosomal abnormality or syndrome.

Pulsed Doppler assessment of umbilical artery blood flow may reveal abnormalities in true cases of IUGR. An increase in the ratio of systolic to diastolic flow in the umbilical artery and an increase in the pulsatility index and resistive index are indicative of increasing placental resistance and poor fetal outcome. Diastolic flow may eventually disappear (Fig. 20-9) or may reverse in direction toward the fetus. Reversed or absent end-diastolic flow in the fetal umbilical artery indicates fetal distress. When an abnormal umbilical artery Doppler waveform exists, further evaluation of the ductus venosus, middle cerebral artery, and intraabdominal umbilical vein is warranted. In severe cases of IUGR, the ductus venosus may demonstrate reversal of flow during the a-wave, the middle cerebral artery may demonstrate reduced flow resistance, and the umbilical vein may become pulsatile.[16]

PREMATURE RUPTURE OF MEMBRANES

PROM is rupture of the amniotic membrane before the onset of labor. When this happens before 37 weeks, it is considered PPROM. Preterm rupture affects approximately 1% to 2% of pregnancies but is associated with 30% to 40% of preterm births.[17] Most women with PROM at term go into spontaneous labor within the first 24 hours. However, when PPROM occurs, the latency period (time from rupture of membranes to labor) may be long. The likelihood of pulmonary hypoplasia depends both on the gestational age at which rupture occurs and on the amount of residual amniotic fluid volume and duration of oligohydramnios. Patients with PPROM have an increased risk for chorioamnionitis, fetal morbidity and death, and having a cesarean delivery.

Sonographic Findings

Sonographic findings associated with PROM are the same as the sonographic findings described earlier in the section on oligohydramnios (see Fig. 20-1). Even when there appears to be convincing evidence of PROM, the fetal urinary bladder should be imaged and documented to exclude renal agenesis as the primary cause.

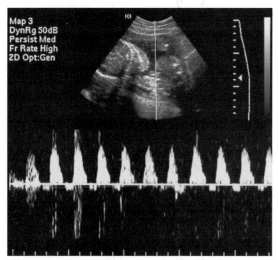

FIGURE 20-9 Doppler demonstrates flow reversal in umbilical artery. This fetus was severely growth restricted and in apparent distress, resulting in early delivery.

SUMMARY

Evaluation of pregnant women referred for size less than dates can sometimes be a challenge for the sonographer and physician. Measurement of the AFV, careful examination of the fetus for congenital anomalies associated with oligohydramnios, a detailed history, and physical examination many times reveal the diagnosis (Table 20-1). Fetal growth restriction is best evaluated with serial sonographic examinations measuring fetal biometric parameters and comparing them with the expected measurements for a given gestational age. When the estimated fetal weight is found to be less than the 10th percentile, IUGR is suspected. IUGR in the presence of AFI less than 5 cm is associated with fetal hypoxia, abnormal Doppler studies and biophysical testing, increased rates of fetal distress in labor, and perinatal mortality.[18] Serial monitoring of fetal growth, AFV, umbilical artery pulsed Doppler evaluation, and nonstress tests are warranted in all cases of IUGR until the age of fetal viability has been reached. In conjunction with clinical data such as severe hypertension, diabetes with vascular disease, or the presence of preeclampsia, a sonographic examination may provide the necessary tools to decide on expectant management of the pregnancy or to proceed with delivery of the fetus.

CLINICAL SCENARIO—DIAGNOSIS

This 39-year-old patient has a long history of type 1 diabetes mellitus. Her age could be a factor in that she is at an increased risk of having a child with a chromosomal abnormality that could be associated with fetal growth restriction. However, that was ruled out by the genetic amniocentesis. No congenital anomalies in the fetus are suspected because a fetal anatomic survey was performed at 16 weeks of gestation. She is a busy professional and may not be ingesting enough water for adequate hydration. This could explain the low AFI of 6.7 cm. However, the most important factors in this patient are her elevated blood pressure, headache, and worsening proteinuria. These findings are consistent with the diagnosis of preeclampsia. The IUGR suggests that the preeclampsia is severe, and delivery of the fetus is indicated.

TABLE 20-1	Causes for Size Less than Dates
Diagnosis	**Sonographic Findings**
Oligohydramnios	MVP, <2 cm; AFI, <5 cm
Renal agenesis	Absence of kidneys and bladder; severe oligohydramnios; absence of renal arteries shown with Doppler
ARPKD	Large echogenic kidneys bilaterally; absence of bladder; severe oligohydramnios
MCDK	Multiple large cysts that do not connect; usually unilateral with normal fluid; when bilateral, associated with severe oligohydramnios and absence of bladder
Hydronephrosis	Dilation of renal collecting system
UPJ obstruction	Dilation of renal collecting system without dilation of ureter; amniotic fluid is usually normal
UVJ obstruction	Dilation of renal collecting system and ureter; may identify ectopic ureterocele; amniotic fluid is usually normal
PUV	Grossly distended bladder; bilateral hydronephrosis and hydroureter; severe oligohydramnios; male gender
IUGR	Fetal weight, <10th percentile
PROM	Oligohydramnios

CASE STUDIES FOR DISCUSSION

1. The Doppler images shown in Figure 20-10 (see Color Plate 21, A-D) were obtained from a 37-week gestational age pregnancy that has an average ultrasound age of 34 weeks. With all the Doppler and growth information obtained, what are the likely diagnosis and outcome for this fetus?

2. A 23-week gestational age fetus has overall biometry measurements consistent with 19 weeks (symmetric). True gestational age is accurate, which was confirmed by an early sonogram. Multiple anomalies, oligohydramnios, and an abnormal Doppler waveform in the umbilical artery are noted (Fig. 20-11; see Color Plate 22). What concern should arise with these findings?

3. A sonogram of a 27-week pregnancy demonstrates anhydramnios (Fig. 20-12; see Color Plate 23). A left hyperechoic kidney is noted with no discernible blood flow. Only an adrenal gland is noted on the right, in a longitudinal lie. What is the likely diagnosis?

4. Normal AFV is noted on a sonogram performed at 23 weeks of gestation. While evaluating the abdomen, a dilated ureter is noted on the left from the renal pelvis all the way to the distal insertion (Fig. 20-13). On further evaluation, the distal ureter is noted connecting inferior to the bladder. What is the probable diagnosis and prognosis for this fetus?

5. Low-normal AFV was noted on this 28-week pregnancy. A large hydroureter was noted, and both kidneys had multiple cystic areas (Fig. 20-14). Other anomalies were also noted in this fetus. What is the likely diagnosis?

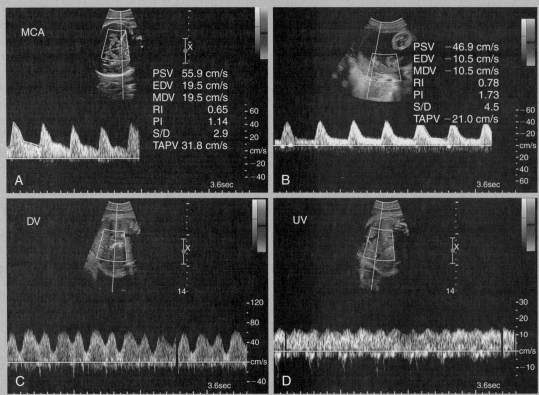

FIGURE 20-10 (A), Middle cerebral artery Doppler demonstrates decreased resistance. **(B),** Umbilical artery demonstrates increased resistance. **(C),** Ductus venosus is pulsatile. **(D),** Umbilical vein is pulsatile.

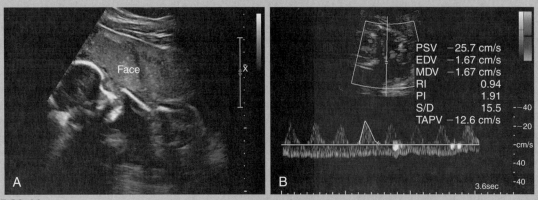

FIGURE 20-11 (A), Minimal fluid is evident around an anomalous fetus. **(B),** Doppler demonstrates abnormal umbilical artery.

CASE STUDIES FOR DISCUSSION—cont'd

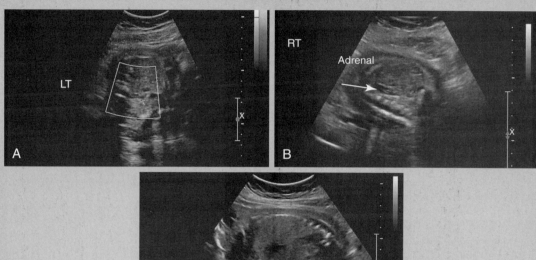

FIGURE 20-12 (A), Hyperechoic left kidney with no discernible blood flow. **(B)**, Note longitudinal lie of right adrenal gland. **(C)**, No discernible amniotic fluid is evident.

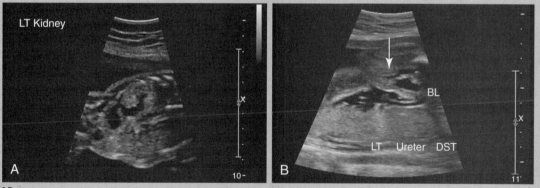

FIGURE 20-13 (A), Note ectatic ureter from the renal pelvis along its entire tract distally. **(B)**, Distal ureter is noted inserting inferior to fetal bladder.

Continued

CASE STUDIES FOR DISCUSSION—cont'd

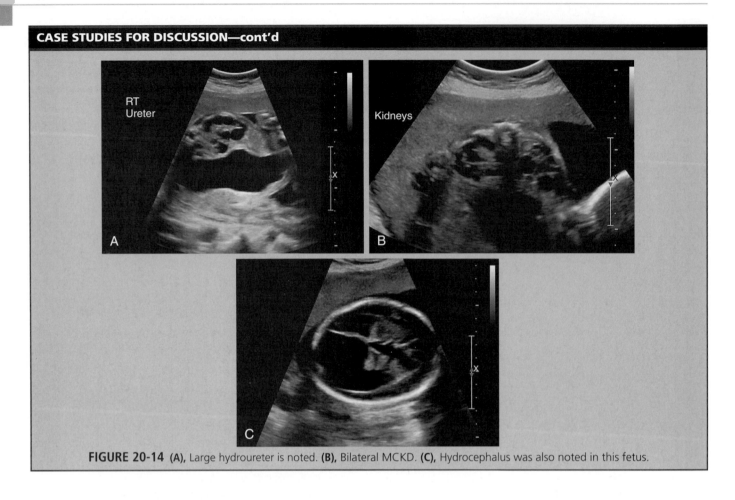

FIGURE 20-14 **(A)**, Large hydroureter is noted. **(B)**, Bilateral MCKD. **(C)**, Hydrocephalus was also noted in this fetus.

STUDY QUESTIONS

1. An AFI measurement was obtained on a 38-week gestational age pregnancy. The AFI was considered within normal limits. A fetal bladder was never demonstrated on imaging. What could be the likely explanation?
   a. There is agenesis of the fetal kidneys
   b. There is no bladder
   c. Patient has PROM
   d. Fetus emptied bladder

2. Severe IUGR is noted on a 30-week fetus. The patient denies having diabetes or lupus, and the fetus appears otherwise normal. What other factor could play a role in the growth of this fetus?
   a. Patient has hypertension
   b. Father of the baby has renal disease
   c. Fetus has a renal anomaly that was not seen sonographically
   d. Fetus has diabetes

3. A detailed sonogram shows a large "keyhole" bladder in the fetus and oligohydramnios. The fetal kidneys are not well visualized, but large tubular structures are seen arising from the bladder. What is the most likely diagnosis?

   a. Renal agenesis
   b. Polycystic kidney disease
   c. PUV
   d. MCDK

4. A gravida 1, para 0 patient comes in at 32 weeks of pregnancy for a sonogram because of decreased fetal movement. Fetal biometry reveals an estimated fetal weight in the 5th percentile. A past sonogram performed at 20 weeks of gestation was normal. At her last monthly visit, the patient's blood pressure was normal, and the fundal height measurement was appropriate. At this visit, her ankles are swollen, and her blood pressure is 150/90 mm Hg. What is the most likely diagnosis?
   a. IUGR secondary to preeclampsia
   b. Macrosomia secondary to diabetes
   c. Normal fetus with preterm labor
   d. Oligohydramnios secondary to fetal renal disease

5. A 28-week gestational age fetus is noted to have severe IUGR. The umbilical artery Doppler waveform shows reversed diastolic flow, and the ductus venosus shows flow reversal of the a-wave. What is the significance of these Doppler findings?
   a. Fetal portal hypertension
   b. Umbilical artery stenosis

c. Fetal respiratory failure

d. Fetal distress

6. When serial sonographic examinations demonstrate the progression of significant IUGR, the clinician needs to try to determine the cause of the problem. A fetal cause that can lead to IUGR is:

a. Hypertension

b. Placental insufficiency

c. Chromosome abnormality

d. Placental chorioangioma

7. A patient presents with a 15-week pregnancy with oligohydramnios. The patient complains that she has had significant bleeding and has lost multiple pregnancies before 20 weeks. The fetus was noted to have a bladder, and no other significant abnormalities were identified. The most likely cause of oligohydramnios is:

a. A maternal condition causing PROM and spontaneous abortions

b. A fetal condition such as renal agenesis

c. Diabetes mellitus

d. Cytomegalovirus

8. A detailed sonogram was obtained of a 23-week fetus whose gestational age was confirmed by a sonogram performed at 13 weeks. The sonogram demonstrates a 19-week fetus with a two-vessel cord, echogenic kidneys, oligohydramnios, and a probable heart defect. The next step should be to:

a. Obtain blood work to determine if the patient is a cystic fibrosis carrier

b. Offer genetic counseling and karyotyping

c. Repeat AFI in 1 week

d. Perform an amniocentesis

9. A large "keyhole"-appearing bladder is noted in a female fetus. A large distended, fluid-filled abdomen is also seen, along with oligohydramnios. The likely prognosis for this 35-week fetus is poor. The likely cause is:

a. PUV

b. Hydronephrosis

c. Urethral atresia

d. Renal agenesis

10. A woman with a 35-week pregnancy is found to have a normal-appearing fetus and AFI of 3 cm. She states she has not felt any more fluid leaking since last week. She has also noticed the baby is not moving like it usually does, and she has had a fever for 2 days. The fetus is at increased risk for what complication?

a. Urinary tract infection

b. Fetal demise

c. IUGR

d. Breech presentation

REFERENCES

1. Sparks T, Cheng Y, McLaughlin B, et al: Fundal height: a useful screening tool for fetal growth? *J Matern Fetal Neonat Med* 24:708–712, 2011.
2. Harman C: Amniotic fluid abnormalities, *Semin Perinatol* 32:288–294, 2008.
3. Magann E, Doherty D, Chauhan S, et al: How well do the amniotic fluid index and single deepest pocket indices (below the 3rd and 5th and above the 95th and 97th percentiles) predict oligohydramnios and hydramnios? *Am J Obstet Gynecol* 190:164–169, 2004.
4. Magann E, Chauhan S, Doherty D, et al: The evidence for abandoning the amniotic fluid index in favor of the single deepest pocket, *Am J Perinatol* 24:549–555, 2007.
5. Cardwell MS: Bilateral renal agenesis: clinical implications, *South Med J* 81:327–328, 1988.
6. Whitehouse W, Mountrose U: Renal agenesis in non-twin siblings, *Am J Obstet Gynecol* 116:880–882, 1973.
7. Avni F, Maugey-Laulom B, Cassart M, et al: The fetal genitourinary tract. In Callen PW, editor: *Ultrasonography in obstetrics and gynecology*, ed 5, Philadelphia, 2008, Saunders, pp 266–296.
8. Gunyay-Aygun M, Avner E, Bacallao R, et al: Autosomal recessive polycystic kidney disease and congenital hepatic fibrosis: summary statement of a first national institutes of health/office of rare diseases conference, *J Pediatr* 149:159–164, 2006.
9. Wool AS, Winyard PJ: Advances in the cell biology and genetics of human kidney malformations, *J Am Soc Nephrol* 9:1114–1125, 1995.
10. Coco C, Jeanty P: Isolated fetal pyelectasis and chromosomal abnormalities, *Am J Obstet Gynecol* 193:732–738, 2005.
11. Wellesley D, Howe D: Fetal renal anomalies and genetic syndromes, *Prenat Diagn* 21:992, 2001.
12. Gramellini D, Fieni S, Caforio E, et al: Diagnostic accuracy of fetal renal pelvis anteroposterior diameter as a predictor of significant postnatal nephrouropathy: second versus third trimester of pregnancy, *Am J Obstet Gynecol* 194:167–173, 2006.
13. Kady S, Gardosi J: Perinatal mortality and fetal growth restriction, *Best Pract Res Clin Obstet Gynaecol* 18:397–410, 2004.
14. Duckitt K, Harrington D: Risk factors for pre-eclampsia at antenatal booking: systematic review of controlled substances, *BMJ* 330:565, 2005.
15. Ness R, Sibai B: Shared and disparate components of the pathophysiologies of fetal growth restriction and preeclampsia, *Am J Obstet Gynecol* 195:40–49, 2006.
16. Mari G: Doppler ultrasonography in obstetrics: from the diagnosis of fetal anemia to the treatment of intrauterine growth-restricted fetuses, *Am J Obstet Gynecol* 200:613. e1-613.e9, 2009.
17. Buchanan S, Crowther K, Levett P, et al: Planned early birth versus expectant management for women with preterm prelabour rupture of membranes prior to 37 weeks' gestation for improving pregnancy outcome, *Cochrane Database Syst Rev* 3:CD004735, 2010.
18. Galan H: Timing delivery of the growth-restricted fetus, *Semin Perinatol* 35:262–269, 2011.

Bleeding with Pregnancy

Charlotte Henningsen, Lennard D. Greenbaum

A 35-year-old woman is seen in the emergency department 10 days postpartum following an uncomplicated delivery at 35 weeks' gestation. She presents with pelvic tenderness and vaginal bleeding.

Clinical evaluation reveals that the patient is febrile with leukocytosis. A pelvic sonogram is ordered revealing the findings in Figure 21-1. What is the most likely diagnosis?

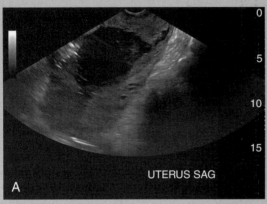
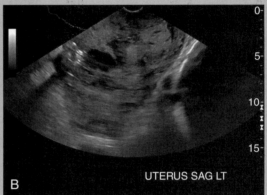

FIGURE 21-1 (A), Midline longitudinal view of the uterus. **(B),** Longitudinal left lateral view of the uterus.

OBJECTIVES

- List the various causes of bleeding with pregnancy.
- Differentiate the most common causes of bleeding in the first trimester of pregnancy from the most common causes of bleeding in the second and third trimesters.
- Explain the β human chorionic gonadotropin levels that are used in diagnosis of ectopic pregnancy, gestational trophoblastic disease, and pregnancy failure.

- List the causes of bleeding in the second and third trimesters of pregnancy, and differentiate the sonographic findings.
- Identify Doppler findings seen with various causes of bleeding with pregnancy.
- Describe the patient symptoms and sonographic findings associated with retained products of conception.

Sonography is a diagnostic tool frequently used in the evaluation of bleeding in pregnant patients. In the first trimester, the viability of the pregnancy is a primary concern; however, patient symptoms and laboratory tests may also lead to a search for an ectopic pregnancy or gestational trophoblastic disease. In the second and third trimesters of pregnancy, the most common causes of bleeding include placenta previa and abruptio placentae, although other conditions, including placenta accreta, may be seen with similar symptoms. Ultrasound examination also may be used in the investigation of abnormal

bleeding after delivery. A thorough search with ultrasound and knowledge of the sonographic findings specific to these various conditions can lead to the correct diagnosis and appropriate treatment.

FIRST-TRIMESTER BLEEDING

Subchorionic Hemorrhage

Subchorionic hemorrhages are low-pressure hemorrhages that occur most commonly in the first trimester of pregnancy. They often result from implantation of the fertilized ovum into the uterus. These areas of hemorrhage are seen between the uterine wall and the membranes and are not associated with the placenta, which distinguishes subchorionic hemorrhage from abruptio placentae. Patients may have spotting or bleeding with or without uterine contractions. Subchorionic hemorrhage may spontaneously regress or may lead to spontaneous abortion (SAB); the prognosis is favorable when the fetal heartbeat is identified in the presence of a small hemorrhage. In addition, hemorrhage in the lower uterine segment has a better prognosis than hemorrhage located at the uterine fundus.[1] Patients who present with bleeding in whom a subchorionic hemorrhage is found have a higher incidence of pregnancy loss than patients with a subchorionic hemorrhage without bleeding.[2]

Sonographic Findings. Sonographic examination of a subchorionic hemorrhage reveals blood, which may initially be echogenic and progressively become anechoic (Fig. 21-2), located adjacent to the gestational sac and at the margin of the placenta. The lack of vascularity identified with color Doppler can help differentiate hematoma from a neoplasm. When the hemorrhage is anechoic, it may resemble a second gestational sac.

Abortion

The incidence of SAB is considered high, occurring in 15% of women with a known pregnancy.[3] Depending on the patient presentation, abortion may be classified as threatened, missed, or complete. Threatened abortion is characterized by bleeding without cervical dilation. Missed abortion is characterized as embryonic death without expulsion of the products of conception. SAB is classified as complete when there is expulsion of the products of conception. Pregnancy loss is often idiopathic but may occur in aneuploid fetuses or as the result of maternal endocrine or vascular disorders, anatomic factors, or immunologic disease. When the pregnancy reaches 12 weeks' gestational age, the SAB rate decreases dramatically.

Correlation between the serum β human chorionic gonadotropin (β-hCG) and the findings in the uterus can be used to confirm whether or not the sonographic milestones of a first-trimester pregnancy are met. The gestational sac may be identified at 4.5 weeks by last menstrual period and should grow about 1 mm per day; additionally, the embryo grows at a rate of 1 mm per day. The size of the gestational sac and the crown-rump length should be consistent with each other. With endovaginal technique, the yolk sac should be visualized by the time the mean sac diameter reaches 8 mm; anomalies of the size, shape, or echogenicity of the yolk sac are associated with a poor prognosis. An embryo should be identified when the gestational sac measures 25 mm, and cardiac motion in the embryo should be visualized when the embryo measures 5 mm.[2] Anembryonic pregnancy should be considered when an empty gestational sac is seen at this point in the gestation (Fig. 21-3). Embryonic bradycardia, defined as less than 85 beats per minute in a gestation less than 7 weeks' gestational age and less than 100 beats per minute from 7 weeks' gestational age forward, is associated with a poor prognosis.[2] Failure to meet any of the milestones in the first trimester of pregnancy can suggest a poor pregnancy outcome. The values assigned to these thresholds have

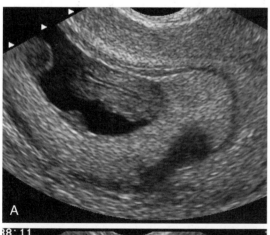

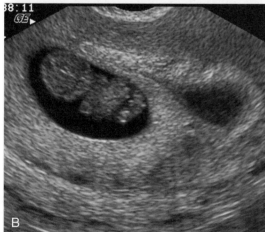

FIGURE 21-2 Subchorionic hemorrhages in 8-week gestation **(A)** and 10-week gestation **(B)**. *(Courtesy GE Medical Systems.)*

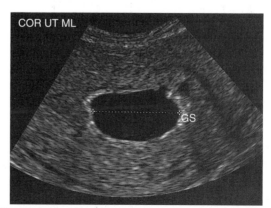

FIGURE 21-3 Uterus demonstrating a large empty gestational sac at 6 weeks' gestation consistent with an anembryonic pregnancy.

changed over time, and the authors are aware that discussion is ongoing regarding increasing the current thresholds; the literature should be monitored for current standards.

Sonographic Findings. A primary role of sonography in the evaluation of pregnancy in the first trimester is confirmation of viability. If the crown-rump length measures 5 mm and cardiac activity is not seen, the diagnosis of embryonic death can be made with confidence.[2] Failure to meet other first-trimester sonographic milestones should be noted. A subchorionic hemorrhage may also lead to pregnancy loss. Ultrasound may be used to follow bleeding with pregnancy to monitor viability, to confirm fetal death, and to determine when dilatation and curettage (D&C) is necessary.

Ectopic Pregnancy

Ectopic pregnancy is defined as a pregnancy located outside of the normal location (Fig. 21-4). It occurs in 2:100 pregnancies in the United States[4] and is a leading cause of maternal death in the first trimester. A history of ectopic pregnancy also affects the future fertility of a patient and increases the risk of a repeat ectopic pregnancy. In addition to a history of ectopic pregnancy, risk factors include a history of pelvic inflammatory disease, tubal surgery, maternal congenital anomalies, late primiparity, defective zygote, fertility treatments, and intrauterine device (IUD) usage. The increased usage of assisted reproductive technology not only has increased the incidence rates of ectopic pregnancies and multiple gestations but also has increased the incidence rate of heterotopic pregnancies.

The most common location of an ectopic pregnancy is in the fallopian tube, with a reported incidence 75% to 80% of ectopic pregnancies specifically in the ampullary portion.[4] Ectopic pregnancies have also been identified in the cervix, ovary, uterine cornu, broad ligament, and abdomen. Interstitial or cornual pregnancy occurs in 2% to 5% of ectopic pregnancies.[5] This type of ectopic pregnancy is located in the interstitial portion of the fallopian tube, which is located in the wall of the uterine cornu, and may result in massive hemorrhage, with rupture leading to serious complications, possible hysterectomy, and death. Ovarian pregnancies occur in 2% of ectopic pregnancies and may be indistinguishable from other ovarian pathologies.[6] Cervical pregnancies are rare but can lead to massive hemorrhage that may necessitate hysterectomy to stop the bleeding. Cervical pregnancy may have an ultrasound appearance that is similar to a SAB because a gestational sac is identified within the cervix. Abdominal pregnancies also are rare and usually occur in the pelvis, although implantations have been reported in the upper abdomen, including in the liver. With the increasing frequency of cesarean section, ectopic pregnancies are also occurring in cesarean section scars. Heterotopic pregnancy (see Fig. 21-4,

D-F) is defined as an intrauterine pregnancy (IUP) with an ectopic pregnancy. This type of ectopic pregnancy is rare, occurring in 1:10,000 to 1:50,000 spontaneous pregnancies but is relatively common in patients undergoing fertility treatment.[6]

The clinical symptoms of ectopic pregnancy include bleeding, pain, and a palpable adnexal mass. These symptoms are nonspecific and may be seen in patients who are not pregnant. In addition, women with an ectopic pregnancy may be asymptomatic or have symptoms more suggestive of a threatened abortion. The ultrasound findings paired with quantitative β-hCG levels assist clinicians in confirmation of an IUP or assessment of the risk of an ectopic pregnancy. The discriminatory zone defines the point at which a normal pregnancy should be identified sonographically, and the values may vary from institution to institution; additionally, these values vary depending on imaging technique. An intrauterine gestational sac should be identified in the uterus when scanning endovaginally if the β-hCG level is 1500 IU/L or greater.[6] The absence of an IUP in the presence of these β-hCG levels suggests an increased risk of ectopic pregnancy. With normal pregnancy, the β-hCG levels should double every 2 days until they plateau. However, in the presence of an ectopic pregnancy, the levels increase more slowly, although a nonviable pregnancy could also be seen with this finding.

Sonographic Findings. The most specific sonographic finding diagnostic of ectopic pregnancy is an extrauterine gestational sac that contains a living embryo (see Fig. 21-4, C). Likewise, ectopic pregnancy is generally excluded in the presence of a living IUP, although heterotopic pregnancy should be considered in patients undergoing assisted reproductive technology. In the absence of an extrauterine embryo, other positive sonographic findings in combination or isolation may suggest ectopic pregnancy.

The uterus may be consistent with a normal nongravid uterus or may have a decidual reaction or pseudogestational sac (see Fig. 21-4, A). A pseudogestational sac does not show the low-resistance, peritrophoblastic flow with Doppler that accompanies a normal IUP. A pseudogestational sac also lacks the "double sac" sign that represents the chorionic villi and endometrial cavity seen with early IUPs.

The adnexa also should be carefully evaluated for signs of ectopic pregnancy. A live extrauterine pregnancy is infrequently identified, but endovaginal sonographic evaluation is able to identify findings suggestive of ectopic pregnancy with confidence. Studies have shown that the correct detection of tubal ectopias specifically has an overall sensitivity of 87% to 99%.[7,8] An echogenic adnexal ring (see Fig. 21-4, F) may be seen with or without the presence of a yolk sac. A peritrophoblastic flow pattern may aid in distinguishing the adnexal ring from an ovarian cyst. However, a corpus luteum may also show a similar flow pattern. A hematosalpinx may be

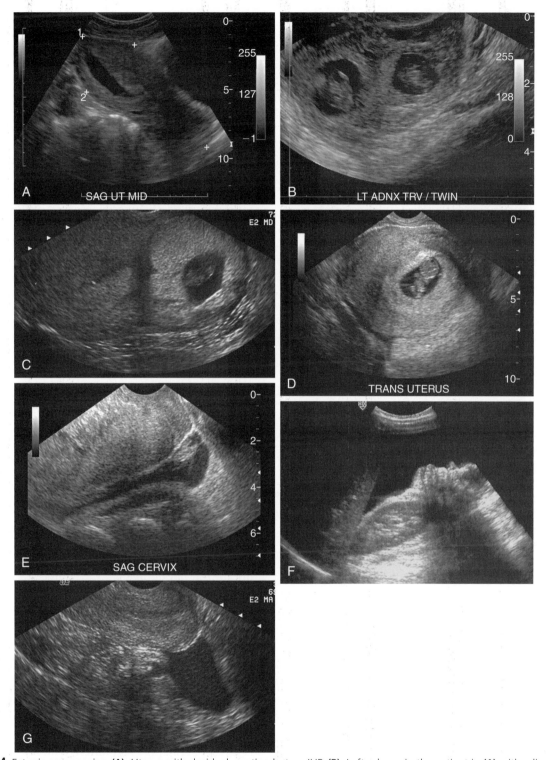

FIGURE 21-4 Ectopic pregnancies. **(A),** Uterus with decidual reaction but no IUP. **(B),** Left adnexa in the patient in **(A)** with a live twin ectopic pregnancy. **(C),** Ectopic pregnancy at 8 weeks located in the left fallopian tube showed heart motion. **(D-F),** IUP seen in a patient with bleeding and severe pain. **(D),** a moderate amount of cul-de-sac fluid identified and adnexal ring sign was seen in the left adnexa consistent with a heterotopic gestation. **(F)** Significant amount of hemoperitoneum seen in patient with an ectopic pregnancy. **(G),** Cul-de-sac fluid is identified in a patient with ectopic pregnancy. **(C** and **G,** Courtesy GE Medical Systems.)

identified if the fallopian tube is distended with blood. An ectopic pregnancy may also be seen as a complex mass (see Fig. 21-18, *B*).

A thorough investigation may reveal an empty uterus and normal-appearing adnexa. Identification of

cul-de-sac fluid (see Fig. 21-4, *G*) is suggestive of ectopic pregnancy, whether or not other positive sonographic findings are present. Hemoperitoneum may appear anechoic, complex, or echogenic. When ultrasound does not show an IUP or a finding suggestive of ectopic pregnancy, clinical correlation determines when surgical, medical, or expectant management is appropriate.

Gestational Trophoblastic Disease

Gestational trophoblastic disease describes a spectrum of diseases of the trophoblast that can be benign, malignant, or malignant/metastatic and includes complete hydatidiform mole, hydatidiform mole with coexistent fetus, partial mole, invasive mole, and choriocarcinoma. Risk factors include maternal age and a previous history of a molar pregnancy, although risk of recurrence is low. **Molar Pregnancy.** A complete hydatidiform mole is of paternal origin and devoid of maternal chromosomes, which results in a 46,XX karyotype without fetal development. This can occur when two X sperm fertilize an empty ovum or one X sperm fertilizes an empty ovum and then duplicates. Partial moles are characterized by triploidy with a 69,XXX or 69,XXY karyotype, of which 23 chromosomes are of the maternal contribution and 46 chromosomes are of the paternal contribution. A partial mole may be accompanied by a fetus or fetal tissue. Although quite rare, a complete hydatidiform mole may also coexist with a normal fetus as the result of a twin gestation.

Because of the availability of sonography, most molar pregnancies are now identified in the first trimester before clinical signs are evident. In these incidences, sonography may suggest a missed abortion, and the diagnosis of molar pregnancy is confirmed by pathologic examination.[9] When symptoms are present, they most commonly include vaginal bleeding; this may prompt evaluation of β-hCG, which is markedly elevated (>100,000 IU/mL[9]) in the presence of molar pregnancy. Maternal serum alpha fetoprotein levels are markedly low in pregnancies complicated by a complete hydatidiform mole. In addition to abnormal laboratory findings, the patient may have symptoms of hyperemesis, preeclampsia, thyrotoxicosis, or respiratory distress. Clinical examination may reveal a uterus that is greater in size than the expected gestational age and bilateral ovarian enlargement owing to theca-lutein cysts.

Molar pregnancies are usually treated with evacuation of the mole followed by serial β-hCG level evaluations to ensure that levels decrease to normal. Increasing β-hCG levels may indicate molar invasion.

Sonographic Findings. A complete hydatidiform mole appears as an echogenic mass within the uterus that contains multiple cystic areas (representing hydropic chorionic villi) and that has been described as having a "snowstorm" appearance (Fig. 21-5, A). In addition, no fetus or fetal parts are identified. Early first-trimester findings may be nonspecific, simulating a missed abortion or anembryonic pregnancy, or may appear as an echogenic mass within the uterus.

A partial mole has an identifiable placenta, although placental enlargement with cystic spaces that represent

the hydropic villi is demonstrated. A fetus or fetal tissue can be identified, but many instances of partial mole spontaneously abort within the first trimester. When a fetus is present, a careful search for structural defects should be performed because of the significant anomalies associated with triploidy, including intrauterine growth restriction (IUGR), heart defects, micrognathia, hand abnormalities such as syndactyly, and ventriculomegaly.

A complete hydatidiform mole with a coexistent fetus (see Fig. 21-5, C) is seen as a normal fetus and placenta with a concurrent molar pregnancy. This entity can be missed in the first trimester because of the presence of a live fetus, and the abnormal echogenicity of the placenta can be mistaken for hemorrhage.[10] Differentiation from a molar pregnancy is important because of the varying malignant potential between these two entities. Although a complete mole with coexistent fetus has the same malignant potential as a solitary hydatidiform mole, a partial mole has a significantly lower malignant potential.

In addition to the findings within the uterus, hyperstimulation of the ovaries may occur as a result of the greatly increased β-hCG levels. Bilateral theca-lutein cysts (see Fig. 21-5, B) are commonly seen in molar pregnancy; however, they are not likely to be seen in the first trimester.[11] These enlarged ovaries may rupture or torque, causing severe pain. The sonographic description of theca-lutein cysts includes enlarged ovaries that contain multiple large cysts, giving them a "soap-bubble" appearance.

Invasive Hydatidiform Mole. Invasive mole occurs when the hydropic villi of a partial or complete mole invade the uterine myometrium and possibly penetrate the uterine wall. Considered an invasive form of gestational trophoblastic disease, invasive mole may occur during the development of a complete or partial mole (although rare with partial mole) or may develop after the evacuation of a mole. Clinical symptoms typically become apparent after the evacuation of a molar pregnancy, when the patient presents with heavy bleeding. Sonography may be used to assist in the diagnosis of this extension of molar pregnancy and may be used to follow the response to treatment.

Sonographic Findings. Sonographic evaluation of the uterus reveals areas of increased echogenicity within the uterus. These focal areas may also appear heterogeneous and contain cystic areas. The uterus and ovaries may also be enlarged.

Choriocarcinoma. Choriocarcinoma is a malignant tumor that arises from the trophoblastic epithelium. Considered a malignant metastatic form of gestational trophoblastic disease, choriocarcinoma may metastasize to the lung, skin, intestines, liver, spleen, heart, and brain; however, the incidence of widespread disease has decreased with the use of effective chemotherapy.[11] Choriocarcinoma may develop after a molar pregnancy; may occur after a normal pregnancy, SAB, or ectopic

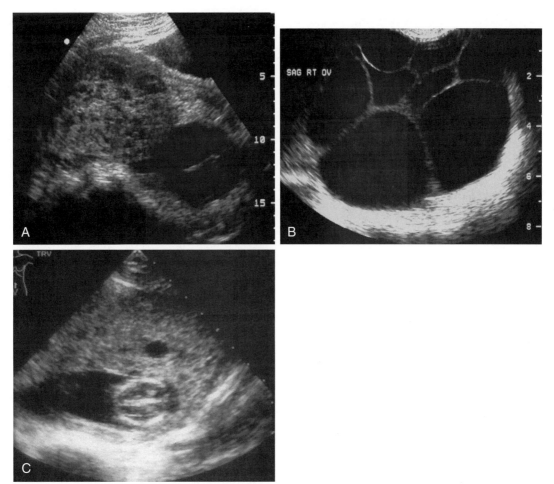

FIGURE 21-5 **(A)**, Complete hydatidiform mole is identified in image. **(B)**, The ovaries were enlarged bilaterally containing theca-lutein cysts as demonstrated in this right ovary. **(C)**, Molar pregnancy with rare coexistent fetus.

pregnancy; and may be seen weeks, months, or several years after a pregnancy. A benign hydatidiform mole and mole with coexistent fetus are considered to have the same malignant potential, whereas a partial mole has a much lower malignant potential. Clinical symptoms most commonly include vaginal bleeding, enlarged uterus and ovaries, and elevated β-hCG levels; patients may also have symptoms related to the site of metastasis.

Sonographic Findings. Sonographic evaluation of these neoplasms often reveals a complex mass because of hemorrhage and necrosis. Metastatic lesions may also be identified. Computed tomography (CT) or magnetic resonance imaging (MRI) may be used in evaluation of the extent of the metastatic disease.

SECOND-TRIMESTER BLEEDING

Placenta Previa

Placenta previa is a common cause of bleeding in late pregnancy and is defined as a placenta that is near or covering the internal cervical os. Placenta previa has been reported in 0.5% or less of term pregnancies and may lead to serious hemorrhage, increasing maternal

morbidity and fetal mortality.[12] Identification of placenta previa is important in prediction of the mode of delivery so that a cesarean section can be scheduled to avoid emergency surgery. Placenta previa has been classified into varying degrees (Fig. 21-6), including low-lying placenta, partial previa, and complete previa. A low-lying placenta is within 2 cm of the internal cervical os, a partial previa partially covers the internal cervical os, and a complete previa extends completely across the internal cervical os. Sonography is used to identify the location of the placenta and to follow patients to monitor for placental "migration."

A low-lying placenta and partial previa may migrate and alleviate the need for cesarean section. This process, which has been defined as trophotropism, describes the atrophy of the placenta in the region of the lower uterine segment with differential growth of other regions of the placenta toward more vascular-rich sites.

Patients who are at increased risk for placenta previa include women with advanced maternal age, multiparous women, and women with a prior history of cesarean section. The most common symptom of placenta previa is painless bleeding in the third trimester, but patients may be asymptomatic.

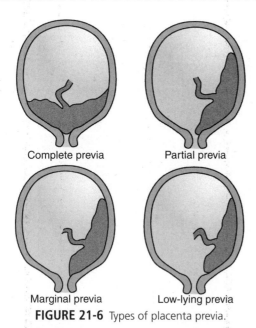

Complete previa   Partial previa

Marginal previa   Low-lying previa

FIGURE 21-6 Types of placenta previa.

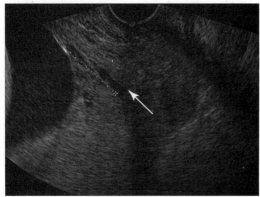

FIGURE 21-7 Placenta is completely covering the internal cervical os *(arrow)* and is delivered by cesarean section.

Sonographic Findings. Three methods exist for imaging of the lower uterine segment to identify the location of the placenta in relationship to the internal cervical os: transabdominal imaging (Fig. 21-7), translabial imaging, and endovaginal imaging. Endovaginal imaging is considered the most accurate for diagnosis of placenta previa.[12] With transabdominal imaging, false-positive results may occur from an overdistended bladder, myometrial contractions, and shadowing of the cervix from the fetal head or other overlying fetal parts.

Vasa Previa

Vasa previa is a condition that describes vessels of fetal origin that completely or partially cover the internal cervical os and occurs in 1:3000 pregnancies.[13] It can lead to devastating consequences, including fetal exsanguination from compression or tearing of the vessels during labor. The most common presentation of vasa previa is dark vaginal bleeding with rupture of the membranes. Associated fetal heart deceleration or demise may also be noted.

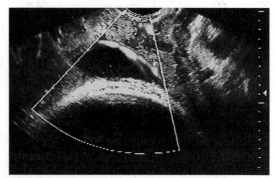

FIGURE 21-8 Vessels are clearly shown covering the internal cervical os and are enhanced with power Doppler imaging.

Vasa previa may arise from velamentous cord insertion or marginal cord insertion or from the connecting vessels of an accessory or bilobed placenta. Vasa previa has also been seen with increased frequency in association with multiple gestations, in vitro fertilization, and low-lying placentas. Prenatal diagnosis can improve fetal and maternal outcome with closer attention to preterm labor, limiting of maternal activity, and planned elective cesarean section. **Sonographic Findings.** An obstetric ultrasound should include visualization of the umbilical cord insertion into the placenta. Endovaginal ultrasound should be used in patients with risk factors for vasa previa, including patients in whom the placental cord insertion is not identified because of the limitations of transabdominal imaging that may be associated with maternal size or position of the maternal bladder. Color or power Doppler (Fig. 21-8; see Color Plate 24) is suggested for evaluation of vasa previa.

Abruptio Placentae

Abruption of the placenta is defined as a placenta that partially or completely prematurely separates, which can lead to preterm delivery, intrauterine growth restriction, and fetal death. Abruptio placentae is primarily a clinical diagnosis and is suspected when a patient has bleeding, significant abdominal pain, trauma, or uterine contractions.[14] Patients may have no symptoms, and the abruption in such patients is noted at the time of visual placental inspection.

Placental abruptions may be classified as marginal or retroplacental. Retroplacental abruptions are considered high-pressure bleeds with the etiology linked primarily to immunologic, inflammatory, and vascular factors.[14] Abruption has been associated with maternal hypertension, vascular disease, placenta previa, smoking, and cocaine abuse. A family history of abruption and previous history of abruption are also risk factors. Conversely, marginal abruptions (Fig. 21-9, *A*) are considered low-pressure bleeds that have mild symptoms or that may be clinically silent.

Sonographic Findings. The sonographic findings suggestive of abruptio placentae include the visualization of

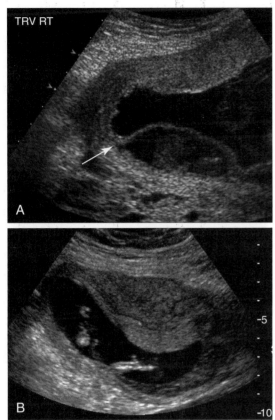

FIGURE 21-9 **(A)**, A patient with subchorionic hemorrhage presented with bleeding. She was placed on bed rest, and the hemorrhage resolved. The remainder of the pregnancy was uneventful. **(B)**, Abruptio placentae occurred in a 31-year-old woman who was seen in the emergency department with abdominal pain, bleeding, and unknown last menstrual period. No fetal heart motion was identified.

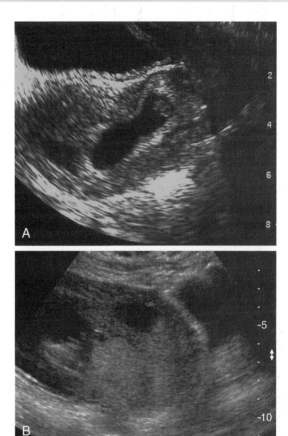

FIGURE 21-10 **(A)**, A 34-year-old patient had a history of two prior cesarean sections and presented with bleeding in the first trimester. Ultrasound shows irregularity in the anterior uterine wall with thinning of myometrium in the region. In the early second trimester, placenta previa was identified. The patient had massive blood loss at the time of delivery owing to placenta accreta. **(B)**, A patient with a history of two prior cesarean sections presented with bleeding. Placenta previa and venous lakes are identified. Placenta accreta was confirmed at the time of delivery.

hemorrhage in the retroplacental region (Fig. 21-9, *B*). Visualization of the hematoma depends on the size, location, and age of the bleed. However, blood may drain through the cervix rather than collecting beneath the placenta, precluding sonographic diagnosis.

Placenta Accreta

Placenta accreta refers to an abnormal placental attachment to the uterus as the result of an abnormal or absent decidua basalis. The three classifications used include placenta accreta, which refers to the attachment of the chorionic villi to the myometrium; placenta increta, which occurs when the villi invade the myometrium; and placenta percreta, which refers to invasion through the myometrium into or through the uterine serosa. Placenta accreta is increasing in frequency with a reported range of 1:533 to 1:2510 pregnancies in the United States.[15] Risk factors include prior cesarean section, placenta previa, multiparity, advanced maternal age, D&C, prior manual removal of the placenta, recurrent SAB, endometritis, adenomyosis, hypertension, smoking, and prior uterine surgery. A history of cesarean section combined with the identification of placenta previa is associated with an

11% chance of placenta accreta, and the risk of placenta accreta increases with a history of more than one cesarean section.[16] Because of the association of placenta previa, patients may have bleeding. Patients with placenta percreta invading the bladder may also have hematuria.

Complications of placenta accreta include significant hemorrhage, which leads to maternal morbidity and mortality and can have a negative impact on the morbidity and mortality of the neonate. Placenta accreta is a major predisposing factor of profound obstetric hemorrhage (Fig. 21-10) leading to pregnancy-related death. In addition, hysterectomy may be necessary in cases of severe blood loss, as may bladder resection in cases where placenta percreta invades the bladder wall.

Sonographic Findings. The sonographic protocol should include a survey of the retroplacental complex when patients have a history of prior cesarean section and placenta previa. In the first trimester, a gestational sac implanted low in the uterus has been identified.[15] The hypoechoic retroplacental complex represents the decidua basalis and uterine myometrium, and placenta accreta is suggested with a thinning or loss of the retroplacental complex. Large venous lakes within the placental substance also may be identified, and a disruption of the linear echogenic interface between the uterine serosa and posterior bladder wall may be shown. Ultrasound may also display the projection of the placenta into or through the bladder wall. Color or power Doppler may be useful in defining the hypervascularity of the venous lakes and the border between the placenta and retroplacental complex.

Short Cervix

The complications surrounding preterm delivery account for 70% of fetal and neonatal deaths; cervical shortening predicts preterm labor.[17] Preterm labor may be diagnosed when the cervix is dilated in the presence of contractions of the uterus between 20 and 37 weeks' gestation. Medical advances in caring for preterm neonates have decreased mortality rates; however, survivors may have long-term chronic lung disease, neurologic deficits, and visual impairment. Risk factors for preterm delivery include a history of preterm delivery, tissue biopsy or excision for cervical dysplasia, congenital uterine anomaly, young maternal age, cigarette smoking, vaginal bleeding, and multiple pregnancy terminations. Other risk factors including multiple gestation, polyhydramnios, diabetes, hypertension, and prior cervical trauma have been documented. Sonography can be used in evaluation of the cervix in women at high risk of preterm delivery.[17,18] The sonographic findings, patient history, and symptoms can be used to develop a management plan, which may include expectant management, cervical cerclage, or bed rest. Intervention with identification of a shortened cervix can improve the perinatal outcome.

Sonographic Findings. Obstetric sonographic protocol includes imaging of the lower uterine segment of the uterus and may include documentation of the cervical length (Fig. 21-11). If transabdominal imaging suggests that the cervix requires additional evaluation, endovaginal imaging should be performed unless contraindicated. Transabdominal imaging of the cervix may be limited; translabial imaging may be preferred for patients with active bleeding or premature rupture of membranes. However, endovaginal imaging is considered the standard approach for evaluation of cervical length. In addition, sonography may be used to follow a patient for evaluation of a cerclage.

Endovaginal sonography should be performed with the patient in a recumbent position with an empty bladder. Measurements of the cervical length should be from the internal to external cervical os. A shortened cervix measures less than 3 cm or may be defined as less than 2.5 cm depending on institutional protocol and imaging method. The application of fundal or suprapubic pressure may aid in identification of patients in whom a shortened cervix otherwise would not be diagnosed. In addition, imaging of the cervix at the beginning of the

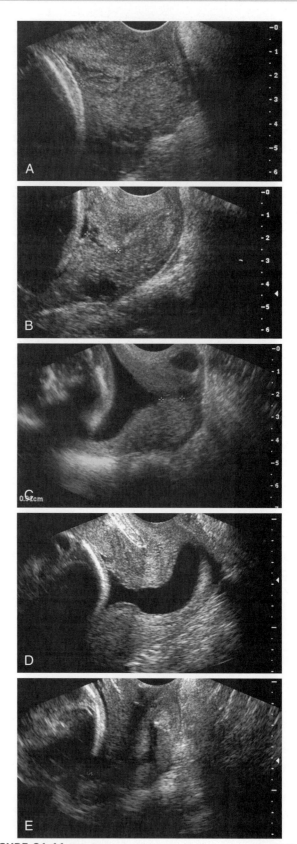

FIGURE 21-11 **(A)**, Example of a normal cervix measuring 3.8 cm imaged with endovaginal technique. **(B)**, Two sets of calipers were used to derive a correct measurement of 4.4 cm of a normal cervix that was not straight. **(C)**, A patient was seen with a cervical length of 0.91 cm. She underwent cerclage placement and was placed on bed rest. **(D)** and **(E)**, A patient was seen with an open cervix. After cerclage placement and bed rest, a closed cervix is identified 1 week later **(E)**.

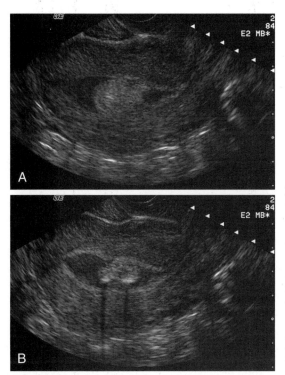

FIGURE 21-12 Retained products of conception. **(A)**, An echogenic mass is identified within the endometrium. **(B)**, Some bony remnants with shadowing are also identified. *(Courtesy GE Medical Systems.)*

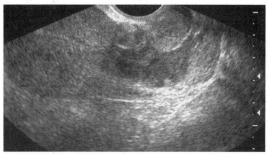

FIGURE 21-13 A patient presented with persistent bleeding after cesarean section. A large hematoma is identified within the uterus and extending into the uterine excision site.

TABLE 21-1	Causes for Bleeding with Pregnancy
Diagnosis	**Sonographic Findings**
Subchorionic hemorrhage	Area of variable echogenicity adjacent to gestational sac
Missed abortion	Embryonic death without expulsion of products of conception
SAB	Uterus devoid of products of conception
Ectopic pregnancy	Variable appearance including absence of normally placed gestational sac, extrauterine live embryo, "ring" sign, cul-de-sac fluid, uterine decidual reaction, hematosalpinx
Complete hydatidiform mole	Echogenic mass with multiple cystic areas in uterus; theca-lutein cysts
Partial mole	Placental enlargement with cystic spaces; fetus or fetal parts
Mole with coexistent fetus	Normal fetus with normal placenta plus large placental mass with cystic spaces
Placenta previa	Placenta partially or completely covering internal cervical os
Vasa previa	Vessels partially or completely covering internal cervical os
Abruptio placentae	Variable amount of blood at margin of placenta or retroplacental; blood may appear echogenic to anechoic
Placenta accreta	Thinning of retroplacental complex; large venous lakes; disruption of uterine serosa; placental mass extending from uterus into bladder; placental hypervascularity

ultrasound examination may identify patients with a cervix that may return to a normal length during the course of an obstetric sonogram. Dynamic cervical changes may occur, and endovaginal imaging should monitor for cervical changes for at least 3 minutes to ensure beaking or funneling of the cervix.

POSTPARTUM BLEEDING

Retained Products of Conception

Postpartum hemorrhage is the most common complication of the uterus after delivery. Abnormal postpartum bleeding may be evaluated sonographically for diagnosis of retained products of conception. In addition, products of conception may be retained after SAB or evacuation by D&C. Complications of retained products include prolonged hemorrhage and infection.[19] The patient may undergo conservative treatment, but when conservative treatment fails, D&C or hysteroscopy may be necessary.
Sonographic Findings. An echogenic mass within the endometrial cavity in a postpartum uterus suggests retained products of conception (Fig. 21-12). Sonographic findings after abortion may also include bony remnants that are highly echogenic and shadow. In addition, increased vascularity using color Doppler may be identified. Retained placental tissue may have a similar appearance to blood clots (Fig. 21-13); a positive finding should be correlated clinically and may be relatively insignificant and resolve without further intervention.

SUMMARY

Sonography can be used to aid in the diagnosis of multiple causes of abnormal bleeding, which vary depending on the gestational age. Sonographic findings can assist in the development of a treatment plan that may prevent further complications and decrease maternal morbidity and mortality and, when feasible, reduce perinatal morbidity and mortality as well. Table 21-1 summarizes the causes for bleeding with pregnancy.

CLINICAL SCENARIO—DIAGNOSIS

The sonogram revealed retained products of conception with air noted in the myometrium, which suggested infection. Based on the correlation with clinical findings, the patient was admitted and given intravenous antibiotics. The pain, bleeding, and infection did not abate, and a hysterectomy was performed.

CASE STUDIES FOR DISCUSSION

1. A 25-year-old woman, gravida 2, para 1, is seen at 22 weeks' gestation with bleeding. Sonographic evaluation reveals the finding in Figure 21-14. What are the important considerations for this patient?

2. A 32-year-old woman is seen with pelvic pain and heavy bleeding following a full-term delivery. The ultrasound findings are shown in Figure 21-15. What is the most likely cause of the bleeding?

3. A 19-year-old woman is seen with significant left lower quadrant pain and bleeding. Clinical assessment also reveals a positive serum pregnancy test. The ultrasound findings are shown in Figure 21-16. What is the most likely diagnosis?

4. A 29-year-old woman, gravida 1, para 0, presents to her obstetrician with a history of irregular periods. She reports that she had an episode of bleeding 6 weeks ago and now has a feeling of fullness in her pelvic region. A sonogram is performed demonstrating a live 13-week fetus. The finding in Figure 21-17 also is noted. What is the most likely explanation for the bleeding 6 weeks ago?

5. A 35-year-old woman, gravida 3, para 2, arrives at the emergency department via ambulance with severe right lower quadrant pain and heavy bleeding. Clinical history reveals that she has had an IUD since the birth of her last child. While waiting for the results of a pregnancy test, a pelvic sonogram is ordered stat. and reveals the findings in Figure 21-18. What is the most likely diagnosis?

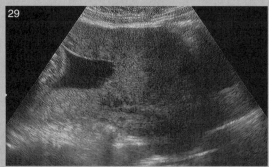

FIGURE 21-14 Longitudinal image of the lower uterine segment shows placenta on the anterior and posterior walls of the uterus.

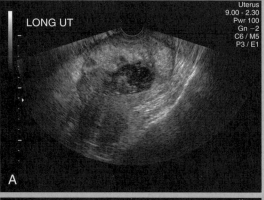

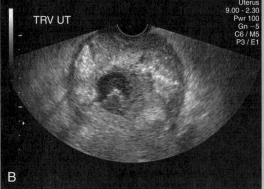

FIGURE 21-15 Longitudinal **(A)** and transverse **(B)** images demonstrate the postpartum uterus.

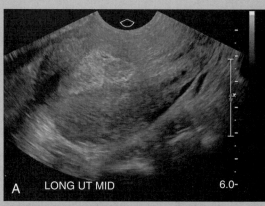

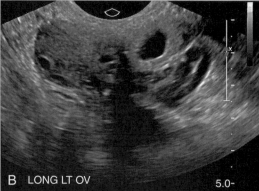

FIGURE 21-16 (A), Longitudinal image of the uterus reveals thickened endometrium and cul-de-sac fluid with debris. **(B),** Right and left ovaries were identified, and a "ring" sign was identified in the left adnexa.

CASE STUDIES FOR DISCUSSION—cont'd

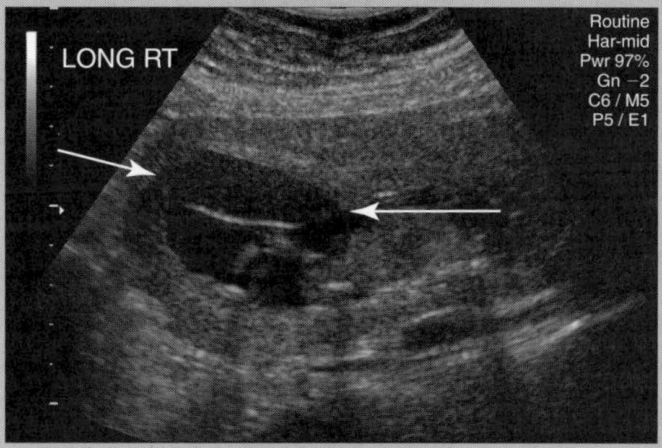

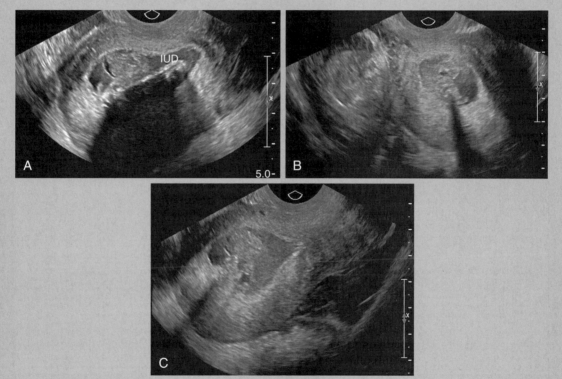

FIGURE 21-17 Ultrasound examination reveals a uterus without evidence of pregnancy. A small amount of fluid is seen in the distal portion of endometrium. A nabothian cyst is incidentally noted in the anterior cervix. Adnexa are unremarkable.

FIGURE 21-18 **(A),** Longitudinal uterus demonstrating IUD with shadowing. **(B),** Transverse view of the uterus and right adnexa show a large right adnexal mass. **(C),** Longitudinal view of the lower uterine segment shows cul-de-sac fluid.

STUDY QUESTIONS

1. A 24-year-old woman with a positive pregnancy test result and pelvic pain is seen for an ultrasound. She has a history of pelvic inflammatory disease. The ultrasound reveals a uterus containing an anechoic sac that lacks a double decidual sac sign with a moderate amount of cul-de-sac fluid. This is most suspicious for which of the following?
   a. Ectopic pregnancy
   b. Missed abortion
   c. SAB
   d. Threatened abortion

2. A 28-year-old pregnant woman presents to the emergency department at 30 weeks' gestation with knifelike abdominal pain following a motor vehicle accident. Her abdomen is tense and hard on palpation. Ultrasound reveals a large hypoechoic collection of fluid in the retroplacental region. This is consistent with which of the following?
   a. Marginal abruption
   b. Placenta previa

c. Placental abruption

d. Subchorionic hemorrhage

3. A 19-year-old woman, gravida 2, para 1, presents to the emergency department at 11 weeks' gestation with vaginal bleeding. Laboratory test results reveal a β-hCG level of 219,000 IU/mL. A sonogram is ordered to confirm which of the following?

a. Ectopic pregnancy

b. Molar pregnancy

c. Placenta previa

d. Threatened abortion

4. A patient is seen with heavy bleeding 7 days after delivery of a 36-week infant. Ultrasound reveals an enlarged postpartum uterus containing an echogenic mass. This suggests which of the following?

a. Partial mole

b. Placenta accreta

c. Retained products of conception

d. Retroplacental hemorrhage

5. An 18-year-old woman is seen by her gynecologist with a 1-week history of spotting. She reports that she had a positive urine pregnancy test result after a missed period 7 weeks ago. Sonographic evaluation reveals an intrauterine sac with an embryo, without a heartbeat, measuring 6 weeks' gestation. This is consistent with which of the following?

a. Abruption

b. Missed abortion

c. SAB

d. Threatened abortion

6. A 41-year-old woman is seen by her obstetrician with vaginal bleeding and hyperemesis. Clinical examination reveals a uterus consistent with a 12-week gestation, which is inconsistent with her predicted 10-week gestation by last menstrual period. An ultrasound is performed and reveals a fetus without heart motion and a crown-rump length consistent with an 8-week gestation. An enlarged placenta is identified containing numerous small cystic lesions. This is most suggestive of which of the following?

a. Complete hydatidiform mole

b. Complete mole with coexistent fetus

c. Invasive mole

d. Partial hydatidiform mole

7. A 35-year-old multiparous woman is seen for an obstetric sonogram with bleeding at 32 weeks' gestation. Endovaginal ultrasound reveals a placenta on the anterior uterine wall, crossing the internal cervical os and extending 2 cm on the posterior uterine wall. This is consistent with which of the following?

a. Complete previa

b. Low-lying placenta

c. Partial previa

d. Placenta accreta

8. A 22-year-old pregnant woman is seen in the sonography department with heavy bleeding and cramping. She had a sonogram 1 week prior because of an episode of spotting, which revealed a 6-week embryo. The current sonogram reveals a uterus without evidence of an embryo or gestational sac. This is most consistent with which of the following?

a. Ectopic pregnancy

b. Missed abortion

c. SAB

d. Threatened abortion

9. A 39-year-old woman, gravida 4, para 3, is seen for an obstetric sonogram at 33 weeks' gestation for late prenatal care. The sonographer identifies placenta previa and observes a cesarean section scar, which is confirmed by the patient. The sonographer should also look for signs suggesting which additional abnormality?

a. Abruptio placentae

b. Placenta accreta

c. Subchorionic hemorrhage

d. Vasa previa

10. A patient presents with pain and spotting at 7 weeks' gestation. Ultrasound confirms a viable IUP consistent with the patient's last menstrual period. An adnexal "ring" sign is imaged in the left adnexal region adjacent to the left ovary. The sonographic finding describes which of the following diagnoses most accurately?

a. Cornual ectopic pregnancy

b. Heterotopic gestation

c. SAB

d. SAB

e. Tubal pregnancy

REFERENCES

1. Dighe M, Cuevas C, Moshiri M, et al: Sonography in first trimester bleeding, *J Clin Ultrasound* 36:352–366, 2008.
2. Arenas JMB, Perez-Medina T, Troyano J: Ultrasonographic signs of poor pregnancy outcome, *Ultrasound Rev Obstet Gynecol* 5:56–68, 2005.
3. Odeh M, Tendler R, Kais M, et al: Gestational sac volume in missed abortion and anembryonic pregnancy compared to normal pregnancy, *J Clin Ultrasound* 38:367–371, 2010.
4. Pereira PP, Cabar FR, Schultz R, et al: Association between ultrasound findings and extent of trophoblastic invasion into the tubal wall in ampullary pregnancy, *Ultrasound Obstet Gynecol* 33:472–476, 2009.
5. Emery A, Buentipo B: Sonographic detection of cornual ectopic pregnancy, *JDMS* 24:252–256, 2008.
6. Farquhar CM: Ectopic pregnancy, *Lancet* 366:583–591, 2005.
7. Kirk E, Daemen A, Papageorghiou AT, et al: Why are some ectopic pregnancies characterized as pregnancies of unknown location at the initial transvaginal ultrasound examination, *Acta Obstet Gynecol* 87:1150–1154, 2008.

8. Condous G: Ectopic pregnancy: challenging accepted management strategies, *Aust N Z J Obstet Gynecol* 49:346–351, 2009.

9. Berkowitz RS, Goldstein DP: Molar pregnancy, *N Engl J Med* 360:1639–1645, 2009.

10. Lee SW, Kim MY, Chung JH, et al: Clinical findings of multiple pregnancy with a complete hydatidiform mole and coexisting fetus, *J Ultrasound Med* 29:271–280, 2010.

11. Madea K, Kurjak A, Varga G: 3D color and power Doppler in the assessment of gestational trophoblastic disease, *Ultrasound Rev Obstet Gynecol* 6:27–44, 2006.

12. Rani PR, Haritha PH, Gowri R: Comparative study of transperineal and transabdominal sonography in the diagnosis of placenta previa, *J Obstet Gynaecol Res* 33:134–137, 2007.

13. Ioannou C, Wayne C: Diagnosis and management of vasa previa: a questionnaire survey, *Ultrasound Obstet Gynecol* 35:205–209, 2010.

14. Tikkanen M: Etiology, clinical manifestations, and prediction of placental abruption, *Acta Obstet Gynecol* 89:732–740, 2010.

15. Ballas J, Pretorius D, Hull AD, et al: Identifying sonographic markers for placenta accrete in the first trimester, *J Ultrasound Med* 31:1835–1841, 2012.

16. Esakoff TF, Sparks TN, Kaimal AJ, et al: Diagnosis and morbidity of placenta accreta, *Ultrasound Obstet Gynecol* 37:324–327, 2011.

17. Madsen AMA: Sonographic methods of evaluating cervical length: a literature review, *J Diag Med Sonography* 19:157–165, 2003.

18. Sung TJ, Lee SY, Ju YS: Effects of maternal cervical incompetence on morbidity and mortality of very low birthweight neonates, *Neonatology* 98:164–169, 2010.

19. Atri M, Rao A, Boylan C, Rasty G, Gerber D: Best predictors of grayscale ultrasound combined with color Doppler in the diagnosis of retained products of conception, *J Clin Ultrasound* 39:122–127, 2011.

Multiple Gestation

Diane J. Youngs, Allan E. Neis

CLINICAL SCENARIO

A 27-year-old woman presents for a follow-up twin obstetric sono-graphic examination at gestational age 19 weeks, 4 days. Previous sonographic assessment performed at 18 weeks of gestation suggested a 5% fetal weight discrepancy between the monochorionic twins and subjective amniotic fluid volume (AFV) disparity. The follow-up sonogram demonstrates an increase in fluid with a single largest pocket measuring 6.9 cm for Twin A and 2.5 cm for Twin B and a weight discrepancy of 17% (Fig. 22-1). Spectral Doppler waveforms show a slightly increased resistance pattern in the umbilical artery of Twin B. Discuss the significance of these findings and the most likely diagnosis.

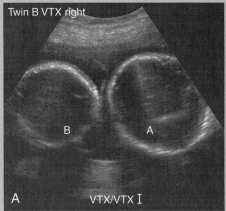
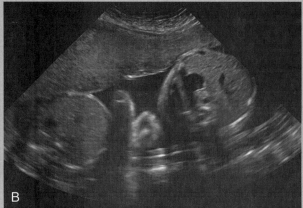

FIGURE 22-1 (A), Fetal heads with membrane in between them. **(B),** Image of fetal abdomens. Twin B *(left)* and twin A *(right)*.

OBJECTIVES

- Discuss the role of sonography in evaluation of a multiple gestation.
- Discuss the embryology and incidence of multiple gestations.
- Describe the sonographic criteria used in evaluation of zygosity, chorionicity, and amnionicity in a multiple gestation.
- List maternal and fetal complications associated with multiple gestations.
- Describe the abnormalities unique to monochorionic multiple gestations.

The incidence rate of twin and higher order multiple gestations has increased steadily through the years, with twin births occurring in the United States at a rate of approximately 32.2 per 1000 births in 2007 compared with 24.8 per 1000 births in 1995.[1] This increase is thought to be the result of the widespread use of assisted reproductive technology (e.g., ovulation induction, in vitro fertilization) and an aging maternal population. The number of higher order multiple births increased 400% from 1980-1998, but the numbers have demonstrated a downward trend since 1998. The more recent decline of higher order multiple gestations has been primarily attributed to the American Society of Reproductive Medicine publishing guidelines that recommend limiting the number of embryos transferred during assisted reproductive technology.[1] Identification of multiple gestations is important because of the significantly increased risk for both the mother and

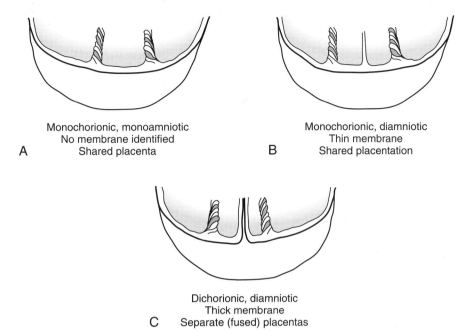

FIGURE 22-2 **(A),** Monochorionic, monoamniotic placentation with no intertwin membrane. **(B),** Monochorionic, diamniotic single placentation with thin intertwin membrane. **(C),** Dichorionic, diamniotic placentation results in separate placentas that may appear fused if close together. The membrane is relatively thick.

the fetus. In the United States in 2007, 3% of twins and 7% of triplets died during infancy compared with less than 1% of all singletons.[1] Early identification of multiple gestations allows careful screening for complications.

EMBRYOLOGY OF TWINNING

Chorionicity and Amnionicity

The number of chorions and amnions that develop in a multiple gestation is referred to as chorionicity and amnionicity; another term for chorionicity is placentation (Fig. 22-2). Two chorions (dichorionic) produce two placentation sites, which presents the least risky form of twinning. Dichorionic twinning accounts for 80% of all natural twinning.[2] The development of one chorion (monochorionic) results in a shared placental site, which places the pregnancy at higher risk. Although monochorionic twinning is less common, this type of placentation accounts for 50% of twin mortalities.[2] The development of a single amnion is termed monoamniotic, and the presence of two amnions is referred to as diamniotic. Monoamniotic twin gestations have the highest incidence of mortality because sharing the amniotic space increases the risk for cord accidents.

Zygosity

The zygosity of twinning refers to the number of zygotes produced at the time of fertilization. Dizygotic twins result when two separate ova are fertilized by two separate sperm cells. Dizygotic, or fraternal, twins are the most common form of twinning, and the incidence

depends on race, geographic area, maternal age, and availability of reproductive technologies. Dizygotic gestations are always dichorionic diamniotic and represent the least risky type of twinning because a placental site is not shared. Dizygotic twins are not genetically identical and can be different genders. Identifying different genders in a multifetal gestation ensures dizygosity.

Monozygotic, or identical, twins result when one ovum is fertilized by a single sperm, and the gestation subsequently splits to form two embryos. The splitting of the embryos is called cleavage. The incidence of monozygotic twins remains steady at 1 in 250 births,[3] representing the least common form of twinning and the most risky. Monozygotic twinning can result in a shared placental site, which can lead to serious complications discussed later in this chapter.

The chorionicity and amnionicity in monozygotic twinning varies and depends on the number of days at which cleavage occurred (Fig. 22-3). If the zygote splits between 0 and 3 days, the gestation is dichorionic, diamniotic. However, most monozygotic twins split between 4 and 8 days resulting in a monochorionic, diamniotic gestation. The later the cleavage, the more that is shared. Cleavage after day 8 results in a pregnancy that is monochorionic and monoamniotic, which places the pregnancy at an even higher risk for complications. Very rarely, cleavage may occur 13 days after conception, resulting in conjoined twins. Conjoined twins are physically fused and often share internal organs.

Although both dizygotic and monozygotic gestations present increased maternal and fetal risks, monochorionic gestations are at the most risk because of shared vasculature between the circulation of the twins.

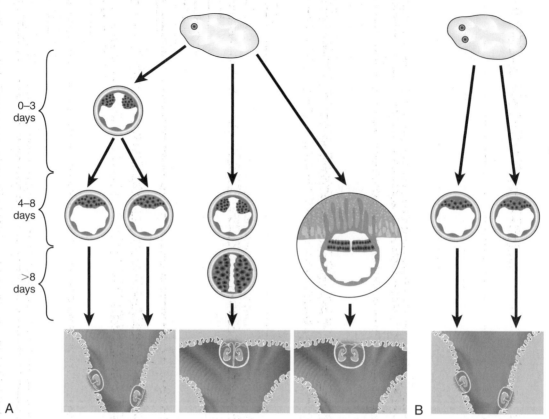

0–3 days

4–8 days

>8 days

A

B

FIGURE 22-3 Embryology of twinning. **(A)**, Monozygotic twinning: Single ovum is fertilized and divides, forming two separate embryos. Division occurring before day 4 results in dichorionic, diamniotic gestation. Division occurring between days 4 and 8 results in monochorionic, diamniotic gestation. Division occurring after day 8 results in monochorionic, monoamniotic gestation. **(B)**, Dizygotic twinning: Two separate ova are released in same cycle and fertilized, resulting in dichorionic, diamniotic gestation.

BOX 22-1	Clinical Signs and Symptoms Associated with Multiple Gestations

Large for dates
Hyperemesis
Hypertension
Increased human chorionic gonadotropin
Increased alpha fetoprotein

Recognizing and identifying chorionicity and amnionicity in a multiple gestation are important concepts and skills for the obstetric sonographer.

CLINICAL SIGNS AND SYMPTOMS

Deliberate evaluation for a multifetal gestation should be initiated whenever a history of ovulation induction exists, a patient measures large for gestational age, hyperemesis is present, preeclampsia develops, or two separate heartbeats are heard (Box 22-1).

Laboratory Values

A multifetal gestation should also be sought in the presence of elevated laboratory screening tests such as β human chorionic gonadotropin and maternal and serum alpha fetoprotein, which are components of the triple and quadruple screen laboratory tests.

COMPLICATIONS

Premature Labor

Prematurity and low birth weight are major contributing factors to the increased morbidity and mortality found in multiple gestations. Premature labor is the most common complication associated with multiple gestations and is thought to occur because of increased uterine volume. Twin pregnancies are five times more likely than singleton pregnancies to be complicated by premature labor, and the risk for triplet gestations is 10 times higher.[2] The role of sonography in these patients includes evaluation of the cervical length for thinning and for evidence of funneling. Transvaginal rather than transabdominal sonography should be considered for monitoring cervical length because it is the most reproducible technique for cervical assessment. As in a singleton pregnancy, either a cervical length of less than 2.5 cm or the presence of funneling at the internal cervical os is considered a significant finding associated with premature delivery (Fig. 22-4).

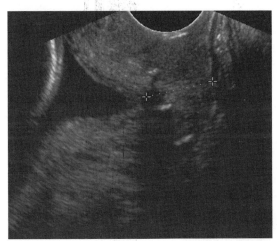

FIGURE 22-4 Cervical incompetence is suggested when cervical length measures less than 2.5 cm or when funneling is present.

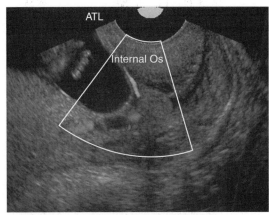

FIGURE 22-5 Vasa previa in a twin gestation. Longitudinal image at the level of the cervix with vessels coursing over the internal cervical os.

Intrauterine Growth Restriction

The birth weight of twins statistically averages 10% less than the birth weight of singletons of comparable gestational age. In 2007, 57% of twins and 96% of triplets born in the United States had low birth weight.[1] Because 14% to 25% of twins are considered to have growth restriction,[3] evaluation of fetal measurements and growth for any discordance is important. A fetal weight less than the 10th percentile is suggestive of intrauterine growth restriction (IUGR), especially in the setting of oligohydramnios and high resistance as demonstrated on the umbilical artery pulsed Doppler waveform. In a multiple gestation, IUGR can be caused by the same conditions as in a singleton pregnancy (e.g., placental insufficiency, fetal anomalies). In addition, IUGR may be the result of an abnormality unique to multiple gestations, such as twin-twin transfusion syndrome. If IUGR is suspected, serial sonography with pulsed Doppler evaluation of the umbilical cord and biophysical profile is generally indicated.

Congenital Anomalies

The incidence of a major fetal anomaly in a multiple gestation is 4% compared with 2% in a singleton pregnancy, including a 4.6% chance of having Down syndrome.[3] First-trimester and second-trimester screening for assessing risk of a fetus with Down syndrome in a twin gestation uses maternal age, serum screening, and sonographic evaluation. Because there is an increased risk for major malformations in multiple gestations, it is critical that all fetuses are sonographically evaluated for structural abnormalities.

Anomalies affecting the central nervous system are the most common in multiple gestations, especially monozygotic twins.[4] Twins and especially triplets are at increased risk for cerebral palsy.

Maternal Complications

Pregnancy-induced hypertension and preeclampsia are common maternal complications associated with multiple gestations. When preeclampsia occurs in a pregnancy with multiple gestations, it typically manifests earlier and is more severe than in singleton pregnancies. Close monitoring in patients with hypertension is necessary in case eclampsia develops. The features of eclampsia include hypertension, edema, proteinuria, and convulsions. Hypertension is also associated with IUGR and placental abruption.

Women with multiple gestations are at higher risk for bleeding complications from preterm labor and placental and cord abnormalities such as placental abruption, placenta previa, and vasa previa (Fig. 22-5; see Color Plate 25). Other maternal disorders observed more often in women with multiple gestations include iron deficiency anemia, hyperemesis gravidarum, and thromboembolism.[5]

SONOGRAPHIC EVALUATION

Chorionicity and Amnionicity

One of the most important features of the sonographic evaluation of a multiple gestation is establishing chorionicity and amnionicity. This evaluation is best accomplished by counting the number of fetuses, placentas, yolk sacs, chorionic sacs, and amniotic sacs. The presence of a single yolk sac suggests a monoamniotic gestation. Determining the number of chorionic and amniotic sacs is easiest during the first trimester because the space between separate implantation sites of a dichorionic pregnancy is evident, and the amnion can be identified separate from the chorion (Fig. 22-6).

Although it is easiest to determine fetal number and placentation during the first trimester, there are some pitfalls to be aware of. Early subchorionic hemorrhage sites can mimic a gestational sac, so it is important to establish

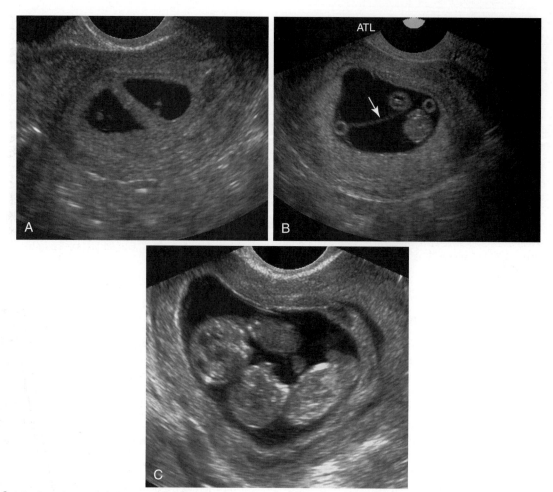

FIGURE 22-6 **(A)**, First-trimester dichorionic, diamniotic gestation with separate implantation sites. Note thick membrane between the gestations. **(B)**, Monochorionic, diamniotic gestation with thin intertwin membrane *(arrow)*. **(C)**, Monochorionic, monoamniotic 10-week twin gestation with no intertwin membrane.

fetal number on the basis of identifiable embryos and not just sacs. Before 6 weeks of gestation, an embryo may not yet be visible, and sonographic evaluation at this time has a greater risk of undercounting gestational number.

Once fetal number has been established, each fetus should be labeled as fetus A, fetus B, fetus C, and so on, with the fetus closest to the cervix labeled as A and the second closest as B. It is important to identify and label the same fetuses on subsequent examinations.

During the second or third trimester, multiple gestations are more difficult to evaluate. Fetal number is best determined by thoroughly scanning the uterus in two planes and counting the number of fetal heads. To evaluate fetal biometry and anatomy, it is important to keep the fetal anatomy separate by beginning at the fetal head and following the fetal trunk to the extremities. Twins should be assessed to ensure they are not conjoined. If the twins demonstrate intertwined limbs or tangled cords, monoamnionicity is present.

Chorionicity and amnionicity may be difficult to determine during the second or third trimester. The sonographer must rely on different sonographic findings than those described for first-trimester evaluation.

Evaluation of Fetal Gender

If one fetus is female and the other male, the gestation is definitely dizygotic and dichorionic. If the twins are the same gender, the gestation could be either monochorionic or dichorionic, and zygosity cannot be determined from this information alone.

Evaluation of Interfetal Membrane and Placental Sites

Sonographic evaluation of the placenta and interfetal membrane during the second or third trimester involves assessing the number and location of the placentas, membrane thickness, and the appearance of the membrane attachment. Sonographic evidence of two placentas in separate locations indicates a dichorionic gestation. Dichorionic pregnancies can also produce two placentas adjacent to each other, which can fuse and appear as one. With identification of only one placenta, the fetal umbilical cords should be followed to where they insert into the placenta. When the two cord insertion sites can be seen in the same plane, one should look for the presence of an

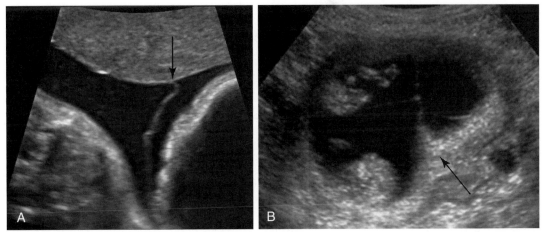

FIGURE 22-7 **(A)**, Second-trimester monochorionic, diamniotic twin gestation with thin membrane meeting the placenta to form a "T" shape *(arrow)*. **(B)**, Dichorionic, diamniotic twin gestation demonstrating a twin peak or lambda sign at the membrane-placental junction *(arrow)*.

interfetal membrane. If no membrane exists between the cord insertion sites, the twins are most likely monochorionic, monoamniotic.

If an interfetal membrane can be found, one should evaluate the thickness and look at the point where the membrane meets the placenta. The intertwin membrane separating twins in a monochorionic pregnancy consists of only two layers of amnion, so it is thin, wispy, and commonly measures less than 1 mm in thickness. Following the membrane to the placenta should reveal a flat, T-shaped attachment (Fig. 22-7, *A*). The dividing membrane in a dichorionic gestation consists of four layers: two chorionic and two amniotic membranes. If the interfetal membrane is greater than 2 mm in thickness, the gestation is most likely dichorionic. Following the membrane to the placenta should reveal a triangular wedge of placenta extending into the membrane, which is commonly referred to as the twin peak sign or the lambda sign (Fig. 22-7, *B*).

Fetal Biometry

The increased incidence of low birth weight and IUGR in multiple gestations emphasizes the importance of assessment of fetal size and growth in these pregnancies. A difference in growth between multiple fetuses is called discordant growth and is often the first sign of complications. The growth of twins is considered discordant if the difference in their birth weights is greater than 20% of the larger twin's weight (Fig. 22-8). Serial biometry provides a more accurate method to recognize discordant growth than a single sonographic evaluation. The greater the discrepancy, the higher the risk for neonatal mortality. Although it may be normal for one twin in a dizygotic gestation to be larger than the other, it is more concerning if the pregnancy is monochorionic because of shared vasculature. Research suggests that early-onset growth discordance (<20 weeks' gestation) in a monochorionic pregnancy indicates unequal placental sharing,

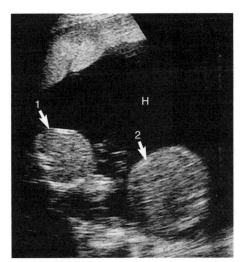

FIGURE 22-8 Discordant growth is shown in comparison of abdominal sizes of twins.

increasing the risk for sudden and significant intertwin transfusion imbalances.[6]

Doppler Evaluation

When the pregnancy is at risk for IUGR, pulsed Doppler evaluation of the umbilical artery may be helpful. The waveform of an umbilical artery in the setting of IUGR may demonstrate a high resistance pattern. Although there are charts for comparing resistive index, pulsatility index, and systolic/diastolic ratio, a Doppler waveform in which diastolic flow is absent or reversed is definitely abnormal. Other vessels that may demonstrate abnormalities in pulsatility in the setting of IUGR include the middle cerebral artery, inferior vena cava, and ductus venosus.

Doppler imaging also provides valuable information when specific twinning abnormalities are present. When a diagnosis of conjoined twins is made, Doppler evaluation can help define vascular connections between the twins. Diagnosing twin transfusion syndromes may benefit from the evaluation of the umbilical artery, such as demonstrating a high resistance waveform in twin-twin transfusion syndrome or reversed arterial flow in twin reversed arterial perfusion (TRAP) sequence.

Cord Entanglement

Monochorionic, monoamniotic twins lack an intertwin membrane, allowing the umbilical cords of the twins to intertwine. Cord entanglement is the main factor contributing to increased mortality rates of monoamniotic twins. Sonographic evidence of entanglement includes the identification of cord knots and the use of Doppler imaging to trace the route of each fetal cord, with demonstration of different fetal heart rates between them. Cord entanglement can be monitored by pulsed Doppler to evaluate for increased arterial and venous velocities and for evidence of high resistance in the umbilical artery.

Amniotic Fluid

Assessment of amniotic fluid begins subjectively by observing whether both amniotic sacs appear to be of equal size, with an adequate amount of amniotic fluid to allow free movement of the membranes during fetal activity. After performing a subjective evaluation, the single pocket method, in which the maximal vertical pocket (MVP) is measured, or the four-quadrant method, in which amniotic fluid index (AFI) is calculated, can be used to evaluate the amount of fluid in each amniotic sac. A quantitative assessment of AFV in a diamniotic gestation is difficult, and the single pocket method and subjective evaluation are the most common methods of evaluating AFV in a multiple gestation.

The terms hydramnios or polyhydramnios are used to describe an excessive accumulation of amniotic fluid. MVP that exceeds 8 cm or AFI exceeding 18 to 20 cm is considered excessive. In a multiple gestation, excess fluid may be a feature of a recipient twin in a gestation with twin-twin transfusion syndrome.

Oligohydramnios refers to a decreased amount of amniotic fluid. Sonographically, MVP less than 2 cm or AFI less than 5 cm suggests this condition. Oligohydramnios can be caused by IUGR, which is a complication associated with the donor twin in gestations with twin-twin transfusion syndrome. The confining amniotic membrane in the presence of reduced fluid restricts fetal movement of the affected twin and causes it to appear "stuck" to the uterine wall.

FETAL DEMISE

With the increased resolution of transvaginal sonography, multifetal pregnancies can be confirmed at 6 weeks of gestation. However, statistically, only 30% to 60% of early twin pregnancies detected sonographically result in the birth of twins, and more than 50% of patients with three or more gestational sacs are at risk for spontaneous reduction before 12 weeks of gestation.[7] The chance of survival of the other fetus is greater if the twin pregnancy is dichorionic, and if cotwin death occurs during the first trimester. In one review, the risk of cotwin death for monochorionic twins was five times higher than for dichorionic twins.[8]

Vanishing Twin

In approximately 21% of twin gestations diagnosed in the first trimester, one twin dies, leaving behind an empty sac.[2] This twin and its gestational sac may be completely reabsorbed, disappearing altogether. This is known as a vanishing twin. Loss of a twin during early pregnancy is often associated with vaginal bleeding, but the outcome for the surviving fetus is good.

Fetus Papyraceus

Fetal papyraceus refers to a twin fetus that has died early in development and has been pressed flat against the uterine wall by the living fetus. Co-twin demise in a diamniotic pregnancy results in reabsorption of the amniotic fluid around the dead twin. Provided that the twins are dichorionic, the surviving twin can continue to grow unaffected.

Sonographic Findings. Sonographically, the dead twin appears as an amorphous structure along the wall of the uterus (Fig. 22-9). Little or no amniotic fluid is seen in the sac surrounding the fetus papyraceus.

Twin Embolization Syndrome

Loss of a twin after 16 weeks of gestation in a monochorionic pregnancy is associated with twin embolization syndrome. One theory for this occurrence is that embolization of thrombus crosses the placental vascular

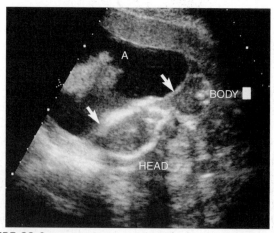

FIGURE 22-9 Death of twin (arrows) resulted in twin being flattened against uterine wall.

anastomosis to the surviving twin. The most current theory suggests loss of blood from the surviving twin to the dead twin, resulting in transient hemodynamic fluctuations leading to ischemic changes of the surviving twin.[8]

Sonographic Findings. Twin embolization syndrome in the surviving twin may manifest as ventriculomegaly, porencephalic cysts, diffuse cerebral atrophy, microcephaly, hepatic and splenic infarcts, gut atresias, renal cortical necrosis, pulmonary infarcts, facial anomalies, and terminal limb defects.[2]

ABNORMAL TWINNING

Conjoined Twins

Conjoined twins are monozygotic twins that are physically united at birth as a result of incomplete division of the embryonic disk. This is a rare anomaly that occurs in only 1 in 100,000 births.[2] Most cases of conjoined twins have symmetry of the joined regions and are classified by the part at which they are joined. For example, twins who are joined at the head are termed craniopagus ("cranio" pertaining to the head, and "pagus" meaning joined or fused). Thoracopagus twins are joined at the thorax, and omphalopagus twins are joined at the anterior mid trunk.

Sonographic Findings. Conjoined twins should be suspected when monoamniotic twins do not move away from each other and is confirmed when fusion of the fetal parts is identified (Fig. 22-10). Evaluation with gray-scale and color Doppler is helpful in the evaluation of the degree of organ sharing and screening for additional malformations. Careful examination is important because monochorionic, monoamniotic twins may become tethered by their cords and appear conjoined.

Twin-Twin Transfusion Syndrome

Twin-twin transfusion syndrome is caused by unbalanced shunting of blood from one twin to the other. Vascular connections are found in virtually all monochorionic twins, and approximately 15% result in twin-twin transfusion syndrome.[9] The "donor" twin pumps blood from its arterial system into the venous system of the "recipient" twin. The donor twin receives less blood and is usually growth restricted, hypovolemic, and anemic. The recipient twin receives too much blood, and although it may be normal in size, it is often macrosomic and hypervolemic. The extra blood flow and work placed on the recipient twin's heart can result in fetal hydrops or heart failure. Monochorionic twins should be evaluated with serial examinations for growth because placental insufficiency and twin-twin transfusion syndrome are often not apparent until later in the gestation.

Sonographic Findings. Sonographic findings suggestive of twin-twin transfusion syndrome include the identification of a true monochorionic pregnancy, a marked discrepancy in fetal size (>20% difference in weight), the smaller donor twin in an oligohydramniotic sac, and the larger recipient twin in a sac with polyhydramnios. In severe cases, the amniotic fluid surrounding the smaller twin is so minimal that the donor twin appears to be stuck to the uterine wall—hence the term "stuck twin" (Fig. 22-11). Turning the mother on her side to see whether the stuck twin drops away from the uterine wall may assist in making the diagnosis. The identification of a fold in the amniotic membrane may also help differentiate a discrepancy in AFV between the twins (Fig. 22-12). There may also be a discrepancy in the size of the urinary bladders, with the donor twin demonstrating a smaller bladder than the recipient twin. Pulsed Doppler assessment of the umbilical cord in the growth-restricted twin to evaluate arterial resistance should also be considered.

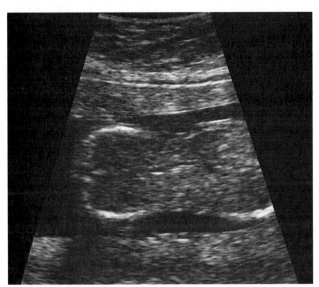

FIGURE 22-10 Image shows conjoining of omphalopagus twins.

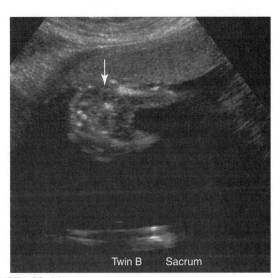

FIGURE 22-11 Twin-twin transfusion syndrome resulting in "stuck" twin (*arrow*). Fetus appears adhered to anterior uterine wall.

Twin Reversed Arterial Perfusion Sequence

TRAP sequence is a rare condition that complicates approximately 1% of monochorionic pregnancies.[2] The exact pathogenesis is unknown, but the condition is thought to occur because of paired artery-to-artery or vein-to-vein anastomosis within the shared placenta. The pump twin, or normal twin, has normal circulation. The recipient twin lacks a functional heart, allowing perfusion pressure of the normal twin to pump blood into the acardiac twin, through the artery-to-artery anastomosis, without passing through a capillary bed for oxygenation. The blood flowing to the acardiac twin through the umbilical arteries and into the internal iliac arteries is retrograde. The limited amount of oxygen and nutrients delivered to the torso and lower extremities of the fetus result in abnormal development, especially of the upper body.

Sonographic Findings. TRAP sequence should be suspected when one twin appears anatomically normal and the other lacks cardiac structures or other upper body structures. Often, the head, cervical spine, heart, and upper limbs are absent or severely malformed with gross skin thickening of the upper trunk and neck areas (Fig. 22-13, A). Clubbing of the feet or absent toes is common (Fig. 22-13, B). Malformations are variable, ranging from a tissue mass without recognizable fetal parts to a twin in which the lower extremities and torso can be seen (and often are moving), but the entire fetus cannot be "laid out," sonographically speaking. Doppler identification of reversed flow in the umbilical arteries and vein of the acardiac twin confirms the diagnosis.

SUMMARY

Multiple gestations are occurring with increased frequency. Because of the higher risk associated with multifetal gestations and the unique complications that affect these pregnancies, proficiency with the unique approach to sonographic evaluation is important. Chorionicity and amnionicity are most accurately determined in the first trimester. Following these pregnancies sonographically throughout the second and third trimesters is important because complications such as IUGR, preterm birth, and fetal anomalies occur at an increased rate in multiple gestations. Careful screening also allows the identification of complications specific to monochorionic twins, such as cord entanglement, twin embolization, conjoined twinning, twin-twin transfusion syndrome, and TRAP sequence (Table 22-1).

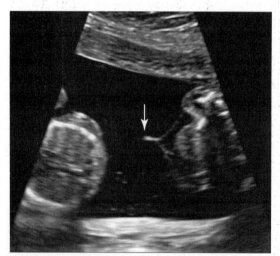

FIGURE 22-12 Difference in fluid volume between oligohydramniotic and polyhydramniotic sacs allows membrane to fold (arrow).

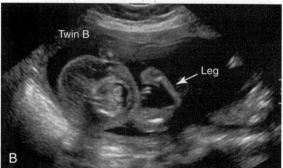

CLINICAL SCENARIO—DIAGNOSIS

The rapid progression and early onset of growth discordance and amniotic fluid discrepancy in monochorionic twins should raise the suspicion of twin-twin transfusion syndrome. The slight elevation in umbilical artery resistance in twin B, the smaller twin, is associated with poor fetal outcome. Although the amniotic fluid measurements were within normal limits at the time of this study, the measurements are approaching oligohydramnios in twin B and polyhydramnios in twin A. The combination of growth discordance and amniotic fluid disturbance in this case represented twin-twin transfusion syndrome.

Within 2 weeks of the initial scan, twin B slowly faltered. After 2 weeks of observation, laser surgery was performed. This procedure uses an operative fetoscope to deliver a laser that seals off the blood vessels on the surface of the shared placenta. Vascular connections between the twins are plugged, allowing no further shared circulation between the twins. The patient delivered at 34 weeks, with no further complications.

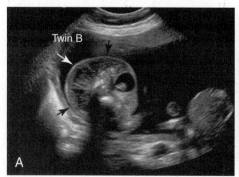

FIGURE 22-13 (A), Acardiac twin with severe skin thickening (arrows) and upper body malformations. **(B),** Clubfoot in same acardiac twin.

TABLE 22-1	Abnormal Twinning	
Abnormality	**Etiology**	**Sonographic Findings**
Vanishing twin	Early embryonic death of one twin	Early multiple gestation confirmed sonographically, with subsequent disappearance of one twin
Fetus papyraceus	Fetal death of one twin in a diamniotic gestation, with reabsorption of amniotic fluid around dead twin	Multiple gestation in which one fetus appears as amorphous structure along wall of uterus; little or no amniotic fluid is seen in sac surrounding fetus; surviving fetus is usually unaffected
Conjoined twins	Monozygotic twins that are physically united at birth; usually results from late and incomplete cleavage	Monochorionic, monoamniotic gestation in which twins do not move away from each other, and fusion of fetal parts can be identified; degree of organ sharing should be assessed along with continued screening for additional fetal malformations
Twin-twin transfusion syndrome	Monochorionic gestation in which there is arteriovenous communication within the placental circulation, resulting in shunting of blood from donor to recipient	Monochorionic gestation with marked discrepancy in AFV and fetal size between the twins; smaller twin shows oligohydramnios and small or absent bladder, and larger twin shows hydramnios with bladder present
Twin reversed arterial perfusion sequence	Monochorionic gestation in which there is paired artery-to-artery and vein-to-vein anastomoses; altered placental circulation leads to reversal of blood flow in umbilical artery with development of malformed recipient twin	Monochorionic gestation in which one twin is acardiac with poorly developed upper body; head, cervical spine, heart, and upper limbs may be absent or severely deformed; lower half of body may show activity; clubbing of feet is common; reversed flow in umbilical vessels of acardiac twin is present

CASE STUDIES FOR DISCUSSION

1. A 41-year-old woman with vaginal bleeding undergoes an obstetric sonogram to evaluate her 9-week twin pregnancy, which was diagnosed at 6 weeks' gestational age. Figure 22-14 is an image from the most current examination. What type of chorionicity is evident, and what is the most likely diagnosis?
2. A 26-year-old woman with a positive pregnancy test and hyperemesis undergoes an obstetric sonogram. Sonographic evaluation reveals a monochorionic twin gestation, with anatomic abnormalities present in twin B (Fig. 22-15) and no abnormalities evident in twin A. In addition, pulsed-wave Doppler in the umbilical artery of the abnormal twin demonstrates reversed flow direction. What is the most likely diagnosis?
3. A 25-year-old woman undergoes a sonogram because she is large for dates. Discuss the risks associated with the sonographic finding in Figure 22-16.

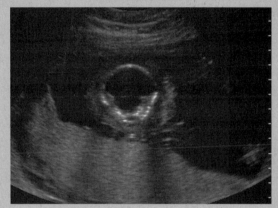

FIGURE 22-15 Image of twin B's head.

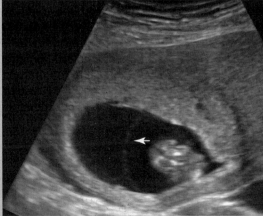

FIGURE 22-14 Follow-up examination of a 9-week pregnancy with a twin gestation diagnosed at 6 weeks.

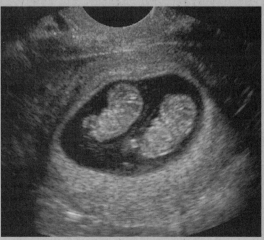

FIGURE 22-16 Image of a 10-week pregnancy.

Continued

CASE STUDIES FOR DISCUSSION—cont'd

4. A 41-year-old woman with a monochorionic twin gestation undergoes a follow-up obstetric sonogram at 20 weeks' gestational age. Twin B is significantly smaller than twin A. Figure 22-17 demonstrates their positions within the uterus and the AFV for twin A. What is the most likely diagnosis?

5. A 27-year-old woman undergoes a follow-up obstetric sonogram at 28 weeks' gestational age to assess fetal growth in her twins. The sonogram reveals twin A is a boy with an abdominal circum-

ference of 18 cm, and twin B is a girl with an abdominal circumference of 24 cm. The pulsed-wave Doppler waveform of twin A's umbilical artery is shown in Figure 22-18 (see Color Plate 26). What is the most likely diagnosis?

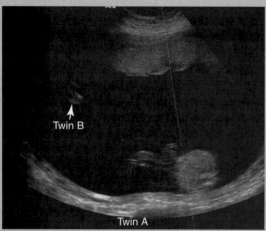

FIGURE 22-17 Twin A in posterior region of uterus. A portion of twin B *(arrow)* is visible near anterior uterine wall.

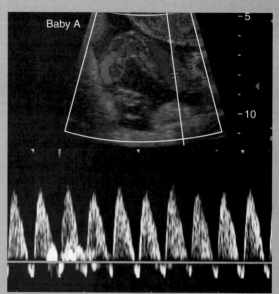

FIGURE 22-18 Pulsed Doppler waveform of twin A's umbilical artery.

STUDY QUESTIONS

1. Which of the following represents the most common complication in a pregnancy with multiple gestations?
   a. Preterm labor
   b. Twin-twin transfusion syndrome
   c. IUGR
   d. Retained placenta

2. Which of the following sonographic findings is associated with twin-twin transfusion syndrome?
   a. Reversed umbilical artery flow
   b. Malformations of the upper body
   c. Different genders with growth discordance
   d. Monochorionicity with unequal distribution of AFV

3. What would you expect to see in the donor twin affected by twin-twin transfusion syndrome?
   a. Enlarged bladder
   b. Hydrops
   c. Double bubble
   d. IUGR

4. Which of the following is a reason for the increased incidence of multiple gestations?

   a. Changes in diet
   b. Environmental factors
   c. Later life pregnancies
   d. Increase in teenage pregnancies

5. Which of the following is a common maternal complication in pregnancies with multiple gestations?
   a. HELLP syndrome
   b. Preeclampsia
   c. Renal stones
   d. Gallstones

6. Which of the following complications related to the death of one twin results in the most danger to the other twin?
   a. Twin embolization syndrome
   b. Heterotopic pregnancy
   c. Fetal papyraceus
   d. Vanishing twin

7. Monozygotic, embryonic division between 0 and 3 days after conception results in which type of placentation?
   a. Monochorionic, monoamniotic
   b. Monochorionic, diamniotic
   c. Dichorionic, diamniotic
   d. Conjoined twins

8. Dizygotic twins are always which type of placentation?
   a. Monochorionic, monoamniotic
   b. Monochorionic, diamniotic
   c. Dichorionic, monoamniotic
   d. Dichorionic, diamniotic

9. Cervical length of less than 2.5 cm and evidence of funneling are associated with which of the following?
   a. Preeclampsia
   b. Preterm delivery
   c. Placenta previa
   d. Vasa previa

10. Which of the following statements describes why monochorionic multiple gestations have the highest fetal mortality?
    a. Placental intertwin vascular anastomoses play a key role in complications associated with monochorionic gestations.
    b. Maternal diabetes is more common in monochorionic pregnancies, and anomalies and growth disturbance are more common.
    c. Monochorionicity delays fetal development.
    d. Placental insufficiency is more common in monochorionic pregnancies.

REFERENCES

1. Martin J, Hamilton B, Sutton P, et al: *Births: final data for 2007. National vital statistics report*, vol 58, no 24, Hyattsville, MD, 2010, National Center for Health Statistics.
2. Mehta T: Multifetal pregnancy. In Rumack CM, Wilson SR, Charboneau JW, editors: ed 4, *Diagnostic ultrasound*, vol. 2, St Louis, 2011, Mosby, pp 1145–1163.
3. Egan J, Borgida A: Ultrasound evaluation of multiple pregnancies. In Callen PW, editor: *Ultrasonography in obstetrics and gynecology*, ed 5, Philadelphia, 2008, Saunders, pp 266–296.
4. Jones K: *Smith's recognizable patterns of human malformation*, ed 6, Philadelphia, 2006, Saunders.
5. American College of Obstetricians and Gynecologists: ACOG Practice Bulletin #56: Multiple gestation: complicated twin, triplet, and high-order multifetal pregnancy, *Obstet Gynecol* 104:869, 2004.
6. Lewi L, Gucciardo L, Huber A, et al: Clinical outcome and placental characteristics of monochorionic diamniotic twin pairs with early-and late-onset discordant growth, *Am J Obstet Gynecol* 199:511, 2008.
7. Dickey R, Taylor S, Lu P, et al: Spontaneous reduction of multiple pregnancy: incidence and effect on outcome, *Am J Obstet Gynecol* 186:77, 2002.
8. Hillman S, Morris R, Kilby M: Co-twin prognosis after single fetal death: a systematic review and meta-analysis, *Obstet Gynecol* 118:928, 2011.
9. Galea P, Jain V, Fisk N: Insights into the pathophysiology of twin-twin transfusion syndrome, *Prenat Diagn* 45:777, 2005.

Elevated Alpha Fetoprotein

Armando Fuentes, Charlotte Henningsen

CLINICAL SCENARIO

A 22-year-old woman with no significant medical history is seen for a sonogram at gestational age 18 weeks, 5 days. The pregnancy has been relatively uncomplicated until now except for one episode of first-trimester spotting; a first-trimester sonogram obtained at the time of spotting confirmed a gestational age of 6 weeks. She had a routine maternal serum alpha fetoprotein (MSAFP) test at 17 weeks' gestation, which was reported as 7.4 multiples of the median. The information was given to her the previous day at her physician's office, and fetal heart tones were auscultated.

Sonographic evaluation reveals the coronal views of the fetal face and spine shown in Figure 23-1. Fetal biometry of the fetal abdomen and femur confirms the established gestational age; in addition, a single umbilical artery is noted. What is the most likely diagnosis?

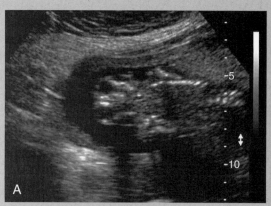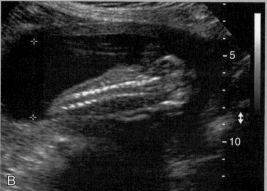

FIGURE 23-1 (A), Coronal image of the fetal face. **(B),** Coronal spine and base of the calvaria.

OBJECTIVES

- Describe the clinical use of serum alpha fetoprotein as a screen for various fetal anomalies.
- Describe the appropriate diagnostic approach to a patient with an elevated alpha fetoprotein value.
- Identify potential pregnancy complications in the setting of an unexplained elevated alpha fetoprotein value.
- Identify the sonographic appearance of neural tube disorders commonly associated with an elevated alpha fetoprotein value.
- Identify fetal abdominal wall anomalies associated with elevated alpha fetoprotein values.
- Describe the sonographic appearance of abdominal wall defects commonly associated with an elevated alpha fetoprotein value.
- Differentiate sonographic features of limb–body wall complex and amniotic band syndrome.

MATERNAL SERUM ALPHA FETOPROTEIN

One of the most common tests routinely offered to pregnant women is serum screening for Down syndrome and neural tube defects (NTD). MSAFP historically has been used to screen for NTDs. Since its discovery, MSAFP screening has been used to identify chromosomal abnormalities, anterior abdominal wall defects, ovarian carcinoma, and various other fetal and maternal conditions. This chapter describes various etiologies for abnormal MSAFP levels.

Alpha fetoprotein is structurally and functionally related to albumin, and genes for both proteins originate on chromosome 4. Alpha fetoprotein is a fetal-specific protein that is synthesized sequentially by the yolk sac, gastrointestinal tract, and liver. Its function is unknown, although there are various theories involving its function, such as immunoregulation during pregnancy or intravascular transport protein. The peak concentration in fetal serum is at the end of the first trimester. As pregnancy progresses, the fetal liver continues to produce a constant amount of alpha fetoprotein until 30 weeks' gestation, which is secreted by the fetal kidneys into the amniotic fluid. Amniotic fluid contains high concentrations of alpha fetoprotein, although it decreases similarly to the fetal serum concentration after 30 weeks. In maternal serum, alpha fetoprotein increases in the second trimester, and the fetal serum alpha fetoprotein decreases. The transfer of alpha fetoprotein to the maternal circulation occurs through the placenta and amniotic fluid.

The optimal period for screening of MSAFP is between 15 and 18 weeks of gestation. MSAFP screening is intended to detect open spina bifida and anencephaly, but other disorders, such as ventral wall defects, tumors, congenital nephrosis, and aneuploidy, can also be identified. The results of MSAFP screening are reported as multiples of the median (MoM) for each gestational age. Measurements of alpha fetoprotein can be affected by laboratory technique. Also, standard deviations may be influenced by the spread of data. MoM reflect an individual patient's value compared with the median. Each laboratory develops its own reference values. Factors that can influence MSAFP results include gestational age, maternal weight, ethnicity, diabetes mellitus, fetal viability, and multiple gestation.

Several studies have demonstrated the reliability of MSAFP screening for NTDs. Wang et al.[1] published a meta-analysis comprising 684,112 patients screened in the second trimester that showed a sensitivity of 75.1 and specificity of 97.7. Detection of anencephaly is even higher. Data from various studies indicate that major fetal anomalies are present in 30% to 58% of patients with MSAFP levels of 5.0 MoM or greater.[2,3] When a cutoff of 2.5 MoM is used, MSAFP screening detects approximately 88% of anencephalic fetuses and 79% of fetuses with open spina bifida. When no explanation can be determined for an elevated alpha fetoprotein value, despite sonographic and chromosomal investigation, 20% to 38% of pregnancies have adverse outcomes. These adverse outcomes include low birth weight, prematurity, intrauterine growth restriction, preeclampsia, and placental abruption.[4]

Sonography has become a very effective tool for detecting NTDs, and it has replaced MSAFP testing as a screening tool in some centers.[5] Sonographic detection of NTDs is influenced by gestational age, maternal body habitus, and type of NTD. First-trimester screenings have reported greater than 90% detection rates for anencephaly and 80% detection rates for encephalocele. In the second trimester, sonographic screening has a detection rate of 92% to 95% for spina bifida.[6]

NEURAL TUBE DEFECTS

Failure of neural tube closure between the third and fourth week of embryologic development results in NTDs. Approximately 18 days after conception, the neural plate folds to form a central neural groove and bilateral neural folds. The neural folds fuse in the midline and begin to form the neural tube. Fusion progresses simultaneously toward the cranial and caudal ends. Closure of the anterior neuropore occurs by day 24, and closure of the posterior neuropore occurs by day 26. The cranial end of the neural tube becomes the forebrain, midbrain, and hindbrain, and failure of closure results in anencephaly. The caudal end of the neural tube becomes the spinal cord, and failure of posterior neuropore closure results in spina bifida.[7]

Several different types of NTDs can occur, which can affect the spinal cord or cranium. The spinal defects are classified as either open or closed; this classification is dependent on whether neural tissue is exposed. Because approximately 20% of spina bifida lesions are closed, not all NTDs are detected with MSAFP screening. Elevations in alpha fetoprotein occur because of communications between the nervous system and amniotic fluid. The most severe elevations are seen in the setting of anencephaly and severe open spinal defects where large areas of neural tissue are exposed.

Most NTDs are either isolated defects or multifactorial. Several factors have been implicated, including folic acid deficiency,[8] medications (valproic acid), genetic factors (MTHFR polymorphism, Meckel-Gruber syndrome),[9] and vitamin B_{12} deficiency.[10] Environmental factors associated with NTDs include hyperthermia, maternal diabetes mellitus, and obesity.[11,12] The incidence of NTDs in the United States is commonly quoted as 1:1000; this is highly dependent on ethnic and geographic variability. The incidence appears to be higher in Hispanic and non-Hispanic whites compared with African Americans and Asians. Higher rates of NTDs have also been seen in the eastern and southern United States compared with the western United States. Additionally, there is an increased risk of recurrence in families with a history of a prior NTD.

The introduction of screening programs and folic acid supplementation has significantly reduced the incidence of NTDs. In 2006, birth data from the United States revealed a combined incidence of anencephaly and spina bifida of 0.3:1000 live births, which is significantly lower than 1:1000 reported in the 1990s.[13]

Anencephaly

Anencephaly, which results in absence of the cranium and brain above the orbits, is the most common NTD. It can also occur as a result of destruction of brain matter exposed to amniotic fluid in fetuses with acrania. It has been identified in 1:1000 pregnancies,[14] but the incidence of live births is significantly lower.

Acrania and anencephaly both have been diagnosed sonographically in the first trimester. Sonography also is highly accurate in the second trimester. Because there is complete communication with the amniotic fluid, alpha fetoprotein values are extremely elevated, which may trigger a sonographic evaluation.

Anencephaly is more common in females and monozygotic twins. Additionally, associated anomalies may be seen in fetuses affected by anencephaly, including spina bifida, cranioschisis, cleft lip/palate, talipes, omphalocele, and aneuploidy (especially when multiple anomalies are seen).

Sonographic Findings. Anencephaly is diagnosed when absence of the calvaria above the orbits and absence of the brain are noted (Fig. 23-2, *A*). It is best seen in the coronal plane where the orbits appear prominent revealing a "frog's eye" appearance (Fig. 23-2, *B*). There may be a small, abnormal remnant of tissue seen above the orbits, known as the cerebrovasculosa. If the fetal head is difficult to visualize because of a low vertex position, an endovaginal sonogram may be necessary. Polyhydramnios is commonly identified in gestations with anencephaly secondary to a decreased swallowing reflex.

Spina Bifida

Spina bifida indicates a cleft in the spinal column. The two main types of spina bifida are spina bifida aperta and spina bifida occulta. Spina bifida occulta is formed when there is failure of the dorsal portions of the vertebrae to fuse with one another, and it is covered by skin and not noticeable unless there is a small tuft of hair or a dimple. In spina bifida aperta, a disruption of the skin and subcutaneous tissues is visible over the area of the spine where the incomplete closure occurs. As a result, the meninges protrude out of the vertebral defect and are exposed to the amniotic fluid. In the absence of nervous tissue extruding into the meningeal sac, the lesion is termed a meningocele and is not related to hydrocephalus or neurologic defects. In most cases, nervous tissue is incorporated into the lesion, and it is termed a meningomyelocele; it is frequently associated with hydrocephalus.

The most common locations for spina bifida anomalies are the thoracolumbar, lumbar, and lumbosacral areas. Also, a wide variation is seen in the size of the lesions, resulting in higher MSAFP values in large defects. Additional anomalies may be seen in association with spinal defects, including microcephaly, cephaloceles, cleft lip/palate, hypotelorism, and hypertelorism.

Sonographic Findings. Complete evaluation of the spine involves viewing of spinous structures in the longitudinal and transverse aspects, from the nuchal origin to the distal sacrum. In the transverse plane, the posterior ossification centers tilt toward the midline. Spina bifida should be considered when the posterior ossification centers assume a splayed "V," "C," or "U" configuration when

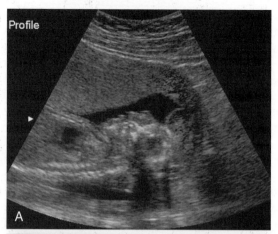
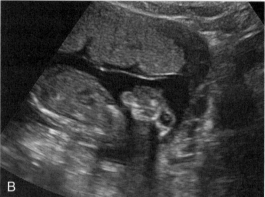

FIGURE 23-2 (A), Fetal profile with absent calvaria with presence of cerebrovasculosa. **(B),** Image of anencephaly shows typical frog-like appearance.

viewed in the transverse plane (Fig. 23-3, *A*). In addition, abnormal curvature of the spine (kyphosis, lordosis, or scoliosis) may be observed. The most superior aspect of vertebral misalignment defines the level of the lesion, which relates to outcome (Fig. 23-4); three-dimensional reconstruction may be useful in clarifying the anatomic level of the defect.[15]

An intracranial anomaly known as Arnold-Chiari malformation often accompanies spina bifida aperta. Arnold-Chiari malformation is characterized by cerebral ventriculomegaly (lateral ventricle >10 mm), decreased intracranial pressure leading to frontal bone collapse (lemon sign), abnormal curvature of the cerebellum as it is impacted into the posterior fossa (banana sign), decreased cerebellar size (which may lead to failure of identification), and obliteration of the cisterna magna (see Fig. 23-3, *B* and *C*).

Cephalocele

Cephalocele or encephalocele is defined as a defect in the cranium through which intracranial tissue protrudes, including meninges with or without brain tissue. The incidence is 0.8:10,000 to 4:10,000 live births.[16] Occipital encephaloceles are usually considered within the NTD group. Associated conditions with occipital

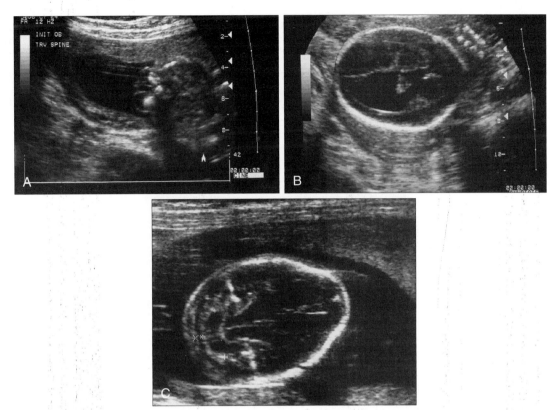

FIGURE 23-3 **(A)**, "V" shape of vertebra is consistent with spina bifida. **(B)**, The fetus shows classic findings of spina bifida, including a sac protruding from the defect containing neural elements and ventriculomegaly. **(C)**, This fetus with spina bifida has a lemon-shaped head with a banana-shaped cerebellum.

encephaloceles include Meckel-Gruber syndrome, amniotic band syndrome (ABS), cerebellar dysgenesis, short limb dysplasia, and warfarin syndrome. Frontal or parietal encephaloceles are not considered a NTD and may be environmental in origin.

MSAFP may not help with the diagnosis because most of these lesions are covered with intact meninges. The outcome is poorer when encephaloceles are associated with hydrocephalus or when significant brain tissue is in the defect.

Sonographic Findings. Sonographically, a cephalocele appears as herniation of the meninges with or without brain through a defect in the calvaria (Fig. 23-5). The sac may appear cystic or solid and can vary in size. Ventriculomegaly is often seen, and traction on the intracranial contents may result in microcephaly. Cephaloceles may also vary in appearance throughout gestation.

Documentation of a cranial defect is necessary for accurate diagnosis of a cephalocele. If a cranial defect cannot be identified, cystic hygroma should be considered.

ABDOMINAL WALL DEFECTS

Abdominal wall defects are described as congenital defects that result in protrusion of intraabdominal contents through an incomplete closure of the ventral wall. The incidence is reported to be less than 1:3000 live

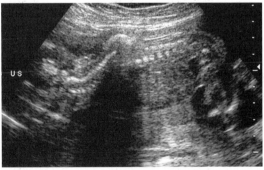

FIGURE 23-4 Large spinal defect involving the thoracic spine. The outcome for this infant was predicted to be extremely poor.

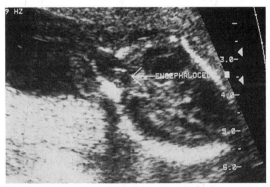

FIGURE 23-5 Brain tissue herniating through a defect in the calvaria is identified in a fetus with encephalocele.

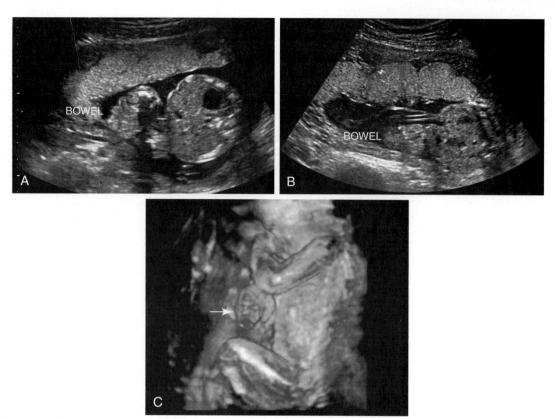

FIGURE 23-6 (A), Free-floating bowel was identified in a patient with an elevated alpha fetoprotein. **(B),** Umbilical cord is inserting adjacent to the defect. **(C),** Three-dimensional imaging demonstrates a gastroschisis.

births.[17] The most common defects are gastroschisis and omphalocele; other rare defects include limb–body wall complex (LBWC), ectopia cordis, pentalogy of Cantrell, and cloacal exstrophy. These defects are the second most common cause of elevated MSAFP. The use of MSAFP screening and sonographic examination has increased the detection of these defects. The assessment of nuchal translucency for Down syndrome has also increased the detection of these defects in the first trimester.

During day 22 to 28 of development, the embryonic disk folds in four planes. The lateral folds ventrally form the abdominal wall. During the sixth week of development, the abdominal contents physiologically protrude into the extraembryonic coelom at the base of the umbilical cord. This herniation invaginates by week 12. The size of the herniation before 12 weeks can assist in determining if it is pathologic. An anterior herniation that measures more than 7 mm at any gestational age suggests a pathologic anomaly.[18]

Gastroschisis

Gastroschisis is a full-thickness abdominal wall defect that occurs in 0.3:10,000 to 2.0:10,000 births.[17] The abdominal wall defect usually lies to the right of the umbilicus and is small in size, with bowel extruding into the amniotic cavity. Because the defect involves all layers of the abdominal wall, an open communication

exists between the amniotic fluid and the intraabdominal space. Herniation of liver or stomach through this defect is uncommon. One consequence is greater extrusion of alpha fetoprotein into the amniotic space and into maternal circulation.

The incidence varies considerably with maternal age, with a higher incidence among younger women. Associated anomalies primarily include gastrointestinal related anomalies and complications. Gastroschisis has not been associated with fetal aneuploidy, and the prognosis overall is considered favorable, with mortality related to prematurity, sepsis, and intestinal complications associated with bowel ischemia.

Sonographic Findings. The hallmark of gastroschisis is free-floating bowel originating from the right of the umbilicus (Fig. 23-6; see Color Plate 27). Early in the course of gastroschisis, bowel appears normal with evidence of peristaltic activity. After prolonged exposure to the caustic effects of urine in amniotic fluid, bowel reacts by thickening and developing what is known as a "peel." Bowel edema and luminal dilation develop later in the clinical course from mechanical obstruction at the site of the defect. The bowel becomes dilated and thickened. Dilation may also occur from atresia at sites of ischemia, necrosis, and stricture formation. As a result, the bowel wall assumes a more hyperechoic appearance, and peristalsis becomes less noticeable. Polyhydramnios is also frequently identified.

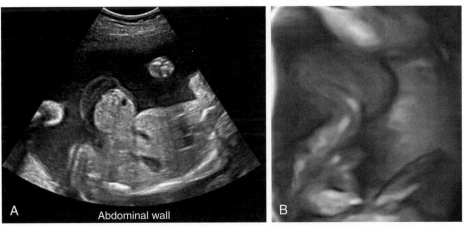

FIGURE 23-7 (A), Sagittal image of a fetus shows a large abdominal wall defect surrounded by a membrane consistent with omphalocele. **(B),** Three-dimensional imaging shows the umbilical cord inserting into the defect. The karyotype was normal.

Omphalocele

Omphaloceles are defects in the abdomen that result in a herniation of the intraabdominal contents into the umbilical stalk covered with peritoneum and amnion. They occur in 1:10,000 to 3:10,000 births.[17] An increased incidence has been seen in women who are older. Because omphaloceles involve herniation into the umbilical stalk, abdominal contents are covered by the cord's structures—the overlying amnion and gelatinous Wharton's jelly. With these protective layers covering the bowel, less alpha fetoprotein extrudes out into the amniotic fluid, and the MSAFP is typically lower than seen with gastroschisis.

Omphaloceles may be differentiated as either liver containing or non–liver containing. Chromosomal abnormalities, such as trisomy 18, trisomy 21, or trisomy 13, can be seen in 35% to 60% of fetuses, and the association with aneuploidy is greater when bowel is included in the herniation.[17] An increased nuchal translucency is identified in most fetuses with an omphalocele and aneuploidy. Anomalies of the cardiovascular, genitourinary, gastrointestinal, and central nervous systems and facial and limb abnormalities may be present. Beckwith-Wiedemann syndrome should be in the differential diagnosis if the karyotype is normal. The prognosis for omphalocele is considered poor, especially when liver is in the defect or when associated with aneuploidy or other anomalies.

Sonographic Findings. The sonographic diagnosis of omphalocele primarily involves identification of a central abdominal mass enclosed in a membrane arising from the midline (Fig. 23-7). The umbilical cord should be identified arising from the defect (see Fig 23-7, *B*; see Color Plate 28). Because the process of normal midgut herniation may not be completed until gestational week 12, diagnosis before this time may be difficult. Liver-containing omphaloceles can be identified before 12 weeks, because the liver is never herniated in physiologic herniation.

Differentiation from gastroschisis may be inferred when ascites is identified because of the presence of a sac encasing the defect. Because no contact exists between the bowel and amniotic fluid, bowel wall does not encounter the caustic urine and does not develop an inflammatory thickened wall. Polyhydramnios can be seen in one-third of fetuses with omphaloceles and is predictive of a poorer prognosis.

Limb–Body Wall Complex

LBWC is a universally fatal condition that results from abnormal body folding during early embryologic development. The incidence rate ranges from 1:14,000 to 1:30,000 pregnancies, but it is probably higher with many spontaneously aborting in early pregnancy.[19] This rare anomaly has been explained by multiple theories, but the exact cause is unknown.

LBWC is characterized by a large, anterior abdominal wall defect with an absent or short umbilical cord with multiple additional anomalies, including skeletal and craniofacial defects. LBWC is also known by other synonyms, including body stalk anomaly, short umbilical cord syndrome, and early amnion rupture sequence; however, there is debate as to whether some of the terms may represent a separate and distinct diagnosis. Regardless of the confusion, these related defects carry a normal karyotype with a grave prognosis.[19] Additionally, MSAFP levels are predictably high given the extent of fetal organ exposure to amniotic fluid.

Sonographic Findings. The primary features of LBWC are a large anterior abdominal wall defect (Fig. 23-8), short or absent umbilical cord, NTD, facial clefting, and limb defects. Scoliosis is frequently seen in addition to severe spinal anomalies. With absence of the umbilical cord, the abdominal wall mass appears to be directly tethered to the placenta; free-floating amniotic bands may also be identified.

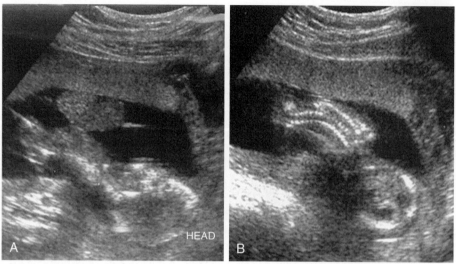

FIGURE 23-8 Abdominal wall defect attached directly to the placenta **(A)** and scoliosis **(B)** are seen in this fetus.

AMNIOTIC BAND SYNDROME

ABS is a developmental disorder in which fibrous remnants of amnion constrict the fetus. Fetal consequences range from simple constriction bands to devastating disruptions that are inconsistent with life. Several synonyms have been used to describe ABS, including ADAM (amniotic deformities, adhesion, mutilation) complex, which defines the severe end of the spectrum.[20] The incidence of ABS is 1:1200 to 1:15,000 live births, and the insult usually occurs between 6 and 18 weeks.[21]

Most commonly, amniotic bands affect limbs and can cause amputations, constrictions with edema, and clubfoot, the latter especially in the setting of oligohydramnios. Severe malformation of fetal structures may also result from adherence to the sticky bands and from slash defects. The prognosis depends on the location of constrictures and the severity of the anomalies.

Sonographic Findings

ABS causes the anomalies that can be seen prenatally and not the actual amniotic band. ABS most commonly results in constrictions but may also result in facial clefting, amputations, and clubfoot deformities. The facial clefting can have unusual demarcations involving the orbits and cranium, including a resemblance to anencephaly (Fig. 23-9). Evidence of edema around the band increases suspicion for ABS, as does identification of asymmetric anomalies. Abdominal and thoracic wall defects may be identified in addition to encephaloceles; rarely, ABS has contributed to fetal decapitation.[21] ABS should be considered when an off-midline encephalocele is identified. Confounding structures that may mimic ABS include uterine synechia, chorioamniotic separation, and subchorionic hemorrhage.

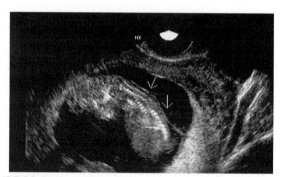

FIGURE 23-9 An amniotic band can be identified extending along the back of a fetus with acrania.

ECTOPIA CORDIS

Ectopia cordis is a very rare defect in which the heart is partially or completely protruding through the thorax. The most common theory for the defect is a failure of fusion of the lateral folds in the thoracic region. The presence of an omphalocele and ectopia cordis should raise the suspicion of pentalogy of Cantrell, which also includes diaphragmatic and pericardial defects, a cardiac anomaly, and a defect of the lower sternum.[22] It is universally lethal; however, there have been reported cases of surgical intervention, particularly in isolated cases of ectopia cordis.

Sonographic Findings

Ectopia cordis is easily diagnosed with visualization of the fetal heart outside of the chest cavity (Fig. 23-10). A wide spectrum of anomalies exists, ranging from a partial eventration of the heart to complete evisceration of abdominal and thoracic contents. When an omphalocele accompanies ectopia cordis (inferring the pentalogy of Cantrell), the abdominal wall defect is usually in the epigastrium. The most common cardiac abnormalities seen are atrial septal defects, ventricular septal defects, and tetralogy of Fallot.[22]

SUMMARY

Elevation in MSAFP can be seen in various fetal anomalies (Table 23-1). The presence of alpha fetoprotein in the fetal circulation and subsequent diffusion into the maternal circulation and detection with sonography has resulted in a very effective screening test. The presence of any disruption of fetal integrity usually results in an elevation of alpha fetoprotein in the mother. Defects involving the spine and abdominal wall have been the earliest anomalies involved in major prenatal screening programs. Sonography and amniocentesis traditionally have been used whenever a positive screen has been reported. However, there is a suggestion that because the presence of NTDs and abdominal wall defects can be accurately detected with a sonogram alone, an amniocentesis may not always be required. When a fetal abnormality is found, sonographic information is valuable in determining prognosis and assisting in prenatal management.

CLINICAL SCENARIO—DIAGNOSIS

This case reveals absence of the brain and calvaria, which explains the elevated MSAFP value. The image in Figure 23-1, **(A)**, demonstrates a froglike appearance of the fetal face. The image in Figure 23-1, **(B)**, shows the coronal spine and the base of the calvaria consistent with a diagnosis of anencephaly. An earlier sonogram confirmed the gestational age used to calculate the alpha fetoprotein level. Because elevation of alpha fetoprotein can also be seen in fetal death, fetal heart tones were auscultated and indicated a live fetus. A single umbilical artery can be associated with isolated fetal anomalies, syndromes, and chromosomal anomalies. In this case, the anencephaly was isolated.

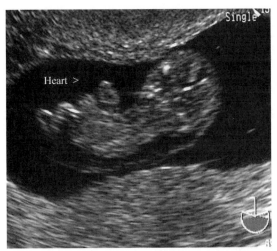

FIGURE 23-10 A beating heart was identified extending into the amniotic cavity in a first-trimester fetus. The indication for sonographic evaluation was recurrent pregnancy losses.

TABLE 23-1	Causes for Abnormal Alpha Fetoprotein Levels	
Elevated		**Decreased**
Wrong dates		Wrong dates
Multiple gestation		Down syndrome
Anencephaly		Trisomy 18
Spina bifida aperta		
Encephalocele		
Gastroschisis		
Omphalocele		
LBWC		
Ectopia cordis		
ABS		
Maternal liver tumors		

CASE STUDIES FOR DISCUSSION

1. A 21-year-old woman is seen for an elevated alpha fetoprotein level at 19 weeks' gestation. Sonographic evaluation reveals a normally growing fetus based on femur length and abdominal circumference. The cranium cannot be visualized as noted in the image of the profile (Fig. 23-11). What is the most likely diagnosis?
2. A 39-year-old woman is seen for sonographic evaluation to confirm gestational age following a slightly elevated MSAFP of 2.8 MoM. The patient reports no complications during the pregnancy and is sure of her last menstrual period. Sonographic evaluation confirms gestational age of 21 weeks, consistent with last menstrual period. It also reveals the umbilical cord inserting into a protrusion on the anterior abdominal wall (Fig. 23-12, **A**). The contents in the protrusion appear to be homogeneous. Three-dimensional sonography is also used to document the anomaly (Fig. 23-12, **B**; see Color Plate 29). What is the diagnosis, and what other anatomic areas are important to visualize?

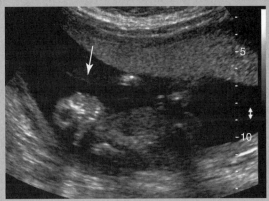

FIGURE 23-11 Fetal profile is identified. Notice lack of visible calvaria.

Continued

CASE STUDIES FOR DISCUSSION—cont'd

3. Sonographic evaluation of a 30-year-old obese woman at gestational age 15 weeks, 4 days is performed for an elevated alpha fetoprotein value. The sonogram is within normal limits. No obvious abnormalities are noted. The gestational age is calculated at 20 weeks, 5 days with all parameters. What is the next step in the management?

4. A sonographic evaluation is performed in a 27-year-old woman to confirm size and dates. A gestational age of 21 weeks is established consistent with last menstrual period. Evaluation of the extremities demonstrates normal upper extremities and a normal right leg and foot (Fig. 23-13, **A**). Evaluation of the left leg and foot reveals the finding in Figure 23-13, **B.** The remainder of the examination is unremarkable. What is the most likely diagnosis?

5. A 26-year-old woman is seen for evaluation of an elevated alpha fetoprotein value of 6.0 MoM. The dating is known to be accurate because a first-trimester sonogram was performed when the patient experienced spotting. Sonographic evaluation is performed at 20 weeks' gestation. Images obtained reveal a large protrusion of the abdominal contents (Fig. 23-14). The umbilical cord is identified in Figure 23-14, **A**. What is the most likely diagnosis?

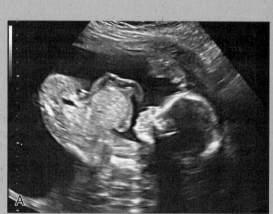
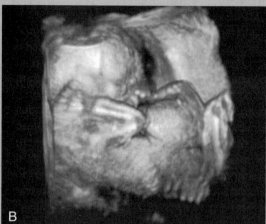

FIGURE 23-12 (A), View of fetus shows defect. **(B),** Three-dimensional imaging clarifies the anomaly further.

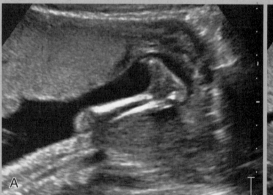
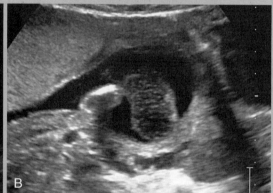

FIGURE 23-13 (A), Right leg and foot. **(B),** Left lower leg and foot.

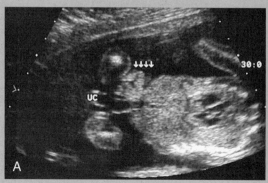
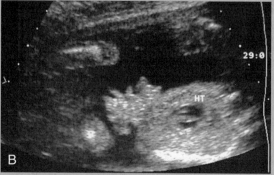

FIGURE 23-14 (A) and **(B),** Anterior abdominal wall defect with umbilical cord insertion noted in **(A).**

STUDY QUESTIONS

1. A 29-year-old woman has an alpha fetoprotein value of 4.2 MoM at 18.5 weeks' gestation. Sonographic evaluation reveals a 24.5-week viable gestation with normal anatomy. What is the most likely explanation?
   a. Laboratory error
   b. Inaccurate dating
   c. Vanishing twin in the first trimester
   d. Macrosomia

2. A 25-year-old woman has a sonogram at an outpatient imaging center that revealed lateral ventricles measuring 14.2 mm and is referred to a maternal-fetal center. The patient declined alpha fetoprotein testing. Sonographic evaluation may reveal which of the following findings?
   a. Ventricular septal defect
   b. Open NTD
   c. Atrial septal defect
   d. Spina bifida occulta

3. A patient is seen for evaluation at 16 weeks' gestation for an alpha fetoprotein of 4.2 MoM. Which of the following sonographic findings would suggest a recalculation of the alpha fetoprotein?
   a. Fetal death
   b. Sonographic dating of 12 weeks
   c. Twin gestation
   d. Sonographic dating of 19 weeks

4. Sonographic evaluation at 19 weeks' gestation reveals an appropriately growing infant with unilateral talipes. Which of the following conditions may be associated with this finding?
   a. Ectopia cordis
   b. Omphalocele
   c. ABS
   d. Gastroschisis

5. A 36-year-old woman is seen for a sonogram for an elevated alpha fetoprotein value at 17 weeks' gestation. A large protrusion of abdominal contents is identified, contained within a membrane. What is the most likely diagnosis?
   a. ABS
   b. Diaphragmatic hernia
   c. Gastroschisis
   d. Omphalocele

6. A 25-year-old woman is seen for an alpha fetoprotein level of 5.7 MoM at 16 weeks' gestation. Sonographic evaluation reveals free-floating bowel anterior to the abdomen. What is the most likely diagnosis?
   a. Omphalocele
   b. LBWC
   c. Gastroschisis
   d. Ectopia cordis

7. Which of the following is not associated with Arnold-Chiari malformation?
   a. Ventriculomegaly
   b. Spina bifida occulta
   c. Lemon sign
   d. Banana sign

8. Which organ produces alpha fetoprotein?
   a. Brain
   b. Lung
   c. Liver
   d. Kidneys

9. A sonographic evaluation at 10 weeks' gestation reveals a small anterior abdominal wall defect. What is the most likely diagnosis at this gestational age?
   a. Gastroschisis
   b. Omphalocele
   c. ABS
   d. Physiologic gut herniation

10. A 32-year-old woman is seen for an elevation of the alpha fetoprotein level at 2.8 MoM. The sonographic evaluation reveals a fetal age consistent with last menstrual period without any anomalies. The placenta has a subchorionic hypoechoic area. What is the most likely explanation for the elevated alpha fetoprotein level?
    a. Spina bifida occulta
    b. Retroplacental clot
    c. Inaccurate dating
    d. Placenta previa

REFERENCES

1. Wang ZP, Li H, Hao LZ, et al: The effectiveness of prenatal serum biomarker screening for neural tube defects in second trimester pregnant women: a meta-analysis, *Prenat Diagn* 29:960–965, 2009.
2. Crandall BF, Robinson L, Grau P: Risks associated with an elevated maternal serum alpha-fetoprotein level, *Am J Obstet Gynecol* 165:581–586, 1991.
3. Larson JM, Pretorius DH, Budorick NE, et al: Value of maternal serum alpha-fetoprotein levels of 5.0 MOM or greater and prenatal sonography in predicting fetal outcome, *Radiology* 189:77–81, 1993.
4. Robinson L, Grau P, Crandall BF: Pregnancy outcomes after increasing maternal serum alpha-fetoprotein levels, *Obstet Gynecol* 74:17–20, 1989.
5. Norem CT, Schoen EJ, Walton DL, et al: Routine ultrasonography compared with maternal serum alpha-fetoprotein for neural tube defect screening, *Obstet Gynecol* 106:747, 2005.
6. Cameron M, Moran P: Prenatal screening and diagnosis of neural tube defects, *Prenat Diagn* 29:402–411, 2009.
7. Moore KL: *The developing human: clinically oriented embryology*, ed 4, Philadelphia, 1988, Saunders.

8. Czeizel AE, Dudas I: Prevention of the first occurrence of neural-tube defects by periconceptional vitamin supplementation, *N Engl J Med* 327:1832–1835, 1992.

9. Wang XW, Luo YL, Wang W, et al: Association between MTHFR A1298C polymorphism and neural tube defect susceptibility: a metaanalysis, *Am J Obstet Gynecol* 206:251.e1–251.e7, 2012.

10. Groenen PM, van Rooij IA, Peer PG, et al: Marginal maternal vitamin B12 status increases the risk of offspring with spina bifida, *Am J Obstet Gynecol* 191:11–17, 2004.

11. Mitchell LE: Epidemiology of neural tube defects, *Am J Med Genet C Semin Med Genet* 135C:88–94, 2005.

12. Rasmussen SA, Chu SY, Kim SY, et al: Maternal obesity and risk of neural tube defects: a metaanalysis, *Am J Obstet Gynecol* 198:611–619, 2008.

13. Martin JA, Hamilton BE, Ventura SJ, et al: Births: final data for 2009, *Natl Vital Stat Rep* 60:1–70, 2011 http://www.cdc.gov/nchs/data/nvsr/nvsr60/nvsr60_01.pdf. Retrieved November 29, 2011.

14. Moore L, Anencephaly: *JDMS* 26:286–289, 2010.

15. Tonni G, Ventura A: Integrating 2D and 3D multiplanar sonography in the prenatal diagnosis of Arnold-Chiari type 2 malformation, *JDMS* 22:24–28, 2006.

16. Ghonge NP, Kanika SS, Poonam B: Familial occipital cephalocele in a fetus at 21 weeks' gestation: imaging demonstration across 3 generations, *J Ultrasound Med* 30:1744–1751, 2011.

17. Bonilla-Musoles F, Machado LE, Bailao LA, et al: Abdominal wall defects, two- versus three-dimensional ultrasonographic diagnosis, *J Ultrasound Med* 20:379–389, 2001.

18. Bowerman RA: Sonography of midgut herniation: normal size criteria and correlation with crown-rump length, *J Ultrasound Med* 5:251–254, 1993.

19. Murphy A, Platt LD: First-trimester diagnosis of body stalk anomaly using 2- and 3-dimensional sonography, *J Ultrasound Med* 30:1739–1743, 2011.

20. Allen LM, Silverman RK, Nosovitch JT, et al: Constriction rings and congenital amputations of the fingers and toes in a mild case of amniotic band syndrome, *JDMS* 23:280–285, 2007.

21. Glass JM: Fetal decapitation associated with amniotic bands, *JDMS* 26:32–34, 2010.

22. Stephenson SR: Sonographic signs of midgut malformations due to ventral wall defects, *JDMS* 20:246–253, 2004.

Genetic Testing

Jane J.K. Burns

A 31-year-old woman, G3 P2002, with late prenatal care is seen at 25 weeks' gestational age for an obstetric sonogram. The sonogram reveals the findings in Figure 24-1 (see Color Plate 30). The patient is referred to a maternal-fetal medicine center for counseling and elects to proceed with an amniocentesis. What does the amniocentesis most likely reveal?

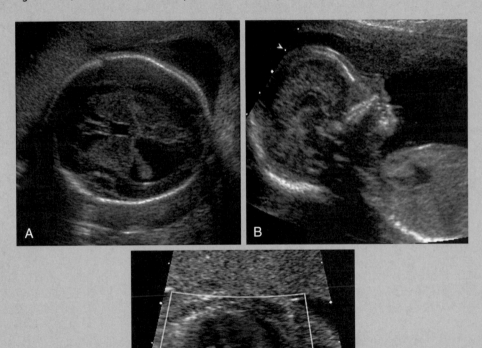

FIGURE 24-1 (A-C), Sonographic findings in a 25-week gestational age fetus. (**C**, See Color Plate 30.)

OBJECTIVES

- Describe the method of noninvasive biochemical testing for assessment of fetal aneuploidy.
- List the methods of invasive testing for chromosomal analysis.
- Describe the anomalies associated with an increased nuchal translucency.
- List the sonographic markers associated with chromosomal anomalies.
- Describe the sonographic findings associated with trisomies 13, 18, 21; Turner syndrome, and triploidy.

MATERNAL SCREENING OPTIONS

Multiple prenatal screening options are available to help identify pregnancies that may be at an increased risk for fetal aneuploidy. Down syndrome, or trisomy 21, is the most common chromosome abnormality seen in live births. A trisomy 21 pregnancy is detected more frequently in older women than in younger women, and the use of maternal age alone helps detect approximately 30% of fetuses with trisomy 21.[1] Incorporation of serum (i.e., blood) screening with early sonographic evaluation has improved detection rates greatly. Offering screening options to all women increases the chance of detecting abnormalities earlier and allows time for counseling and referral for women in need of a targeted sonographic evaluation (level II) or diagnostic testing (e.g., amniocentesis). With advances in ultrasound technology, it is now possible to assess fetuses in greater detail at an earlier gestational age.

Detailed sonographic evaluation along with current serum screening tests can provide a noninvasive alternative to search for aneuploidy. The biochemical markers that are evaluated depend on the gestational age at the time of screening. In the first trimester, pregnancy-associated plasma protein A (PAPP-A) and β human chorionic gonadotropin (hCG) are used. In the second trimester, various combinations of alpha fetoprotein (AFP), hCG, unconjugated estriol (uE3), and dimeric inhibin A (DIA) are evaluated. These biochemical markers are produced by the fetus and placenta and cross into the maternal blood. The most important step before drawing blood work for any screen is confirmation of correct gestational age, cardiac activity, and the number of fetuses present. A discrepancy of 7 days can have a large impact on the serum results. Inaccurate dating or an undiagnosed multiple gestation is the most common cause of an abnormal serum screening result.

Serum tests and sonography cannot diagnose chromosome abnormalities. Although results of both serum tests and sonography may increase suspicion of a problem, the definitive diagnostic tests are chorionic villus sampling (CVS) and amniocentesis. A review of serum screening in conjunction with the targeted sonogram can reveal a new risk for aneuploidy in a patient. The patient can be counseled regarding prognosis, treatment, and pregnancy options.

MATERNAL SERUM SCREENING

First-Trimester Screening

PAPP-A is a first-trimester biochemical marker produced by the placental trophoblast and found in maternal serum. Pregnancies affected by trisomy 21 and trisomy 18 have a decreased PAPP-A. Free β hCG is a glycoprotein hormone derived from the placenta that peaks at 8 to 10 weeks' gestational age and then decreases to

TABLE 24-1	First-Trimester Multiple Marker Screening	
	Down Syndrome	**Trisomy 18 and Trisomy 13**
Free β hCG	↑	↓
PAPP-A	↓	↓
NT	↑	↑

a plateau. Free β hCG is increased in pregnancies with trisomy 21 and decreased in pregnancies with trisomy 18 (Table 24-1). The use of the two analytes in conjunction with maternal age and sonographic evaluation of nuchal translucency (NT) has an estimated detection rate of 85% for trisomy 21.[2] Additionally, it has been noted that an unexplained low PAPP-A is associated with an increased frequency of adverse obstetric outcomes.[3,4]

The sequential screen and the integrated screen are two tests currently available that combine the first-trimester screen with second-trimester analytes to provide better detection rates for trisomy 21 and trisomy 18. The sequential screen incorporates the first screen with a second blood draw at 15 to 21 weeks of gestation that looks at AFP, hCG, uE3, and DIA. A preliminary result is given 1 week after the first blood draw with the final result available 1 week after the second blood draw. The sequential screen has a detection rate of trisomy 21 and trisomy 18 of approximately 90%.[4] The integrated screen also follows the two blood draws protocol and uses the same analytes as the sequential screen, but no preliminary result is given, and the final result is available 1 week after the second blood draw. The integrated screen has a slightly better trisomy 21 detection rate (approximately 92%); the trisomy 18 detection rate remains at 90%. It is helpful to have the patient meet with a genetic counselor to review all of the testing options available; this allows patients to make an informed decision regarding which test would best meet their needs.

Second-Trimester Screening

Four blood tests are currently available for fetal genetic screening in the second trimester: maternal serum AFP test, triple screen, quadruple (quad or tetra) screen, and penta screen. Blood work should be drawn between 15 and 21 weeks of gestation, but guidelines and requirements may vary among laboratories. The maternal blood work and information regarding fetal gestational age and number, maternal age, ethnicity, family history, maternal weight, and diabetic status are evaluated to give a fetal risk assessment for neural tube defects, trisomy 21, and trisomy 18. These results are expressed as a numeric value or odds ratio. The odds ratio assigns a risk value for open neural tube defect, Down syndrome risk, and trisomy 18 risk. Current second-trimester screening cannot provide a risk assessment for trisomy 13, Turner

TABLE 24-2 Draw Times and Detection Rates

	Blood Drawn	Results	Detection Rates		
			Down Syndrome	Trisomy18	Open Neural Tube Defect
First trimester	11-13 wk	1 wk	~83%	~80%	None
Sequential (with 1st trimester)					80%
1st	11-13 wk	Preliminary-1 wk	~70%	~70%	
2nd	15-21 wk	Final-1 wk after 2nd draw	~90%	~90%	
Integrated (with 1st trimester)					80%
1st	11-13 wk	No preliminary	None	None	
2nd	15-21 wk	Final-1 wk after 2nd draw	~92%	~90%	
Triple	15-21 wk	1 wk	~60%	~60%	80%
Quad/tetra	15-21 wk	1 wk	~75-80%	~60-70%	80%
Penta	15-21 wk	1 wk	~83%	~60-70%	80%
Maternal serum AFP	15-21 wk	1 wk	None	None	80%

All screens have an approximate 5% false-positive rate.

TABLE 24-3 Maternal Serum Screening

Screen Test	Markers and Analytes							
	NT	PAPP-A	β hCG	AFP	hCG	uE3	DIA	H-hCG
First trimester	X	X	X					
Sequential (with 1st trimester)	X	X	X	X	X	X	X	
Integrated (with 1st trimester)	X	X	X	X	X	X	X	
Maternal serum AFP				X				
Triple				X	X	X		
Quad/tetra				X	X	X	X	
Penta				X	X	X	X	X

H-hCG, Hyperglycosylated human chorionic gonadotropin.

syndrome, or congenital heart defects. Table 24-2 lists the draw times and detection rates and Table 24-3 lists the analytes assayed for each maternal serum screening test discussed.

Maternal Serum Alpha Fetoprotein. Maternal serum AFP is a biochemical test that measures the amount of AFP within the maternal serum. AFP is an oncofetal protein produced by the fetal liver and yolk sac. Maternal serum AFP results are expressed in multiples of the median (MoM), using a normal range of 0.25 to 2.50. Some laboratories use 2.0 as their upper MoM cutoff. Maternal serum AFP was the first prenatal screening test developed in the late 1970s for the detection of neural tube defects. Shortly afterward, it was recognized that fetuses with trisomy 21 had lower levels of serum AFP (<0.74 MoM). Elevated levels of AFP have been associated with open neural tube defects, open ventral wall defects, multiple gestations, placental abnormalities, and numerous fetal structural defects and disorders. In the presence of a normal targeted sonogram, an unexplained elevation in the maternal serum AFP has been associated with preeclampsia and an increased frequency of adverse obstetric outcomes.[4]

Triple Screen. The triple screen is a biochemical test that evaluates AFP, hCG, and uE3 in the maternal serum. uE3 is a steroid hormone produced by the fetal liver and placenta. Low levels of uE3 have been seen in association with Down syndrome, Smith-Lemli-Opitz syndrome, and steroid sulfatase deficiency.[4]

The combination of elevated hCG and decreased AFP and uE3 yields an increased risk for trisomy 21 in that pregnancy. The triple screen has a detection rate of trisomy 21 of approximately 70%.[4] When hCG, AFP, and uE3 all are decreased, there is an increased risk for trisomy 18 in that pregnancy. An increased frequency of adverse obstetric outcomes is associated with an unexplained elevation in maternal serum AFP (>2.5 MoM) or hCG (>3.0 MoM), or both, or a decreased level of maternal serum AFP (<0.25 MoM) or uE3 (<0.5 MoM), or both.[3,4]

Quadruple Screen. The quad screen adds DIA to the analytes used in the triple screen. DIA is produced in the placenta and increases the detection rate of Down syndrome to 75% to 80%. An unexplained elevation in DIA (≥2.0 MoM) is associated with an increased frequency of adverse obstetric outcomes.[4] In contrast to the serum markers used in the triple test, DIA values are independent of gestational age. However, the quad screen includes hCG, AFP, and uE3, so it is imperative that an accurate gestational age be assigned. An analyte pattern of decreased maternal serum AFP and uE3 with an elevation of hCG and DIA yields an increased risk for Down syndrome. In pregnancies with trisomy 18, AFP, uE3, and hCG all are decreased. DIA does not contribute to the detection of trisomy 18.

Penta Screen. The penta screen uses the four previous maternal biochemical markers in conjunction with hyperglycosylated hCG. Some laboratories refer to hyperglycosylated hCG as invasive trophoblast antigen. This addition increases the detection of trisomy 21 slightly to 83%.[5] The penta screen is the newest screen and not yet as proven as the quad screen.

INVASIVE DIAGNOSTIC AND GENETIC TESTING

Genetic testing in pregnancy is performed to identify the presence or absence of a normal karyotype. A normal human karyotype contains 46 chromosomes: 22 pairs of autosomes and 1 pair of sex chromosomes. The chromosome analysis of a normal male fetus reveals 46,XY, and analysis of a normal female fetus reveals 46,XX. Chromosome analysis may detect additions, deletions, breaks, translocations, and other arrangements in the karyotype. Chromosome analysis also detects mosaicism, a condition in which genetic defects are found in a portion of the cells with other portions appearing normal.

Genetic disorders may be dominant, recessive, or X-linked. In a dominant genetic disorder, usually only one parent is affected, but it carries a 50% risk of transmission to the fetus. In a recessive genetic disorder, usually both parents are carriers, with a 25% risk of transmission to the fetus. X-linked disorders are transmitted by the mother with a 50% risk to a male fetus.

Genetic testing in pregnancy is accomplished via CVS, amniocentesis, or cordocentesis. This testing is performed with ultrasound guidance using sterile technique.

Chorionic Villus Sampling

CVS is a technique that extracts the chorionic villi from the trophoblast in the placenta with either transabdominal or transvaginal sonographic guidance. CVS is usually performed at a gestational age of 10 to 13 weeks. A sonogram should be obtained before the procedure for confirmation of gestational age and cardiac activity. Test results are usually available in 7 to 10 days. An advantage of CVS compared with amniocentesis is earlier access to fetal genetic information. Earlier intervention in the pregnancy may help to decrease the complication rate for any termination procedures and help reduce the maternal psychological burden.

Chromosome analysis from CVS can be used to identify genetic abnormalities, although they may be confined just to the placenta. When mosaicism is identified, an amniocentesis may be necessary to determine whether the abnormal chromosome pattern is also in the fetus. In addition, CVS does not evaluate AFP and cannot screen for open neural tube defects. Fetal limb-reduction abnormalities have been associated with CVS performed before 10 weeks' gestational age. Fetal loss rates are similar to loss rates associated with second-trimester amniocentesis.[6,7]

Amniocentesis

An alternative to CVS is early amniocentesis, which may be performed between 12 and 15 weeks' gestational age. Although early amniocentesis alleviates the risk of an additional invasive procedure for placental mosaicism, failed attempts may occur when tenting of the amniotic membranes results from the lack of fusion of the amnion to the chorion. This tenting of the membranes does not allow the needle to enter the amniotic cavity to draw the amniotic fluid. Testing of amniotic fluid AFP is impossible until after 15 weeks' gestational age. The fetal loss rate may vary with gestational age, although studies have found the loss rate to be increased over that of second-trimester amniocentesis.[7] Early amniocentesis has also been associated with talipes equinovarus.[6] Early and midtrimester amniocentesis procedures are performed in a similar manner.

Midtrimester amniocentesis to rule out genetic abnormalities is usually performed between 15 and 18 weeks' gestational age. The current fetal loss rate is stated to be 0.5%.[7] The procedure usually includes a sonogram to screen for abnormalities and check gestational age, fetal number, and cardiac activity. An amniocentesis is performed transabdominally under direct ultrasound guidance. Results of the chromosomal analysis are usually available in 7 to 14 days and are considered the "gold standard" for detection of chromosomal abnormalities.

Conventional chromosomal analysis of the amniotic fluid may require 2 weeks to culture and evaluate the chromosomes (Fig. 24-2, *A*). This time could add additional stress to patients who are at increased risk for aneuploidy based on maternal serum screening, advanced maternal age, or sonographic findings. Fluorescence in situ hybridization (FISH) allows for limited analysis of uncultured amniotic fluid or chorionic villi, with results available within 24 hours. The FISH assay typically evaluates for numeric abnormalities of chromosomes 13, 18, 21, X, and Y by adding a probe labeled with fluorescent dye to the fetal cells. The number of colored signals (Fig. 24-2, *B* and *C*; see Color Plate 31) represents the number of copies of select chromosomes. The information obtained is more limited than with a cultured analysis, but the results regarding the most common aneuploidies can be obtained more quickly. A conventional cultured analysis should be completed to confirm the findings.

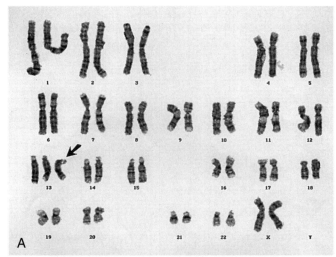

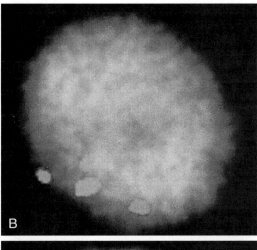

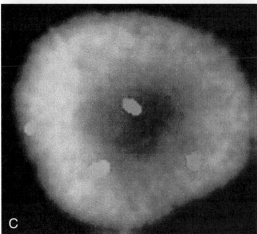

FIGURE 24-2 (A), Chromosomal analysis reveals a female with trisomy 13. **(B)** and **(C),** FISH analysis shows two copies of X chromosome coded in green and two copies of chromosome 18 coded in blue **(B)**; two copies of chromosome 21 are coded in red, and three copies of chromosome 13 are coded in green **(C)**.

In addition to genetic analysis, second-trimester and third-trimester amniocentesis can evaluate amniotic fluid AFP; this helps in the assessment of spina bifida and open ventral wall defects. The most sensitive test for open neural tube defects is acetylcholinesterase. TORCH

(*t*oxoplasmosis, *o*ther [congenital syphilis, viruses] *r*ubella, *c*ytomegalovirus, *h*erpes simplex virus) titers on the amniotic fluid are helpful in the evaluation of fetal infections. Amniocentesis may also be used to drain off excess amniotic fluid in patients with severe polyhydramnios to help prevent preterm delivery. In the third trimester, amniocentesis may be used to assess lung maturity before cesarean section or induction of labor. Whenever an invasive procedure is performed on an Rh-negative mother, $Rh_O(D)$ immune globulin (RhoGam) should be administered to help prevent sensitization in future pregnancies.

NONINVASIVE PRENATAL TESTING FOR ANEUPLOIDY

The most recent advance in maternal screening has been the development of noninvasive prenatal testing using cell-free fetal DNA found in maternal plasma.[8] Identification and subsequent research of cell-free fetal DNA in the maternal plasma began in the late 1990s. The goal was to provide an alternative to invasive testing in the high-risk population, termed noninvasive prenatal diagnosis. This new test uses a technique called massively parallel sequencing to sequence millions of maternal and fetal cell-free DNA fragments from a sample of maternal blood. If a specific chromosome is substantially overrepresented in the DNA sequence, this indicates the fetus has extra copies of that chromosome, and underrepresentation of sequence indicates a monosomy.[8] The two commercial tests currently offered are the MaterniT21 test, which is designed to detect Down syndrome pregnancies, and the MaterniT21 Plus, which tests for trisomies 21, 13, and 18. The MaterniT21 tests are manufactured by Sequenom Center for Molecular Medicine in San Diego, CA, and Grand Rapids, MI. Other laboratories are likely to offer DNA testing in the near future, with each test being given a name specific to that laboratory or developer.

The current debate around noninvasive prenatal diagnosis is in the use of the word "diagnostic." The term "diagnostic" could describe a test that has 100% sensitivity and 100% specificity or could signify a test whose performance characteristics are high enough to allow a definitive diagnosis without serious concern for an erroneous clinical conclusion. So far, the results with massively parallel sequencing fail to fulfill either definition of "diagnostic" with a detection rate of 99.1% and a false-positive rate of 0.3%.[9] All trials that have been published so far have been done on a high-risk population, and it is unknown what the detection rates would be in a low-risk population.[10] In the future, current screening protocols will be challenged and revised to incorporate this prenatal blood test into practice.

SONOGRAPHIC MARKERS

The sonographic evaluation of a fetus may identify an anomaly that should precipitate a thorough search for

TABLE 24-4	Abnormalities Associated with an Increased Nuchal Translucency in Normal Karyotype	
Congenital Heart Defects	**Genetic Syndromes**	**Skeletal Dysplasias**
Ventricular septal defect	Akinesia deformation	Thanatophoric dysplasia
Atrioventricular septal defect	Noonan syndrome	Achondrogenesis
Ebstein's anomaly	Smith-Lemli-Opitz syndrome	Asphyxiating thoracic dystrophy
Pulmonary stenosis/pulmonary atresia	Jarcho-Levin syndrome	Camptomelic dysplasia
Aortic stenosis/aortic atresia	Beckwith-Wiedemann syndrome	Nance-Sweeney syndrome
Hypoplastic left heart	Fryns syndrome	Roberts syndrome
Hypoplastic right heart	Zellweger syndrome	VATER association*
Various other heart defects	Spinal muscular atrophy	

*VATER association refers to *v*ertebral defects, imperforate *a*nus, *t*racheoesophageal fistula, *r*adial and *r*enal dysplasia.

additional anomalies. An aneuploid fetus may have structural abnormalities, growth delay, or "soft" sonographic markers. These "soft" markers are considered controversial because they are often transient, nonspecific findings that frequently can be seen in the normal fetus. The most common soft markers for aneuploidy in the first or second trimester include choroid plexus cysts, echogenic intracardiac focus (EIF), renal pyelectasis, shortened long bones, and hyperechoic (echogenic) bowel.[11] More established sonographic markers associated with fetal aneuploidy include increased NT, nuchal fold (NF) thickening, and hypoplastic or absent nasal bone. When detection of these sonographic markers occurs with abnormal maternal serum screening, advanced maternal age (≥35 years old), or additional sonographic findings, genetic counseling or amniocentesis for chromosomal analysis should be offered.

Nuchal Translucency

NT is the translucent space in the posterior fetal neck apparent during the first trimester. The presence of NT is normal in the first trimester, but NT may become distended in association with several abnormalities. Increased NT has been seen with multiple syndromes, congenital heart defects, and skeletal dysplasias (Table 24-4). NT may be increased with renal anomalies, cardiac anomalies, and aneuploidy (trisomies 13, 18, and 21; Turner syndrome; and triploidy). The most common aneuploidy seen with an abnormal NT is trisomy 21. Abnormal NT may spontaneously resolve, and resolution does not affect the associated risks for anomalies. Increased NT may be isolated or part of "spacesuit" hydrops, where the skin line is elevated from the body by fluid over the entire body. "Spacesuit" hydrops suggests an increased risk of aneuploidy. Increased NT that contains septations or has increased echogenicity has an increased association with aneuploidy.[12] In the absence of identifiable structural defects and normal chromosomes, increased NT has been associated with a poor pregnancy outcome, including spontaneous abortion and fetal death.[13]

Sonographic Findings. NT can be reliably measured from 11 to 14 weeks' gestational age. Measurement of NT in the correct midsagittal plane is paramount to its accuracy and reliability. The head and chest must be in a neutral position without flexion or extension. An image must be obtained with the fetus away from the amnion to ensure that it is not included in the NT measurement. A high-resolution transducer (≥6 MHz) should be used with calipers (+) that have the ability to measure structures to 0.001 mm. The image should be magnified so that the fetal head and chest occupy two-thirds of the image. The measurement calipers should be placed on the inner borders of the fluid-filled space ("on-to-on"), perpendicular to the long axis of the fetus (Fig. 24-3).

NT is dependent on gestational age, so the 95th percentile varies with the fetal crown-rump length measurement, and the correct charts should be used. NT is abnormal if it is greater than the 95th percentile for assigned gestational age by crown-rump length. Increased NT can be confirmed when the lucency measures 3 mm or more.[13] Specialized training and certification for sonographers is required before test results are processed for this screening test.

Nuchal Fold

Similar to NT in the first trimester, the thickness of the NF is a sonographic observation that may help detect a trisomy 21 fetus during the second trimester.

Sonographic Findings. The NF measurement should be taken at the back of the neck at the level of the transcerebellar measurement, or occipital fossa view (Fig. 24-4). Adjusting the transducer so that it is perpendicular to the back of the fetal head increases the accuracy of the measurement. Similar to NT, the cutoff for NF varies with gestational age. From 15 to 18 weeks, NF 5.0 mm or greater is abnormal. From 18 to 21 weeks, NF 6.0 mm or greater is abnormal.

Fetal Nasal Bone

One of the first articles published about sonographic evaluation of the fetal nasal bone in the first-trimester fetus was by Cicero in 2001.[14] A high association of an absent nasal bone in fetuses with trisomy 21 was noted. A subsequent series in

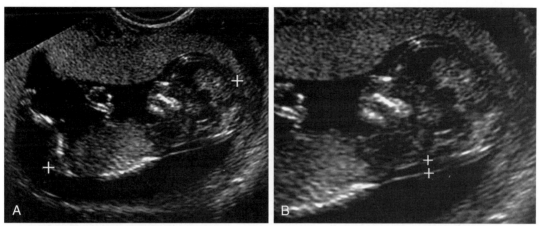

FIGURE 24-3 Measurement of NT. **(A),** Crown-rump length should confirm that the gestation is between 11 and 14 weeks' gestational age. **(B),** Obtain NT measurements on a magnified image in the true midsagittal plane with the transducer parallel to the nasal bone. Measurement calipers are placed "on-to-on" in relation to the borders.

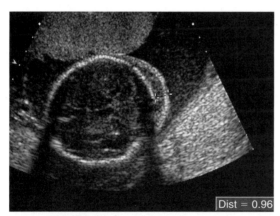

FIGURE 24-4 Increased NF (>5 mm).

2002 evaluated the nasal bone during the second trimester and found that an absent or shortened nasal bone (<25th percentile for gestational age) has an increased association with trisomy 21.[15] More recent studies have shown that the nasal bone is as sensitive as NF thickening in screening for trisomy 21. The optimal time for nasal bone assessment is between 12 and 13.5 weeks of gestation.[16] Including the nasal bone in screening sonograms can increase the sensitivity rate for the detection of aneuploidy.[17]

Sonographic Findings. The nasal bone should be evaluated in a midsagittal plane with an angle of insonation close to 45 degrees (Fig. 24-5). The head should be in a neutral position, not hyperflexed or hyperextended. The nasal bone is actually a pair of bones usually of equal size. Scanning is performed through the midface to identify the greatest nasal bone length. The nasal bone should appear as a linear echogenic structure beneath and separate from the fetal skin. The fetal nasal bone increases linearly with advancing gestational age. Some ethnic groups may normally have a shorter nasal bone, specifically the Asian population. The percentiles for nasal bone length depend on gestational age, so correlation with a graph or chart is required.[17]

An alternative to using the graph is obtaining a biparietal diameter-to-nasal bone length ratio (BPD/NBL ratio). The nasal bone is shorter and the BPD/NBL ratio is greater (≥10) in fetuses with trisomy 21.[17] The advantages of using the BPD/NBL ratio is that it is a quick calculation that does not require a chart, and its sensitivity is independent of gestational age and maternal age. The nasal bone measurement and BPD/NBL ratio can be used throughout pregnancy.

Choroid Plexus Cysts

Choroid plexus cysts have been identified in 0.4% to 3.6% of pregnancies and are usually an insignificant finding that resolves spontaneously. Choroid plexus cysts have been associated with aneuploidy, most specifically trisomy 18.[11] If choroid plexus cysts (Fig. 24-6) are identified, a targeted sonogram to search for additional anomalies should be performed. A new risk for aneuploidy can be given that combines the targeted scan and serum screen with maternal age and family history; this allows the patient to make an informed decision in regard to CVS or amniocentesis.

Echogenic Intracardiac Focus

EIF is a common finding identified in 5% to 10% of fetuses.[18] Although generally considered a normal variant, EIF has also been associated with trisomy 21 and trisomy 13. In most instances, the EIF is located in the left ventricle (Fig. 24-7), which may be less significant than when identified in the right ventricle or seen bilaterally. The EIF is identified on the four-chamber view of the heart, with the apex toward the transducer, and should have a similar echogenicity to fetal bone.[18,19] As with choroid plexus cysts, other factors, such as maternal age, maternal serum testing, family history, and presence of other anomalies, should be considered when deciding whether further testing is appropriate.

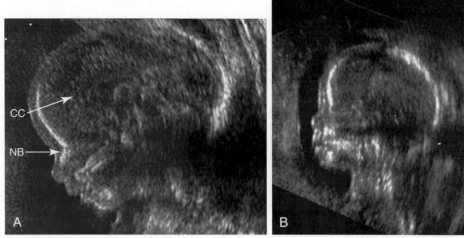

FIGURE 24-5 (A), Fetal profile demonstrates the presence of a normal nasal bone *(NB)*. Corpus callosum *(CC)* ensures a midline scanning plane. **(B),** Absent nasal bone.

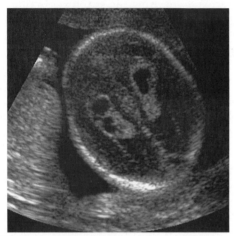

FIGURE 24-6 Bilateral choroid plexus cysts in a fetus with trisomy 18.

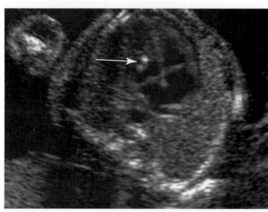

FIGURE 24-7 Four-chamber cardiac view demonstrating two left EIF.

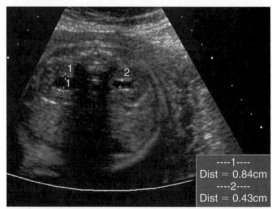

FIGURE 24-8 Fetal kidneys demonstrate mild pyelectasis, which is associated with trisomy 21. In isolation, this finding is not significant.

Renal Pyelectasis

Mild renal pyelectasis is another common finding that has questionable significance, although it has been associated with trisomy 21. Mild pyelectasis (Fig. 24-8) is defined as a dilated renal pelvis of 4.0 mm or more in the anteroposterior diameter.[20] Many cases resolve by the third trimester. Multiple studies have shown that approximately 25% of fetuses with trisomy 21 have pyelectasis; however, as an isolated finding, pyelectasis generally does not warrant amniocentesis.[21]

Shortened Long Bones

Fetuses with Down syndrome tend to have slightly shorter long bones than normal fetuses. Sonographic criteria for a mildly shortened femur or humerus (<0.9 femur length-to-biparietal diameter ratio) overlap with the range observed in unaffected fetuses, making it necessary for laboratories to establish criteria based on their own population.[21] Long bones less than the 5th

percentile are associated with early-onset intrauterine growth restriction (IUGR) or skeletal dysplasia.

Echogenic Bowel

Echogenic bowel refers to hyperechoic bowel that is the same as or brighter than the surrounding bone

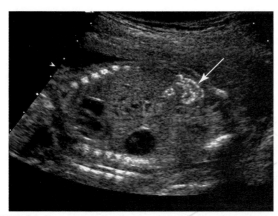

FIGURE 24-9 Sagittal image through the fetal body and thorax demonstrates hyperechoic (echogenic) bowel, which is associated with trisomy 21, cystic fibrosis, and other abnormalities.

BOX 24-1	Trisomy 21: Sonographic Findings
Increased NF	Absent or short nasal bone
Shortened long bones	Brachycephaly
EIF	Congenital heart defects
Clinodactyly	Short or absent fifth midphalanx
Duodenal atresia	Hyperechoic (echogenic) bowel
Cystic hygroma	Pyelectasis
Ventriculomegaly	Sandal gap toes
Flat facies	

(Fig. 24-9). It may be an isolated finding with no significance, but echogenic bowel has been associated with aneuploidy (most commonly trisomy 21), cystic fibrosis, intrauterine infections, and intestinal obstructions.[11] In addition, echogenic bowel has been identified with pregnancies affected by IUGR, placental insufficiency, and perinatal death. Echogenic bowel also has been identified in pregnancies with a history of bleeding and echogenic foci noted within the amniotic fluid. It is believed that the bowel may have areas of increased echogenicity secondary to swallowed blood. Results of maternal infection titers and cystic fibrosis carrier testing should be factored into the decision to offer amniocentesis.

CHROMOSOMAL ABNORMALITIES

Trisomy 21

Trisomy 21, or Down syndrome, is most commonly characterized by an extra chromosome 21. The remaining cases manifest as either mosaic, in which only part of the cell line has the extra 21 chromosome, or a translocation, in which part of chromosome 21 is located on another chromosome. Trisomy 21 is the most common chromosome abnormality in live births, occurring at a rate of 1 in 504.[22] Infants with trisomy 21 have a characteristic appearance that includes epicanthal folds, a round head, flattened nasal bridge, small ears, redundant skin at the back of the neck, and a protruding tongue. Children with Down syndrome have mild to moderate mental retardation and various other anomalies. Approximately 40% to 50% have some form of a cardiac anomaly. An increased risk exists in women who are of advanced maternal age, but trisomy 21 may affect fetuses in women of any age.

Sonographic Findings. Sonographic evaluation of a fetus with suspected trisomy 21 is challenging because many of the findings are nonspecific, and approximately 50% of fetuses with trisomy 21 demonstrate no markers or findings. The two most sensitive sonographic markers for trisomy 21 are increased NF and shortened or absent nasal bone. The most common congenital heart defects seen are atrioventricular canal defect and ventricular septal defect. Duodenal atresia, which manifests as a double bubble sign, is also associated with trisomy 21, although it may not be seen until after 26 weeks' gestational age. Although shortened long bones are a feature associated with trisomy 21, a shortened humerus length is more sensitive than a shortened femur length. The "sandal gap toes" appearance to the foot is caused by syndactyly of the second and third digits, which causes a gap between the first and second digits. Numerous other soft findings may suggest trisomy 21, including renal pyelectasis, echogenic bowel, EIF, low-set ears, clinodactyly, and single umbilical artery (SUA) (Box 24-1).[21] However, in isolation, these findings are generally insignificant. Other anomalies that may be identified are limb anomalies, cystic hygroma, renal anomalies, omphalocele, and gastrointestinal defects.

The sensitivity of sonographic detection of trisomy 21 in experienced hands is reported to be 59.2% to 91.0%.[23] Women of all ages choose to screen for trisomy 21 by using a combination of sonographic evaluation and maternal serum screening along with family history and maternal age.

Trisomy 18

Trisomy 18, or Edwards syndrome, is a severe anomaly characterized by an extra chromosome 18 that occurs in approximately 1 in 5000 live births.[22] Trisomy 18 is associated with defects that affect multiple organ systems and is seen in increased frequency in women of advanced maternal age. Many fetuses with trisomy 18 spontaneously abort, and approximately 80% of infants die within the first year of life.[22] Survivors have profound mental and physical disabilities.

Sonographic Findings. The two most common sonographic findings seen with trisomy 18 are persistently clenched hands and choroid plexus cysts. The second digit of the hand may overlap the remaining digits (Fig. 24-10, A). Trisomy 18 is the most common aneuploidy to have a SUA.[24] Sonographic findings associated with trisomy 18 are evident in 77% to 97% of fetuses. Other findings

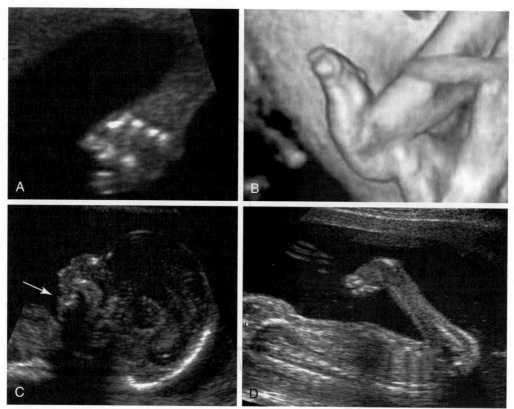

FIGURE 24-10 Findings associated with trisomy 18. **(A)**, Clenched hand. **(B)**, Rocker-bottom foot. **(C)**, Micrognathia *(arrow)*. **(D)**, Abnormal arm and hand posturing.

BOX 24-2	Trisomy 18: Sonographic Findings
Clenched hands	Choroid plexus cysts
Congenital heart defects	SUA
IUGR	Neural tube defects
Rocker-bottom feet	Diaphragmatic hernia
Radial ray anomalies	Agenesis of corpus callosum
Clubfoot	Micrognathia
Cystic hygroma	Strawberry-shaped skull
Polyhydramnios	Ocular anomalies

that may be identified include rocker-bottom feet, omphalocele, congenital heart defects, micrognathia, strawberry-shaped head, talipes, radial ray defects, hydronephrosis, agenesis of corpus callosum, and congenital diaphragmatic hernia (Fig. 24-10, *B-D*). Anomalies of the gastrointestinal, genitourinary and central nervous systems may also be seen with trisomy 18. Severe IUGR, hydrops, and polyhydramnios may be present (Box 24-2).

Trisomy 13

Trisomy 13, or Patau syndrome, is a severe anomaly characterized by an extra chromosome 13 occurring in 1 in 8000 births.[22] Women who are of advanced maternal age are at an increased risk for a fetus with trisomy 13. This chromosomal anomaly is characterized by multiple anomalies that occur across most organ systems. Many fetuses spontaneously abort, and most live-born

infants die within the first month. Survivors have severe mental and physical deficits and have a high rate of seizure disorders.

Sonographic Findings. Characteristic features suggestive of trisomy 13 include holoprosencephaly, facial anomalies, polydactyly (Fig. 24-11), heart defects, and omphalocele. Various anomalies of the cardiovascular, gastrointestinal, genitourinary, and central nervous systems may also occur. Sonographic identification of trisomy 13 has a sensitivity of 90% to 100%. Other sonographic findings include talipes, microcephaly, agenesis of corpus callosum, meningocele, renal anomalies, cystic hygroma, omphalocele, EIF (often bilateral), and SUA. Mild ventriculomegaly and polyhydramnios may also be found (Box 24-3).

Turner Syndrome

Turner syndrome is characterized by the absence of a sex chromosome and always results in a female fetus (45,X). The occurrence rate of Turner syndrome is 1 in 2000 to 5000 births and is not associated with advanced maternal age.[22] Many fetuses spontaneously abort. Live-born infants usually have normal intelligence. Infants have a characteristic webbed neck, are short in stature, and are infertile.

Sonographic Findings. The most common sonographic findings associated with Turner syndrome are listed in Box 24-4. Fetuses with Turner syndrome often have

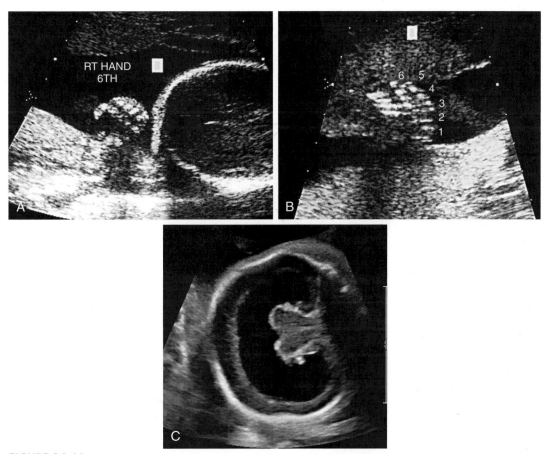

FIGURE 24-11 Findings associated with trisomy 13. **(A)** and **(B)**, Postaxial polydactyly. **(C)**, Holoprosencephaly.

BOX 24-3	Trisomy 13: Sonographic Findings
Holoprosencephaly	Polydactyly
Congenital heart defects	Facial clefts
Microcephaly	EIF
Neural tube defects	IUGR
Ocular anomalies	Polycystic kidneys
Cystic hygroma	Omphalocele
Ventriculomegaly	SUA

BOX 24-5	Triploidy: Sonographic Findings
Early-onset IUGR	Syndactyly (third and fourth digits)
SUA	Prominent forehead
Cleft lip and palate	Micrognathia
Omphalocele	Dysplastic cranial bones
Hypertelorism	Asymmetric development
Macroglossia	Low-set malformed ears
Microphthalmia	Cystic placenta (paternal origin)

BOX 24-4	Turner Syndrome: Sonographic Findings
Cystic hygroma	Congenital heart defects
IUGR	Hydrops
Horseshoe kidney	Fetal tachycardia
Other renal anomalies	SUA
Bone dysplasia	

large cystic hygromas (Fig. 24-12) and have a high association of hydrops.[12,13] Congenital heart defects, specifically coarctation of the aorta; short femurs; and renal anomalies may also be identified. Tissue edema over the entire fetal body, which is termed anasarca, occurs in many cases.

Triploidy

Triploidy is a profoundly severe anomaly characterized by an extra set of chromosomes that is most commonly caused by two sperm fertilizing one ovum (69,XXX, 69,XXY). Triploid fetuses frequently abort spontaneously and are often associated with a partial mole (see Chapter 21).

Sonographic Findings. Multiple anomalies involving the gastrointestinal tract, genitourinary tract, cardiovascular system, and central nervous system (e.g., holoprosencephaly, hydrocephalus) may be identified. Facial anomalies (clefts), SUA, and abnormalities of the extremities (syndactyly, talipes) may also be noted (Fig. 24-13; see Color Plate 32). Severe IUGR, oligohydramnios, and a large placenta containing multiple cystic spaces may be present as well. This is a lethal condition and is rarely reported in live births. The most common features seen with triploidy are listed in Box 24-5.

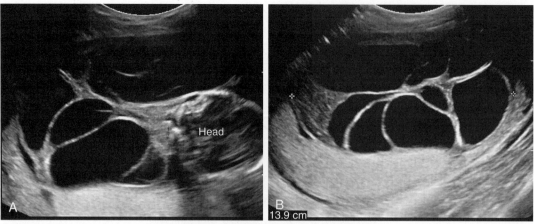

FIGURE 24-12 Images of large cystic hygroma seen in the transverse **(A)** and sagittal **(B)** scanning planes in a fetus with Turner syndrome.

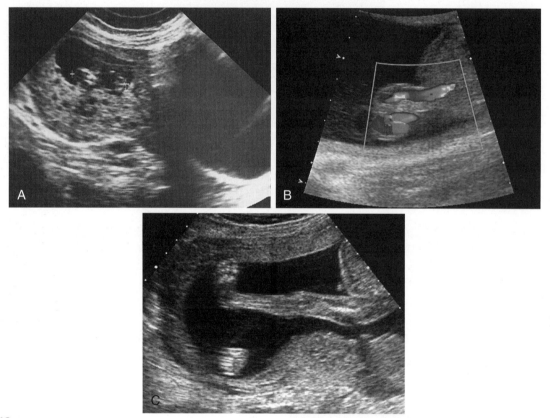

FIGURE 24-13 Fetuses with triploidy. **(A)**, Partial mole with a fetus with severe growth restriction. **(B)**, Omphalocele with SUA. **(C)**, Talipes and other extremity anomalies are commonly seen with triploidy. **(B,** See Color Plate 32.)

SUMMARY

By using a combination of serum screening and sonographic evaluation, the detection of fetal aneuploidy has increased. With improved sensitivity of sonographic equipment, many fetal abnormalities can be detected in greater detail at an earlier gestational age. The greatest challenge remains in continuing education and keeping up-to-date with advances in technology.

CLINICAL SCENARIO—DIAGNOSIS

The amniocentesis revealed trisomy 21 (Down syndrome). The combination of sonographic findings of absent nasal bone, ventriculomegaly, and congenital heart defect (ventricular septal defect) is highly suspicious for Down syndrome. The patient was followed with routine care and presented at 38 weeks' gestational age with decreased fetal movement for 2 days; a subsequent sonogram confirmed intrauterine fetal demise. The sonogram obtained at 25 weeks' gestation demonstrated findings consistent with trisomy 21: ventriculomegaly (Fig. 24-1, *A*), an absent nasal bone (Fig. 24-1, *B*), and a ventricular septal defect (Fig. 24-1, *C*).

CASE STUDIES FOR DISCUSSION

1. A 20-year-old woman experiencing spotting in the first trimester undergoes a sonogram. A large septate fluid collection surrounding the nuchal region is identified along with the findings shown in Figure 24-14. An amniocentesis is recommended. What is the most likely diagnosis?

2. A 32-year-old woman with no prior serum screening is referred for a sonogram at 20 weeks' gestational age. The significant sonographic findings are shown in Figure 24-15. What is the primary concern for this pregnancy?

3. A 21-year-old woman is referred for a targeted sonogram because she measures small for dates and facial anomalies were identified on a sonogram performed elsewhere. The current sonogram reveals a 17-week gestational age fetus with polydactyly, delayed growth, and the findings shown in Figure 24-16. What is the most likely diagnosis?

4. A 41-year-old woman presents for a genetic sonogram at 19 weeks, 2 days gestational age. The sonogram shows the findings in Figure 24-17. By the third trimester, duodenal atresia and polyhydramnios are evident. What chromosome abnormality is suggested by these findings?

5. A 29-year-old woman presents for a targeted sonogram because outside studies suggest a small fetal chin and a fetus small for gestational age. The patient has no significant family history of congenital birth defects, so she declined serum screening. She does have a history of two previous first-trimester losses. Images of the fetal face and feet are shown in Figure 24-18. What chromosome abnormality is most likely present?

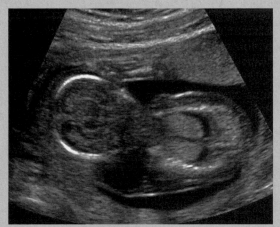

FIGURE 24-14 First-trimester fetus.

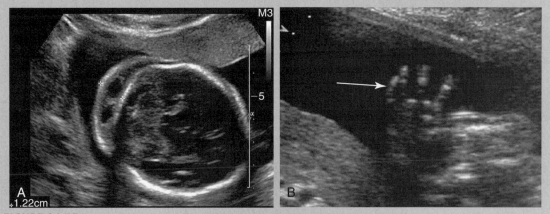

FIGURE 24-15 **(A),** Posterior fossa view of fetal head. **(B),** Image of fetal hand, specifically the fifth digit *(arrow).*

Continued

CASE STUDIES FOR DISCUSSION—cont'd

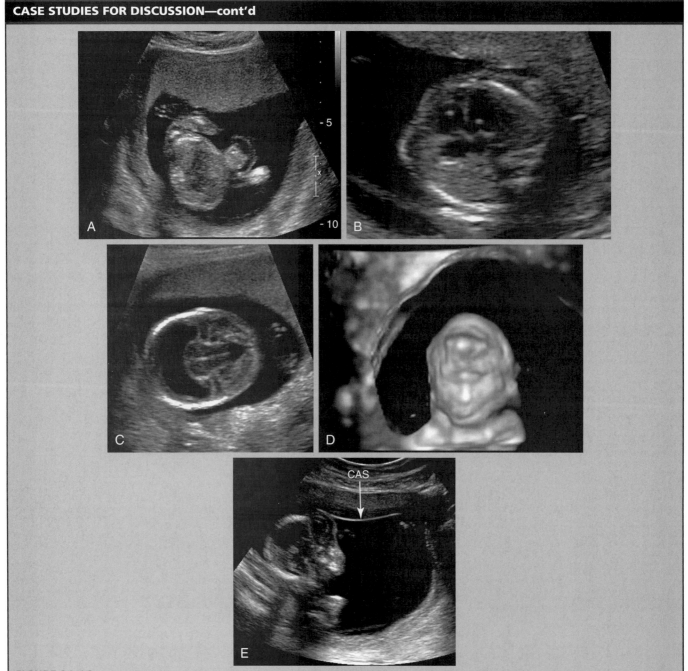

FIGURE 24-16 Images of a 17-week fetus. **(A)**, Transverse image of fetal abdomen. **(B)**, Four-chamber view of the heart. **(C)**, Fetal brain. **(D)**, Three-dimensional image of the fetal face. **(E)**, Chorioamniotic separation *(arrow)*.

CASE STUDIES FOR DISCUSSION—cont'd

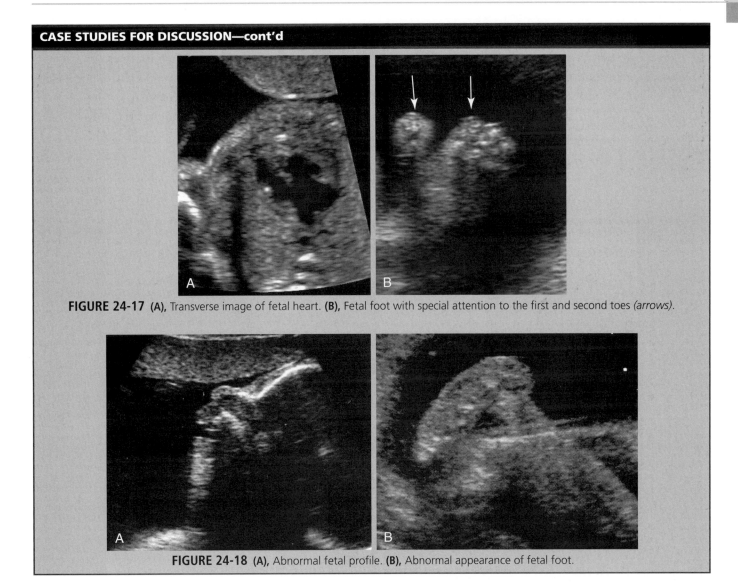

FIGURE 24-17 **(A)**, Transverse image of fetal heart. **(B)**, Fetal foot with special attention to the first and second toes *(arrows)*.

FIGURE 24-18 **(A)**, Abnormal fetal profile. **(B)**, Abnormal appearance of fetal foot.

STUDY QUESTIONS

1. A 32-year-old woman is seen for an obstetric sonogram with an abnormal triple screen. hCG, uE3, and AFP all were decreased. Which abnormality is most likely to be seen on the sonogram?
   a. Clenched hands
   b. Cystic hygroma
   c. Polydactyly
   d. Syndactyly

2. Which of the following genetic markers is considered as sensitive as a thickened NF in screening for Down syndrome?
   a. Congenital heart defect
   b. Clinodactyly
   c. Absent nasal bone
   d. Sandal gap toes

3. What test result is available in 24 hours for anomalies of chromosomes 13, 18, 21, X, and Y?
   a. CVS
   b. Cultured amniotic cells
   c. Fetal fibronectin
   d. FISH

4. Which chromosome abnormality is a lethal condition and is rarely reported in live births?
   a. Trisomy 13
   b. Triploidy
   c. Trisomy 18
   d. Turner syndrome

5. A 23-year-old woman had increased NT on her first-trimester screen. She chose not to proceed with CVS or early amniocentesis. At the time of her targeted sonogram, polydactyly, microcephaly, and a renal abnormality were identified. What chromosome abnormality is most likely to be seen in this case?
   a. Trisomy 13
   b. Triploidy
   c. Trisomy 18
   d. Turner syndrome

6. Which of the following is the most common chromosome abnormality to have a SUA?
   a. Trisomy 13
   b. Triploidy
   c. Trisomy 18
   d. Trisomy 21

7. Echogenic bowel has an association with all of the following except for which one?
   a. Trisomy 21
   b. Trisomy 18
   c. Cystic fibrosis
   d. Swallowed blood

8. A 28-year-old woman presents for a sonogram at 28 weeks' gestational age with a history of no prenatal care and a recent fall. The sonographic examination demonstrates an atrioventricular canal defect, BPD/NBL ratio of 12.2, and polyhydramnios. What is the most likely diagnosis?
   a. Patau syndrome
   b. Triploidy
   c. Edwards syndrome
   d. Down syndrome

9. A 31-year-old woman with a quadruple screen analyte pattern of decreased maternal serum AFP and uE3 and elevated hCG and DIA is referred for a genetic sonogram at 19 weeks' gestational age. You would expect to see all of the following markers except for which one?
   a. Polydactyly
   b. Clinodactyly
   c. Absent nasal bone
   d. Dilated renal pelves

10. A cystic hygroma may be seen in association with many chromosomal abnormalities; however, it is most often associated with which syndrome?
    a. Edwards syndrome
    b. Turner syndrome
    c. Down syndrome
    d. Patau syndrome

Acknowledgment

Special thanks to Rachel Clark, MS, CGC. Thank you for sharing your vast knowledge about genetics and for the time and energy you put into this project. You are a great teacher and friend!

REFERENCES

1. Cicero S, Bindra R, Rembouskos G, et al: Integrated ultrasound and biochemical screening for Trisomy 21 using fetal nuchal translucency, absent nasal bone, free beta-hCG and PAPP-A at 11 to 14 weeks, *Prenat Diagn* 23:306–310, 2003.
2. Palomaki G, Lambert-Messerlian G, Canick J: A summary analysis of Down syndrome markers in the late first trimester, *Adv Clin Chem* 43:177, 2007.
3. Gagnon A, Wilson RD, Audibert F, Allen VM, et al: Society of Obstetricians and Gynaecologists of Canada Genetics Committee: Obstetrical complications associated with abnormal maternal serum marker analytes, *J Obstet Gynaecol Can* 30:918–932, 2008.
4. Dugoff L: Society for Maternal-Fetal Medicine: First- and second-trimester maternal serum markers for aneuploidy and adverse obstetric outcomes, *Obstet Gynecol* 115:1052, 2010.
5. Palomaki G, Neveux L, Knight G, et al: Maternal serum invasive trophoblast antigen (hyperglycosylated hCG) as a screening marker for Down syndrome during the second trimester, *Clin Chem* 50:1804–1808, 2004.

6. Caughey A, Hopkins L, Norton M: Chorionic villus sampling compared with amniocentesis and the difference in the rate of pregnancy loss, *Am Coll Obstet Gynecol* 108:612–616, 2006.

7. Tabor A, Vestergaard C, Lidegaard O: Fetal loss rate after chorionic villus sampling and amniocentesis: an 11-year national registry study, *Ultrasound Obstet Gynecol* 34:19–24, 2009.

8. Chitty L, Hill M, White H, et al: Noninvasive prenatal testing for aneuploidy—ready for primetime, *Am J Obstet Gynecol* 206:269–275, 2012.

9. Benn P, Cuckle H, Pergament E: Non-invasive prenatal diagnosis for Down syndrome: the paradigm will shift, but slowly, *Ultrasound Obstet Gynecol* 39:127–130, 2012.

10. Bianchi D, Platt L, Goldberg J, et al: Genome-wide fetal aneuploidy detection by maternal plasma DNA sequencing, *Obstet Gynecol* 119:890–901, 2012.

11. Rochon M, Eddleman K: Controversial ultrasound findings, *Obstet Gynecol Clin North Am* 31:61–99, 2004.

12. Kharrat R, Yamamoto M, Roume J, et al: Karyotype and outcomes of fetuses diagnosed with cystic hygroma in the first trimester in relation to nuchal translucency thickness, *Prenat Diagn* 26:369–372, 2006.

13. Molina F, Avgidou K, Kagan K, et al: Cystic hygromas, nuchal edema, and nuchal translucency at 11-14 weeks of gestation, *Obstet Gynecol* 107:678–683, 2006.

14. Cicero S, Curcio P, Papageorghiou A, et al: Absence of nasal bone in fetuses with trisomy 21 at 11-14 weeks of gestation: an observational study, *Lancet* 358(9294):1665–1667, 2001.

15. Cicero S, Sonek J, McKenn D, et al: Nasal bone hypoplasia in trisomy 21 at 15-22 weeks' gestation, *Ultrasound Obstet Gynecol* 21(1):15–18, 2003.

16. Ville Y: What is the role of fetal nasal bone examination in the assessment of risk for trisomy 21 in the clinical practice? *Am J Obstet Gynecol* 195:1–3, 2006.

17. Sonek J, Cicero S, Neiger R, et al: Nasal bone assessment in prenatal screening for trisomy 21, *Am J Obstet and Gynecol* 195:1219–1230, 2006.

18. Borgida A, Maffeo C, Gianferarri E, et al: Frequency of echogenic intracardiac focus by race/ethnicity in euploid fetuses, *J Matern Fetal Neonatal Med* 18:65–66, 2005.

19. Bethune M: Time to reconsider our approach to echogenic intracardiac focus and choroid plexus cysts, *Aust N Z J Obstet Gynaecol* 48:137–141, 2008.

20. Coco C, Jeanty P: Isolated fetal pyelectasis and chromosomal abnormalities, *Am J Obstet Gynecol* 193:732–738, 2005.

21. Benacerraf B: The role of second-trimester genetic sonogram in screening for fetal Down syndrome, *Semin Perinatol* 29:386–394, 2005.

22. Bromley B, Benacerraf B: Chromosomal abnormalities. In Rumack C, Wilson S, Charboneau J, et al, editors: *Diagnostic ultrasound*, vol. 1, ed 4, Philadelphia, 2011, Mosby, pp 547–612.

23. Breathnach F, Fleming A, Malone F: The second trimester genetic sonogram, *Am J Med Genet C Semin Med Genet* 145C:62, 2007.

24. Granese R, Coco C, Jeanty P: The value of single umbilical artery in the prediction of fetal aneuploidy: findings in 12,672 pregnant women, *Ultrasound Q* 23:117–121, 2007.

25

Fetal Anomaly

Charlotte Henningsen

CLINICAL SCENARIO

A young woman is seen for a sonogram for late prenatal care. The sonogram reveals a single, live fetus at 34 weeks' gestation. In addition to the findings in Figure 25-1, a single umbilical artery and an absent stomach bubble are noted. What is the most likely diagnosis and prognosis?

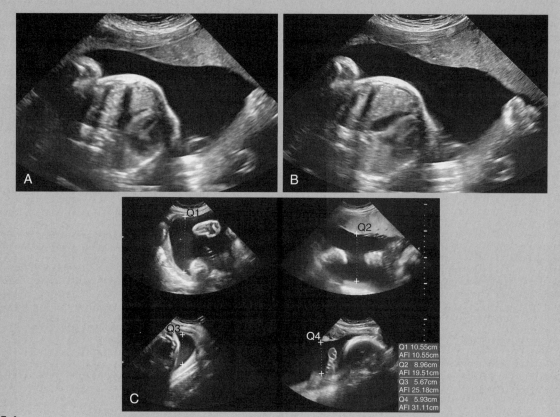

FIGURE 25-1 Transverse images of the fetal thorax showing the heart **(A)** and cystic structure **(B)** and amniotic fluid index of 31.1 cm **(C)**.

OBJECTIVES

- Describe anomalies that may be identified with prenatal sonography.
- Identify the sonographic features that differentiate fetal anomalies.
- List anomalies that may benefit from in utero treatment.
- Identify anomalies that are incompatible with survival after birth.
- List other methods of fetal evaluation used in the diagnosis of anomalies.

Patients may be referred for an obstetric sonogram for a suspected fetal anomaly. With little additional information, the sonographer must survey the fetus carefully to identify and clarify the nature of the abnormality. Sonographers must be familiar with a variety of fetal anomalies. Proper documentation and subsequent diagnosis must be made for a meaningful discussion with the patient of pregnancy, treatment, and delivery options. This chapter presents many of the fetal anomalies that are identified with sonography (Table 25-1). Other chapters review renal anomalies (see Chapter 20), neural tube and abdominal wall anomalies (see Chapter 23), chromosomal anomalies (see Chapter 24), and fetal heart defects (see Chapter 26).

FETAL BRAIN

Hydrocephaly

Hydrocephalus is defined as a dilated ventricle with enlargement of the head, and ventriculomegaly is dilation of the ventricles without enlargement of the head, although these terms are sometimes used interchangeably. Hydrocephalus occurs in 0.5:1000 to 3:1000 live births and is associated with high morbidity and mortality rates.[1] Hydrocephalus may be the result of a congenital anomaly or acquired; when hydrocephalus leads to intracranial pressure, brain parenchyma may also be compromised. In addition, ventricular enlargement may result from compensation for atrophy or abnormal development of brain parenchyma. The outcome is variable depending on the associated anomalies and the severity of the ventricular enlargement.

The multiple causes of hydrocephalus include holoprosencephaly, spina bifida, encephalocele, Dandy-Walker malformation (DWM), aqueductal stenosis, arachnoid cysts, and agenesis of the corpus callosum (ACC). Hydrocephalus or ventriculomegaly may be identified in fetuses with congenital infections, neoplasms, and musculoskeletal anomalies and may be identified as an isolated finding. Ventriculomegaly may also be associated with aneuploidy.

Sonographic Findings. The diagnosis of ventriculomegaly can be made when the atrium of the lateral ventricle exceeds 10 mm (Fig. 25-2) in the second and third trimesters of pregnancy. When ventriculomegaly is identified, an evaluation of all fetal measurements can help to determine the degree of ventriculomegaly and whether fetal head enlargement is present. A thorough sonographic evaluation should also be performed in a search for associated anomalies.

TABLE 25-1	Fetal Anomalies
Diagnosis	**Sonographic Findings**
Hydrocephaly	Enlarged head; atrium of lateral ventricle >10 mm
Holoprosencephaly	Single ventricle, fused thalami, absent cavum septi pellucidi and corpus callosum, absent falx; facial anomalies (clefts, hypotelorism, cyclopia, proboscis)
Hydranencephaly	Liquefaction of brain parenchyma; brainstem may be identified
DWM	Posterior fossa cyst with enlarged cisterna magna, splaying of cerebellar hemispheres with absent or dysplastic vermis; commonly associated with hydrocephalus
ACC	Absent cavum septi pellucidi, mild ventriculomegaly with dilated occipital horns; lateral displacement of lateral ventricles and superior displacement of third ventricle; dilated third ventricle
Cleft lip	Disruption of soft tissue of upper lip; bilateral cleft may appear to have premaxillary mass
Micrognathia	Recessed chin
CDH	Abdominal contents, usually in stomach, in thorax; malposition of fetal heart; absence of intraabdominal stomach
CCAM	Type I, multiple large cysts; type II, visible cysts <1 cm; type III, large echogenic mass in thorax
Pulmonary sequestration	Echogenic mass, may be triangular; separate blood supply from aorta
PE	Fluid collection surrounding lungs; unilateral or bilateral
Duodenal atresia	Dilated stomach and proximal duodenum appearing as double bubble, polyhydramnios common
Bowel obstruction	Dilated loops of bowel proximal to obstruction
Meconium peritonitis	Calcifications on peritoneal surfaces; meconium pseudocyst; associated ascites or polyhydramnios may be identified
Ascites	Collection of fluid in fetal abdomen outlining organs and bowel
Abdominal cysts	Usually round, thin-walled anechoic structure; location and gender should be noted to identify origin
SCT	Heterogeneous or complex mass extending from fetal sacrum
Thanatophoric dysplasia	Significant micromelia, narrow thorax with protuberant abdomen, bowed limbs, macrocephaly with frontal bossing, trilobular skull may be identified
Achondrogenesis	Extreme micromelia, variable degrees of ossification of spine and calvaria, narrow thorax and ribs, rib fractures may be noted
Achondroplasia	Rhizomelia, trident hand, macrocephalus with frontal bossing, depressed nasal bridge
SRPS	Micromelia, narrow thorax, short ribs, polydactyly, cleft lip and palate may be identified
OI	Decreased ossification of bones, compressible calvaria, narrow ribs, short limbs, multiple fractures

Holoprosencephaly

Holoprosencephaly encompasses a range of severity characterized by incomplete or lack of cleavage of the forebrain. The condition has been identified in 1:10,000 to 1:20,000 births,[2] and many affected fetuses spontaneously abort in the first trimester. The most severe form, alobar holoprosencephaly, manifests with a complete failure of separation of the forebrain with subsequent fusion of the thalami, a single ventricle, and fusion of the cerebral hemispheres. Absence of the falx, corpus callosum, olfactory bulbs, and optic tracts is also noted. Semilobar holoprosencephaly is seen with partial cleavage of the forebrain and absence of the corpus callosum and olfactory bulbs. Identification of the mildest form, lobar holoprosencephaly, may be difficult because separation of the cerebrum is evident, but fusion of the lateral ventricles and absence of the corpus callosum may be noted. The outcome is variable depending on the severity, but the most severe forms of holoprosencephaly carry an extremely poor prognosis.

Holoprosencephaly is associated with severe facial anomalies, including cyclopia, ethmocephaly, cebocephaly, and facial clefts. Holoprosencephaly is also associated with multiple chromosomal anomalies, most commonly trisomy 13. In addition, holoprosencephaly may be identified in many syndromes, including Edwards' syndrome (trisomy 18), Smith-Lemli-Opitz syndrome, and Pallister-Hall syndrome.[3] Holoprosencephaly may also

be transmitted through autosomal dominant, autosomal recessive, and X-linked modes. There is a 2:1 female-to-male prevalence and a 13% risk of recurrence.[2] Also, several teratogenic effects have been linked to holoprosencephaly, including hyperglycemia (in diabetes) and maternal infections.

Sonographic Findings. Sonographic identification of holoprosencephaly is easier in its most severe form, and identification of a single ventricle (Fig. 25-3, A) surrounded by brain parenchyma is diagnostic. The thalami appear fused, and the falx is absent, as are the cavum septi pellucidi and corpus callosum. In semilobar holoprosencephaly (Fig. 25-3, B and C), variable fusion may be identified, and lobar holoprosencephaly may be difficult to distinguish from ACC, which should be suspected when the cavum septi pellucidi is not identified. When enlargement of the ventricle is identified, holoprosencephaly may be difficult to differentiate from hydranencephalus or severe hydrocephalus, unless the characteristic facial anomalies are also identified.

When holoprosencephaly is identified, the face should be meticulously surveyed for the presence of associated anomalies (Fig. 25-3, C-G), including facial clefts, hypotelorism, a nose with a single nostril, a proboscis, and cyclopia. Other anomalies, such as a heart defect, polydactyly, or encephalocele, may suggest association with a chromosomal anomaly or syndrome.

Hydranencephaly

Hydranencephaly is characterized by destruction of the brain parenchyma with replacement by cerebrospinal fluid. It may result from vascular compromise leading to occlusion of the internal carotid artery[4]; however, other causes including congenital infections and cocaine abuse have been linked. The destruction to the brain usually occurs in the second trimester of pregnancy and may be preceded by a normal sonographic evaluation. Hydranencephaly is a rare anomaly with a grave outcome.

Sonographic Findings. The sonographic findings of hydranencephaly (Fig. 25-4) include liquefaction of the brain parenchyma with replacement by cerebrospinal fluid. The brainstem is intact and visible on sonographic evaluation. The head may be normal or large in size. Hydranencephaly can be differentiated from severe hydrocephaly by a lack of surrounding brain parenchyma.

Dandy-Walker Malformation

DWM is characterized by absence or dysplasia of the cerebellar vermis and maldevelopment of the fourth ventricle with replacement by a posterior fossa cyst. It occurs in 1:30,000 births[5] and is frequently associated with ventriculomegaly. A less severe form, referred to as the Dandy-Walker variant, may occur with dysplasia of the cerebellar vermis without enlargement of the posterior fossa. DWM may be isolated or associated with

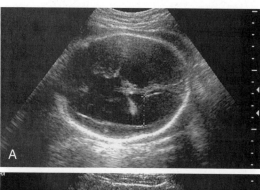
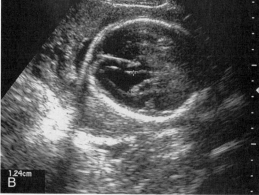

FIGURE 25-2 **(A),** Lateral ventricle of fetus measured 24 mm. DWM was also identified. **(B),** Lateral ventricle measured 12 mm and was associated with Down syndrome.

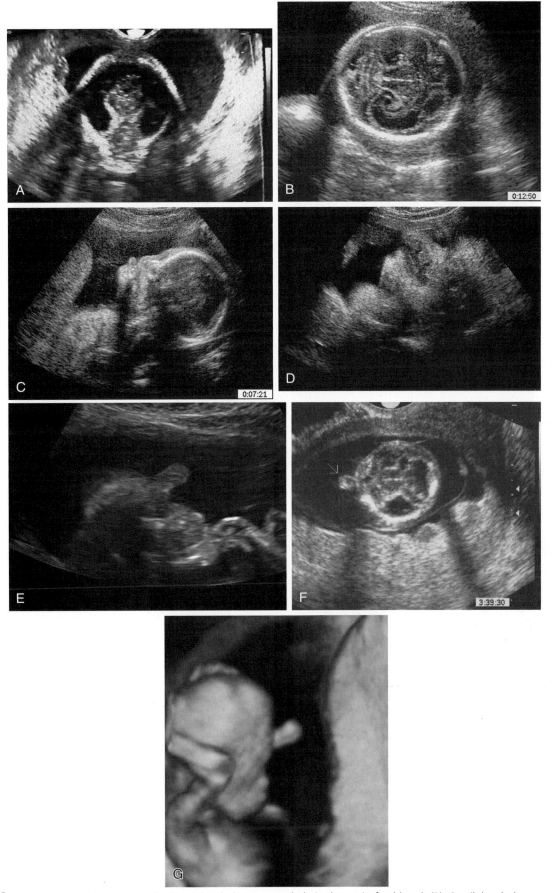

FIGURE 25-3 (A), Monoventricle associated with alobar holoprosencephaly is shown in fetal head. **(B),** Semilobar holoprosencephaly was suspected in fetus with normal chromosomes. Anterior portion of brain was abnormal, and absent cavum septi pellucidi was noted. Abnormal profile **(C)** and bilateral cleft lip **(D)** were also identified. Semilobar holoprosencephaly was confirmed at birth, and the infant died within the first few days of birth. Other facial anomalies may be identified in association with holoprosencephaly, including proboscis **(E)** and hypotelorism **(F).** Fetus shown in **(F)** also had microphthalmos and trisomy 13. **(G),** Proboscis is demonstrated using three-dimensional technology.

syndromes, aneuploidy, and maternal infections.[6] DWM also has been linked to other intracranial anomalies, including ACC. Of infants who survive, 40% to 70% are intellectually impaired.[5]

Sonographic Findings. The diagnosis of DWM can be made with the identification of a posterior fossa cyst, with a resultant enlarged cisterna magna and splaying of the cerebellar hemispheres (Fig. 25-5) from the abnormal development of the cerebellar vermis. Hydrocephalus (see Fig. 25-2, A) frequently accompanies DWM. A thorough search for additional anomalies may assist in determination of whether DWM is isolated or associated with a chromosomal anomaly or syndrome.

Agenesis of the Corpus Callosum

ACC is considered relatively common occurring in 0.3% to 0.7% of the general population and affecting 2% to 3% of individuals with mental retardation,[7] although the condition may go undiagnosed. The corpus callosum connects the cerebral hemispheres and aids in learning and memory. ACC may be found in isolation but is often associated with other anomalies of the central nervous system, a variety of chromosomal anomalies, syndromes, and metabolic diseases.[7] The outcome is variable depending on the association and severity of other anomalies, but ACC can be asymptomatic or have a grave prognosis when severe anomalies are identified.

Sonographic Findings. The diagnosis of ACC should be suspected when the cavum septi pellucidi is absent (Fig. 25-6) because the corpus callosum develops with the cavum septi pellucidi. In addition, colpocephaly, defined as mild ventriculomegaly with dilation of the occipital horns, giving the ventricle a teardrop appearance, may be identified. The lateral ventricles are also displaced laterally, and the third ventricle may appear

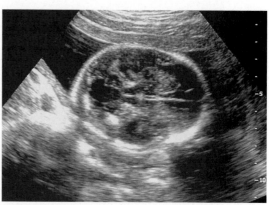

FIGURE 25-5 Splaying of cerebellar hemispheres is identified in posterior fossa of fetus with DWM.

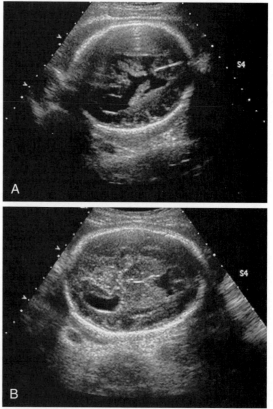

FIGURE 25-6 (A), ACC was diagnosed in fetus. Cavum septi pellucidi was also absent. **(B),** Occipital horns of lateral ventricles were dilated. *(Courtesy Melissa Spagnuolo, Fetal Diagnostic Center of Orlando.)*

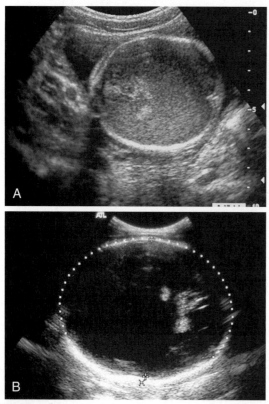

FIGURE 25-4 Hydranencephaly. A young woman with poorly controlled diabetes was seen for a sonogram for late prenatal care. The fetal head was disproportionately large compared with abdominal circumference and femur length. **(A),** Normal head anatomy was not seen, and homogeneous echogenic matter was identified swirling within calvaria. **(B),** Follow-up examinations showed fetal head filled with anechoic fluid. The fetus died in utero near term.

dilated and displaced superiorly. The sonographic examination should include a thorough search for additional anomalies that would suggest a more extensive central nervous system anomaly, aneuploidy, or syndrome.

FETAL FACE

Cleft Lip

Cleft lip or cleft palate is characterized by a defect in the upper lip or palate in the roof of the mouth. These anomalies constitute the most common congenital defects of the face, with occurrence of 1:700 to 1:1000.[8] Cleft palate occurs in approximately 80% of cases of cleft lip[8] and can be difficult to detect sonographically, especially in isolation. Cleft lip may be unilateral, bilateral, and median in location (Fig. 25-7). Unilateral clefts more commonly are left-sided. Median clefts and bilateral clefts frequently have an associated cleft palate with an increased frequency of associated anomalies, including aneuploidy, skeletal anomalies, and syndromes.

Sonographic Findings. Sonographic evaluation for a facial cleft includes imaging the soft tissue of the lips and nose in the coronal plane. A fetal profile may also show the cleft, especially bilateral clefts, which may appear as a premaxillary mass. Three-dimensional sonography of the face may improve the identification and characterization of the cleft.

Micrognathia

Micrognathia is defined as a small or recessed chin. Micrognathia has been associated with aneuploidy, skeletal anomalies, and multiple syndromes. The most common anomaly associated with micrognathia is trisomy 18.[9] The outcome for fetuses with micrognathia depends on the associated anomalies.

Sonographic Findings. Micrognathia may be identified sonographically in the sagittal plane. A recessed chin (Fig. 25-8) may be identified in visualization of the fetal profile. Polyhydramnios may also be identified in association with the micrognathia.

FETAL THORAX

Congenital Diaphragmatic Hernia

Congenital diaphragmatic hernia (CDH) is a herniation of abdominal contents into the thorax through a defect in the diaphragm; it has an incidence of 3:10,000 to 5:10,000 births.[10] The cause is unknown, although genetic and teratogenic factors have been associated. This uncommon malformation is most commonly left-sided and is associated with a high morbidity and mortality rate with a survival rate of 60%.[10] Although associated anomalies influence the outcome, isolated defects also are associated with significant mortality secondary to respiratory complications from pulmonary hypoplasia.

CDH has been associated with chromosomal anomalies; in addition, defects of the central nervous system and heart have been identified, as have other structural defects. Sonographic examination and karyotyping assists in patient counseling so that pregnancy options and surgical management, including prenatal surgery, can be discussed.

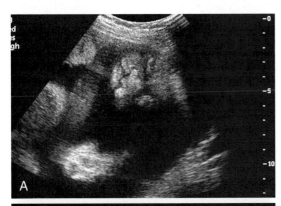

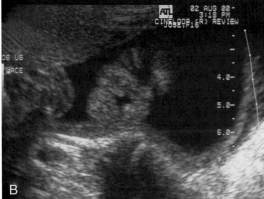

FIGURE 25-7 Cleft lip may be unilateral, bilateral **(A)**, or median **(B)**. Bilateral and median clefts are more frequently associated with other anomalies.

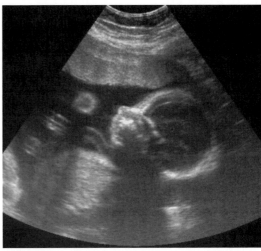

FIGURE 25-8 Micrognathia. Recessed chin was identified in fetus with Edwards' syndrome.

Sonographic Findings. Because left-sided defects occur more frequently, the most common sonographic finding is identification of the stomach above the diaphragm (Fig. 25-9). The intestines may also be identified in the thorax, and the heart is malpositioned in the chest. Identification of the absence of an intraabdominal stomach is important to differentiate between CDH and cystic lung defects. Right-sided defects may show the liver and gallbladder within the thoracic cavity. Polyhydramnios and hydrops may also be identified in association with CDH. A thorough search for additional anomalies that may affect pregnancy management is imperative.

Congenital Cystic Adenomatoid Malformation

Congenital cystic adenomatoid malformation (CCAM) is a rare lung abnormality characterized by an overgrowth of terminal bronchopulmonary tissue occurring in 1:25,000 to 1:35,000 pregnancies.[11] Five classifications have been defined, based on pathologic findings and cyst size. Type 0 is described as an acinar dysplasia. Types I and II are macrocystic masses that consist of multiple large cysts (type I) or a single large cyst and smaller cysts less than 1 cm (type II). Type III is a microcystic variety that appears as a large echogenic mass. Type IV is characterized as a peripheral cyst.[11] CCAM is usually unilateral, involving one lobe of the lung. There is no gender prevalence.

CCAM may be associated with hydrops, polyhydramnios, and pulmonary hypoplasia, all of which are associated with a poor outcome. Some lesions identified in the prenatal period may involute spontaneously, although they may become symptomatic after birth from infection or hemorrhage; malignant transformation has also been reported. Early diagnosis is important for management of pregnancy and delivery. Delivery at a hospital with a neonatal intensive care unit should be arranged because newborns may require respiratory support or surgery or both. Asymptomatic infants should have a chest radiograph, even if the CCAM appears to regress in the

perinatal period, and evaluation with computed tomography (CT) should be considered in light of the fact that a normal chest radiograph may be seen in infants with an abnormal CT.[12]

Sonographic Findings. The sonographic appearance of CCAM type I is one or more large cysts in the thorax, type II appears as multiple small cysts, and type III (Fig. 25-10) appears as a large echogenic mass. Displacement of the fetal heart, polyhydramnios, and hydrops may also be identified. Sonography may be used to monitor for possible regression of the lesion.

Pulmonary Sequestration

Pulmonary sequestration is a rare abnormality characterized by a mass of lung tissue (Fig. 25-11) that does not connect with the tracheobronchial tree and has a separate blood supply that usually originates from the abdominal aorta. Intralobar and extralobar varieties are seen, with extralobar pulmonary sequestration representing most anomalies. The extralobar variety may also appear above or below the diaphragm.[13]

Although pulmonary sequestration may regress in utero and may be asymptomatic after birth, it has been

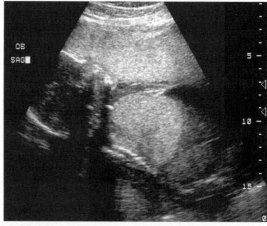

FIGURE 25-10 CCAM may have cystic appearance or solid echogenic mass appearance as identified in fetus with type III.

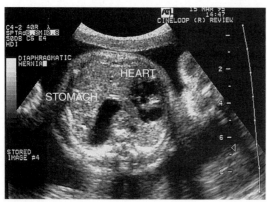

FIGURE 25-9 CDH most commonly manifests with intrathoracic stomach and malpositioned heart as seen in this fetus.

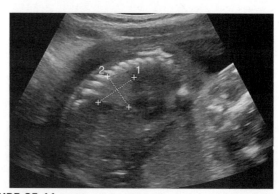

FIGURE 25-11 Wedge-shaped lesion characteristic of pulmonary sequestration is identified in a fetus.

associated with mediastinal shift, pleural effusion (PE), and hydrops. Polyhydramnios may also develop and initiate preterm labor. The outcome for pulmonary sequestration is variable. Fetuses may die in utero, and newborns may die of pulmonary hypoplasia or be completely asymptomatic and need respiratory support or surgery to resect the sequestered lung. In utero intervention to decrease polyhydramnios or drain pleural fluid may improve the outcome.

Sonographic Findings. The sonographic appearance of pulmonary sequestration is an echogenic mass that may be triangular. Differentiation of this lesion from other echogenic thoracic lesions can be made with demonstration of the aberrant blood supply with color Doppler. Serial sonographic examinations may be used to monitor the fetus for lesion regression or the development of polyhydramnios, PE, or hydrops.

Pleural Effusion

PE, also known as hydrothorax, is a rare entity characterized by an abnormal accumulation of fluid in the fetal thorax occurring in 1:15,000 neonates.[14] PE may be unilateral or bilateral and isolated or a component of a generalized fluid overload (hydrops). PE may resolve spontaneously, lead to pulmonary hypoplasia, or progress to hydrops and fetal death.

PE may be associated with other abnormalities of the thorax, including CCAM, pulmonary sequestration, CDH, and cardiac defects. PE may also be associated with chromosomal anomalies and other structural defects. Fetal thoracentesis, thoracoamniotic shunting, or early delivery may improve outcome in fetuses without associated anomalies; these options would preclude intervention and should be reserved for severe cases of PE.

Sonographic Findings. Sonographic diagnosis of PE can be made when fluid is identified in the fetal thorax surrounding lung tissue. A survey for associated findings provides the information necessary to explore pregnancy management and treatment options.

FETAL ABDOMEN

Duodenal Atresia

Duodenal atresia is characterized by stenosis, atresia, or development of webs that obstruct the distal duodenum. An increased familial inheritance and a strong association with aneuploidy are also seen, most specifically trisomy 21, which has been identified in one-third of cases of duodenal atresia. It may rarely be seen with concomitant esophageal atresia, in which case an increased risk for aneuploidy exists.[15]

Sonographic Findings. Sonographic evaluation of duodenal atresia reveals a dilated stomach and proximal duodenum that gives the characteristic double-bubble sign (Fig. 25-12). Polyhydramnios is commonly associated

with duodenal atresia. This anomaly may not be evident until after 20 weeks' gestation. When duodenal atresia is identified, sonography may also be used for amniocentesis guidance for evaluation for chromosomal anomalies.

Esophageal Atresia

Esophageal atresia is the result of a congenital blockage of the esophagus and may be associated with a fistula connecting the esophagus and trachea. Esophageal atresia may be associated with chromosomal anomalies, especially trisomies 21 and 18, and the VACTERL association. The outcome depends on the severity of associated abnormalities.

Sonographic Findings. Prenatal diagnosis of esophageal atresia is difficult. The most suggestive sonographic finding is an absent stomach, detected by a failure of amniotic fluid to pass from the esophagus to the stomach. When a tracheoesophageal fistula is present, a normal or small stomach may be visualized. Atypically, sonography may show the fluid-filled esophagus coming to a blind end. Polyhydramnios (Fig 25-13) may also be identified because of the inability to swallow effectively.

Bowel Obstruction

Obstruction of fetal bowel may occur anywhere along the length of the small or large bowel. The more proximal the level of obstruction, the more likely polyhydramnios will be identified in association with this anomaly. Obstructions may occur with malrotation, atresia, volvulus, and peritoneal bands; they may be isolated or associated with cystic fibrosis, ascites, meconium peritonitis, or other anomalies.

Sonographic Findings. Obstructed bowel appears as dilated loops (Fig. 25-14) to the level of obstruction. Proximal obstructions are more likely to appear fluid-filled. Dilated bowel may also be hypoechoic or hyperechoic,

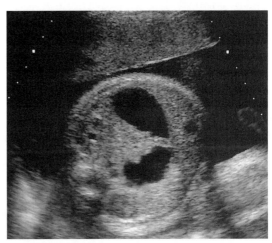

FIGURE 25-12 Characteristic double bubble sign is seen in fetus with duodenal atresia.

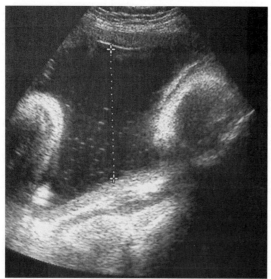

FIGURE 25-13 Polyhydramnios was diagnosed in a fetus with amniotic fluid index of 24 cm. Stomach bubble was not identified on multiple examinations. Amniocentesis confirmed trisomy 21. Esophageal atresia was suspected and confirmed at birth.

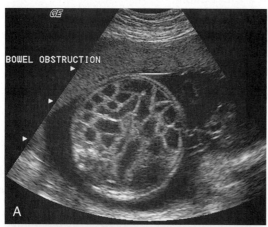

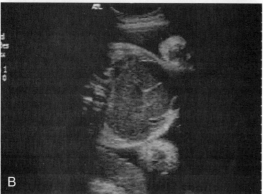

FIGURE 25-14 (A), Dilated loops of bowel are identified in fetus with bowel obstruction. **(B)**, Bowel obstruction was identified in fetus with later diagnosis of cystic fibrosis. (*A, Courtesy GE Medical Systems.*)

and peristalsis may be seen on real-time imaging. Serial sonographic examinations should be ordered to monitor fetal well-being. Changes in echogenicity and a lack of peristalsis may indicate that torsion of the bowel has occurred.

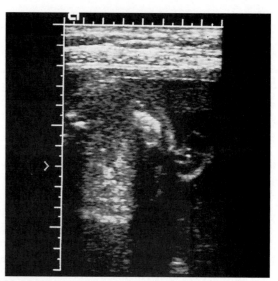

FIGURE 25-15 Echogenic shadowing may be identified in fetuses with meconium peritonitis.

Meconium Peritonitis

Meconium peritonitis is rare and is a complication in fetuses with perforation of a bowel obstruction. It may be associated with atresia, stenosis, volvulus, hernia, or ileus or a sequela of maternal infection.[16] This sterile chemical peritonitis may further result in an inflammatory reaction and formation of a meconium pseudocyst. Polyhydramnios may also be identified in fetuses with meconium peritonitis.
Sonographic Findings. Sonographic examination may reveal calcifications (Fig. 25-15) in the fetal abdomen on the peritoneal surfaces and in the scrotum in male fetuses. Ascites or bowel dilation may also be identified in the abdomen, and polyhydramnios may be noted.

Ascites

Fetal ascites is the result of fluid collection in the fetal abdomen. The condition may be associated with bowel or bladder perforations or fetal hydrops. Fetal ascites also has been associated with congenital infections and fetal abdominal neoplasms.
Sonographic Findings. The sonographic evaluation of fetal ascites should show fluid outlining the abdominal organs and the fetal bowel (Fig. 25-16). The hypoechoic muscle adjacent to the fetal skin line should not be confused with fluid in the fetal abdomen.

Abdominal Cysts

Numerous cystic lesions within the fetal abdomen rarely may be identified prenatally (Fig. 25-17). The focus of the sonographic examination of a cystic lesion is identification of the origin of the cyst and determination of the gender of the fetus because many cystic lesions identified in female fetuses are ovarian in origin. Serial sonographic examinations may also document resolution

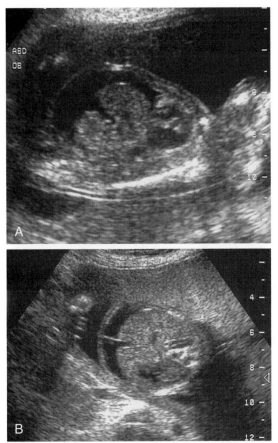

FIGURE 25-16 **(A)** and **(B)**, Fluid can be identified surrounding fetal abdominal organs and bowel.

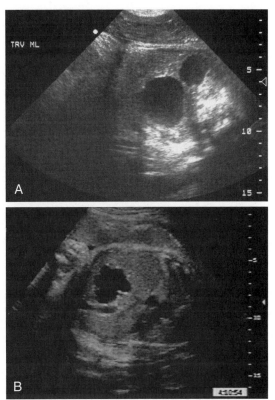

FIGURE 25-17 Fetal abdominal cysts. **(A)**, Ovarian cyst was confirmed in female fetus with cystic lesion identified adjacent to bladder. **(B)**, Irregular cyst was identified in liver of fetus, and diagnosis of choledochal cyst was made after infant was delivered.

or a change in size or a change in echogenicity of these lesions. Cystic lesions that are located in the liver or right upper quadrant include choledochal cysts, hepatic cysts, and gallbladder duplication. Urachal cysts are located between the bladder and umbilicus. Duplication cysts may be identified anywhere along the gastrointestinal tract and may show the muscular layers of gut rather than a thin wall. Mesenteric, omental, renal, and adrenal cysts may be identified, in addition to cystic lesions of other origins.[17]

Sacrococcygeal Teratoma

Sacrococcygeal teratoma (SCT) is rare occurring in 1:40,000 births and is the most common congenital neoplasm, with a female-to male ratio of 4:1.[18] This neoplasm arises from the three germ cell layers (ectoderm, endoderm, and mesoderm) and is usually benign. SCTs are primarily external tumors, but they may have intrapelvic extension or arise entirely within the pelvis or abdomen. In addition, teratomas may arise anywhere in the fetus (Fig. 25-18), including the liver and brain.

The outcome for a fetus with SCT is generally poor because of the development of fetal hydrops, cardiac failure, anemia, tumor hemorrhage or rupture, and premature delivery from polyhydramnios. Prenatal diagnosis allows pregnancy options to be considered, including termination, amniotic fluid reduction, and delivery with cesarean section. In utero invasive procedures also have been performed successfully. Infants can have successful resection of these tumors, although there is still an increase in neonatal morbidity and mortality.

Sonographic Findings. SCT most commonly appears as a mass extending from the sacral region (see Fig. 25-18, B-D) of the fetus. The tumor may vary greatly in size and echogenicity. Heterogeneous or complex tumors are frequently noted, and color Doppler may show the increased vascularity of this mass. Placentomegaly and cardiomegaly may also be seen. Evaluation of tumor size and identification of hydrops, urinary obstruction, and polyhydramnios should be noted because these findings have an increased fetal mortality rate.

FETAL SKELETON

Skeletal dysplasias are a rare group of anomalies that involve abnormal development of bone and cartilage. The occurrence rate is 3.2:10,000 live births,[19] and the most common of the skeletal dysplasias are thanatophoric dysplasia, achondrogenesis, achondroplasia, osteogenesis imperfecta (OI), and short rib–polydactyly syndrome (SRPS). Fetal skeletal anomalies can be a challenge to diagnose accurately because of the overlap of similar

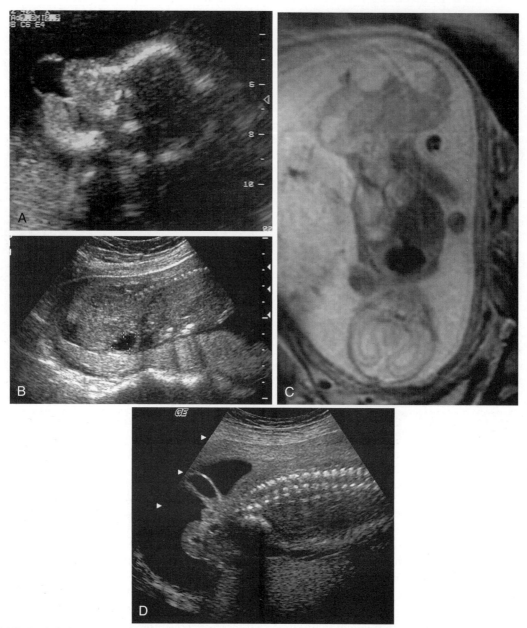

FIGURE 25-18 (A), Cystic lesion appeared to be attached to roof of fetal mouth. Near term, the lesion had a more complex appearance, and polyhydramnios developed. Surgical excision was performed shortly after delivery, and benign cystic teratoma was confirmed. **(B)**, Complex SCT is identified extending from sacral region of fetus. **(C)**, Magnetic resonance imaging is also used to show characteristics of mass. **(D)**, SCT had more cystic characteristics. *(D, Courtesy GE Medical Systems.)*

sonographic findings. The imaging protocol should be adjusted when a skeletal dysplasia is suspected to aid in the diagnosis and determination of chances for survival after birth. In addition to sonographic evaluation, fetal radiographs, chromosomal analysis, and genetic testing may be used to assist in an accurate diagnosis.

The sonographic evaluation should include imaging and measurement of all long bones because some skeletal dysplasias are associated with shortening or absence of a specific bone or segment of the extremities, as in thrombocytopenia–absent radius syndrome, which manifests with an absent radius. Bones should also be evaluated for shape and for fractures. The hands and feet should be assessed for abnormal posturing and polydactyly, which

may help in the diagnosis of certain dysplasias, such as diastrophic dysplasia, which manifests with a hitchhiker thumb, and SRPS. The fetal thorax should be analyzed for narrowing, associated with pulmonary hypoplasia, which is a feature of many lethal skeletal dysplasias. The absence or presence of other associated anomalies, such as facial clefts, hydrocephalus, and heart defects, may also lead to a specific diagnosis.

Thanatophoric Dysplasia

Thanatophoric dysplasia, although rare, is the most common lethal skeletal dysplasia occurring in 1:20,000 to 1:40,000 live births.[20] It is usually a sporadic anomaly, although a 2% risk of recurrence is seen.[21] The condition is divided into two types, I and II, based on characteristic features. Both types of thanatophoric dysplasia have been linked with a mutation of the *FGFR3* gene. Infants born with thanatophoric dysplasia usually die shortly after birth of pulmonary hypoplasia and respiratory distress.

Type I thanatophoric dysplasia is the more common of the two types and is characterized by micromelia, curved femurs, and a narrow thorax. Type II is characterized by micromelia, straight femora, a narrow thorax, and a cloverleaf skull.

Sonographic Findings. The sonographic features of thanatophoric dysplasia (Fig. 25-19) include significant

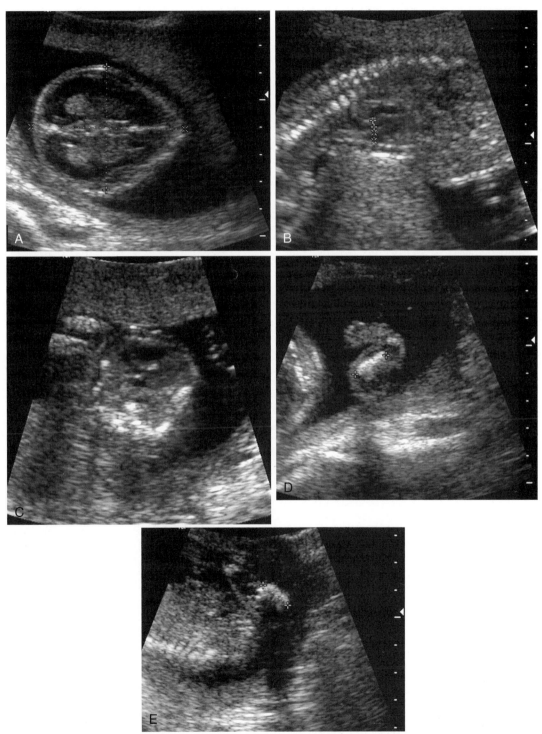

FIGURE 25-19 A patient was seen for sonographic confirmation of gestational age of 18 weeks, 1 day. **(A),** Fetal head measurements were within tolerance, although fetal head shape was unusual. **(B)** and **(C),** Fetal abdomen was very narrow, and abdomen appeared protuberant. **(D)** and **(E),** Humeral and femoral lengths were consistent with 13-week gestation. The patient was counseled that the fetus appeared to have lethal skeletal dysplasia resulting from narrow thorax, and pregnancy was terminated. Thanatophoric dysplasia was confirmed.

shortening of the extremities and a narrow thorax with a protuberant abdomen. Long bones may appear bowed with a "telephone receiver" appearance, and macrocephaly with frontal bossing may be evident. A trilobular appearance of the skull suggests type II, although this cloverleaf appearance may be identified in other anomalies, including homozygous achondroplasia and camptomelic dysplasia. Other anomalies that have been identified with thanatophoric dysplasia include ventriculomegaly and other central nervous system anomalies and renal and cardiovascular defects.[20]

Achondrogenesis

Achondrogenesis is a lethal skeletal dysplasia caused by a defect in cartilage formation that leads to abnormal bone formation and hypomineralization of the bones. The condition occurs in 1:40,000 live births and is usually transmitted in an autosomal recessive manner or as a new sporadic mutation.[22] The two types of achondrogenesis are classified based on histologic and radiologic characteristics.

Type I achondrogenesis (Parenti-Fraccaro) is the more severe of the two types and is characterized by severe micromelia, a lack of ossification of the spine and calvaria, and fractured ribs. Type II achondrogenesis (Langer-Saldino) is the more common of the two types and is characterized by micromelia and variable ossification of the spine and calvaria.

Sonographic Findings. The sonographic findings (Fig. 25-20) associated with achondrogenesis include extreme shortening of the extremities. Variable degrees of ossification may be noted of the spine and calvaria. The thorax and ribs may be shortened, and the ribs may appear to have multiple fractures. Polyhydramnios and a pseudohydropic appearance also may be identified in association with achondrogenesis.[22]

Achondroplasia

Achondroplasia is the most common of the nonlethal skeletal dysplasias, occurring in 5:100,000 to 15:100,000 births.[23] This condition occurs from abnormal endochondral bone formation that results in rhizomelia. The phenotypic appearance also includes a large head with a prominent forehead, a depressed nasal bridge, and marked lumbar lordosis. Individuals with this skeletal dysplasia can have a normal life expectancy, unless they have the uncommon severe complications of this disorder, including brainstem or cervical spinal cord compression, severe hydrocephalus, or spinal stenosis.

Achondroplasia is transmitted through an autosomal dominant mode, although most instances are the result of spontaneous mutation. There are heterozygous and homozygous forms of achondroplasia, and the homozygous form is rare and lethal.

Sonographic Findings. The sonographic findings of achondroplasia include long-bone shortening, especially of the proximal segment of the extremities, although limb shortening may not be obvious until the third trimester.[23] An additional finding of the trident hand may be documented when the hand is extended and the fingers appear shortened and of similar lengths. Macrocephalus with frontal bossing and a depressed nasal bridge may also be noted. The homozygous form of achondroplasia is indistinguishable from thanatophoric dysplasia.

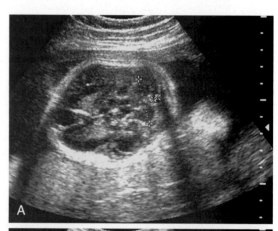

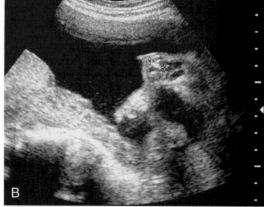

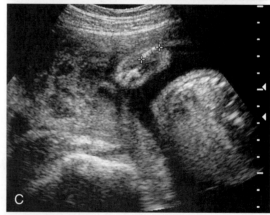

FIGURE 25-20 Fetus was diagnosed with achondrogenesis at birth and died within hours. **(A)**, Fetal head was poorly ossified as shown by compression of calvaria with transducer pressure. At 24 weeks' gestation measurements of femur **(B)** and humerus **(C)** correlated with approximately 13 weeks.

Short Rib–Polydactyly Syndrome

SRPS is an autosomal recessive skeletal dysplasia characterized by the presence of short limbs and ribs and polydactyly. The narrow thorax associated with this syndrome is of a lethal nature because most infants die shortly after birth of pulmonary hypoplasia. The four types of SRPS may be classified based on radiologic and pathologic findings; however, there is overlap of the clinical features that can cause differentiation to be challenging. Type I is also known as Saldino-Noonan syndrome, type II is also known as Majewski syndrome, type III is also known as Verma-Naumoff syndrome, and type IV is also known as Beemer-Langer syndrome.[24]

Sonographic Findings. The typical sonographic features of SRPS are micromelia, a narrow thorax with short ribs, and polydactyly (Fig. 25-21). Cleft lip and palate may also be identified, and numerous other anomalies have been identified in association with the various types.

Osteogenesis Imperfecta

OI is a rare disorder of connective tissue that leads to brittle bones (Fig. 25-22) and affects the teeth, ligaments, skin, and blue sclera. Four types of OI are seen, with types I and IV as the mildest forms transmitted through autosomal dominant modes of inheritance. Type III is a severe form transmitted through autosomal dominant or recessive modes. Type II is the most severe and lethal form of OI and may be transmitted through autosomal dominant or recessive modes or the result of a spontaneous mutation. Type II is the most likely to be diagnosed prenatally. Infants with type II OI usually die shortly after birth of pulmonary complications.

Sonographic Findings. The sonographic features (Fig. 25-23) of OI type II include decreased ossification of the bones, including the skull and multiple fractures, shortening, and bowing of the long bones.[25] Hypomineralization of the bones may be identified with noting that the bones are decreased in echogenicity with decreased attenuation. The fetal head structures may be seen exquisitely well,

and the reverberation artifact typically identified in the proximal hemisphere is absent. The calvaria may also be compressible with slight transducer pressure. The thorax appears narrow, and the limbs are shortened and may show marked deformities from the numerous fractures. Polyhydramnios may also be identified. OI type III may be diagnosed prenatally, although sonographic findings are less severe. An increased nuchal translucency has also been identified in the first trimester.[25]

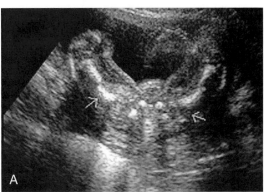

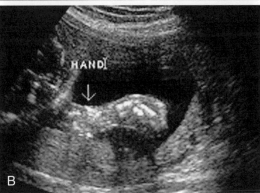

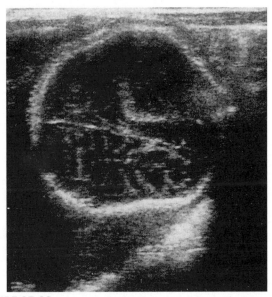

FIGURE 25-22 Multiple fractures of the femurs **(A)** and arms **(B)** can be seen. Concave, fractured ribs and a compressible calvaria were also noted in a fetus with OI type II.

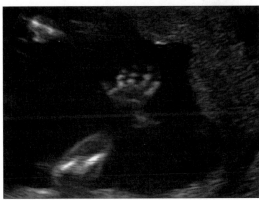

FIGURE 25-21 Polydactyly coupled with narrow thorax and micromelia suggests SRPS.

FIGURE 25-23 Poorly ossified calvaria is associated with OI type II.

VACTERL ASSOCIATION

The VACTERL association is characterized by a group of anomalies that occur in concert and include vertebral anomalies, anal atresia, cardiac defects, tracheoesophageal fistula, renal anomalies, and limb defects. The condition usually occurs spontaneously and is of unknown etiology. The VATER association is a more narrow classification of anomalies that includes vertebral anomalies, imperforate anus, tracheoesophageal fistula, and radial and renal dysplasias. The diagnosis of these spectra of fetal anomalies can be made with the identification of three features of the association. A single umbilical artery and polyhydramnios may also be identified.

This association is considered nonlethal, although morbidity and mortality are affected by the severity of the anomalies and the presence of polyhydramnios, which may lead to premature labor and delivery. Most infants need significant neonatal care and surgical treatment. Accurate diagnosis with sonographic evaluation may assist in adequate planning for pregnancy management and delivery and treatment options.

Limb Anomalies

Limb abnormalities are numerous and may occur in isolation or as a feature of a chromosomal anomaly, skeletal dysplasia, or syndrome. When a limb anomaly is identified sonographically, a thorough evaluation for additional anomalies should ensue.

Talipes, also known as clubfoot (Fig. 25-24, *A*), involves abnormalities of the foot and ankle. The condition may be unilateral or bilateral, and a male prevalence is seen. Most cases are isolated and idiopathic in nature. Talipes may be associated with oligohydramnios and chromosomal anomalies, skeletal dysplasias, and other syndromes. It has also been identified in multiple gestations and with spina bifida and some teratogens.

Rocker-bottom foot can be identified when the bottom of the foot is convex. This condition has been found in association with syndromes and chromosomal anomalies, especially trisomy 18.

Polydactyly (extra digits) may involve the hands or feet (see Fig. 25-21) and may be isolated or associated with syndromes or chromosomal anomalies. Abnormal posturing, including clenched hands (Fig. 25-24, *B*) or overlapping digits, may also be associated with chromosomal anomalies or syndromes, and clenched hands specifically has a high association with trisomy 18. Absence of all or part of an extremity may be the result of an amputation associated with amniotic band syndrome. Fusion of extremities or digits may be associated with a variety of syndromes.

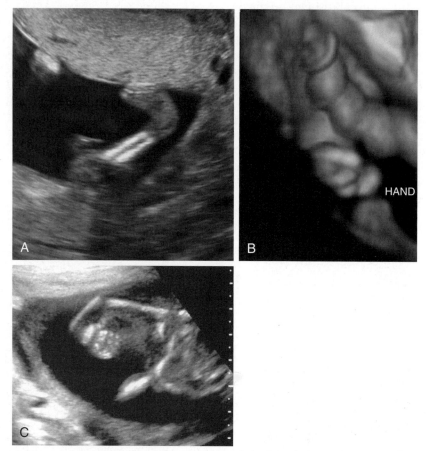

FIGURE 25-24 Limb abnormalities may be isolated or part of a syndrome, skeletal dysplasia, or chromosomal anomaly. **(A)**, Isolated clubfoot. **(B)**, Clenched hand was associated with trisomy 18. **(C)**, Clubhand deformity may be identified with absent radius.

Absence or hypoplasia of the radius is termed a radial ray defect and has been associated with skeletal dysplasias, chromosomal anomalies, and syndromes. The hand turns back toward the arm (Fig. 25-24, C), giving a characteristic clubhand appearance that may be identified sonographically.

SUMMARY

Obstetric sonography is challenging when a fetal anomaly is identified. An understanding of the many associated anomalies and completion of a thorough survey of the fetus are essential. Accurate diagnosis of an abnormality provides the patient and the physician with the information necessary to make decisions regarding pregnancy management, treatment, and delivery options.

CLINICAL SCENARIO—DIAGNOSIS

The fetal heart is malpositioned to the right, and a cystic structure is identified in the thorax, above the diaphragm. Combined with absence of an intraabdominal stomach bubble, a diagnosis of CDH can be assumed. Additionally, polyhydramnios and a two-vessel cord were noted. Because of the association with aneuploidy, an amniocentesis was performed to guide delivery and neonatal decisions. The karyotype was normal; however, CDH still has high morbidity and mortality rates secondary to pulmonary hypoplasia.

CASE STUDIES FOR DISCUSSION

1. A 32-year-old woman, gravida 1, para 0, is seen for sonographic evaluation for growth at 35 weeks' gestation. A prior sonogram at 20 weeks' gestation was within normal limits. The sonographic evaluation shows a head circumference (Fig. 25-25, A) appropriate for fetal age; however, the femur length (which was difficult to obtain) measures 28 weeks, 4 days (Fig. 25-25, B). Other long bones are also consistent with micromelia. What is the most likely diagnosis?

2. A 25-year-old woman, gravida 2, para 1, is seen for a sonogram at the maternal-fetal center at 24 weeks' gestation for evaluation of the fetal thorax. A single live fetus is identified with the finding in Figure 25-26. What is the most likely diagnosis?

3. A 36-year-old woman, gravida 3, para 2, is seen for a sonogram because of advanced maternal age at 18 weeks' gestation. Sonographic evaluation reveals the finding in Figure 25-27. The rest of the examination is within normal limits. What is the most likely diagnosis?

4. A sonographic evaluation is performed for size and dates. The sonogram shows the finding in Figure 25-28 in addition to a bilateral cleft lip and multiple echogenic foci in the heart. What is the most likely diagnosis?

5. A 39-year-old woman is seen for late prenatal care. The sonogram reveals the finding in Figure 25-29. The remainder of the examination is unremarkable. What is the most likely diagnosis?

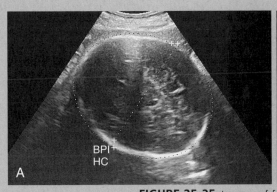
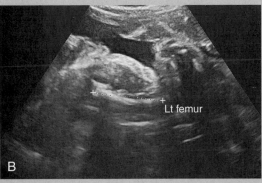

FIGURE 25-25 Images of fetal head **(A)** and femur **(B)**.

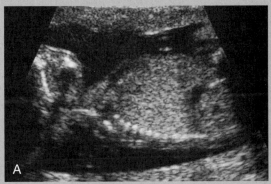
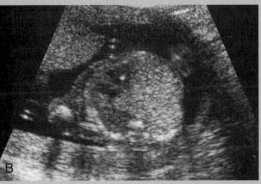

FIGURE 25-26 Longitudinal **(A)** and transverse **(B)** views of the fetal thorax.

Continued

CASE STUDIES FOR DISCUSSION—cont'd

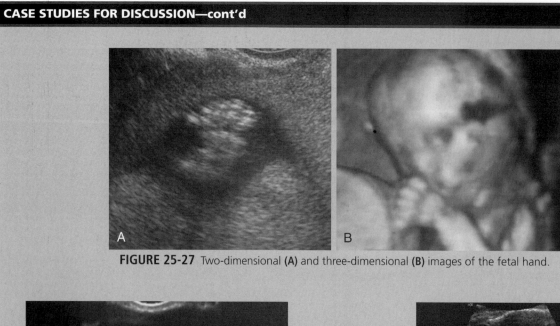

FIGURE 25-27 Two-dimensional **(A)** and three-dimensional **(B)** images of the fetal hand.

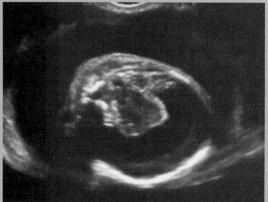

FIGURE 25-28 Fetal head.

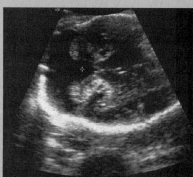

FIGURE 25-29 Image of fetal head shows cerebellum and region of cisterna magna.

STUDY QUESTIONS

1. A sonographic evaluation of a 29-week gestation reveals that the lateral ventricle has a teardrop shape with asymmetric enlargement of the occipital horn, and the fetal head measurement is consistent with established due date. The remainder of the examination is unremarkable. This is consistent with which of the following?
   a. Colpocephaly
   b. Hydranencephaly
   c. Hydrocephaly
   d. Ventriculomegaly

2. A 35-year-old woman is seen for a sonographic evaluation for advanced maternal age. The examination reveals polyhydramnios and absence of the stomach. This is most suggestive of which of the following anomalies?
   a. CDH
   b. Cystic fibrosis
   c. Duodenal atresia
   d. Esophageal atresia

3. Sonographic evaluation of a fetal head reveals hypotelorism with a midline facial cleft. Severe microcephaly is present, preventing adequate visualization of fetal head anatomy. On the basis of the findings that are evident, what is the most likely diagnosis?
   a. DWM
   b. Holoprosencephaly
   c. Hydranencephaly
   d. Hydrocephaly

4. Which of the following describes the decreased length of the entire extremity?
   a. Mesomelia
   b. Micromelia
   c. Phocomelia
   d. Rhizomelia

5. A 35-year-old woman is seen for an obstetric sonogram, late prenatal care, and an uncertain last menstrual period. The sonogram establishes a gestational age of 27 weeks, 4 days. Polyhydramnios and the presence of two stomachs in the fetal abdomen

are identified. This is suggestive of which of the following anomalies?
a. CDH
b. Duodenal atresia
c. Esophageal atresia
d. Tracheoesophageal fistula

6. A transverse image of a fetal thorax shows a cystic structure adjacent to a malpositioned fetal heart. A normally placed stomach is not visualized in the fetal abdomen. This is most suggestive of which of the following anomalies?
a. CCAM
b. CDH
c. Esophageal atresia
d. Pulmonary sequestration

7. A cystic lesion is identified in the fetal abdomen adjacent to the bladder. No other anomalies are identified. A normal stomach and gallbladder are seen; the gender is female. This is most suggestive of which of the following?
a. Duplication cyst
b. Mesenteric cyst
c. Ovarian cyst
d. Urachal cyst

8. A 31-year-old woman is seen for a sonogram for an anatomy scan at 30 weeks' gestation for size greater than dates. The examination shows an approximately 31-week gestation based on fetal head measurement. The femoral measurements are consistent with 18 weeks' gestation, and the humeral lengths are consistent with 19 weeks' gestation. The fetal spine is almost translucent without any shadowing, the brain is extremely well visualized, and the thorax is extremely small compared with the abdominal circumference. Polyhydramnios is also noted. This would be most consistent with which of the following?
a. Achondrogenesis
b. Achondroplasia
c. OI
d. Thanatophoric dysplasia

9. Clenched hands are identified in a fetus that has a heart defect. Which of the following is most likely?
a. VACTERL association
b. Trisomy 13
c. Trisomy 18
d. Trisomy 21

10. A sonographic evaluation reveals a fetus with short, bowed limbs with multiple fractures and a compressible skull. This would be most suggestive of which of the following?
a. Achondrogenesis
b. Diastrophic dysplasia

c. OI type II
d. Thanatophoric dysplasia

REFERENCES

1. Durfee SM, Kim FM, Benson CB: Postnatal outcome of fetuses with the prenatal diagnosis of asymmetric hydrocephalus, *J Ultrasound Med* 20:263–268, 2001.
2. Diawara FM, Diallo M, Camara M, et al: Sonographic detection of holoprosencephaly with cyclopia and proboscis, *JDMS* 26:28–31, 2010.
3. Kagan KO, Staboulidou I, Syngelaki A, et al: The 11-13-week scan: diagnosis and outcome of holoprosencephaly, exomphalos and megacystis, *Ultrasound Obstet Gynecol* 36:10–14, 2010.
4. Counter SA: Brainstem mediation of the stapedius muscle reflex in hydranencephaly, *Acta Otolaryngol* 127:498–504, 2007.
5. Zalel Y, Gilboa Y, Babis L, et al: Rotation of the vermis as a cause of enlarged cisterna magna on prenatal imaging, *Ultrasound Obstet Gynecol* 27:490–493, 2006.
6. Lee W, Vettraino IM, Comstock CH, et al: Prenatal diagnosis of herniated Dandy-Walker cysts, *J Ultrasound Med* 24:841–848, 2005.
7. Volpe P, Paladini D, Resta M, et al: Characteristics, associations and outcome of partial agenesis of the corpus callosum in the fetus, *Ultrasound Obstet Gynecol* 27:509–516, 2006.
8. Gillham JC, Anand S, Bullen PJ: Antenatal detection of cleft lip with or without cleft palate: incidence of associated chromosomal and structural anomalies, *Ultrasound Obstet Gynecol* 34:410–415, 2009.
9. Teoh M, Meagher S: First-trimester diagnosis of micrognathia as a presentation of Pierre Robin syndrome, *Ultrasound Obstet Gynecol* 21:616–618, 2003.
10. Knox E, Lissauer D, Khan K, et al: Prenatal detection of pulmonary hypoplasia in fetuses with congenital diaphragmatic hernia: a systematic review and meta-analysis of diagnostic studies, *J Matern Fetal Neonatal Med* 23:579–588, 2010.
11. Sanz-Cortes M, Raga F, Bonilla-Musoles F: Prenatal diagnosis of congenital cystic adenomatoid malformation using three-dimensional inversion rendering: a case report, *J Obstet Gynaecol Res* 34:631–634, 2008.
12. Tran H, Fink MA, Crameri J, et al: Congenital cystic adenomatoid malformation: monitoring the antenatal and short-term neonatal outcome, *Aust N Z J Obstet Gynaecol* 48:462–466, 2008.
13. York D, Swartz A, Johnson A, et al: Prenatal detection and evaluation of an extralobar pulmonary sequestration in the posterior mediastinum, *Ultrasound Obstet Gynecol* 27:214–216, 2006.
14. Ruano R, Ramlho AS, de Freitas RCM, et al: Three-dimensional ultrasonographic assessment of fetal total lung volume as a prognostic factor in primary pleural effusion, *J Ultrasound Med* 31:1731–1739, 2012.
15. Mitani Y, Hasegqwa T, Kubota A, et al: Prenatal findings of concomitant duodenal and esophageal atresia without tracheoesophageal fistula (gross type A), *J Clin Ultrasound* 37:403–405, 2009.
16. Amagada JO, Premkumar G, Arnold JM, et al: Prenatal meconium peritonitis managed expectantly, *J Obstet Gynaecol* 24:311–312, 2004.
17. Sepulveda W, Dickens K, Casasbuenas A, et al: Fetal abdominal cysts in the first trimester: prenatal detection and clinical significance, *Ultrasound Obstet Gynecol* 32:860–864, 2008.
18. Shannon SA, Henningsen C: Sacrococcygeal teratoma, *JDMS* 20:351–354, 2004.
19. Ruono R, Molho M, Roume J, et al: Prenatal diagnosis of fetal skeletal dysplasias by combining two-dimensional and three-dimensional ultrasound and intrauterine and three-dimensional helical computer tomography, *Ultrasound Obstet Gynecol* 24:134–140, 2004.

20. Tsai P-Y, Chang C-H, Yu C-H, et al: Thanatophoric dysplasia: role of 3-demensional sonography, *J Clin Ultrasound* 37:31–34, 2009.

21. Bekdache GN, Begum M, Al-Gazali L, et al: Prenatal diagnosis of thanatophoric dysplasia and obstetrical challenges, *J Obstet Gynaecol* 30:628–630, 2010.

22. Taner MZ, Kurdoglu M, Taskiran C, et al: Prenatal diagnosis of achondrogenesis type I: a case report, *Cases J* 1:406, 2008.

23. Chitty LS, Griffin DR, Meaney C, et al: New aids for the non-invasive prenatal diagnosis of achondroplasia: dysmorphic features, charts of fetal size and molecular confirmation using cell-free DNA in maternal plasma, *Ultrasound Obstet Gynecol* 37:283–289, 2011.

24. Taori KB, Shardidre KG, Krishnan V, et al: Diagnosis of short rib polydactyly syndrome type IV (Beemer-Langer syndrome) with cystic hygroma: a case report, *J Clin Ultrasound* 37:406–409, 2009.

25. Hiseh CT-C, Yeh G-P, Wu H-H, et al: Fetus with osteogenesis imperfecta presenting as increased nuchal translucency thickness in the first trimester, *J Clin Ultrasound* 36:119–122, 2008.

26

Abnormal Fetal Echocardiography

Sandra Hagen-Ansert

CLINICAL SCENARIO

A 33-year-old patient who is pregnant with her third child is seen for her first visit with the obstetric service at 24 weeks. Her first child died shortly after birth of hypoplastic left heart syndrome (HLHS). Her second child is 4 years old and is undergoing evaluation for a systolic ejection murmur. The mother has a history of a bicuspid aortic valve and underwent a balloon valvulotomy nearly 20 years ago. Because of this high risk for congenital heart disease, she was referred to pediatric cardiology for further fetal echocardiographic evaluation.

A complete fetal echocardiogram was performed. The aortic valve was thickened with reduced cusp excursion. The ascending aorta measured 2.1 mm, and the pulmonary artery measured 4.1 mm. The left ventricle was thicker and smaller than the right ventricle, measuring 6.7 mm compared with the right ventricular measurement of 8.0 mm. The velocity taken at the root of the aorta was increased at 2.5 m/s. What conclusions may be drawn from the fetal echocardiogram? What is the risk of congenital heart disease in this fetus?

OBJECTIVES

- Describe the echocardiographic protocol for evaluating the fetal heart.
- List the various septal defects and their sonographic appearances.
- Differentiate between a complete and a partial atrioventricular septal defect.
- Name the echocardiographic findings in the tetralogy of Fallot.
- List the echocardiographic findings in a fetus with critical aortic stenosis.
- Describe the sonographic characteristics of hypoplastic left heart syndrome.
- Identify the risk factors associated with congenital heart disease.
- Describe how the sonographer may identify transposition of the great arteries.

The evaluation of the fetal heart has become a routine addition to the perinatal sonographic evaluation. This chapter provides a guideline for the sonographer to become better acquainted with the cardiologist's view of the fetal heart. The fetal heart protocol is presented, followed by a brief introduction to some common congenital heart defects (i.e., atrial septal defect [ASD], ventricular septal defect [VSD], atrioventricular septal defect [AVSD], tetralogy of Fallot [TOF], transposition of the great arteries [TGA], and HLHS) the sonographer may encounter during the routine fetal sonographic evaluation. In general practice, once a fetal heart abnormality has been observed, the patient is referred to a specialty center with a pediatric cardiologist experienced in congenital heart disease to provide ongoing care, counseling, and surgical options for the patient.

INCIDENCE OF CONGENITAL HEART DISEASE IN THE FETUS

Congenital heart disease in the fetus represents the most common major congenital malformation with an incidence of 8:1000 live births. This figure encompasses all types of heart disease (e.g., tiny secundum ASD, mild valvular pulmonary stenosis, patent ductus arteriosus, and small muscular or membranous VSDs).

RISK FACTORS INDICATING FETAL ECHOCARDIOGRAPHY

Specific risk factors indicate the fetus is at a higher than normal risk for congenital heart disease to warrant a structured fetal echocardiography evaluation. These risk factors may be divided into the following three categories: fetal, maternal, and familial risk factors.

Fetal Risk Factors

Fetal risk factors include abnormal visceral or cardiac situs; abnormal four-chamber view or outflow tracts; cardiac arrhythmia; aneuploidy (50% of infants with trisomy 21 have congenital heart disease); two-vessel umbilical cord; extracardiac structural malformation; intrauterine growth restriction; abnormal amniocentesis indicating a chromosomal anomaly; abnormal amniotic fluid collections; abnormal heart rate; twins; increased nuchal translucency thickness; and other anomalies as detected with the sonogram, such as hydrops fetalis.

Maternal Risk Factors

Maternal risk factors include the previous occurrence of congenital heart disease in siblings or parents; a maternal disease known to affect the fetus, such as diabetes mellitus or connective tissue disease (i.e., lupus erythematosus); viral syndrome (mumps, coxsackievirus, influenza, rubella, cytomegalovirus); teratogen exposure; or maternal use of drugs such as lithium or alcohol.

Familial Risk Factors

Familial risk factors include genetic syndromes or the presence of congenital heart disease in a sibling. If a sibling has one of the most common cardiovascular abnormalities (VSD, ASD, patent ductus arteriosus, TOF), the risk of recurrence ranges from 2.5% to 3%. When one parent has one of the common congenital heart defects, the risk of recurrence ranges from 2.5% (ASD) to 4% (VSD, patent ductus arteriosus, TOF). Other syndromes include DiGeorge, long QT, Noonan, Marfan, and Williams syndromes. Tuberous sclerosis tumors may also be found within the fetal heart.

SONOGRAPHIC EVALUATION OF THE FETAL HEART

Fetal Cardiac Rhythm

The fetal heart undergoes multiple changes during the embryologic stages. One of these stages is the progression of the cardiac electrical system, which matures at the end of fetal life to cause a normal sinus rhythm in the cardiac cycle. The pacemaker of the heart is the sinoatrial node, which fires 60 to 100 electrical impulses each minute. From the sinoatrial node, the electrical activity travels to the atrioventricular node, across the bundle of His to the ventricles, and down the right and left bundle branches, before being distributed to the rest of the cardiac muscle. This electrical activity precedes the ventricular contraction of the heart.

During this developmental stage, deceleration of the normal fetal heart rate from 150 beats per minute to a bradycardia stage (<55 beats per minute), or even a pause of a few seconds, is common during the course of a fetal echocardiogram. This deceleration may occur if the fetus is lying on the umbilical cord or if the transducer pressure is too great. The fetus should be given a recovery time to bring the heart rate to a normal sinus rhythm, which is usually done by changing the position of the mother (i.e., rolling to her left side to release pressure from inferior vena cava compression) or by releasing the pressure from the transducer.

Normally, the fetal heart should have a baseline rate of 110 to 160 beats per minute. Some variability may be seen in rhythm and acceleration. Abnormal rate and rhythm may lead to fetal asphyxia, and early recognition of "normal" versus "abnormal" is critical. Short episodes of sinus bradycardia may be common in early pregnancy. However, if the bradycardia (<100 beats per minute) continues for several minutes, it is abnormal. Likewise, sinus tachycardia (>160 beats per minute) is common in later stages of pregnancy and may be associated with fetal movement. This rate becomes abnormal when it exceeds 200 beats per minute or has frequent "dropped" beats (premature ventricular contractions).

The sonographer should evaluate the fetus for normal cardiac structure and signs of cardiac failure (enlarged right ventricle, hydrops, ascites, edema, pleural effusion, or pericardial effusion) and perform a simultaneous M-mode study with the transducer perpendicular through the atrial and ventricular cavities. Every ventricular contraction should be preceded by an atrial contraction. Alterations in the rhythm pattern seen during fetal development may result from premature atrial contractions and premature ventricular contractions, supraventricular tachycardia, tachycardia, or atrioventricular block.

Fetal Echocardiogram

Ideally, a clear redundant view of the cardiac anatomy occurs when the fetus is at least 20 to 22 weeks of gestational age. Although reports in the literature have demonstrated some congenital heart defects with transvaginal sonography in the first trimester,[1] it is difficult to image all of the cardiac anatomy clearly. In addition, some cardiac lesions may not show changes until much later in fetal development (e.g., HLHS).

A fetal echocardiogram always begins with the determination of fetal lie, fetal number, activity level, location and size of the placenta, evaluation of the umbilical cord, gestational age, and fluid assessment. The visceroatrial situs should be determined. A transverse view of the abdomen reveals the aorta anterior and to the left of the spine (closest to the left atrium); the inferior vena cava is anterior and to the right with drainage into the

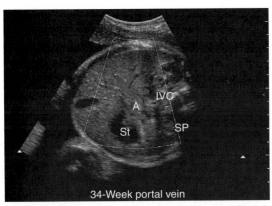

FIGURE 26-1 Fetal situs is normal. Heart position is in the left chest, and the apex of the heart points to the left; stomach *(ST)* is to the left; aorta is anterior and to the left of the spine; and inferior vena cava is anterior and to the right of the spine. (See Color Plate 33.)

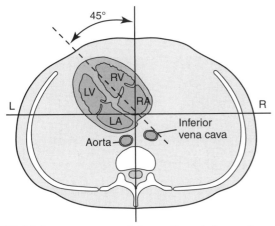

FIGURE 26-2 Measurement of the cardiac axis from a four-chamber view plane of the fetal chest. The apex of the heart should not exceed a 45-degree angle from the line drawn perpendicular to the fetal spine. *LA,* Left atrium; *LV,* left ventricle; *RA,* right atrium; *RV,* right ventricle.

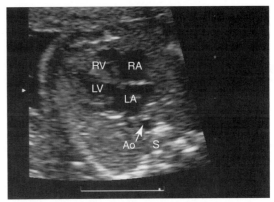

FIGURE 26-3 Normal fetal heart lies horizontal in the fetal thorax, with the apex pointing to the left hip. As the transducer is angled cephalad, the four-chamber view of the heart is seen within the thorax. The spine *(S)* is posterior to the aorta *(AO)*. The left atrium *(LA)* lies directly anterior to the aorta. *LV,* Left ventricle; *RA,* right atrium; *RV,* right ventricle.

right atrium (Fig. 26-1; see Color Plate 33). The stomach should be anterior and leftward.

Four-Chamber View. The four-chamber view provides the groundwork for the cardiac examination. The normal position of the fetal heart is in the left thorax with the apex directed about 45 degrees to the left (Fig. 26-2). The size of the heart should be less than one-third of the area of the thorax, and the heart circumference should be less than half of the thoracic circumference. Four chambers of the heart should be clearly present with the right-sided chambers slightly larger than the left-sided chambers (Fig. 26-3).

Venous Drainage. The venous drainage of the heart is through the coronary sinus, which may be seen coursing from left to right just superior to the mitral groove. Enlargement of the coronary sinus may prompt evaluation for an abnormality known as left-sided superior vena cava. Four pulmonary veins drain into the left atrium (two upper and two lower). These veins deliver oxygenated blood flow from the lungs to the heart after

birth. Usually at least two or three of these veins may be identified as they drain into the left atrium (Fig. 26-4). Color Doppler imaging may aid in their visualization.

Atrial and Ventricular Septa. The four chambers should be divided by the interatrial septum and interventricular septum to separate the right from the left side. In the fetus, a communication exists between the right and left atrial cavities known as the foramen ovale. This is found in the center of the atrial septum, and the "flap" of the foramen moves slightly during the cardiac cycle with greater movement toward the left atrium. The sonographer should be able to identify atrial septal tissue superior and inferior to this foramen ovale flap. The ventricular septum is thicker than the atrial septum. This septum has two anatomic descriptors, the membranous (thin) and muscular (thicker) septa. The ventricular septum is approximately the same thickness as the posterior myocardial wall of the left ventricle. Septal defects may occur anywhere along the ventricular septum with membranous defects slightly more visible than muscular defects.

Ventricles. The right and the left ventricles should extend to the cardiac apex, and both ventricles should squeeze simultaneously during systole (Fig. 26-5). There is a bright linear structure near the apex of the trabeculated right ventricle, which is the moderator band. The blood leaves the right ventricle through the pulmonary artery via the right and left pulmonary arteries to their respective lung. The left ventricle is smooth-walled compared with the right ventricle. The aorta delivers blood from the left ventricle to the rest of the body.

Atrioventricular Valves. The two atrioventricular valves separate the filling chambers (atria) from the pumping chambers (ventricles). The septal leaflet of the tricuspid valve is slightly more apical than the left-sided mitral valve leaflets. These leaflets should be thin, pliable structures that open fully with ventricular diastole and close completely during systole. Doppler evaluation

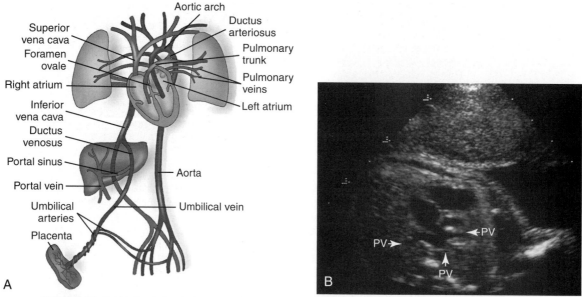

FIGURE 26-4 **(A)**, Fetal circulation. **(B)**, Three of the four pulmonary veins *(PV)* enter the left atrial cavity.

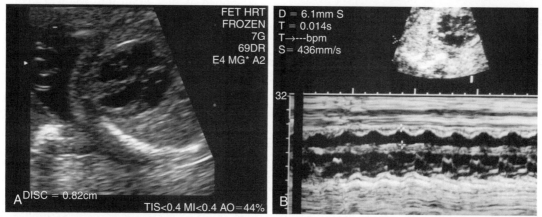

FIGURE 26-5 **(A)**, Left ventricle is measured at the level of the mitral anulus. **(B)**, M-mode measurements may also be made at the level of the anulus for the right ventricle and left ventricle.

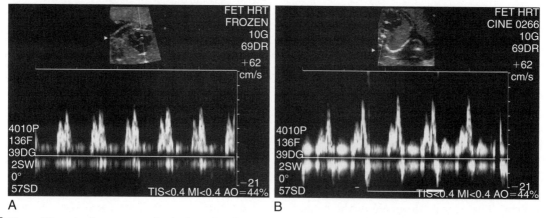

FIGURE 26-6 Normal Doppler flow patterns in the four-chamber view of the mitral **(A)** and tricuspid **(B)** leaflets. The smaller first peak is the *e* wave; the second higher peak is the *a* wave.

of the atrioventricular valves shows a biphasic motion as the valve opens in diastole and closes in systole (Fig. 26-6).

Semilunar Valves and Great Arteries. The pulmonary anulus should be at least the same size, if not slightly larger, as the aortic anulus (Fig. 26-7; see Color Plate 34). The long-axis view is best to image the base of the aorta, ascending aorta, and sometimes the arch. The normal aorta should be seen in the "center" of the heart, arising from the base of the left ventricle. Continuity between

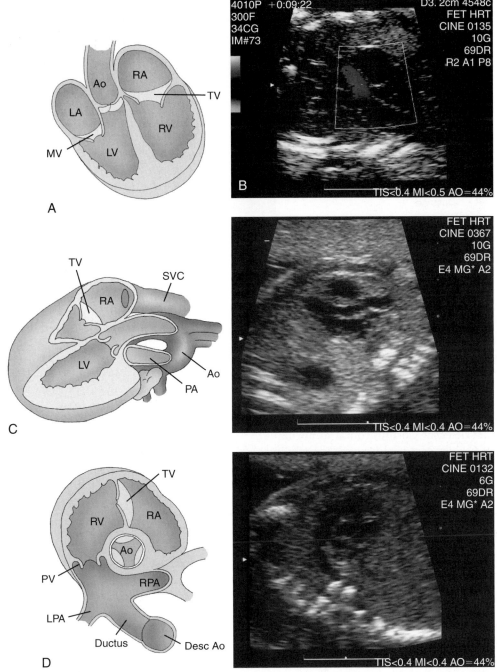

FIGURE 26-7 (A), Four-chamber view. **(B),** Aortic outflow is shown in red in this four-chamber view. (See Color Plate 34.) **(C),** Long-axis view of the left ventricular outflow tract shows the crescent left ventricle *(LV)*, the interventricular septum and its continuity with the anterior wall of the aorta *(Ao)*, and the posterior wall of the aorta with its continuity with the anterior leaflet of the mitral valve. The fetal echocardiogram was imaged at early diastole, with the mitral valve open fully and aortic valve closed. **(D),** High, short-axis view of the great vessels. The right ventricular outflow tract wraps around anterior to the aorta. The pulmonary artery arises from the right ventricle and bifurcates into right and left branches. The ductal insertion occurs midway between the bifurcation of the pulmonary vessels. The great vessel diameters may be measured at the level of the cusps. *Desc Ao,* Descending aorta; *LA,* left atrium; *LPA,* left pulmonary artery; *LV,* left ventricle; *PV,* pulmonary vein; *RA,* right atrium; *RPA,* right pulmonary artery; *TV,* tricuspid valve.

the anterior wall of the aorta with the interventricular septum is normal; continuity between the posterior wall of the aorta and anterior leaflet of the mitral valve should be present. The pulmonary artery is anterior and to the right of the aorta as it arises from the right ventricular cavity. The main pulmonary artery bifurcates into right and left pulmonary artery branches that drain into the

lungs. The semilunar valves should be thin, lunar-shaped cusps that open fully in systole.

Ductal Arch. The ductal arch may be seen best on the high short-axis view or sagittal view (Fig. 26-8). This short-axis view demonstrates the trifurcation of the main pulmonary artery into the right pulmonary artery (which wraps around the aorta in the short-axis view), the left

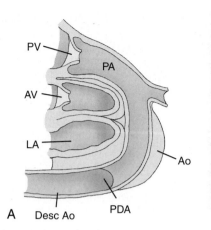
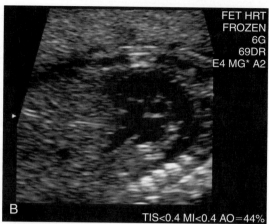

FIGURE 26-8 **(A),** The ductal arch is found slightly inferior to the aortic arch. **(B),** Short-axis view shows the main pulmonary artery and ductal arch as it empties into the descending aorta *(Desc Ao)*. *Ao,* Aorta; *AV,* aortic valve; *LA,* left atrium; *PA,* pulmonary artery; *PDA,* patent ductus arteriosus; *PV,* pulmonary valve.

pulmonary artery, and the large ductus arteriosus. The sagittal view shows the ductus resembling a "hockey stick" as it drains into the descending aorta.

CONGENITAL HEART ANOMALIES

The most common type of congenital heart disease is VSD, followed by ASDs and pulmonary stenosis. Environmental factors may influence the development of congenital heart disease. Chromosomal abnormalities also have a higher association with congenital heart disease (e.g., fetuses with trisomy 21 have a 50% incidence rate of congenital heart disease, specifically AVSDs).

Atrial Septal Defects

ASDs are usually not recognized during fetal life, unless a large part of the atrial septum is missing. The embryologic development of the atrial septum evolves in several stages; interruption of any of these stages could lead to the formation of an ASD. A natural communication exists between the right and left atria during fetal life. This communication (foramen ovale) is covered by the flap of the foramen ovale that remains open in the fetal heart until after birth, when the pressures from the left heart become greater than the pressures in the right heart to force the foramen to close completely. After birth, a remnant of the foramen ovale, now closed, is a thin depression known as fossa ovalis. Failure of the foramen to close may result in one type of ASD, the secundum defect.

The area of the foramen ovale is thinner than in the surrounding atrial tissue; it is prone to signal dropout during sonographic evaluation, particularly in the apical four-chamber view when the transducer is parallel to the septum. Any break in the atrial septum in this view must be confirmed with the short-axis or perpendicular four-chamber view (subcostal view) in which the septum is

more perpendicular to the transducer. Because of beam-width artifact, the edges of the defect may be slightly blunted and appear brighter than the remaining septum.

In utero, the natural flow is right to left across the foramen because the pressures are slightly higher on the right. A small reversal of flow may be present. The flap of the foramen should open into the left atrial cavity. The flap should not be so large as to touch the lateral wall of the atrium; when this redundancy of the foramen occurs, the sinoatrial node may become agitated in the right atrium and cause fetal arrhythmias. The sonographer should sweep inferior to superior along the atrial septum to identify the three parts of the septum: the primum septum (near the center or crux of the heart), the foramen ovale (middle of the atrial septum), and the septum secundum (base of the heart, near the right upper pulmonary vein and superior vena cava).

Secundum Atrial Septal Defect. Secundum ASD is the most common atrial defect and occurs in the area of the foramen ovale (Fig. 26-9; see Color Plate 35). Usually an absence of the foramen ovale flap is noted, with the foramen ovale opening larger than normal. The size of the normal foramen should measure at least 60% of the aortic diameter (i.e., if the aorta measures 4mm, the foramen should be at least 2.4mm).

Doppler tracings of the septal defect with the sample volume placed at the site of the defect show a right-to-left flow with a velocity of 20 to 30 cm/s. The flow patterns of the mitral and tricuspid valves are slightly increased with the increased shunt flow.

Primum Atrial Septal Defect. The ostium primum ASD occurs at the base of the atrial septum. This defect may be an isolated defect or may have an abnormal "cleft" mitral valve as an associated anomaly. This defect is best imaged in the four-chamber view with the cardiac chamber perpendicular to the transducer (Fig. 26-10).

Sinus Venosus ASD. The sinus venosus ASD is technically more difficult to visualize. This defect lies in the superior portion of the atrial septum (Fig. 26-11), close

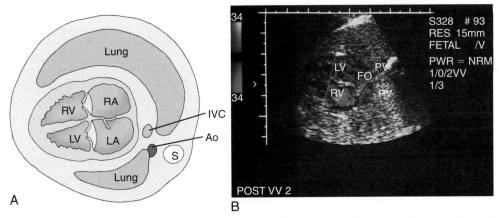

A   **B**

FIGURE 26-9 **(A)**, The most common type of ASD occurs in the area of the foramen ovale, known as the secundum defect. **(B)**, In the fetus, normal flow should occur at the level of the foramen ovale *(FO)*. (See Color Plate 35.) *Ao*, Aorta; *IVC*, inferior vena cava; *LA*, left atrium; *LV*, left ventricle; *PV*, pulmonary vein; *RA*, right atrium; *RV*, right ventricle.

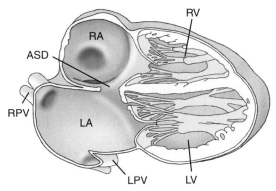

FIGURE 26-10 Ostium primum *ASD* in four-chamber view. *LA*, left atrium; *LPV*, left pulmonary vein; *LV*, left ventricle; *RA*, right atrium; *RPV*, right pulmonary vein; *RV*, right ventricle.

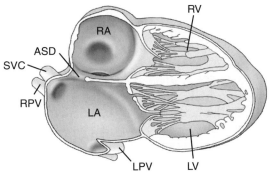

FIGURE 26-11 Sinus venosus *ASD* near the entrance of the superior vena cava *(SVC)* and right upper pulmonary vein *(RPV)*. *LA*, Left atrium; *LPV*, left pulmonary vein; *LV*, left ventricle; *RA*, right atrium; *RV*, right ventricle.

to the inflow pattern of the superior vena cava, and is best visualized with the four-chamber view. If signs of right ventricular volume overload are present, with no ASD obvious, care should be taken to study the septum in search of a sinus venosus type of defect.

Partial anomalous pulmonary venous drainage of the right pulmonary vein is usually associated with this type of defect; identification of the entry site of the pulmonary veins into the left atrial cavity is important. Color-flow

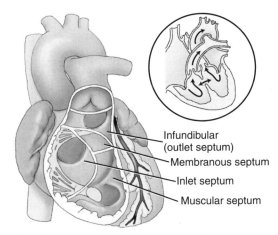

FIGURE 26-12 VSD. Portions of the ventricular septum showing the infundibulum (outlet septum), membranous septum, inlet septum, and muscular septa.

mapping is useful for this type of problem because the sonographer can visualize the venous return to the left atrium and a flow pattern crossing into the right atrial cavity.

Ventricular Septal Defect

VSD is the most common congenital lesion of the heart, accounting for 30% of all structural heart defects. The septum is divided into two basic segments: the thin membranous and the thicker muscular septum (Fig. 26-12). Septal defects may be found in numerous sites within the septum. Muscular defects are usually very small and may be multiple. These smaller defects often close spontaneously shortly after birth. The prognosis is good for a patient with a single VSD. However, the association of other cardiac anomalies, such as TOF, single ventricle, TGA, and endocardial cushion defect, is increased when a VSD is found.

Membranous Septal Defect. Membranous defects are more common and may be found just inferior to the aorta or in the roof of the right ventricular septum

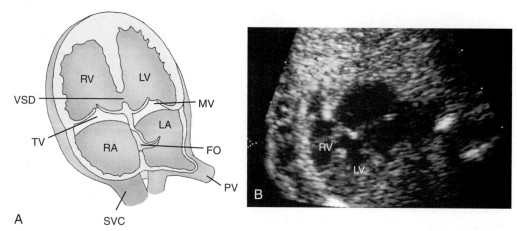

FIGURE 26-13 **(A),** Membranous septal defect is shown in four-chamber view. The defect is located in the inflow of the ventricles. The muscular defect in this four-chamber view may be large, small, or multiple along the thicker part of the septum. **(B),** Large isolated membranous septal defect shown in four-chamber view. The edges of the defect are slightly brighter than the rest of the septum. *FO,* Foramen ovale; *LA,* left atrium; *LV,* left ventricle; *MV,* mitral valve; *PV,* pulmonary vein; *RA,* right atrium; *RV,* right ventricle; *SVC,* superior vena cava; *TV,* tricuspid valve; *VSD,* ventricular septal defect.

(perimembranous or supracristal) (Fig. 26-13). The perimembranous VSD may be classified as membranous, aneurysmal, or supracristal. The significant anatomic landmark is the crista supraventricularis ridge. The defect lies either above or below this ridge. Defects that lie above are supracristal. These defects are located just beneath the pulmonary orifice with the pulmonary valve forming part of the superior margin of the interventricular communication. Defects that lie below the crista are infracristal and may be found in the membranous or muscular part of the septum. These are the most common defects.

The lesion may be partially covered by the septal leaflet of the tricuspid valve, and careful evaluation of this area with spectral Doppler and color flow tracings is necessary. The membranous defect is found just inferior to the aortic leaflets; sometimes the aortic leaflet is sucked into this defect. The presence of an isolated VSD in utero usually does not change the hemodynamics of the fetus. Septal defects must be at least half the size of the aorta to be imaged; defects smaller than 2mm are not detected with fetal echocardiography. Malalignment (override) of the anterior wall of the aorta with the septum is a sign that a septal defect may be present. While performing the four-chamber view, the sonographer should carefully sweep the transducer posterior to record the inlet part of the septum and sweep anterior to record the outlet part of the septum.

Muscular Septal Defect. A less common infracristal defect is located in the muscular septum. These defects may be large or small, single or multiple fenestrated holes. Multiple defects are more difficult to repair, and their combination may have the same ventricular overload effect as a single large communication. Pressures between the right and left heart are different in utero, and a small defect probably would not show a flow velocity change.

Atrioventricular Septal Defect

The septum primum and endocardial cushions should fuse during the normal development of the fetal heart. Failure of the fusion may result in abnormalities that may cause a defect in the primum septum or membranous septum or maldevelopment of the atrioventricular valves (Fig. 26-14). AVSD is subdivided into complete or partial forms. The defect occurs at the crux (center) of the heart. AVSD is associated with an increased incidence rate of Down syndrome.

Partial Atrioventricular Septal Defect. A fetus with a partial AVSD shows failure of the septum primum to fuse with the endocardial cushion. In addition, there is usually a cleft abnormality with the anterior leaflet mitral valve, which may lead to regurgitation into the atrial cavity. A cleft mitral valve means that the anterior part of the leaflet is divided into two parts: medial and lateral. When the leaflet closes, blood leaks through this hole into the left atrial cavity. The leaflet is usually malformed, causing further regurgitation into the atrium. The absence of the atrioventricular septum results in the absence of the normal apical displacement of the septal leaflet of the tricuspid valve, and the sonographer may note the tricuspid and mitral valves insert onto the ventricular septum at the same level.

The crux of the heart is carefully analyzed in the four-chamber view by sweeping the transducer anteroposteriorly to record the outlet and inlet portions of the membranous septum. Spectral Doppler and color flow are extremely useful in determining the direction and degree of regurgitation present in the atrioventricular valves and the direction of shunt flow. Increased right heart pressure causes a right ventricular-to-left atrial shunt in the fetus.

The best views to search for abnormalities in the atrioventricular valves (e.g., the presence of a cleft) are

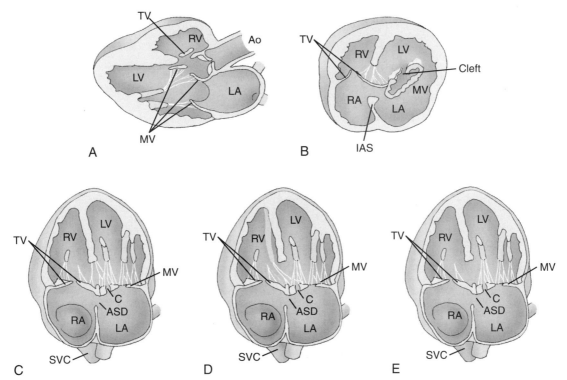

FIGURE 26-14 AVSD. **(A)**, Long-axis view shows discontinuity of the anterior leaflet of the mitral valve *(MV)* with the posterior wall of the aorta *(Ao)*. The membranous septal defect is seen. **(B)**, Short-axis view through the atrioventricular valves shows the cleft in the anterior leaflet of the mitral valve. The primum septal defect is seen. **(C)**, Four-chamber view showing the Rastelli type A large defect in the center (crux) of the heart. Membranous and primum septal defects are seen with the cleft mitral valve. There is a common leaflet from the anterior mitral leaflet to the septal tricuspid leaflet. **(D)**, Rastelli type B defect shows chordal attachments from the medial portion of the cleft mitral leaflet related to the papillary muscle on the right side of the septal defect. **(E)**, Rastelli type C defect shows a free-floating common atrioventricular leaflet *(C).ASD*, atrial septal defect; *IAS*, interarterial septum; *LA*, left atrium; *LV*, left ventricle; *RV*, right ventricle; *SVC*, superior vena cava; *TV*, tricuspid valve.

the long-axis and short-axis views. To search for chordal attachment or overriding or straddling of the valves and to identify the defect in the primum atrial septum, the four-chamber view is the best.

Complete Atrioventricular Septal Defect. A complete AVSD is present when the endocardial cushions fail to fuse and the septum primum fails to fuse with the endocardial cushions. This lack of fusion leaves a hole in the middle of the heart, with the primum atrial septum and membranous atrial septum both absent. There may be a cleft in the mitral leaflet and overriding of the atrioventricular leaflets or chordal structures or both. When this occurs, the anterior and posterior leaflets are on both sides of the interventricular septum, which causes the valve to override or straddle the septum. This abnormality is best seen on the four-chamber view (Fig. 26-15; see Color Plate 36). The sweep from posterior to anterior demonstrates the complexity of the atrioventricular valve apparatus and the chordal attachments. Color Doppler should be used to demonstrate the amount of regurgitation present from the abnormal atrioventricular valves into the atrial cavity.

This abnormality is more complex to repair because the defect is larger, and the single atrioventricular valve is more difficult to manage clinically, depending on the amount of regurgitation. Complete AVSDs are frequently associated with malpositions of the heart (mesocardia and dextrocardia) and atrioventricular block, which is caused by distortion of the conduction tissues. AVSDs are frequently associated with other cardiac defects, including truncoconal abnormalities, coarctation of the aorta, and pulmonary stenosis or atresia. Occasionally, complete absence of the interatrial septum is noted in the four-chamber view. With color flow, the atria are completely filled throughout systole and diastole; this is termed common atria.

Tetralogy of Fallot

TOF is the most common form of cyanotic heart disease and the most common major congenital heart disease associated with a totally normal four-chamber view (Fig. 26-16). The severity of the disease varies according to the degree of pulmonary stenosis present. A large septal defect with mild to moderate pulmonary stenosis is classified as acyanotic disease, whereas a large septal defect with severe pulmonary stenosis is considered cyanotic disease ("blue baby" at birth). This disease is associated with maternal diabetes, trisomy 21, DiGeorge syndrome, omphalocele, and pentalogy of Cantrell.

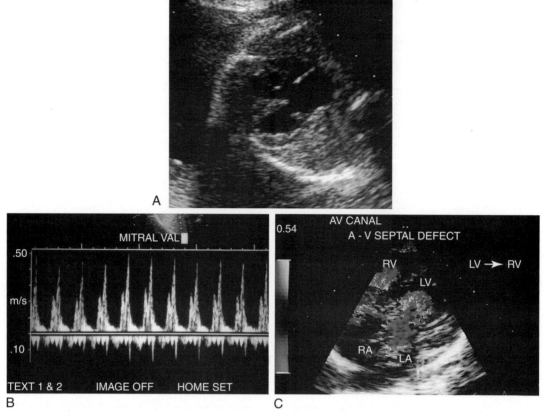

A

B

C

FIGURE 26-15 **(A),** A patient with trisomy 21 had 2:1 heart block secondary to a complete AVSD, which included the membranous and atrial septa. **(B),** Prominent inflow velocities are seen across the mitral valve. There is a small regurgitant flow into the left atrium *(LA)* seen as flow reversal at the end of diastole below the baseline. **(C),** Color flow imaging is helpful to map the flow across the defect and to track regurgitation into the atria. *LV,* Left ventricle; *RA,* right atrium; *RV,* right ventricle. (See Color Plate 36.)

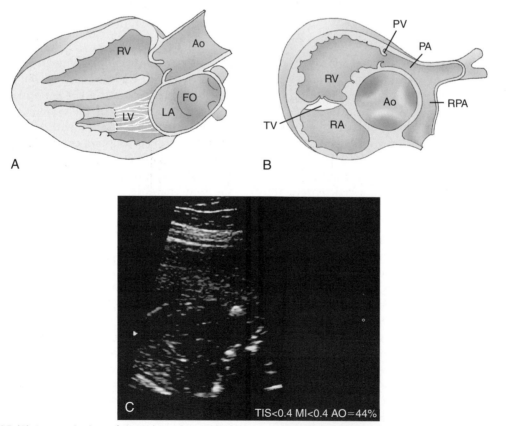

A

B

C

FIGURE 26-16 TOF. **(A),** Long-axis view of the enlarged aorta *(Ao)* as it overrides the interventricular septum. The amount of aortic enlargement depends on the degree of pulmonary stenosis or atresia present. **(B),** Short-axis view of the small pulmonary artery *(PA)* displaced anteriorly by the enlarged aorta. **(C),** Long axis of the heart shows the aorta as it overrides the septum. *FO,* Foramen ovale; *LA,* left atrium; *LV,* left ventricle; *PV,* pulmonary valve; *RA,* right atrium; *RPA,* right pulmonary artery; *RV,* right ventricle; *TV,* tricuspid valve.

TOF is characterized by the following sonographic findings:

1. High membranous VSD
2. Large anteriorly displaced aorta, which overrides the septal defect
3. Pulmonary stenosis
4. Right ventricular hypertrophy, which is not seen in fetal life because it occurs after birth when pulmonary stenosis causes increased pressures in the right ventricle.

Many other cardiac malformations tend to occur in patients with pulmonary stenosis and VSD, including (1) right aortic arch, (2) persistent left superior vena cava, (3) anomalies of the pulmonary artery and its branches, (4) absence of the pulmonary valve, (5) regurgitation of the aortic valve, and (6) variations in coronary arterial anatomy.

The demonstration of TOF is distinguished on the long-axis view. The large aorta is seen to override the ventricular septum. If the override is greater than 50%, the condition is called double-outlet right ventricle, in which both great vessels arise from the right heart. A septal defect is present and may vary in size from small to large.

The short-axis view shows the small hypertrophied right ventricle (if significant pulmonary stenosis is present). The pulmonary artery is usually small, and the cusps may be thickened and domed or difficult to image well. A sample Doppler volume should be obtained in the high parasternal short-axis view to determine the turbulence of the right ventricular outflow tract and the degree of pulmonary valve stenosis.

Color flow is helpful in this condition for actual delineation of the abnormal high-velocity pattern and for directing the sample volume into the proper jet flow. If the VSD is large, increased flow may be seen in the right heart (increased tricuspid velocity, right ventricular outflow tract velocity, and increased pulmonic velocity).

Transposition of the Great Arteries

TGA is an abnormal condition that exists when the aorta arises from the right ventricle and the pulmonary artery arises from the left ventricle (Fig. 26-17). The atrioventricular valves are normally attached and related. Two major types of transposition are "dextro" (D-TGA) and "levo" (L-TGA).

Transposition occurs because of an abnormal completion of the "loop" in embryonic development. The great vessels originate as a common truncus and undergo rotation and spiraling; if this development is interrupted, the great arteries do not complete their spiral, and transposition occurs. Usually, the aorta is anterior and to the right of the pulmonary artery (Fig. 26-18). In the fetal heart, no hemodynamic compromise is seen in the fetus when the great arteries are transposed. Problems occur in the

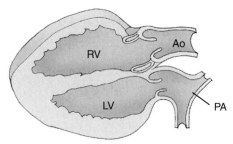

FIGURE 26-17 TGA. The aorta *(Ao)* arises anteriorly from the right ventricle *(RV)*, and the pulmonary artery *(PA)* arises posteriorly from the left ventricle *(LV)*.

neonatal period with inadequate mixing of oxygenated and unoxygenated blood.

D-Transposition of the Great Arteries. In D-TGA, the visceral situs is normal (with the stomach on the left and liver on the right), and the ventricular looping is normal (D-looped). The aortic valve is usually anterior and rightward of the pulmonary valve. The systemic venous return passes from right atrium to right ventricle to aorta, and pulmonary venous return passes from left atrium to left ventricle to pulmonary artery. This fetus may or may not have a VSD.

The short-axis view is the key for imaging of the great arteries and their normal relationship. In the normal fetus, the right ventricular outflow tract and pulmonary artery with its bifurcation should be seen anterior to the aorta in the parasternal short-axis view. In a fetus with TGA, this relationship would not be present; it would be impossible to show the bifurcation of the pulmonary artery because the aorta would be the anterior vessel. Often, the double circles of the great arteries can be seen in this view, as opposed to the normal fetus with a central circle (aorta) and crescent anterior chamber (right ventricular outflow tract and pulmonary artery).

On the modified long-axis view, the crisscross pattern obtained from a normal fetal echocardiogram occurs when the transducer is swept from the left ventricular outflow tract anterior and medial into the right ventricular outflow tract. In a fetus with TGA, this crisscross sweep of the great arteries is impossible. Instead, parallel great arteries may be seen in this view as they arise from the ventricles.

Other associated cardiac anomalies include ASDs, anomalies of the atrioventricular valves, and underdevelopment of the right or left ventricles.

L-Transposition of the Great Arteries. In L-TGA, the heart has normal visceral situs, L-looped ventricles, and TGA. The aorta is anterior and leftward of the pulmonary artery. The systemic venous return passes from the right atrium to left ventricle to pulmonary artery, and the pulmonary venous return passes from left atrium to right ventricle to aorta. This has also been called "congenitally corrected transposition."

Corrected transposition is a cardiac condition in which the right and left atria are connected to the morphologic

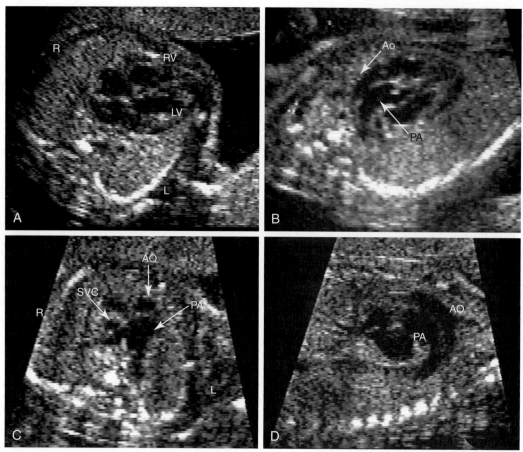

FIGURE 26-18 D-TGA. **(A),** Four-chamber view and cardiac axis are usually normal. **(B),** Sweeping to the outflow tracts, the great arteries arise in a parallel fashion so that both can be imaged in their long axis in the same plane. **(C),** In the three-vessel view, the aorta *(AO)* is the most anterior structure, and the pulmonary artery *(PA)* is posterior and to the left. **(D),** Both arches can be demonstrated in a single plane as a result of the parallel proximal origins of the great arteries. *L,* Left; *LV,* left ventricle; *R,* right; *RV,* right ventricle.

left and right ventricles, respectively, and the great arteries are transposed. These two defects cancel each other out without hemodynamic consequences. L-TGA is demonstrated on sonography with an abnormal four-chamber view and abnormal outflow tracts. The four-chamber view shows the left ventricle anterior and rightward of the posterior and leftward right ventricle. The right ventricle may be identified by the moderator band and coarse apical trabeculations. The tricuspid valve inserts slightly more apically than the mitral valve.

As the sonographer images the outflow tracts, absence of the normal crisscross of the aorta and pulmonary artery is noted. The aortic valve arises anterior and leftward of the pulmonary valve and gives rise to the aorta, which heads superiorly. The pulmonary valve arises posterior and rightward of the aortic valve and gives rise to the pulmonary artery, which bifurcates and heads posteriorly. Stenosis of the pulmonary valve may be seen with two-dimensional imaging as increased thickening and with color Doppler imaging as turbulence. The presence of a VSD should be seen on four-chamber view or outflow tract views. If the defect is more anterior, it is more likely to be identified with imaging of the outflow tracts.

Corrected transposition is associated with malpositions of the heart and sometimes with situs inversus. A ventricular perimembranous septal defect may be present in half of the fetuses. The pulmonary artery may be seen to override the septal defect, with pulmonary stenosis in 50%. Abnormalities of the atrioventricular valves, such as an Ebstein type of malformation and straddling of the tricuspid valve, may be present. Because of the atrial switch, the regurgitant jet from the abnormal tricuspid valve is directed into the left atrial cavity. Heart block may also be associated with L-TGA.

Hypoplastic Left Heart Syndrome

HLHS is a heterogeneous collection of various forms of congenital heart disease in which underdevelopment of the left heart is present. Most cases of HLHS also are associated with an increased risk for congenital or acquired central nervous system abnormalities or aneuploidy. The most classic form of HLHS is characterized by a small, hypertrophied left ventricle with dysplastic aortic or mitral atresia. HLHS has been found to be an autosomal recessive condition. If a couple has had one child with HLHS, the recurrence rate is 4%; if two

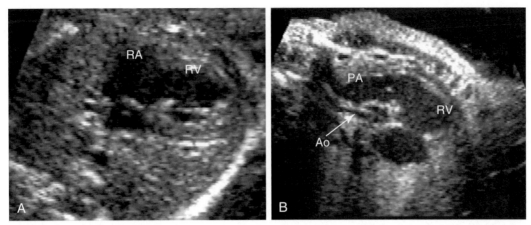

FIGURE 26-19 HLHS. **(A)**, Typical four-chamber view seen in this disease with a very small left atrium and left ventricle and prominent right atrium *(RA)* and right ventricle *(RV)*. **(B)**, Sagittal image demonstrates large pulmonary artery *(PA)* arising from the RV and a very diminutive ascending aorta *(Ao)*.

siblings have been affected, the recurrence rate increases to 25%.

The cause of HLHS is unknown but is thought to be decreased filling and perfusion of the left ventricle during embryologic development. When this closure occurs, the blood cannot cross the foramen to help the left ventricle grow. A real-time image shows a reduction in the size of the foramen ovale (the foramen should measure at least 0.6 multiplied by the diameter of the aortic root). Premature closure of the foramen would also show increased velocities across the interatrial septum (approximately 40 to 50cm/s). Restriction to flow across the foramen ovale may lead to pulmonary venous congestion and irreversible pulmonary vascular disease. This reduction in flow may be apparent until the third trimester. Retrograde filling of the aortic arch may occur through the patent ductus arteriosus.

Atresia of the mitral or aortic valve may occur at any time during fetal development. Changes may be subtle, such as slight thickening of the valvular apparatus or slightly diminished growth of the aorta compared with the pulmonary artery. Subtle changes in the size of the left ventricle compared with the right ventricular cavity may need to be monitored with serial sonographic examinations.

The right ventricle supplies both the pulmonic and the systemic circulations. The pulmonary venous return is diverted from the left atrium to the right atrium through the interatrial communication. Through the pulmonary artery and ductus arteriosus, the right ventricle supplies the descending aorta, along with retrograde flow to the aortic arch and the ascending aorta. Overload on the right ventricle may lead to congestive heart failure in utero with the development of pericardial effusion and hydrops.

A fetus that has had a major disturbance in the development of the mitral valve or aortic valve would show dramatic changes in the development of the left ventricle (Fig. 26-19). The amount of hypoplasia would depend on when the left-sided atresia developed in the valvar area. If mitral atresia is the cause, the blood cannot fill the left ventricle to provide volume, and the aortic valve

would become atretic as well, with concentric hypertrophy of the small left ventricular cavity. If the cause is aortic stenosis, the myocardium shows extreme hypertrophy from the increased pressure overload.

SUMMARY

Echocardiographic evaluation of a fetus with a suspected congenital heart problem has been a tremendous aid to the obstetrician and pediatric cardiologist in the management of the mother and fetus. For the mother of a child with congenital heart disease, a normal fetal echocardiogram in subsequent pregnancies is reassuring. A new diagnosis of congenital heart disease in utero may allow time for the pediatric cardiologist and surgeon to discuss possible options for the fetus after delivery. It also allows time to arrange the delivery in a medical center equipped to manage congenital heart problems.

CLINICAL SCENARIO—DIAGNOSIS

When a mother has given birth to a child with congenital heart disease, the risk increases for subsequent pregnancies. In the case of left-sided heart disease, the risk is slightly greater with each subsequent pregnancy. Because the first child had HLHS, the chance of the second child having left-sided heart disease increases to 4%. If the second child also has left-sided congenital heart disease, the risk for a third pregnancy increases to 25%. In addition, because the mother is known to have aortic valve disease, the risk further increases for each pregnancy.

This patient needs to be followed closely to evaluate for the presence of left-sided heart disease that may lead to HLHS. This patient was seen at 24 weeks' gestation, but typically the initial sonographic evaluation may occur by 16 weeks to look for symmetry between the ventricular sizes. The fetus should again be scanned at 20 to 22 weeks for a detailed cardiac anatomy study. The last scan should be made at the beginning of the third trimester, at about 28 weeks. At that time, the ventricular growth pattern should be established, with the right ventricle being only slightly larger than the left. Any variation of more than 5 to 10 mm in growth pattern between the ventricles is suspicious for the development of HLHS.

CASE STUDIES FOR DISCUSSION

1. A 36-year-old woman presents at 22 weeks' gestation for a fetal echocardiogram. An obstetric scan performed at 18 weeks' gestation revealed a possible cardiac anomaly on the four-chamber view. A genetic amniocentesis was performed, and the fetus has trisomy 21. Which heart abnormality is most specifically linked with trisomy 21, and what will the sonographer identify to make this diagnosis?

2. A 28-year-old woman presents for a fetal echocardiogram after an obstetric sonogram revealed chamber asymmetry on the four-chamber view. The woman was counseled that her fetus may have Ebstein's anomaly. Identify which cardiac structures should be closely evaluated, and describe the classic sonographic findings of Ebstein's anomaly.

3. During an echocardiogram on a 25-week fetus, the apical four-chamber view demonstrates an area of dropout in the atrial septum. What additional view should the sonographer obtain to differentiate between the foramen ovale and an ASD?

4. An echocardiogram demonstrates a single muscular septal defect with no other cardiac anomalies identified. What is the prognosis for the newborn?

5. Asymmetry of the four-chamber view is seen with the left ventricle and aortic arch small and difficult to image. What is the differential consideration?

STUDY QUESTIONS

1. Which of the following statements regarding fetal cardiac rhythm is false?
   a. The normal fetal heart should have a baseline rate of 110 to 160 beats per minute.
   b. Ventricular contraction precedes electrical activation.
   c. Bradycardia is less than 55 beats per minute.
   d. Sinus tachycardia may be common in later stages of pregnancy.

2. A 36-year-old woman is seen for a routine obstetric examination at 28 weeks' gestation, and the fetus is noted to have an arrhythmia. An echocardiogram is ordered. To assess fetal cardiac rhythm adequately, an M-mode tracing should be performed simultaneously through which cardiac structures?
   a. Right atrium, left atrium
   b. Right atrium, left ventricle
   c. Left atrium, pulmonary artery
   d. Tricuspid valve, right ventricle

3. While performing a fetal echocardiogram, the sonographer cannot identify the foramen ovale flap and notes the foramen ovale opening is larger than normal. The ventricular septum is intact. What abnormality is most likely present?
   a. Secundum ASD
   b. Sinus venosus ASD
   c. Primum atrial defect
   d. Atrioventricular canal malformation

4. A fetus is diagnosed with TOF. On which of the following does the prognosis depend?
   a. Type of VSD
   b. Degree of anterior displacement of the overriding aorta
   c. Degree of pulmonary stenosis
   d. Size of aortic arch

5. A fetal echocardiogram demonstrates a small left ventricular cavity. Which of the following abnormalities is associated with this finding?
   a. Mitral atresia
   b. Tricuspid atresia
   c. Pulmonary stenosis
   d. Pulmonary atresia

6. A fetus is diagnosed with a complete atrioventricular heart block (AVSD). Which of the following statements regarding the infant's prognosis or treatment or both is true?
   a. Repairing an endocardial cushion defect is impossible, making this a uniformly lethal abnormality.
   b. AVSDs typically close on their own shortly after birth, so no surgical intervention is required.
   c. AVSDs are more complex to repair and are frequently associated with other cardiac defects.
   d. A single atrioventricular valve rarely demonstrates regurgitation, and intervention is seldom necessary.

7. L-TGA is best described as:
   a. Normal visceral situs, L-looped ventricles, and TGA
   b. Situs inversus, L-looped ventricles, and TGA
   c. Situs solitus, L-looped ventricles, and single great artery
   d. Normal visceral situs and aorta is anterior and rightward of pulmonary valve

8. HLHS involves which structures?
   a. One great artery, which arises from the base of the heart
   b. The great arteries, which are reversed
   c. The left ventricle, mitral valve, and aorta
   d. The pulmonary artery and the coronary sinus

9. The most common site for a VSD is:
   a. Subpulmonic
   b. Membranous
   c. Muscular
   d. Infracristal

10. On the modified long-axis view, the sonographer was unable to view the normal crisscross pattern

when evaluating the outflow tracts. The great vessels appeared to arise from the ventricle in parallel. This finding is associated with which cardiac abnormality?

a. Ebstein's anomaly
b. TOF
c. AVSD
d. TGA

REFERENCES

1. Smrcek J, Berg C, Geipel A, et al: Detection rate of early fetal echocardiography and in utero development of congenital heart defects, *J Ultrasound Med* 25:187–196, 2006.

BIBLIOGRAPHY

Rychik J, Ayres N, Cuneo B, et al: American Society of Echocardiography guidelines and standards for performance of the fetal echocardiogram, *J Am Soc Echocardiogr* 17:803–810, 2004.

Fink BW: *Congenital heart disease*, ed 3, St Louis, 1991, Mosby.

Hagen-Ansert SL: Fetal echocardiography, *Textbook of sonography*, vol II, St Louis, 2012, Mosby.

Hoffman JE, Kaplan S: The incidence of congenital heart disease, *J Am Coll Cardiol* 3:1890–1900, 2002.

Quartermain MD, Cohen MS, Dominguez TE, et al: Left ventricle to right ventricle size discrepancy in the fetus: the presence of critical heart disease can be reliably predicted, *J Am Soc Echocardiogr* 22:1296–1301, 2009.

Sklansky M: Fetal cardiac malformations and arrhythmia: detection, diagnosis, management, and prognosis. *Creasy and Resnick's Maternal fetal medicine: principles and practice*, 2011, Saunders.

PART IV

Superficial Structures

27

Breast Mass

Dana Salmons, Charlotte Henningsen

CLINICAL SCENARIO

An 11-year-old African American, menstrual-age girl is seen in the emergency department with rapidly increasing breast size, with the left breast noticeably larger than the right. She is referred for a sonogram the following day. According to the patient's mother, the girl wore a size 36A bra 2 months previously and now wears a size 36D on the right and a 36DD on the left. She went to her family physician 1 week previously for this condition and was told that this was part of the girl's normal breast development.

The day of the sonogram, the patient has no pain and is not febrile. The clinical breast examination is negative for discrete masses, but the breasts feel hard, similar to encapsulated breast implants, with a foamlike, spongy consistency. The skin and nipples are stretched taut, but the nipples are not displaced. The sonographic examination shows little to no normal-looking tissue. Homogeneous branching tissue is seen beneath both areolae with a positive Doppler signal. Ductal ectasia is noted bilaterally. Multiple lobular areas are seen with a lacy heterogeneous "Swiss cheese" appearance. The patient also undergoes a left breast magnetic resonance imaging (MRI) examination that reveals a 13-cm neoplasm (Fig. 27-1, **A** and **B**). What is the most likely diagnosis?

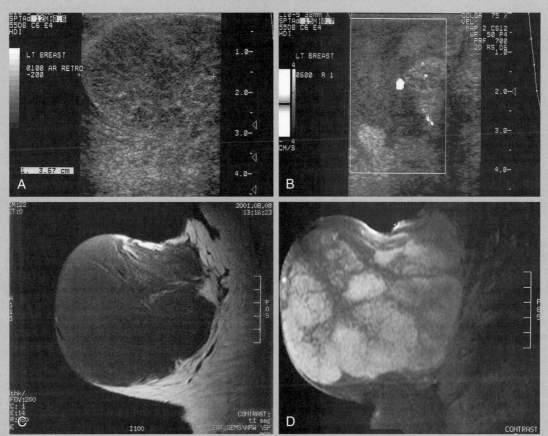

FIGURE 27-1 (A), Ultrasound of an 11-year-old girl with bilateral breast enlargement. **(B),** Color Doppler of lesion. **(C)** and **(D),** MRI of lesion.

OBJECTIVES

- Describe the sonographic appearance of common cystic masses of the breast.
- Describe the sonographic appearance of common benign neoplasms of the breast.
- Describe the sonographic appearance of common malignant neoplasms of the breast.
- Describe the sonographic appearance of an augmented breast.
- Describe the sonographic appearance of an inflamed breast.
- Describe the sonographic appearance of an injured or postsurgical breast.
- Describe the sonographic appearance of a male breast.

The two most common indications for breast sonography are a palpable breast mass and the need for more information regarding a lesion seen with another method. Other indications for breast sonography include evaluation of dense breasts and areas of asymmetry not well visualized with mammography, evaluation of implant integrity, follow-up on either accidentally or surgically traumatized breasts, and serial sonogram evaluation of tumor size. In addition, sonographic guidance is often advantageous in invasive procedures, such as cyst aspiration, abscess drainage, needle localization, lymphoscintigraphy, and core biopsy.

With the improvement in resolution of sonography, there is a growing movement toward screening breast sonograms; however, sonography is not to be used as a replacement for mammography. Sonography cannot consistently detect microcalcifications that are often an indicator of breast cancer.

BREAST

Sonography Scanning Planes

The preferred method for breast sonography uses radial and antiradial planes (Fig. 27-2, A). Multiple ducts start at the nipple and radiate out toward the periphery of the breast parenchyma. With radial and antiradial scanning, ductal involvement of a mass is more readily seen. Turning on the lesion is important so that all aspects of the lesion are evaluated.

Breast Sonography Annotation

Documentation of the location within the breast that is being imaged is imperative. Documentation proves that the area of interest was evaluated, and it facilitates relocation of any discovered pathology for follow-up.

The preferred method of annotation uses a quasigrid pattern. First, the breasts are viewed as a clock face. Directly above the nipple on either breast is 12:00. Right medial breast and left lateral breast are 3:00. Directly below the nipple bilaterally is 6:00. Right lateral breast and left medial breast are 9:00

(Fig. 27-2, B). Next, the distance the image is taken from the nipple is documented in centimeters from nipple (CMFN). The pathology in Fig. 27-2, C, would be labeled as follows: RT BREAST, 5:00 1 CMFN rad (radial) or arad (antiradial); LT BREAST, 1:00 4 CMFN rad or arad.

Location of a Mass with Mammographic Images

With a search for a mass first seen on mammogram, isolation of the quadrant of interest is essential. An understanding of mammographic images is vital to correlation of sonographic findings.

A craniocaudal (CC) mammogram is used to discover whether a mass is in the medial or lateral portion of the breast. A CC mammogram is acquired with placement of the film inferior to the breast, and the radiograph beam is directed superiorly to inferiorly (Fig. 27-2, D). The CC marker is placed just outside the lateral breast border. If the mass is located between the nipple and the CC marker, the mass is in the lateral portion of the breast. If the mass is located between the nipple and the contralateral side of the CC marker, the mass is medial. Superior and inferior mass location is determined with a mediolateral oblique (MLO) mammogram. A MLO mammogram is acquired with placement of the film at an oblique angle that is lateral and slightly inferior to the breast. The radiograph beam is directed mediolaterally at the same obliquity as the film (see Fig. 27-2, D). Because this is not a true mediolateral image, masses on the lateral breast are slightly lower than masses that appear in the image. Masses in the medial breast are slightly higher.

Normal Sonographic Anatomy

Normal human breasts are two modified sweat glands on the upper anterior portion of the chest, lying anterior to the pectoralis major. The areola and nipple are centrally located on each breast. Each adult female breast has a conic formation with a "tail" that extends toward the associated axilla (Fig. 27-3). The function is to produce and release milk during reproduction. The breasts are composed of fatty, glandular, and fibrous connective tissues, all with differing echogenicities. Proportions of these tissues vary from patient to patient and can vary within the breast of the same patient. The normal sonographic appearance is quite variable.

The normal skin thickness overlying the breast is less than 2mm. Beneath the skin are three layers of mammary tissue. Starting superficially, the subcutaneous layer located just under the skin is mainly fat and, in the breast, is sonographically hypoechoic. The middle mammary layer contains the ducts, glands, and stroma of the breast and is relatively echogenic. The deep retromammary layer is also composed of hypoechoic fat and is the portion of the breast that lies superficial to the pectoralis major. Traversing through these layers are hyperechoic Cooper's ligaments (Fig. 27-4).

CYSTIC MASSES

Cysts are fluid-filled masses that form at the terminal ductal-lobular unit or from an obstructed duct and are the most common breast masses in women 40 to 50 years old. They are frequent findings in perimenopausal women and often fluctuate with the menstrual cycle.

Patients with cysts may have firm, smooth, mobile, or palpable masses. Cysts are often painful and hard when they are full of fluid and the walls are stretched taut; however, the patient may be asymptomatic. Cysts typically regress after menopause but may persist or be new findings in postmenopausal women undergoing hormone replacement therapy. They may be singular or multiple, ranging in size from a few millimeters to multiple centimeters. Sonographically, they may be classified further as simple or complex.

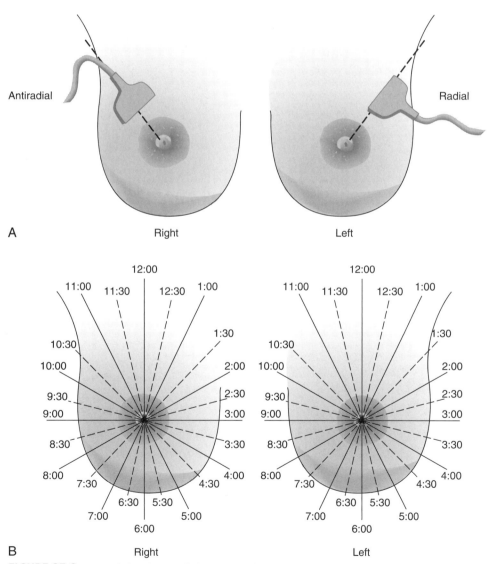

FIGURE 27-2 (A), Radial and antiradial scanning planes. **(B),** Annotation uses clock face technique.

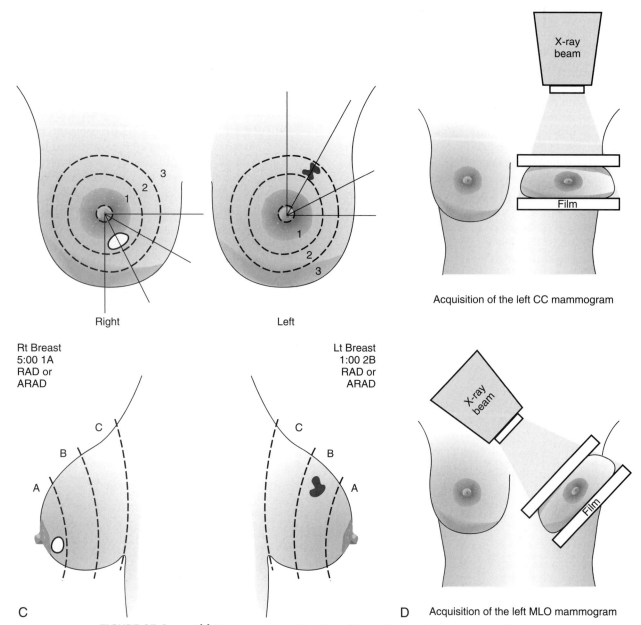

Right

Left

Rt Breast
5:00 1A
RAD or
ARAD

Lt Breast
1:00 2B
RAD or
ARAD

C

B

A

C

C

B

A

D

Acquisition of the left CC mammogram

X-ray
beam

Film

X-ray
beam

Film

Acquisition of the left MLO mammogram

FIGURE 27-2, cont'd (C), Annotation of location of breast lesion. **(D),** Mammographic views.

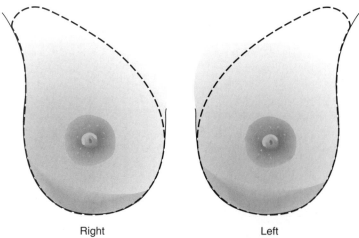

Right   Left

FIGURE 27-3 Shape of normal adult female breasts.

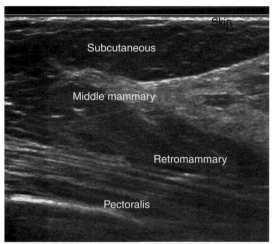

FIGURE 27-4 Sonogram of normal breast tissue.

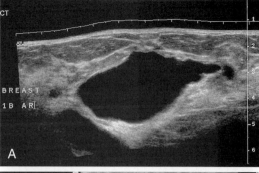

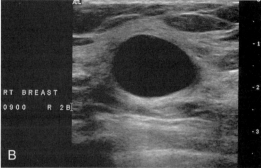

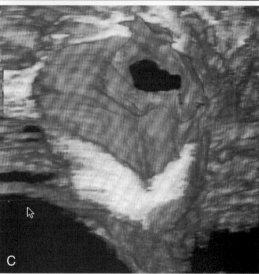

FIGURE 27-5 Simple cyst measuring 5.6 cm in a 50-year-old woman. Antiradial **(A)** and radial **(B)** views show lesion. **(C),** Three-dimensional image of same cyst shows smooth walls.

Aspiration of a cyst is generally done for one of three reasons: (1) the cyst is painful, (2) the cyst is radiographically or sonographically abnormal in appearance, or (3) the cyst obscures the diagnostic quality of a mammogram because of its size. Simple cysts do not become malignant and are usually left alone.

Simple Cyst

Sonographic Findings. A simple cyst must have certain sonographic qualities to be considered simple. The mnemonic STAR may assist in identification of a simple cyst. (Fig. 27-5, A and B). A simple cyst should be: S, smooth and thin-walled; T, through transmit; A, anechoic; and R, round or oval.

Interior echoes within a cyst can be the result of improper gain or power settings or anterior reverberation artifact, or they may be real and considered complex. Newer ultrasound machines are better at depicting debris within cysts. This debris may be seen and yet not be considered worrisome for malignant disease. In these cases, some radiologists use the term "benign-appearing" instead of "simple-appearing" cyst (Fig. 27-6).

Complex Cyst

Complex cysts are cysts that do not meet the criteria of STAR, meaning they are cystic with a solid component. The reasons for a cyst to be classified as complex are multiple. Just as skin sloughs its cells, so do the cyst walls; this causes layering debris within the cyst. Cysts may also have internal echoes from infection, hemorrhage, mass, or abscess. Seromas may also be considered complex if they have septations and irregular walls.

Sonographic Findings. A cyst that deviates from STAR is considered complex. It may have thick, irregularly shaped walls or internal echoes or lack through transmission (Fig. 27-7).

Oil Cyst

Oil cysts are the liquefaction of injured fat, usually from trauma or surgery. Clinically, when palpable, they appear as smooth masses. Galactoceles resolve to oil cysts because of their fatty milk properties.

Sonographic Findings. Oil cysts are usually anechoic but can have hyperechoic internal echoes. They appear as round or oval, well-marginated masses (Fig. 27-8).

Galactocele

During pregnancy or lactation, a milky cyst may form from an obstruction of the lactiferous ducts. Galactoceles are considered rare, but when galactoceles are present,

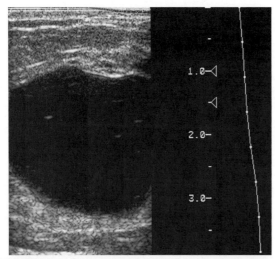

FIGURE 27-6 Benign-appearing cyst with internal floating debris.

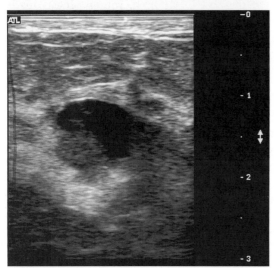

FIGURE 27-7 Complex cyst in a 48-year-old woman.

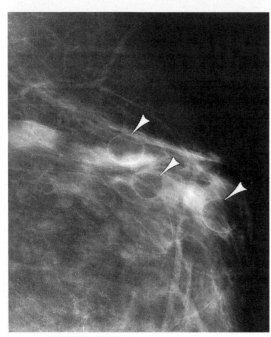

FIGURE 27-8 Oil cysts *(arrowheads)*.

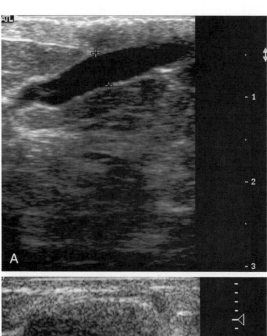

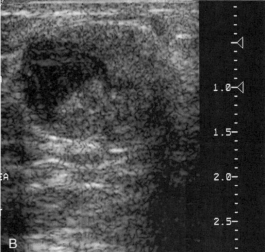

FIGURE 27-9 (A), Dilated lactiferous ducts. **(B),** Galactocele in a postpartum woman.

patients usually have periareolar palpable masses. As expected, ductal ectasia may be present (Fig. 27-9, *A*). Abnormalities associated with galactoceles are mastitis and abscess.

Sonographic Findings. Galactoceles appear as well-marginated, round or oval masses. They typically contain echoes from fatty, milky material and can demonstrate fat-fluid levels. They resolve to oil cysts because of their composition and usually change from a complex cyst to one with a more anechoic appearance. Limited through transmission may be visualized. Doppler evaluation should be negative for internal blood flow (Fig. 27-9, *B*).

Sebaceous Cyst

Sebaceous cysts are not specific to the breast. A sebaceous cyst is a retention cyst that occurs from the blockage of a sebaceous gland in the skin. Sebaceous cysts can become infected, containing thick, white material on drainage. Patients usually have a small, superficial, smooth, mobile, palpable mass.

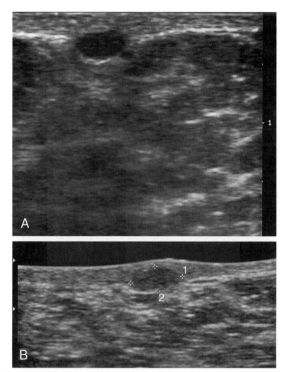

FIGURE 27-10 **(A)**, Palpable area in a 57-year-old woman that has been present for several years representing a sebaceous or inclusion cyst. **(B)**, Another example of an inclusion cyst.

Sonographic Findings. A sebaceous cyst is a well-marginated mass that arises from the skin. The appearance may be variable from anechoic to echogenic with through transmission. The skin line should be visualized posterior to this superficial mass (Fig. 27-10).

BENIGN NEOPLASMS

When benign lesions are palpable clinically, they are usually discrete, mobile, and compressible masses. Several types of benign neoplasms that can occur in the breast are described.

General Sonographic Findings

The general sonographic characteristics of benign breast lesions are smooth or macrolobulated masses with well-marginated borders. They are homogeneous and oval-shaped and have a wide rather than tall formation. They do not attenuate the ultrasound beam and have no posterior shadowing. However, they can demonstrate through transmission. Benign neoplasms displace rather than infiltrate surrounding tissue. Doppler evaluation either is negative or shows some peripheral flow.

Fibroadenoma

Fibroadenoma is the most common benign mass in premenopausal women and is more common in black women. About 50% of all breast biopsies result in a fibroadenoma tissue diagnosis. Fibroadenomas are stimulated by estrogen and are frequently identified in women of reproductive age, usually women younger than 30 years.[1] Because they are hormonally stimulated, they can grow rapidly in pregnant women. New fibroadenomas rarely are found in postmenopausal women with or without hormone replacement therapy. These masses, as with any new solid mass in a postmenopausal woman, should be considered highly suspicious for cancer, and tissue diagnosis is essential.

Fibroadenomas are composed of the normal tissues of the breast but in an abnormal formation; they can have carcinoma within them. However, the risk of cancer within a fibroadenoma is no greater than the risk within other breast tissue.

Clinically, the patient usually has a firm, rubbery, mobile mass when palpable. Fibroadenomas are found more frequently in the upper outer breast quadrants. Bilateral and multiple masses are found in 10% of cases.[2] If small and proven to be a fibroadenoma via core biopsy, these masses may be left within the breast and followed with serial sonograms. When fibroadenomas are large, surgical removal is usually recommended. Fibroadenoma variants consist of giant fibroadenomas and juvenile fibroadenomas. There is no standard measurement a fibroadenoma must reach before it is considered giant, but the term is usually reserved for fibroadenomas measuring 6 to 8cm or greater.

Juvenile fibroadenomas are found in adolescents and can have extremely rapid growth, to the point of deforming the breast and causing nipple displacement. They may be multiple and bilateral. Sonographically, they are indistinct from other fibroadenomas. When large, these masses can concurrently be called juvenile and giant.

Sonographic Findings. Fibroadenomas are smooth or macrolobulated masses that have a wide rather than tall formation. They usually measure less than 3cm. These lesions displace rather than infiltrate surrounding tissue, making them well-marginated masses. They are typically homogeneous with low-level internal echoes but can show areas of cystic necrosis if they outgrow their blood supply. Through transmission may or may not be seen (Fig. 27-11, A and B). Peripheral vascularity may be visualized with Doppler. "Popcorn" calcifications can form; sonographically, these masses may completely attenuate the ultrasound beam, producing significant posterior shadowing. A sonogram may not be helpful in these cases (Fig. 27-11, C).

Cystosarcoma Phylloides

Cystosarcoma phylloides are also called phylloides tumors, proliferative fibroadenomas, or periductal stromal tumors. The peak age for cystosarcoma phylloides is 30 to 40 years, roughly 10 years after the peak age for fibroadenomas. Cystosarcoma phylloides are rare but when seen are usually unilateral. Approximately 10%

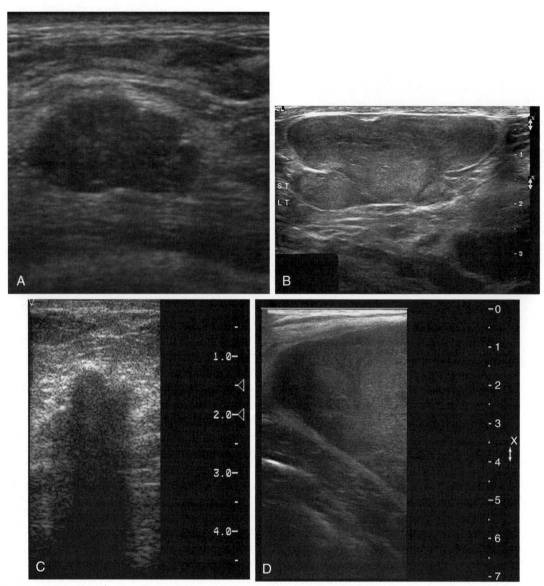

FIGURE 27-11 **(A)**, A 46-year-old woman with a fibroadenoma. **(B)**, A 4.2-cm palpable mass in a 51-year-old woman representing a fibroadenoma. **(C)**, Calcified fibroadenoma in a 75-year-old woman. **(D)**, Large juvenile fibroadenoma.

of cystosarcoma phylloides are malignant and have the potential for metastases, usually to the lung.[3] Malignant phylloides tumors tend to grow faster and larger than benign phylloides tumors. Sonography cannot differentiate between benign phylloides tumors, malignant phylloides tumors, or fibroadenomas.

Sonographic Findings. The sonographic appearance is similar to fibroadenoma. Cystosarcoma phylloides show rapid growth on serial imaging examinations. They often contain cystic spaces from hemorrhage, necrosis, and mucinous fluid. Calcifications are atypical (Fig. 27-12).

Intraductal Papilloma

An intraductal papilloma is a proliferation of epithelial tissue within a duct or cyst that produces a mural nodule. Tumors are typically small and retroareolar. They are often undetectable but sometimes palpable. Intraductal

papilloma is the most common cause of unilateral, spontaneous, bloody nipple discharge. This discharge can also be clear, serous, white, or dark green. Patients are typically late reproductive age or postmenopausal, between the ages of 30 and 55 years.

Sonographic Findings. Unless some ductal ectasia is seen, intraductal papilloma is difficult to show and may result in a negative sonogram. Radial scanning to elongate ducts is essential. When visible, intraductal papilloma demonstrates a solid mass or solid tissue mural nodule within a duct or cyst. The nodule may be round, oval, or tubular following the contour of the duct or cyst (see also the description of papillary carcinoma) (Fig. 27-13).

Lipoma

Lipomas are not specific to the breast. Patients with lipomas are usually middle-aged and older. Clinically,

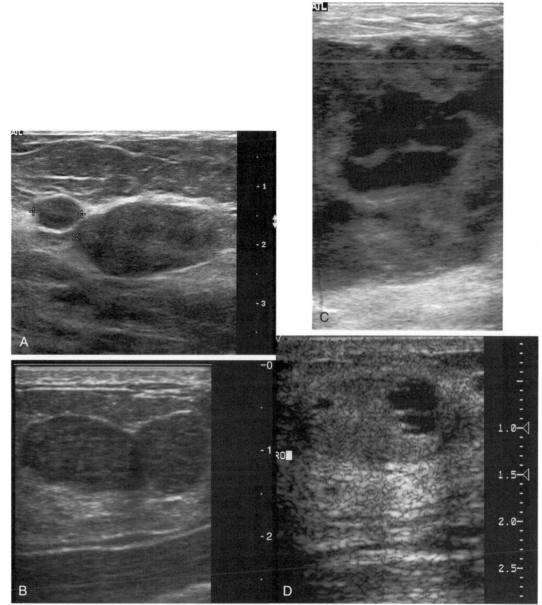

FIGURE 27-12 (A-D), Variable appearances of benign cystosarcoma phylloides.

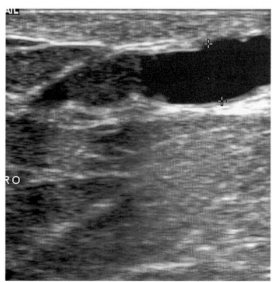

FIGURE 27-13 Intraductal papilloma surgically removed from a 32-year-old woman.

the patient either is asymptomatic or has a soft, mobile, compressible, palpable mass. Lipomas are usually unilateral and are often incidental findings.

Sonographic Findings. Lipomas can be hypoechoic or hyperechoic, but usually they are isoechoic to surrounding tissue. They are discrete, and palpation during scanning may be necessary to locate these masses (Fig. 27-14). Calcifications may be present.

Hamartoma

Also known as fibroadenolipomas, hamartomas are composed of fibrous, glandular, and fat tissue. They are normally found in the breast but are in a disorganized format surrounded by a pseudocapsule. Hamartomas are not specific to the breast, and tissue types are normal to the organ within which they are located. Clinically, hamartomas are large, soft, mobile, painless masses if palpable. Patients are typically in their mid-30s or older.

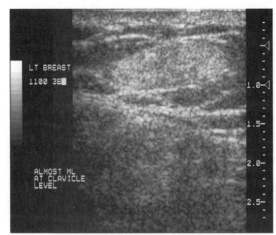

FIGURE 27-14 Incidental finding in a 47-year-old woman representing a lipoma.

Sonographic Findings. Hamartomas have a varying appearance depending on the prominent tissue component. Generally, they appear ovoid, heterogeneously hypoechoic, without posterior attenuation.

BREAST CANCER

Breast cancer is not one disease. There are several types of breast cancers that have differing sonographic and clinical findings. Different types of breast cancers can occur concurrently.

Clinically, most patients with breast cancer are either asymptomatic or have a hard, immobile mass. Pain is a rare indicator of breast cancer. Advanced malignant diseases with lymphatic and neurologic invasion are often more painful. Patients may also have skin changes, such as discoloration, usually red; edema with skin thickening; peau d'orange (Fig. 27-15); or inversion of the nipple. Nipple discharge is a common symptom but is rarely associated with breast cancer because it is found in only about 3% to 9% of cases.[4] Sanguineous nipple discharge is of more concern for breast carcinoma but still has a stronger association with benign breast processes. The chance of breast carcinoma with nipple discharge increases as the age of the patient increases. Other skin changes include asymmetry and contour change, bulging, dimpling, and retraction.

Breast cancers metastasize to the lymph node, liver, lung, bone, and brain.

General Sonographic Findings

Malignant breast masses generally are hypoechoic and inhomogeneous. They often attenuate the ultrasound beam and cause posterior shadowing. Breast cancer usually infiltrates tissue rather than displacing it and has a tall rather than wide formation. These masses are generally spiculated, and borders can be poorly marginated or microlobulated. In addition, microcalcifications may be present and may or may not be detectable with

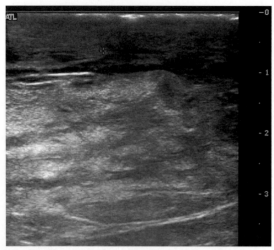

FIGURE 27-15 Skin thickening seen on a patient with invasive breast carcinoma.

sonography. Neovascularity is necessary for a cancer to grow. Doppler evaluation typically shows an increase in blood flow in malignant masses.

Invasive Ductal Carcinoma

Invasive ductal carcinoma has many types of malignant diseases and accounts for 65% to 80% of all breast cancers.[5] The peak age for this cancer is 50 years. With symptomatic disease, patients usually have a palpable mass. Focal breast tenderness and nipple discharge are possible symptoms. Depending on how advanced the lesion is, skin changes may also be noted. Invasive ductal carcinoma originates in the lactiferous ducts of the breast.
Sonographic Findings. Invasive ductal carcinoma manifests as a hypoechoic, spiculated mass with finger-like extensions into dilated ducts. Sharp angulations may be identified with posterior shadowing and a tall rather than wide formation (Fig. 27-16).

Invasive Lobular Carcinoma

Invasive lobular carcinoma accounts for 5% to 10% of all breast cancers.[5] The peak age range is 55 to 70 years, and young women are rarely affected. Invasive lobular carcinoma is bilateral in about 21% of cases and is often multicentric.[6] Clinically, palpation of a discrete mass is rare with invasive lobular carcinoma because it is typically diffusely infiltrating. Patients may have an area of breast thickening and focal breast tenderness. The survival rate with early discovery is better than the survival with invasive ductal carcinoma.

Microcalcifications are uncommon, and mammography has difficulty in detecting these masses, resulting in a higher incidence rate of false-negative reports than with other invasive cancers. Occasionally, lobular carcinoma may appear as an area of distortion seen only on the CC image. However, the mammogram can still look negative even in retrospect, which can explain why these masses

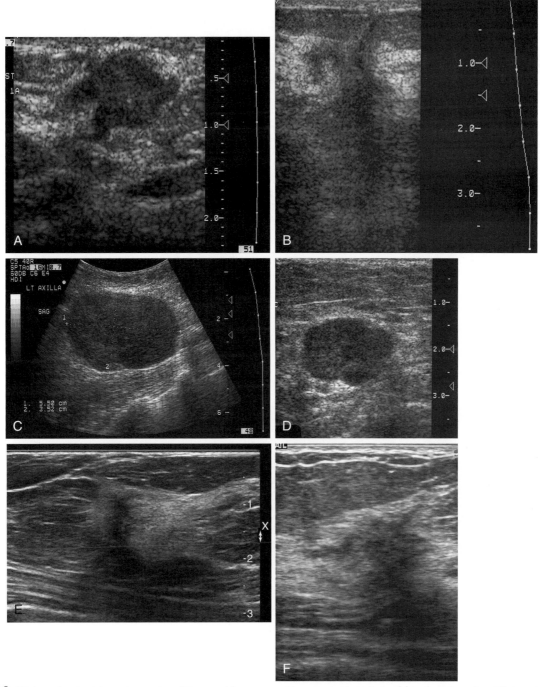

FIGURE 27-16 **(A)**, Invasive ductal carcinoma in a 54-year-old woman with metastases to two of four lymph nodes. **(B)**, Invasive ductal carcinoma in a 44-year-old woman with no evidence of metastasis. **(C)**, Invasive ductal carcinoma in a 75-year-old woman who is not a candidate for surgery. Mass measures 5.5 cm. **(D)**, Same patient as in (C), 12 months after chemotherapy. Mass now measures 2.3 cm. **(E)**, Invasive ductal carcinoma in a 50-year-old woman with metastasis to one of seven lymph nodes. **(F)**, Invasive ductal and lobular carcinoma within same lesion.

are sometimes large when they are finally detected and already have lymph node involvement. There is often more underestimation than overestimation in size of these masses.

Sonographic Findings. These masses are often spiculated, infiltrating, and rarely discrete, and demonstration of borders may be difficult. There may be hypoechoic areas with significant posterior shadowing, but there may also be an area that simply appears distorted (Fig. 27-17).

Colloid Carcinoma

Colloid carcinoma is also known as mucinous or gelatinous carcinoma and accounts for less than 3% of breast cancer.[7] This disease is more prevalent in women 60 to 70 years old. These are slow-growing lesions with a fairly good prognosis. Clinically, these masses manifest as soft and discrete when palpable. This lesion does not typically produce skin or nipple changes.

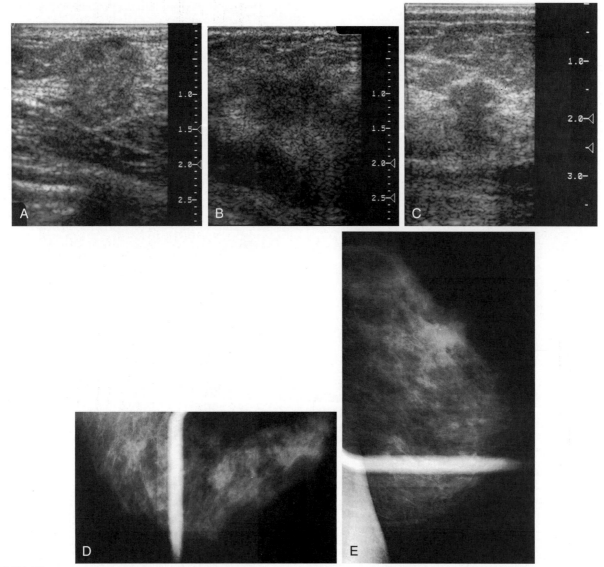

FIGURE 27-17 (A), Palpable mass that was pathologically proven to be invasive lobular carcinoma. **(B),** Bilateral palpable masses. Invasive lobular carcinoma was diagnosed in left breast, and invasive ductal carcinoma was diagnosed in right breast. **(C),** Invasive lobular carcinoma in a 52-year-old woman; sonographically, mass measured 1.3 cm. Pathology documented lesion to be 4.5 cm. Mammograms of this patient document lesion in craniocaudal **(D)** and mediolateral oblique **(E)** views.

Sonographic Findings. These masses can appear benign. They may look well circumscribed, microlobulated, round or oval, and smooth. They are usually hypoechoic. Because of their high cellular fluid content, sonographically they may show through transmission (Fig. 27-18).

Medullary Carcinoma

Medullary carcinoma accounts for about 5% of all breast cancers.[8] The peak age group is premenopausal. Although these are fast-growing cancers, the prognosis is good. Clinically, these cancers manifest as discrete, mobile masses.
Sonographic Findings. These masses are usually hypoechoic, round, and well marginated and can be mistaken for fibroadenomas. Necrosis can produce a cystic

component to this mass. Calcifications are atypical (Fig. 27-19).

Papillary Carcinoma

Papillary carcinoma represents 1% to 2% of breast cancers.[9] It is more prevalent in older women, with a peak age of 63 to 67 years. These are slow-growing malignant diseases. Of papillary carcinomas, 50% are found in the retroareolar area and can be associated with bloody nipple discharge.[10] Skin changes also may be noted.
Sonographic Findings. Sonographically, these intraductal mural masses are as challenging to find as their benign counterpart, intraductal papilloma, and they cannot be differentiated from a papilloma without tissue diagnosis. Microcalcifications may be present (Fig. 27-20).

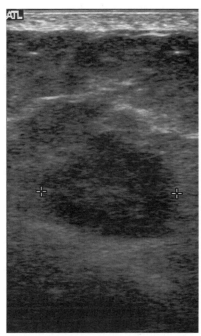

FIGURE 27-18 Colloid carcinoma in a 66-year-old woman with no metastasis.

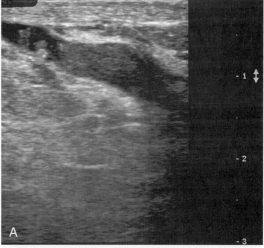

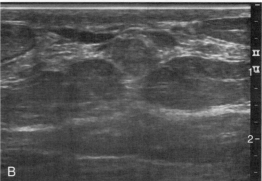

FIGURE 27-20 (A), Mural nodule seen within cyst pathologically proven to be papillary carcinoma. **(B),** Papillary carcinoma.

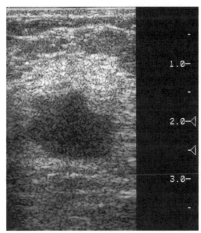

FIGURE 27-19 Medullary carcinoma surgically removed from a 39-year-old woman.

METASTASES

Metastases to the Breast

Metastatic disease to the breast occurs in approximately 0.5% to 6.6% of cases and is considered uncommon.[11] Diagnosis of the primary lesion is essential because treatment for metastatic breast cancer can be quite different from treatment for primary breast cancer. Mastectomy is not normally necessary. Primary cancers that metastasize to the breast are non-Hodgkin's lymphoma, melanoma, lung cancer, ovarian cancer, cervical cancer, prostate cancer, and bladder cancer.

Clinically, these are singular or multiple, round, palpable breast masses. They are hard but mobile and grow rapidly. They can occur bilaterally and with

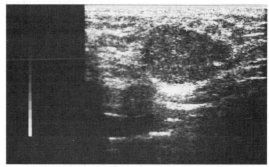

FIGURE 27-21 Metastases to breast.

lymphadenopathy. Mammographically, these lesions are nonspiculated and discrete with slightly irregular margins. Usually there are no microcalcifications.

Sonographic Findings. Sonographically, metastatic breast disease appears as a discrete solid breast mass. It does not typically infiltrate surrounding tissue and can appear relatively indistinguishable from some well-marginated primary breast cancers (Fig. 27-21).

Elastography

An elastogram is an imaging tool that uses the principle that most malignant masses are harder and more fixed into position because of their infiltrated nature than benign masses, which usually displace rather than infiltrate tissue planes. Using an external force, measurements are obtained relating to the stiffness of a mass. Elastography can assist noninvasively in the reduction of unnecessary biopsies. Elastography also has applications in magnetic resonance imaging (MRI) and computed tomography (CT).

AUGMENTATION

Approximately 300,000 breast augmentation procedures are performed in the United States annually.[12] In the augmented breast, the imaging role of sonography includes surveying for breast tissue abnormalities and implant integrity. The tissue abnormalities may or may not be related to the implant.

The most successful methods for identification of implant rupture are MRI and sonography. Because of the cost of MRI, the patient typically has a sonogram first, and if the examination is equivocal, MRI is ordered next. MRI is also the best way to evaluate the area around the chest wall. Mammographically, implants can still obscure a reported 35% to 40% of breast tissue, even with the use of the Eklund maneuver. Nevertheless, mammography is still important for these patients to assess the breast tissue for abnormalities, unless all breast tissue was removed before reconstruction.

In the United States, augmentation prostheses currently are placed in either the subglandular or the subpectoral position. Some countries inject silicone directly into the tissue, resulting in a difficult and confusing sonogram because of granuloma formation (Fig. 27-22, A).

Complications of implants in addition to rupture include hematoma, abscess, implant displacement, and autoimmune disease. Clinically, a patient with suspected implant rupture has a palpable mass, pain or burning, a contour change, increase or decrease of breast fullness, or a compromised autoimmune system.

Sonographic Findings

There are several types of implants with varying sonographic findings. The following is a description of double-lumen silicone implants.

Sonographically, implants should be anechoic internally with three echogenic rings surrounding the implant. From inner to outer, these rings are the inner surface of the implant shell, the outer surface of the implant shell, and the body's reactive fibrous capsule (Fig. 27-22, B and C). The sonographic signs for implant rupture are the "stepladder" sign and the "snowstorm" sign. The "stepladder" sign is parallel echogenic lines within the interior of the implant and indicates an intracapsular rupture. The "stepladder" sign correlates with the "linguine" sign on MRI. The "snowstorm" sign is described as echogenic noise with dirty shadowing similar to the

appearance of bowel gas. These sonographic signs may be noted concurrently (Fig. 27-22, D-F).

INFLAMMATION

Mastitis

Mastitis is inflammation of the breast. Mastitis can occur at any age, but most cases occur during lactation, usually in the second or third postpartum week. It is usually caused by a bacterial infection. Mastitis can begin with a crack on the nipple or a skin wound and may lead to abscess formation. It may also be caused by a foreign body, parasite, or disease, or be the result of an infected cyst. Clinically, patients have warm, red, swollen, and tender breasts. They may be febrile. There may be associated purulent discharge or a clogged lactiferous duct. Compression during mammography may be difficult because of the patient's skin edema and pain. Antibiotics may resolve mastitis.

Inflammatory carcinoma, which can have a similar patient presentation as mastitis, accounts for 1% of breast cancers. Differentiation between these two conditions is essential.

Sonographic Findings. The sonographic evaluation of mastitis may appear normal or reveal diffuse edema with an increase in tissue echogenicity. Skin thickening measuring greater than 2mm and inspissated material within dilated ducts sometimes can be seen. Visualization of reactive lymph nodes is possible (Fig. 27-23).

Abscess

An abscess is a localized area of pus and can form anywhere in the body. Within the breast, an abscess is usually retroareolar. Abscesses form in a small percentage of patients from mastitis, usually in lactating or weaning women. An abscess can also be a by-product of an infected cyst. Clinically, the patient usually has a palpable lump and tender, enlarged lymph nodes, in addition to symptoms of mastitis. Drainage or surgical removal may be necessary.

Sonographic Findings. An abscess is usually a complex mass with irregular thick walls. Debris levels and septations are common. Edema, skin thickening, and reactive lymph nodes are also common findings (see Figs. 27-15 and 27-23, C and D). As the abscess ages, the walls become more discrete (Fig. 27-24).

HEMATOMA

Breast hematomas typically form after an accidental or surgical trauma. Clinically, these patients often have a painful, palpable mass. Depending on the age of the hematoma, skin bruising and edema may also be noted. A seroma is similar to a hematoma except it contains serous fluid. The term "seroma" is usually used for a postsurgical fluid cavity.

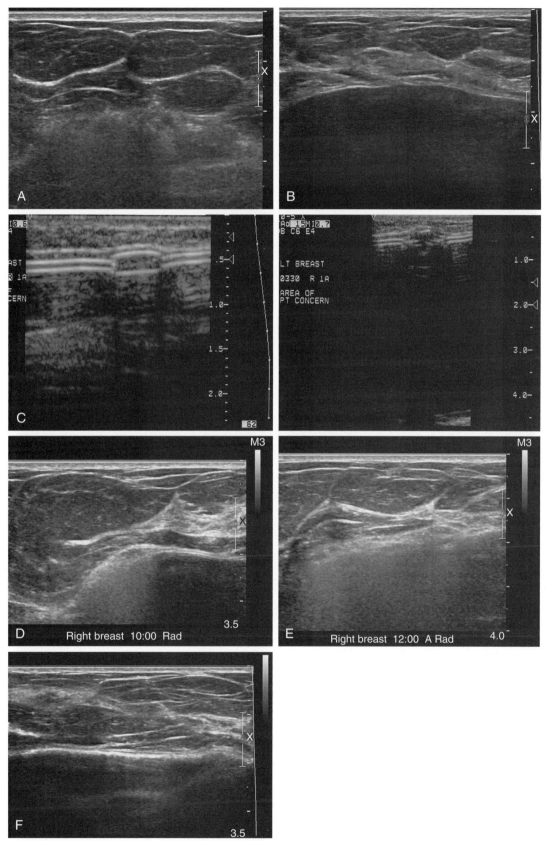

FIGURE 27-22 (A), Palpable granuloma in a 58-year-old woman with a history of implant rupture and removal. **(B)**, Normal-looking breast implant. **(C)**, A palpable area in a 26-year-old woman with breast implants proved to be a normal valve on implant. Implants with "snowstorm" sign **(D)** and "stepladder" sign **(E)**, indicating implant rupture. **(F)**, "Stepladder" sign.

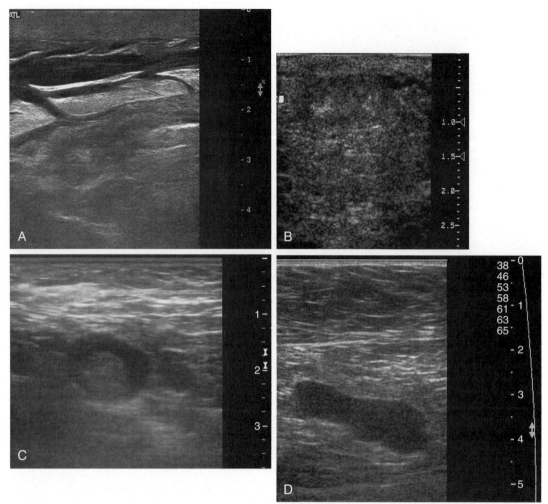

FIGURE 27-23 (A), A woman at 13 days postpartum with signs of mastitis. **(B),** Inspissated material seen within duct of a 35-year-old nursing woman. The patient was seen with a palpable lump and had decreased milk flow from this breast. **(C),** Normal appearance of lymph node, reniform in shape with echogenic fatty hilum. **(D),** Reactive lymph node in a patient with HIV.

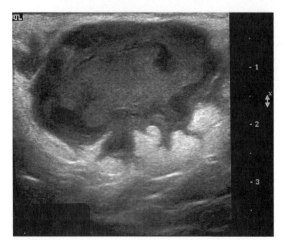

FIGURE 27-24 Palpable abscess in a woman at 39 weeks' gestation.

Sonographic Findings

Depending on the age and amount of blood within the fluid, a hematoma may appear as an anechoic and well-marginated mass or as a complex mass with thick walls and layering debris. Hematomas can decrease in size with age. Sonographically, they may regress and show no abnormality, or they may become a scar with some tissue distortion. Associated edema can look like a general area of increased echogenicity. Sonographically, a hematoma and a seroma may be indistinguishable (Fig. 27-25).

MALE BREAST DISEASES

Gynecomastia

All breast anomalies found in the female breast can also be found in the male breast with reduced incidence. The most common male breast anomaly is gynecomastia, which is enlargement from benign ductal and stromal proliferation. It typically occurs at three age periods: transiently at birth; again at puberty, declining in the late teens; and at adulthood, between 50 and 80 years old. Gynecomastia may be idiopathic but has been associated with estrogen excess; androgen deficiency; increased age; Klinefelter's syndrome; testicular failure; renal failure; cirrhosis; AIDS; and certain drugs, including marijuana, digitalis, heroin, and steroids. Gynecomastia can regress

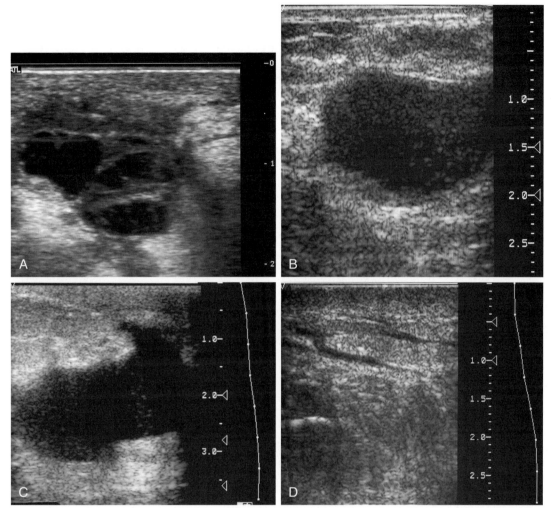

FIGURE 27-25 Hematoma and seroma. **(A),** Hematoma and seroma in lumpectomy site 2 weeks postoperatively. **(B),** Decreasing hematoma on serial sonograms in a patient with a history of an automobile accident. **(C),** A 5-year-old seroma in a patient with a history of lumpectomy and radiation therapy. **(D),** Edema in a patient 8 days after needle core biopsy.

on its own, but treatment depends on the cause. Clinically, it manifests as unilateral or bilateral breast enlargement with a tender or nontender retroareolar mass.
Sonographic Findings. Gynecomastia manifests sonographically as normal-appearing fibroglandular breast tissue with a triangular-shaped pattern. Occasionally, the ducts may also be appreciated (Fig. 27-26).

Male Breast Cancer

Male breast cancer is rare, representing 0.5% to 1% of all breast cancers. It usually occurs between 60 and 70 years of age. The most common form, representing about 80% of occurrences, is invasive ductal carcinoma.[13] Male breast cancer has been associated with Klinefelter's syndrome, family history, testicular injury, cryptorchidism, and advancing age. Clinically, breast cancer is usually palpated in the retroareolar region and feels similar to breast cancers in women. Nipple discharge is rare in male patients, and it is a strong indicator of malignancy when present.[14]

Sonographic Findings. Sonographically, male breast cancers look the same as female breast cancers (Fig. 27-27).

SUMMARY

Sonography is an essential diagnostic tool used to define better the characteristics of a mass by quantifying its size, shape, and location. Sonography is dynamic, making it uniquely qualified for invasive procedures and examinations involving the breast. Patient comfort is not usually compromised in the process. Performance of a sonogram can help reduce the number of unwarranted surgeries. Tables 27-1 to 27-3 are summaries of the pathologies of the breast.

CLINICAL SCENARIO—DIAGNOSIS

The patient was sent to a breast surgeon and was diagnosed with bilateral juvenile fibroadenomas. The fibroadenomas in this case are sonographically atypical. Fibroadenomas are usually discrete masses. The patient underwent bilateral breast reductions.

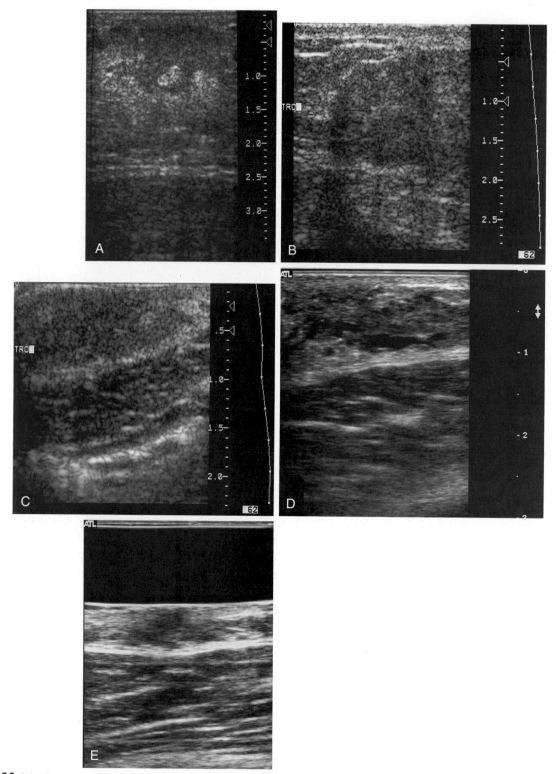

FIGURE 27-26 (A), A 43-year-old HIV-positive man with gynecomastia. **(B),** A 5-cm area of fibroglandular tissue in a 58-year-old man with palpable breast mass. Tissue diagnosis was gynecomastia. **(C),** Gynecomastia in a 12-year-old boy with nipple discharge. **(D),** Left unilateral gynecomastia in a 49-year-old man. **(E),** Normal-appearing right nipple complex in same patient as in *(D).*

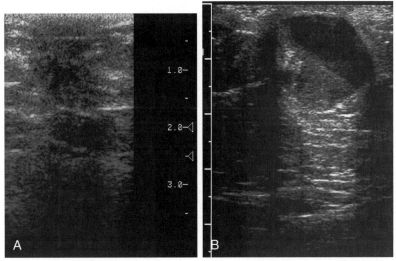

FIGURE 27-27 (A), Invasive ductal breast cancer in a man with palpable abnormality. **(B),** Papillary carcinoma in a 55-year-old man.

TABLE 27-1	Cysts of Breast	
Pathology	**Symptoms**	**Sonographic Findings**
Simple cyst	Asymptomatic, tender, palpable mass	Round or oval, anechoic, thin-walled, through transmission
Complex cyst	Asymptomatic, tender, palpable mass	Irregular or thick-walled, hypoechoic, may lack through transmission
Oil cyst	Usually result of surgical or accidental trauma; smooth, palpable mass; asymptomatic	Usually anechoic, may have hyperechoic internal echoes
Galactocele	Pregnancy or lactating; usually periareolar; palpable mass; associated with mastitis and abscess	Anechoic, complex, fat-fluid level, may have through transmission
Sebaceous cyst	Smooth, superficial, palpable mass	Anechoic to echogenic, through transmission

TABLE 27-2	Benign Neoplasms of Breast	
Pathology	**Symptoms**	**Sonographic Findings**
Fibroadenoma	Firm, rubbery, mobile mass; asymptomatic	Smooth, macrolobulated, usually homogeneous, hypoechoic, wide rather than tall
Cystosarcoma phylloides	Palpable, firm, mobile, rapidly enlarging mass	Similar to fibroadenoma, often contains cystic spaces
Papilloma	Nipple discharge; retroareolar when palpable; asymptomatic	Small solid mass within cyst or dilated duct
Lipoma	Soft, mobile, compressible mass; asymptomatic	Usually isoechoic
Hamartoma	Soft, mobile, compressible mass; asymptomatic	Usually heterogeneously hypoechoic

TABLE 27-3	Carcinoma of Breast	
Pathology	**Symptoms**	**Sonographic Findings**
Invasive ductal carcinoma	Hard, fixed, palpable mass; skin changes; asymptomatic	Hypoechoic, spiculated mass, posterior shadowing, tall rather than wide
Invasive lobular carcinoma	Breast thickening; usually not palpable; asymptomatic shadowing, indiscrete borders	Areas of distortion with heavy posterior
Colloid or mucinous carcinoma	Soft mass; skin changes are atypical; asymptomatic	Hypoechoic, microlobulated, well-defined mass, may have through transmission
Medullary carcinoma	Discrete, mobile, rapidly enlarging mass	Hypoechoic round mass
Papillary carcinoma	Nipple discharge; retroareolar; palpable mass; asymptomatic	Cystic or intraductal solid mass
Metastatic carcinoma	Hard, round, mobile, rapidly enlarging mass or masses	Hypoechoic discrete mass or masses
Inflammatory carcinoma	Mastitis	Diffuse increase in tissue echogenicity, skin thickening

CASE STUDIES FOR DISCUSSION

1. A 32-year-old woman in her first trimester of pregnancy presents for a breast sonogram because of a palpable lump. The sonogram reveals a large, predominately cystic mass with multiple mural nodules (Fig. 27-28). What is the most likely diagnosis?
2. A 12-year-old girl presents with breast asymmetry and a large, palpable mass in her right breast (Fig. 27-29). What is the likely diagnosis?
3. A 49-year-old woman who is HIV positive undergoes a sonogram that shows a small mass (Fig. 27-30, *A*) with multiple, enlarged axillary nodes (Fig. 27-30, *B*). What is likely causing the lymph node abnormality?

4. A 65-year-old man presents for a mammogram and sonogram of a palpable retroareolar mass (Fig. 27-31). What is the likely diagnosis?
5. A 64-year-old woman presents with the breast pathology shown in Figure 27-32, *A*. What is the likely diagnosis?

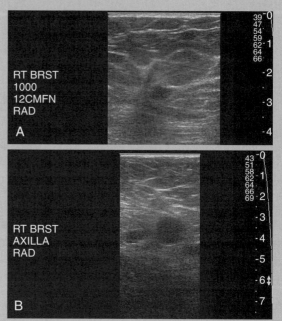

FIGURE 27-30 (A), Small mass with attenuation is noted. **(B),** Multiple, enlarged lymph nodes are demonstrated in the same patient.

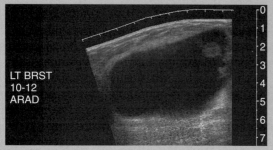

FIGURE 27-28 Large, predominantly cystic mass with mural nodules.

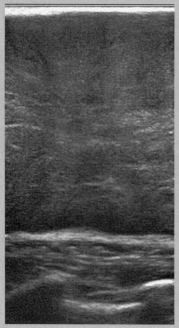

FIGURE 27-29 Very large, solid breast mass.

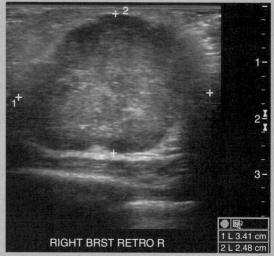

FIGURE 27-31 Large, solid, lobulated lesion is demonstrated.

CASE STUDIES FOR DISCUSSION—cont'd

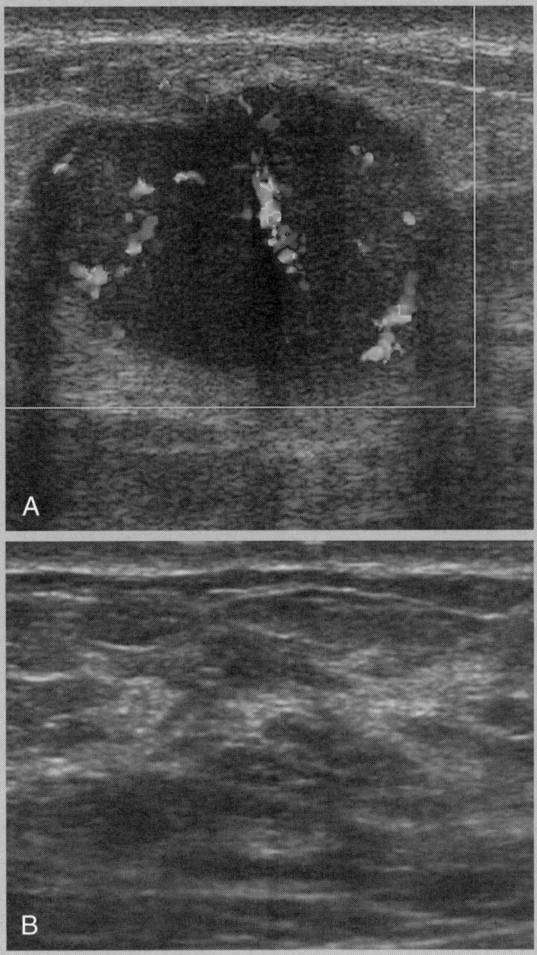

FIGURE 27-32 (A), Large, irregular breast lesion is demonstrated with prominent vascularity. **(B)**, Follow-up image of lesion after chemotherapy.

STUDY QUESTIONS

1. A 53-year-old woman is sent for a breast sonogram because of an abnormality seen only on one view of her recent mammogram. The sonogram reveals an area of distortion with thickened Cooper's ligaments and lymphadenopathy but does not show a discrete mass. The findings are most consistent with which of the following?
   a. Fibrocystic breast tissue
   b. Cystosarcoma phylloides
   c. Invasive lobular carcinoma
   d. Papillary carcinoma
   e. Metastases to the breast

2. A 30-year-old woman with a history of a breast reduction is sent to the sonography department for imaging of palpable masses along the surgical scar. A sonogram reveals three round, smooth, anechoic masses. The findings are most consistent with which of the following?
   a. Hematomas
   b. Granulomas
   c. Papillomas
   d. Oil cysts
   e. Papillary carcinoma

3. A 65-year-old man presents to the sonography department with a palpable right upper outer quadrant breast mass. Sonographically, a solid mass with posterior shadowing is seen at 10:00 3 CMFN. The findings are most consistent with which of the following?
   a. Invasive ductal carcinoma
   b. Lobular carcinoma
   c. Gynecomastia
   d. Lymphadenopathy
   e. Lipoma

4. A 38-year-old pregnant woman presents to the sonography department with a rapidly enlarging, retroareolar, palpable mass. Sonographically, a microlobulated mass with internal blood flow is identified. The findings are most consistent with which of the following?
   a. Galactocele
   b. Fibroadenoma
   c. Invasive ductal carcinoma
   d. Papillary carcinoma
   e. Mastitis

5. A 50-year-old woman with augmented breasts presents to the sonography department complaining of newly occurring asymmetry of breast size, right smaller than left. Sonographically, the right breast has long, echogenic lines within the internal portion of the implant. Shadowing, resembling bowel gas, is also seen along the external periphery of the implant. The findings are most consistent with which of the following?
   a. Right breast intracapsular rupture only
   b. Left breast extracapsular rupture only
   c. Right breast extracapsular rupture only
   d. Right breast "stepladder" and "snowstorm" signs
   e. Right breast "linguine" and "snowstorm" signs

6. Which of the following is not considered a mass of the breast tissue?
   a. Oil cyst
   b. Inclusion cyst
   c. Lipoma
   d. Hematoma
   e. Galactocele

7. A 16-year-old girl presents to the sonography department with a breast mass that has been palpable for 6 months. Sonographically, a 7-cm, smooth, oval, gently lobulated mass is seen. The findings are most consistent with which of the following?
   a. Fibroadenoma
   b. Phylloides tumor
   c. Giant fibroadenoma
   d. Proliferative fibroadenoma
   e. Lipoma

8. Which of the following would be the most worrisome sonographic finding?
   a. A hypoechoic oval mass with a hyperechoic center found in the breast of a 45-year-old woman
   b. A macrocalcified mass seen in the breast of a 38-year-old woman
   c. A hard, mostly cystic mass seen 2 months postoperatively, posterior to a mastectomy scar
   d. A 4-cm, smooth, oval mass with cystic areas in the breast of a 55-year-old woman
   e. A cystic mass seen in the breast of a postmenopausal woman receiving hormone replacement therapy

9. A 50-year-old woman palpates a compressible, mobile mass in her left breast. Sonographically, the mass, although palpable, is indistinguishable from the surrounding breast tissue. What would be the most likely diagnosis?
   a. Fibroadenoma
   b. Lymph node
   c. Lobular carcinoma
   d. Papilloma
   e. Lipoma

10. A 55-year-old woman undergoes a sonogram that reveals a retroareolar, solid mass within dilated ducts. She has evidence of skin edema and complains of unilateral pink nipple discharge. What would be the most likely diagnosis?
    a. Invasive ductal carcinoma
    b. Papillary carcinoma
    c. Papilloma
    d. Galactocele
    e. Abscess

REFERENCES

1. Fibroadenoma. mayoclinic.com/health/fibroadenoma/DS01069. Retrieved May 12, 2013.
2. Stephan P: Breast fibroadenomas, breastcancer.about.com/od/mammograms/p/fibroadenomas.htm. Retrieved May 12, 2013.
3. Phyllodes tumors, hopkinsmedicine.org/avon_foundation_breast_center/breast_cancers_other_conditions/phyllodes_tumors.html. Retrieved May 12, 2013.
4. Richards T, Hunt A, Courtney S, et al: Nipple discharge: a sign of breast cancer? *Ann R Coll Surg Engl* 89:124–126, 2007.
5. Maeda R: Types of breast cancer, medicinenet.com/script/main/art.asp?articlekey=21902. Retrieved May 12, 2013.
6. Arpino G, Bardou V, Clark G, et al: Infiltrating lobular carcinoma of the breast: tumor characteristics and clinical outcome, *Breast Cancer Res* 6:R149–R156, 2004.
7. Stephan P: Mucinous (colloid) carcinoma of the breast, breastcancer.about.com/od/types/p/mucinous_ca.htm. Retrieved May 13, 2013.
8. Stephan P: Medullary carcinoma - invasive breast cancer, breastcancer.about.com/od/types/p/medullary_ca.htm. Retrieved May 13, 2013.
9. Griggs JJ, Hudis C: IDC Type: papilary carcinoma of the breast. breastcancer.org/symptoms/types/rare_idc/papillary.jsp. Retrieved May 13, 2013.
10. papilary carcinoma of the breast, cancercenter.com/breast-cancer/types/papillary-carcinoma.cfm. Retrieved May 12, 2013.
11. Vaughan A, Dietz J, Moley J, et al: Metastatic disease to the breast: the Washington University experience, *World J Surg Oncol* 5:74, 2007.
12. Breast augmentation, plasticsurgeryguide.com/breast-augmentation-implants.html.
13. Breast cancer in men, cancer.org/Cancer/BreastCancerinMen/DetailedGuide/breast-cancer-in-men-what-is-breast-cancer-in-men. Retrieved May 12, 2013.
14. Farooq A, Horgan K: Male breast cancer presenting as nipple discharge, *Case Reports in Surgery*, 2011:804843, 2011. Retrieved May 12, 2013.

Scrotal Mass and Scrotal Pain

Duane Meixner

CLINICAL SCENARIO

A previously healthy, 29-year-old man reports 12 days of fatigue and malaise with occasional nausea. On physical examination, a small tender palpable nodule is discovered on the lower pole of the right testis. Sonographic evaluation demonstrates a small cystic mass in the area of the palpable abnormality and a mostly solid complex mass occupying most of the right testicle (Fig. 28-1; see Color Plate 37). Discuss possible causes for the sonographic findings.

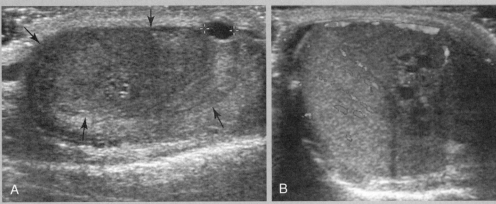

FIGURE 28-1 **(A)**, Small tunical cyst *(calipers)* represents the palpable abnormality. A mostly hypoechoic mass *(arrows)* occupies most of the testis. **(B)**, Transverse view shows cystic components and internal blood flow (see Color Plate 37).

OBJECTIVES

- Describe the sonographic appearance of the normal scrotal contents.
- Identify the clinical signs and symptoms of benign processes in the scrotum.
- Describe the sonographic appearance of benign findings in the scrotum.
- Identify the clinical signs and symptoms of clinically significant processes in the scrotum.
- Describe the sonographic appearance of common clinically significant pathologies of the scrotum.

Sonography can display the scrotal contents in exquisite detail and is the imaging method of choice for evaluating the scrotum. When a patient presents with scrotal pain, or a scrotal mass is discovered or suspected clinically, a sonogram should be the first imaging test ordered. Not only are abnormalities within the testicle easily seen with ultrasound imaging, but also other conditions of the scrotum can be characterized, such as epididymal masses, fluid collections, and infectious processes. Along with clinical and laboratory findings, sonography can provide valuable information for the diagnosis and treatment planning of abnormalities in the scrotum.

SCROTUM

The scrotum is an outpouching of the lower abdominal wall, with layers derived from the muscles and connective tissues. The structures contained within the scrotum are the testicles, the epididymides, and the proximal spermatic cords (Fig. 28-2). The testicles are two ovoid spermatogenic endocrine glands separated from each

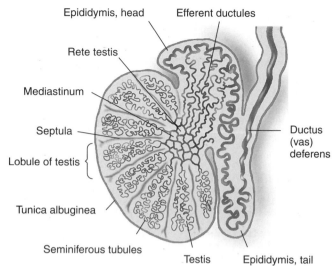

FIGURE 28-2 Anatomy of testis and epididymis.

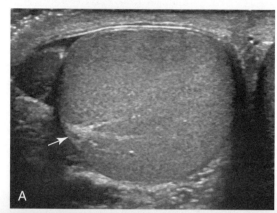

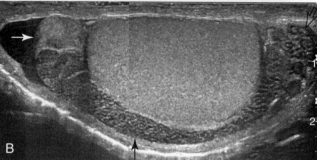

FIGURE 28-3 (A), Transverse view of the testis shows the echogenic mediastinum *(arrow)* with septa radiating toward the capsule. **(B)**, Dual, longitudinal image of normal scrotal contents. The epididymal head *(white arrow)*, body *(black arrow)*, and tail *(open black arrow)* lie adjacent to the homogeneous testis.

other within the scrotum by the scrotal septum. Each testicle has a capsule of fibrous connective tissue called the tunica albuginea. At the posterior aspect of the testicle, the tissue of the tunica albuginea enters the testicle to form the mediastinum testis and then extends toward the outer capsule as numerous septa, which create lobules that house the spermatogenic seminiferous tubules. The seminiferous tubules converge at the mediastinum to form the rete testis, a network of microtubules, which gives off several efferent ductules. The epididymal head comprises the convoluted efferent ductules that transport spermatozoa out of the testis into the epididymis. The ductules of the head converge to become a single coiled duct, the epididymal body and tail, passing next to the testis from the upper pole toward the lower pole. Near or at the inferior pole of the testis, the duct turns back toward the upper pole, deconvolutes, and enlarges slightly to become the ductus deferens, which exits the scrotum as part of the spermatic cord. Each scrotal compartment, or hemiscrotum, is lined by tunica vaginalis, a serous membrane that also covers the testicle and epididymis and encloses the potential peritesticular space.

Sonographic Findings

Normal testicles are homogeneous and mildly echogenic except for the mediastinum testis, which is hyperechoic, is of variable thickness, and runs along the posterolateral side of the testicle in a craniocaudal orientation (Fig. 28-3, *A*). Each testicle is approximately 5 cm × 3 cm × 2 cm in size. The peritesticular spaces normally contain small amounts of serous fluid. The normal epididymis may have a perceptible tubular appearance and has an echogenicity that is less than the testicle, although the head may be more echogenic than the rest of the epididymis (Fig. 28-3, *B*).

EXTRATESTICULAR MASS

Many abnormalities that occur in the scrotum do not involve the testes. Any scrotal abnormality discovered by the patient or his physician may precipitate sonographic evaluation. Extratesticular masses are nearly always benign.

Cysts and Fluid

Epididymal Cysts and Spermatoceles. Epididymal cysts are serous fluid–filled cysts that occur anywhere in the epididymis. Spermatoceles are cystic dilations of the epididymal ductules containing spermatozoa and other debris and usually occur in the head. Both lesions are common. If large enough to be palpable, cysts and spermatoceles are discernible as a nodule separate from the testis, although larger lesions may manifest as generalized painless scrotal enlargement.

Sonographic Findings. Epididymal cysts and spermatoceles are indistinguishable sonographically. Both may appear as anechoic simple cysts (Fig. 28-4) or may contain fine low-level echoes, sometimes with precipitative layering. Scrotal cysts can be several centimeters in diameter and can be mistaken for a large hydrocele. Neither epididymal cyst nor spermatocele is of clinical significance unless large enough to be symptomatic. Spermatoceles tend to be solitary, whereas epididymal cysts are often multiple.

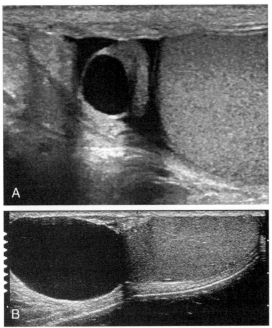

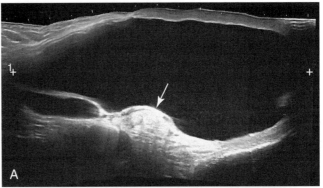

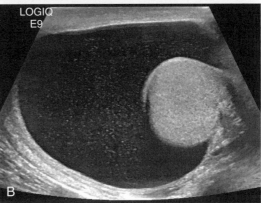

FIGURE 28-4 (A), Palpable upper pole abnormality is an epididymal cyst or spermatocele. **(B),** Large epididymal cyst displaces testis inferiorly. (*B, Courtesy Cindy Rapp, Radiology Imaging Associates, Greenwood Village, Colorado.*)

FIGURE 28-5 (A), Extended field of view image of a massive hydrocele (*calipers*). The testis (*arrow*) is compressed at its attachment to the inner scrotal wall. It is unusually hyperechoic because of acoustic enhancement. **(B),** Moderate to large hydrocele with internal echoes.

Hydrocele. A hydrocele is an abnormal amount of serous fluid in the peritesticular space. Hydroceles may be unilateral or bilateral and can occur at any age. Congenital hydroceles are common in newborn boys because the processus vaginalis, the passage between the abdomen and scrotum, may not obliterate for some time after delivery. Acquired hydroceles can occur at any age and have many causes, including trauma, infection, infarction, torsion, and testicular neoplasms. The patient usually has unilateral painless scrotal enlargement, from minimal to large enough to alter gait. Most hydroceles transilluminate on clinical examination.

Sonographic Findings. A hydrocele appears as a fluid collection next to or around the testis, sometimes with septations. It might be seen as a relatively small amount of free paratesticular fluid, or it might be massive, enlarging the hemiscrotum greatly and compressing the testis against the inner scrotal wall. Large hydroceles are better demonstrated with dual imaging or an extended field of view (Fig. 28-5). In chronic hydroceles, echoes may be seen within the fluid; documenting acoustic streaming within such a hydrocele confirms the diagnosis. A very large hydrocele can be confused with a massive extratesticular cyst.

Varicocele. A varicocele is a network of veins, the pampiniform plexus, dilated owing to increased venous pressure. It may be palpated as a sometimes painful cluster of tubular structures next to or superior to the testis. Varicoceles are predominantly found on the left because the left testicular vein is longer and enters the left renal vein at a right angle creating greater resistance to flow. Most varicoceles are extratesticular, but they

can also extend into the testicular parenchyma. Varicoceles can be primary, caused by incompetent valves in the internal spermatic veins, or secondary, caused by compression of the testicular vein by an extrinsic process such as a retroperitoneal mass. Primary varicocele can occur at any age and is a correctable cause of male infertility.

Sonographic Findings. Varicoceles appear as dilated fluid-filled tubular structures in the posterolateral aspect of the scrotum measuring greater than 2 mm.[1] Echogenic blood may be seen moving slowly through the veins, but color Doppler is essential in the diagnosis of a varicocele (Fig. 28-6; see Color Plate 38). Increased flow is identified within the prominent veins when the patient performs the Valsalva maneuver and is scanned while the patient is standing. Measuring the vein diameter should be done during the Valsalva maneuver also. If a large or unilateral right-sided varicocele is discovered, the right upper and lower quadrants should be investigated for external compression of the right testicular vein.

Hematocele. A hematocele is a collection of blood in the peritesticular space. Hematoceles are similar to hydroceles on clinical examination and must be considered in patients with a history of recent trauma, including torsion or scrotal and inguinal surgical procedures.

Sonographic Findings. A hematocele is seen as a complex collection around the testis, usually with

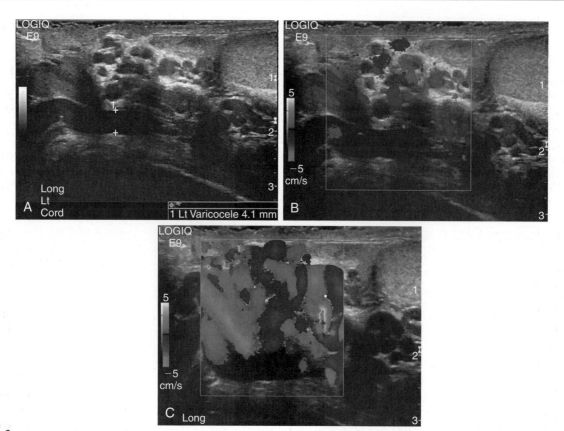

FIGURE 28-6 (A), Gray-scale image of the spermatic cord shows a vein of the pampiniform plexus dilated to 4.1 mm. **(B),** Longitudinal color Doppler image shows minimal blood flow with normal respiration (see Color Plate 38). **(C),** Increased flow with Valsalva maneuver (see Color Plate 38).

septations and varying amounts of cystic versus solid contents depending on the age of the hematoma.

Pyocele. A pyocele is a collection of peritesticular pus in patients with an inflammatory scrotal condition or who have sustained scrotal trauma. A patient with pyocele presents with an enlarged scrotum of varying degrees and may exhibit pain, redness, and localized warmth. If the patient has an active infection, he is likely to have an elevated white blood cell count and low-grade fever.

Sonographic Findings. A pyocele appears as a complex, sometimes septate fluid collection surrounding the testis (Fig. 28-7; see Color Plate 39). Unusual presentations include relatively homogeneous and echogenic material around the testis or a discrete mass near the testis. Gentle transducer pressure sometimes creates visible movement of the pyocele echoes. Similar to other peritesticular fluid collections, they can be of any size but rarely achieve several centimeters in greatest dimension.

Solid Lesions

Scrotal Pearls. Scrotal pearls are calcifications within the peritesticular space. They are thought to be caused by epididymitis, testicular torsion, torsion of the appendix testis or appendix epididymis, inflammation, or a chronic hydrocele. They are usually silent but can sometimes be palpated.

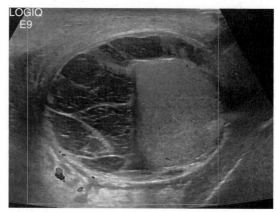

FIGURE 28-7 Complex septate paratesticular collection in a man 13 days after vasectomy, which was a pyocele at surgical exploration (see Color Plate 39).

Sonographic Findings. Scrotal pearls are highly echogenic and sometimes have a less echogenic fibrous "rind" or concentric rings of varying echogenicity (Fig. 28-8). They are more likely to be seen in the presence of a hydrocele and may not be noticeably mobile. Although calcified, they may not shadow.

Adenomatoid Tumor. Adenomatoid tumor is a very commonly found solid mass in the epididymis. It is benign and manifests as a hard, discrete extratesticular nodule, usually at the tail. It typically appears in the third to fifth decade of life.[1]

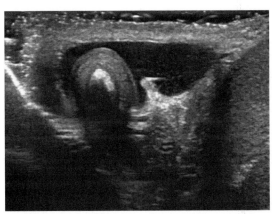

FIGURE 28-8 Scrotal pearl demonstrating the sometimes seen concentric appearance of a hypoechoic outer layer surrounding a calcified core.

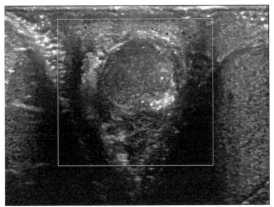

FIGURE 28-9 A 1.5-cm sperm granuloma at the tail of the epididymis, which is heterogeneous with no internal blood flow.

Sonographic Findings. Adenomatoid tumors most commonly appear as a well-circumscribed extratesticular solid mass with echogenicity ranging from hypoechoic to hyperechoic. Most are less than 2 cm in size but can be 5 cm.[1]

Sperm Granuloma. Sperm granulomas are discrete extratubular collections of granulomatous spermatozoa that occur at the epididymis or rete testis in men who have had a vasectomy or, less frequently, trauma. On physical examination, a sperm granuloma is palpable as a usually painless firm epididymal nodule.

Sonographic Findings. Sperm granulomas are usually less homogeneous than adenomatoid tumors and may have areas of particularly bright echoes (Fig. 28-9). A sperm granuloma in the rete testis appears as an intratesticular lesion.

Scrotal Hernia. Scrotal hernias are inguinal hernias that enter the scrotum. These may contain serous fluid contained by peritoneum, small bowel, colon, mesentery, or omentum. The abdominal contents are able to enter the scrotum because the processus vaginalis persists after birth or recanalizes later. There are two types of hernias—indirect and direct. Indirect hernias are more common than direct hernias, but in either case the patient

has a swollen scrotum of variable size that contains a palpable mass. Incarceration occurs when the abdominal structures are no longer able to pass between the abdomen and scrotum, potentially causing the blood supply of the herniated tissue to be compromised. An incarcerated hernia is likely to be painful, and if timely surgery is not performed, the incarcerated tissue becomes ischemic, then infarcted, and finally necrotic and gangrenous.

Sonographic Findings. Sonography reveals a mass of greatly variable echogenicity and echotexture depending on what structures are herniated to the scrotum (Fig. 28-10). There may be variably echogenic fluid with or without a visible hernia sac or a solid mass of varying complexity. Shadowing from air may be identified. If peristaltic motion is identified, the diagnosis of scrotal hernia is confirmed. Gentle transducer pressure may demonstrate reduction of a hernia in the proximal scrotal space, and a Valsalva maneuver may force a hernia deeper into the hemiscrotum; both can aid in the diagnosis. Sonography is not dependable for differentiating indirect from direct hernias.

CYSTIC TESTICULAR MASS

Every solid intratesticular mass must be considered malignant until proven otherwise. Scrotal sonography approaches 100% accuracy in distinguishing a solid mass from a cystic mass, but it is poor for distinguishing whether a solid intratesticular mass is malignant or benign.

Tunica Albuginea Cyst

Tunica albuginea cysts form in the tunica albuginea and are typically present in men 30 to 50 years old. They range in size from 2 mm to 3 cm, but most are less than 1 cm in diameter.[1] They are painless and palpable at the testicular surface as a classic "BB" or "pea" presentation. **Sonographic Findings.** These lesions appear as well-defined round or ovoid anechoic areas at the peripheral edge of the testis with or without deep enhancement.

Testicular Cyst

Purely cystic lesions seen within the testicle are true cysts, most likely originating in the rete testis. They can be tiny and barely perceptible, or they can nearly replace the testicular tissue. Most are not appreciated on physical examination and are identified incidentally. **Sonographic Findings.** These lesions appear as well-defined anechoic areas with smooth distinct walls and deep acoustic enhancement (Fig. 28-11).

Tubular Ectasia of Rete Testis

Epididymal obstruction from various causes, including vasectomy and trauma, can result in cystlike dilation of the rete testis.

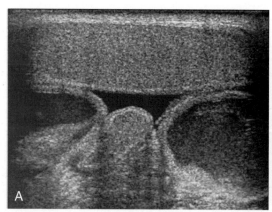
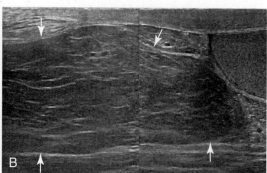

FIGURE 28-10 (A), Deep to the testis (seen at the top of the image) lie herniated loops of bowel, some fluid-filled. Active peristalsis was noted in real time. **(B),** Dual image of a large mesenteric hernia *(arrows)* superior to the testis. On Valsalva, the mass protruded farther into the scrotum.

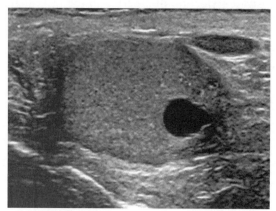

FIGURE 28-11 Intratesticular simple cyst.

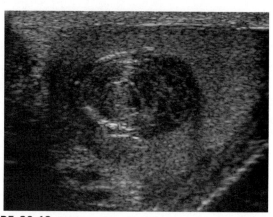

FIGURE 28-12 Epidermoid cyst demonstrating whorled "onion-skin" lamellar appearance.

Sonographic Findings. Rete testis ectasia appears at the mediastinum as innumerable small cysts. Image optimization and careful interrogation is imperative to confirm the cystic nature of rete testis ectasia to avoid mistaking this for a hypoechoic solid lesion.

Epidermoid Cyst

Epidermoid cysts account for only about 1% of testicular neoplasms. They are benign keratin-containing cysts with an "onion-skin" lamellar architecture. They most commonly are discovered as a well-circumscribed, painless testicular mass in postpubertal boys and men 40 years old or younger.[1]

Sonographic Findings. Epidermoid cysts manifest as well-defined hypoechoic round or oval masses, and although they are cysts, acoustic enhancement is absent (Fig. 28-12). The concentric laminar architecture within these lesions sometimes generates a whorled appearance that is suggestive of the diagnosis. Also suggestive is the absence of internal vascularity on Doppler examination. If these characteristics are seen in a testicular mass, it must be reported so that surgical planning can allow for the possibility of a testis-sparing enucleation.

SOLID TESTICULAR MASS

Germ Cell Tumors

Most solid intratesticular masses are malignant, and half of the tumors are of primary germ cell origin. Germ cell testicular cancer can be seminomatous or nonseminomatous germ cell tumors, including embryonal cell carcinoma, teratoma, and choriocarcinoma. Pure nonseminomatous germ cell tumors are uncommon, whereas mixed germ cell tumors, containing at least two of the types, are second only to seminoma in incidence.[1] All types are usually discovered as a hard testicular mass or as firm testicular enlargement on physical examination. Earlier discovery of retroperitoneal or mediastinal metastases often precipitates the discovery of nonpalpable primary testicular germ cell tumors. Patients younger than 50 years old account for nearly all presentations of testicular germ cell tumors. The serum tumor markers alpha fetoprotein, human chorionic gonadotropin (hCG), and lactate dehydrogenase can be helpful in decisions regarding management of testicular cancers but not for screening asymptomatic patients.[2] Although some testicular cancers cause pain, most do not.

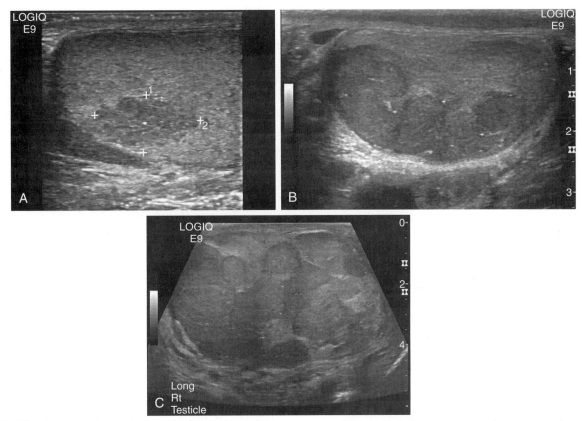

FIGURE 28-13 **(A),** Discrete hypoechoic mass in the upper pole is a seminoma. **(B),** Lobular, heterogeneous seminoma occupying most of the testis. Note the presence of scattered microlithiasis. **(C),** Multifocal seminoma completely replaces testicular tissue.

Seminoma

Seminomas are the most common germ cell tumor, accounting for approximately half of tumors. Seminomas readily metastasize to retroperitoneal lymph nodes, and a significant number of these tumors are found only after the discovery of the distant disease. Despite their metastatic tendency, seminomas respond well to therapy and are the most likely germ cell tumor to be successfully treated.

Sonographic Findings. Seminomas usually manifest as a hypoechoic mass that is homogeneous, although scattered hyperechoic areas may occasionally be identified (Fig. 28-13). Seminomas are usually unilateral and may be very small in size, or they may completely replace normal testicular parenchyma, in which case they tend to be heterogeneous or appear multilobular. The presence of microlithiasis, tiny nonshadowing echogenic foci, in a testis with a solid tumor is suggestive of seminoma, although screening with sonography in asymptomatic men with no risk factors for seminoma has not been shown to be beneficial.[3]

Embryonal Cell Carcinoma

Embryonal cell carcinoma typically occurs in men 20 to 40 years old and is the second most common testicular cancer, found in pure or mixed form in 40% of primary

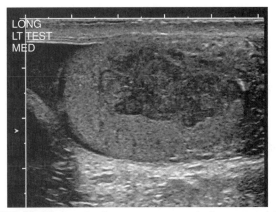

FIGURE 28-14 Irregular heterogeneous testicular mass, which is embryonal cell cancer, invading the epididymis via the rete testis *(upper right)*. The patient also had retroperitoneal adenopathy.

testicular neoplasms.[2] Metastasis can occur through the bloodstream and lymphatics. These cancers are more aggressive than seminomas.

Sonographic Findings. Embryonal cell cancer usually is seen as a hypoechoic, inhomogeneous mass in the testicle (Fig. 28-14). The tumor may distort the normal contour of the testicle when invasion of the tunica albuginea occurs. If calcifications are present, they tend to be bulkier than microlithiasis and may shadow.

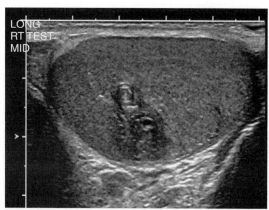

FIGURE 28-15 Mixed germ cell tumor with cystic and brightly echogenic components was predominately teratoma.

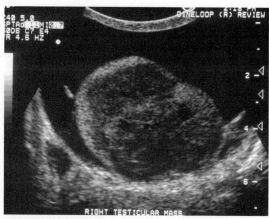

FIGURE 28-16 Heterogeneous intratesticular mass is shown in addition to a hydrocele. The pathology report revealed choriocarcinoma. *(Courtesy Cindy Rapp, Radiology Imaging Associates, Greenwood Village, Colorado.)*

Teratoma

Teratomas may contain hair, bone, teeth, and other tissue types. They are generally seen in neonates, prepubertal boys, and men 25 to 35 years old. When found in younger patients, teratoma is usually benign; however, in older patients, almost 30% are malignant.[4] Prognosis in patients with malignant teratoma is less favorable than in patients with either seminoma or embryonal cell tumors.

Sonographic Findings. Teratomas are usually well differentiated histologically. Depending on which tissue components are present, these masses may be hyperechoic, hypoechoic, or complex and often demonstrate shadowing and cystic areas (Fig. 28-15).

Choriocarcinoma

Pure choriocarcinomas are the rarest germ cell tumors. Choriocarcinoma is more often part of a mixed tumor, found in about 23% of that kind of germ cell tumor, and the most common age group is 10 to 30 years of age.[1] Elevated levels of hCG are found in 100% of men with choriocarcinomas making gynecomastia a common sign. However, men with any type of malignant testicular neoplasm can have breast enlargement from elevated hCG levels. Whether found in its pure form or as part of a mixed germ cell tumor, the presence of choriocarcinoma is associated with the least favorable prognosis for long-term survival.

Sonographic Findings. Tumors that include choriocarcinoma usually manifest as a mass with mixed echogenicity (Fig. 28-16) not only because of the mixed histologic nature of these tumors but also because of the possible presence of hemorrhage, necrosis, and calcifications.

Stromal Tumors

Stromal cell tumors arise from Leydig cells between the seminiferous tubules and Sertoli cells within the seminiferous tubule walls. Leydig cell and Sertoli cell tumors are usually benign.

Leydig Cell Tumor

Leydig cell tumors are also called interstitial cell tumors. Of these tumors, 15% are malignant, which makes them the most common non–germ cell cancer of the testis. They most commonly occur from the third through the sixth decade of life and may produce excessive amounts of either estrogen or testosterone causing feminization or virilization.[1] Determination of whether such tumors are benign or malignant with histopathologic examination alone is often difficult, and the presence of metastatic disease may reveal the malignant nature of a Leydig cell tumor. Patients normally have painless enlargement of the testicle or a palpable mass.

Sonographic Findings. Leydig cell tumors appear as a solid intratesticular mass and are usually hypoechoic. Hemorrhage and necrosis are common, so cystic areas may be seen. Although most Leydig cell tumors are benign, sonography cannot distinguish benign from malignant tumors.

Sertoli Cell Tumor

Similar to Leydig cell tumors, Sertoli cell tumors are usually benign; however, in contrast to Leydig cell tumors, they occur equally at all ages.[1] Patients normally have painless enlargement of the testicle or a palpable mass. Sertoli cell tumors, especially when malignant, can secrete estrogens, causing some patients to have gynecomastia.

Sonographic Findings. The sonographic appearance of Sertoli cell tumors is nearly identical to Leydig cell tumors.

INFILTRATING TESTICULAR DISEASE

The infiltrative testicular processes lymphoma and leukemia are nearly always metastatic manifestations of advanced disease. They are rare, accounting for a very

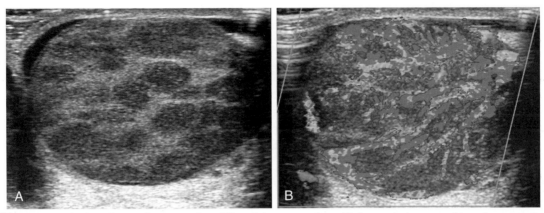

FIGURE 28-17 (A), Testicular lymphoma demonstrating diffuse inhomogeneity, with hypoechoic areas of invasion surrounded by normal testicular tissue. **(B),** Transverse color Doppler view of the same patient demonstrates the typical finding of undistorted vasculature (see Color Plate 40).

small proportion of solid intratesticular masses. Lymphoma is the most commonly occurring testicular cancer in elderly men, whereas testicular leukemia is often seen in children with the disease. Testicular lymphoma is commonly bilateral. Advanced stages of these diseases can cause general enlargement of the testicle.

Sonographic Findings

Malignancies that infiltrate the testicles are most often hypoechoic and do not disrupt the vasculature or anatomic architecture of the testicles (Fig. 28-17; see Color Plate 40). Lymphoma and leukemia are likely to be hypervascular on color Doppler, and absence of pain aids in ruling out inflammation.

INGUINAL MASS

Cryptorchidism

Cryptorchidism manifests as the absence from the scrotum of one or both testicles. In a normal fetus, the testicles descend through the processus vaginalis into the scrotal sac before delivery, and failure of either to arrive in the scrotum is cryptorchidism. The location of the undescended testicles can be anywhere along the path, from the renal pedicle in the retroperitoneum to the distal inguinal canal; 80% are palpable in the inguinal canal.[1] If descent stops in the inguinal canal, the testicle can be felt as a firm, sometimes mobile mass superior to the scrotum. Surgical correction of inguinal cryptorchidism, called orchiopexy, moves the undescended testicle to the scrotal sac and attaches it there. Several conditions are associated with a history of cryptorchidism, including infertility, cancer, and scrotal hernia.
Sonographic Findings. An inguinal undescended testicle is identified as an ovoid soft tissue mass in the inguinal canal, often recognizable as the testis and epididymis (Fig. 28-18; see Color Plate 41). An inguinal testicle is typically smaller than a normally located testicle. The

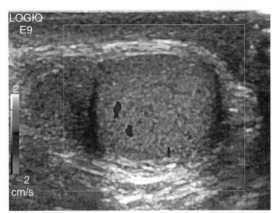

FIGURE 28-18 Otherwise normal testis and epididymis seen in the inguinal canal of a 5-year-old boy (see Color Plate 41).

echotexture of a normal undescended testicle is homogeneous and hypoechoic, and color Doppler usually reveals diminished blood flow, especially in prepubescent boys. Retroperitoneal and pelvic cryptorchidism is not visible sonographically.

SCROTAL PAIN

Scrotal pain is nearly always the result of inflammation or torsion. Inflammation typically results from retrograde progression of a urinary tract infection but can also be caused by trauma. Torsion is the result of twisting mechanical forces on scrotal structures. In addition to torsion and inflammation, trauma can cause hematoma, hematocele, and testicular rupture.

Epididymitis and Epididymo-orchitis

Epididymitis accounts for most acute inflammatory disease of the scrotum. Painful swelling, redness, skin warmth and thickening, and hydrocele are strongly suggestive of inflammation. Patients with acute epididymitis have excruciating pain and may have urethral discharge because the most frequent etiology of epididymitis is bacterial urinary tract infection; however, epididymitis may also be viral in origin. The patient's white blood cell count is likely to be elevated. It is usually a unilateral condition but may be bilateral.

Orchitis is inflammation of the testis. It usually occurs as progression into the testicle of untreated epididymitis resulting in epididymo-orchitis. Initially, a localized area of testis may be inflamed, with the entire gland eventually becoming involved. Viral causes of orchitis include mumps, influenza, and tonsillitis. Patients with orchitis may have fever, nausea, and vomiting. If the disease is left untreated, areas of necrosis or abscess may develop.
Sonographic Findings. In the earliest stages, the tail of the epididymis is enlarged, and color Doppler analysis shows markedly increased flow in the affected area. With progression, the entire epididymis enlarges and becomes hyperemic, and a reactive hydrocele may develop (Fig. 28-19). If the infection becomes chronic, the epididymis becomes thickened and focally echogenic, and calcifications may be evident. In the acute phase of orchitis, the involved areas of the testis appear less echogenic than normal testicle. Hyperemia develops throughout the testis; later, the scrotal wall may be thickened and hyperemic (Fig. 28-20; see Color Plate 42). In long-term chronic orchitis, the testicle becomes atrophic and heterogeneous.

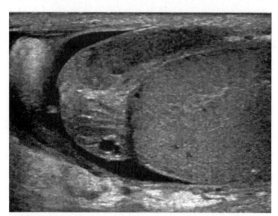

FIGURE 28-19 Epididymitis with enlarged epididymis and hydrocele.

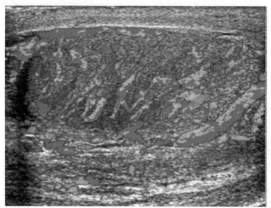

FIGURE 28-20 Color Doppler image showing hyperemia of epididymo-orchitis, including in the scrotal skin (see Color Plate 42).

Abscess

Intratesticular abscesses are uncommon and usually result from epididymo-orchitis, although other causes have been reported. Clinically, the patient has a swollen and tender testis from epididymo-orchitis, and the abscess is discovered incidentally.
Sonographic Findings. An intratesticular abscess may appear as a homogeneous hypoechoic or anechoic area or may be complex and irregular with increased blood flow outside of the abscess on color Doppler (Fig. 28-21; see Color Plate 43). A concurrent pyocele is possible.

Torsion

Testicular torsion results when the testis rotates within the scrotum, twisting the spermatic cord. This twisting compresses or occludes the testicular vessels and results in decreased or lost blood flow to and from the testis. The two types of testicular torsion are intravaginal and extravaginal. Extravaginal torsion is rare and is

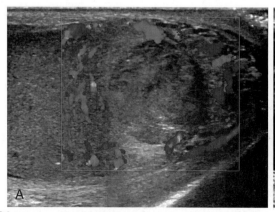
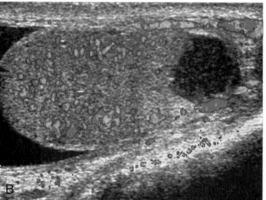

FIGURE 28-21 **(A),** Rounded complex intratesticular mass in a patient with acute scrotal pain is avascular but surrounded by hyperemia, suggesting epididymo-orchitis abscess instead of neoplasm (see Color Plate 43). **(B),** Follow-up examination in 2 weeks shows the mass to be shrinking and with continued avascularity, confirming the diagnosis (see Color Plate 43).

seen most frequently in newborns. Intravaginal torsion occurs most commonly in adolescents and adults. Most testicular torsion occurs when the testicle is suspended within the hemiscrotum by a stalk of spermatic cord rather than having the typical broad attachment—the so-called bell-clapper anomaly. Patients with testicular torsion experience sudden severe pain during strenuous physical activity or sleep. Some patients have nausea and vomiting. The involved testicle may be oriented horizontally in the scrotum. The timing of diagnosis and correction is critical to the prognosis. A salvage rate of 80% to 100% is found in patients who undergo detorsion and orchiopexy within 5 to 6 hours of pain onset. The viability rate decreases to 70% after 6 to 12 hours and 20% if surgery is delayed greater than 12 hours.[1] Appendix testis and appendix epididymis torsion are the most common causes of acute scrotal pain in prepubescent boys, and clinically it manifests the same as testicular torsion. It is not considered a surgical emergency and is treated conservatively with nonsteroidal antiinflammatory drugs and rest.

Sonographic Findings. Gray-scale and Doppler findings can vary depending on the duration and degree of rotation. Early or partial torsion occludes venous outflow before arterial inflow causes venous congestion and edema. Sonography reveals an enlarged hypoechoic testis with diminished high-resistance arterial flow on Doppler. A "whirlpool sign" is seen 96% of the time above or posterior to the affected testis, appearing as a spiral or doughnut shape on gray-scale or color Doppler imaging.[5] If uncorrected or with greater rotation, arterial inflow is absent (Fig. 28-22, *A*; see Color Plate 44). The testicular blood supply in preadolescent boys is normally minimal, so optimization of Doppler settings for low flow is imperative for demonstrating the presence of normal testicular flow in these patients. A hydrocele may be seen, hypoechoic or heterogeneous areas of infarction can develop, and eventually complex or cystic areas of necrosis are seen. A small inhomogeneous or hypoechoic testicle can be seen with chronic torsion.

In appendix testis and appendix epididymis torsion, a septate hydrocele is almost always present, and the torqued appendage is enlarged, has variable echogenicity,[6] and does not have internal blood flow (Fig. 28-22, *B*; see Color Plate 44). To ensure proper management, it is imperative to make the distinction between testicular torsion and appendiceal torsion when evaluating an acutely painful scrotum, especially in younger patients.

Testicular Hematoma

Any trauma to the scrotum can cause bleeding within a testicle. The scrotum is likely to be painful.

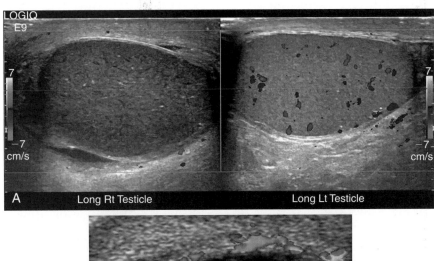

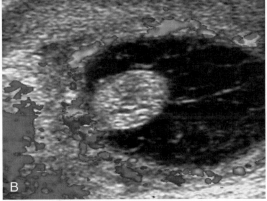

FIGURE 28-22 (A), Dual bilateral image of right testicular torsion. The affected testis is enlarged, is hypoechoic, and lacks blood flow, and there is a small hydrocele (see Color Plate 44). **(B),** Hyperechoic mass within a complex hydrocele is a torqued appendix testis. Hyperemic tissue surrounds the abnormality (see Color Plate 44). The testicle was normal.

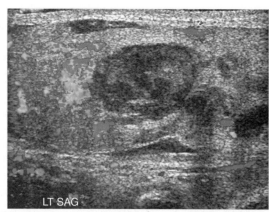

FIGURE 28-23 Testicular hematoma resulting from motorcycle straddle injury does not have blood flow within it (see Color Plate 45).

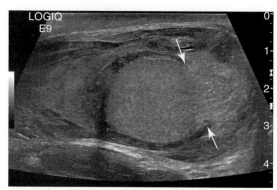

FIGURE 28-24 Longitudinal image of testicular rupture of the right testis after a motorcycle crash. Testicular contents are seen extravasated outside the tunica albuginea inferior to the testis, and the absence of tunica albuginea is apparent at the inferior pole (*between arrows*). Hematoma is seen superior to the testis.

Sonographic Findings. Unless scanned immediately, an intratesticular hematoma is heterogeneous, and septations may be present (Fig. 28-23; see Color Plate 45).

Infarct

Infarction occurs in a testis after focal or diffuse ischemia from various etiologies. Typically, there is a history of torsion or trauma, and there is no palpable abnormality.
Sonographic Findings. If the sonographic examination is done soon after the precipitating event, an infarct appears as a focal hypoechoic mass of any size, including complete involvement of the testis, indistinguishable from a true neoplastic mass. In contrast to most testicular masses, they become smaller over time and do not have vascularity on Doppler interrogation. Close attention to the patient's history combined with these findings can make conservative management reasonable.

Testicular Rupture

Rupture of the testicle, sometimes called testicular fracture, results when the tunica albuginea is ripped or cut by blunt or sharp trauma; blunt trauma is more common. Damage to the capsule allows testicular tissue to be pushed into the peritesticular space. Clinical examination reveals a scrotum extremely tender to the touch, usually with edema, making physical examination difficult. If untreated, the patient can develop gangrene and may endure chronic scrotal pain. Testicular rupture is a urologic emergency because prompt surgical intervention salvages 90% of ruptured testes.[1]
Sonographic Findings. A ruptured testicle has an irregular outline and tissue outside the tunica that is hyperechoic or isoechoic to normal testicular tissue. The intratesticular appearance can be complicated by hematoma replacing seminiferous contents. On careful examination, the tunical rent may be seen (Fig. 28-24). Color Doppler may indicate absent or decreased intratesticular blood flow or localized hyperemia from the trauma.

SUMMARY

Sonography plays a vital role in the evaluation of patients with scrotal masses or scrotal pain. Dubinski stated, "There is no doubt that sonography is ideally suited for evaluation of the testicles, and there is near-universal consensus about this."[7] The sonographer must be familiar with the normal sonographic appearances of scrotal structures and be able to recognize appearances associated with scrotal abnormalities (Table 28-1). Sonography is very accurate in distinguishing extratesticular from intratesticular masses and cystic from solid lesions, which is valuable in characterizing palpable scrotal abnormalities. Most extratesticular processes are benign, whereas most intratesticular findings are malignant. However, sonography can rarely distinguish benign from malignant solid lesions, meaning all solid intratesticular masses are considered significant. Even extratesticular solid masses should be followed, either with repeat sonographic examination or clinically. Sonography is also helpful for characterizing processes in painful and posttraumatic scrotum. The sonographic difference between inflammation and torsion is clear, and recognizing it is vital for appropriate treatment.

CLINICAL SCENARIO—DIAGNOSIS

The small palpable nodule is a benign tunica albuginea cyst, an incidental finding. The significant finding is the complex intratesticular mass, which is highly suggestive of carcinoma. Because the patient is 29 years old and the hypoechoic mass includes cystic components, this mass would most likely be a malignant teratoma, but other neoplasms cannot be definitively ruled out. His presenting symptoms of fatigue and nausea can be accounted for by the discovery of metastatic liver disease and retroperitoneal lymphadenopathy, which fit the pathologic diagnosis of mixed germ cell tumor, predominantly teratoma and including choriocarcinoma components.

TABLE 28-1	Pathology of Scrotum	
Pathology	**Symptoms and Clinical Signs**	**Sonographic Findings**
Abscess	Scrotal pain, fever, nausea and vomiting, history of UTI, possibly elevated WBC count	Round or oval with irregular wall; hypoechoic, anechoic, or mixed
Adenomatoid tumor	Painless extratesticular nodule	Small, solid, hypoechoic to hyperechoic
Choriocarcinoma	Elevated hCG level with or without palpable mass	Intratesticular mass with mixed echogenicity
Cryptorchidism	Palpable mass in inguinal canal	Homogeneous ellipsoid mass in inguinal canal
Embryonal cell carcinoma	Palpable testicular mass, rarely painful; possibly elevated hCG	Hypoechoic, may have echogenic areas or shadowing calcification
Epidermoid cyst	Palpable testicular mass	Solid hypoechoic intratesticular mass, usually with concentric hyperchoic layers
Epididymal cyst	Painless extratesticular scrotal mass	Round or oval lesion predominately anechoic, with enhancement, possible layering; possibly multiple
Epididymitis	Scrotal pain, possible fever, discharge, usually elevated WBC count, UTI	Enlarged epididymis with decreased echogenicity, hyperemia, hydrocele
Hernia	Swollen scrotum, pain	Scrotal mass with variable echogenicity pattern; peristaltic motion may be identified
Hydrocele	General scrotal enlargement	Fluid collection anterolateral to or surrounding testis
Infarction	Testicular pain; history of inflammation, torsion, or trauma	Focal hypoechoic lesion or entire testis
Lymphoma/leukemia	Enlarged testicle with or without palpable mass, known disease	Hypoechoic area or enlarged testicle with possible anechoic portions
Orchitis	Pain, fever, nausea and vomiting, exquisitely tender scrotum, elevated WBC, UTI, or trauma	Decreased echogenicity, possible hydrocele, increased blood flow; testicular atrophy in chronic orchitis
Rupture	Painful to touch, recent trauma, scrotal edema	Irregular testicular outline with hypoechoic or hyperechoic areas, extratesticular soft tissue
Seminoma	Palpable testicular mass, rarely painful, possible microlithiasis	Solid hypoechoic homogeneous mass
Testicular cyst	Usually asymptomatic, occult, incidental	Round or oval, anechoic, thin-walled, acoustic enhancement
Spermatocele	Painless extratesticular scrotal mass	Round or oval lesion predominately anechoic, with enhancement, possible layering
Stromal tumor	Painless testicular mass or enlargement	Solid hypoechoic intratesticular mass
Teratoma	Palpable testicular mass, rarely painful	Hypoechoic to hyperechoic usually complex mass, possible shadowing
Torsion	Sudden severe testicular pain, nausea and vomiting	Initially, enlarged hypoechoic testicle with diminished or absent blood flow
Varicocele	Prominent scrotal vessels, especially with standing, infertility	Increased blood flow in prominent veins with Valsalva, usually on left; vessels >2 mm

UTI, Urinary tract infection; *WBC*, white blood cell.

CASE STUDIES FOR DISCUSSION

1. A 57-year-old man presents with general malaise and unintentional weight loss. An abdominal computed tomography scan reveals retroperitoneal masses. He has no palpable scrotal abnormalities, but a sonographic examination is ordered, which reveals the findings seen in Figure 28-25. What is the most likely diagnosis?

2. A 40-year-old man is seen after being involved in an explosion accident. A sonographic evaluation is ordered because of a contusion on the right hemiscrotum; the results are shown in Figure 28-26. What is the most likely diagnosis?

3. A 16-year-old boy is seen in the emergency department after being awakened by severe scrotal pain in the early morning hours, approximately 4 hours earlier. The sonographic examination reveals an enlarged, slightly hypoechoic left testicle compared with the right. Initial color Doppler of the left testis is shown in Figure 28-27, A (see Color Plate 46), and Doppler evaluation performed 11 minutes later at the end of the examination is shown in Figure 28-27,

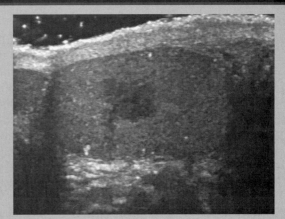

FIGURE 28-25 Irregular hypoechoic testicular lesion and microlithiasis.

Continued

CASE STUDIES FOR DISCUSSION—cont'd

B (see Color Plate 46). What is the most likely explanation of the findings?

4. A 72-year-old man is seen in the emergency department with swelling and pain in the right hemiscrotum of 2 days' duration. His scrotum is red and warm to the touch. Sonography reveals the findings in Figure 28-28 (see Color Plate 47). What is the most likely diagnosis?

5. A 39-year-old man is seen with right-sided painless scrotal swelling. Sonographic examination reveals the appearance shown in Figure 28-29. What is the most likely explanation for this appearance? Where else should the sonographer investigate?

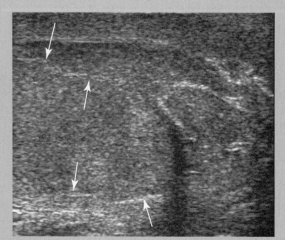

FIGURE 28-26 Longitudinal view shows that the capsule of the testis is irregular *(arrows)*, and there is a collection of extratesticular tissue similar in appearance to the testis.

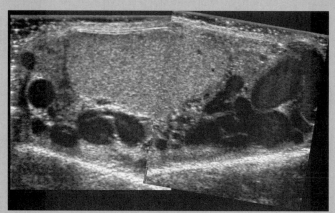

FIGURE 28-29 Composite image of right hemiscrotum showing greatly dilated blood vessels.

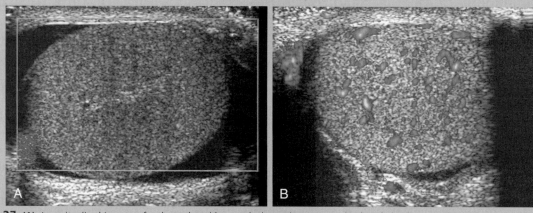

FIGURE 28-27 **(A),** Longitudinal image of enlarged and hypoechoic testis was acquired early in the examination. Spectral Doppler at that time showed diminished, high-resistance blood flow (see Color Plate 46). **(B),** Image of the same testis at the end of the examination shows normal perfusion (see Color Plate 46). Spectral Doppler measurements at this time showed normal resistive index.

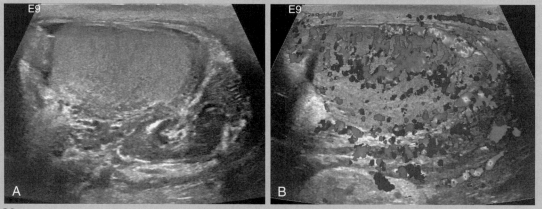

FIGURE 28-28 **(A),** Longitudinal image of testicle and epididymis. **(B),** Longitudinal color Doppler image of testicle and epididymis (see Color Plate 47).

STUDY QUESTIONS

1. A 10-year-old boy is referred for scrotal sonography because on clinical examination only one of his testicles was palpable within the scrotal sac. A homogeneous ovoid mass is identified within the left inguinal canal. Surgical repair is recommended because this condition is associated with an increased risk for which of the following?
   a. Testicular rupture
   b. Testicular torsion
   c. Orchitis
   d. Cancer

2. A 52-year-old man is diagnosed with epididymo-orchitis after a sonographic evaluation. His clinical signs and symptoms most likely include which of the following?
   a. Painless palpable testicular mass
   b. Painless scrotal enlargement
   c. Painful enlargement of the scrotum
   d. Small, hard mass palpable near the testicular surface

3. A 25-year-old man has a sudden onset of scrotal pain during a soccer game. During examination in the emergency department, the right hemiscrotum is still painful. A sonogram reveals slight enlargement of the right testicle, and on color Doppler examination, no blood flow can be found in the right testicle. What is the most likely diagnosis?
   a. Epididymo-orchitis
   b. Varicocele
   c. Abscess
   d. Testicular torsion

4. A 43-year-old man is seen with a mobile painless mass at the upper pole of his right testis. Sonographic examination reveals a 1.5 cm, round anechoic lesion that demonstrates acoustic enhancement. No other abnormalities are apparent. This probably represents a:
   a. Varicocele
   b. Spermatocele
   c. Focal epididymitis
   d. Teratoma

5. A 30-year-old man undergoes sonographic examination for a painless mass in the right hemiscrotum. The sonogram reveals multiple punctate hyperechoic nonshadowing foci and a hypochoic mass within the right testis. What is the most likely diagnosis?
   a. Seminoma with microlithiasis
   b. Orchitis with microlithiasis
   c. Leydig cell tumor
   d. Varicocele with clotted blood

6. A 32-year-old man undergoes evaluation for infertility, and his physician orders a sonogram. The examination shows a collection of vessels measuring 2.0 to 2.5 mm in the left hemiscrotum. What Doppler findings within this collection of vessels would suggest a primary varicocele?
   a. Substantial decrease in flow velocity with and without Valsalva maneuver
   b. Further dilation and increased blood flow during Valsalva maneuver
   c. Increased resistance and velocity while standing
   d. Decreased resistance and tardus parvus waveform

7. A 15-year-old boy is seen in the emergency department after falling and straddling a bicycle cross-bar. He has pain and swelling of the scrotum. The sonogram demonstrates heterogeneity of the right testicle and hypervascularity on color Doppler examination. An area of echogenic material is seen just outside the upper margin of the right testicle. What is the most likely diagnosis?
   a. Testicular torsion
   b. Scrotal hernia
   c. Testicular rupture
   d. Complicated hydrocele

8. A 28-year-old man undergoes clinical evaluation for a palpable mass in the left testicle. A sonogram reveals a solid, mostly hypoechoic mass including a shadowing calcification within the left testicle. A small amount of fluid also surrounds the left testicle. These findings are most suggestive of:
   a. Scrotal hernia
   b. Epididymitis
   c. Embryonal cell carcinoma
   d. Epididymal cyst
   e. Teratoma

9. A 61-year-old man is seen with intermittent pain and swelling of the right scrotum, radiating to the right inguinal canal. A sonogram is ordered because a scrotal hernia is suspected. Which of the following sonographic findings is suggestive of a scrotal hernia?
   a. Inguinal mass
   b. Hypoechoic areas within the testicles
   c. Increased peritesticular vascularity
   d. Tubular structures that demonstrate peristalsis within the scrotum

10. A 30-year-old man with gynecomastia, elevated hCG, and no palpable scrotal mass presents for a sonogram. The most significant sonographic finding includes a 1.5 cm heterogeneous mass within the right testicle. After orchiectomy, the prognosis remains poor because this type of cancer does not

respond well to radiation and chemotherapy. The clinical and sonographic findings suggest which type of cancer?

a. Choriocarcinoma
b. Seminoma
c. Embryonal cell tumor
d. Lymphoma

REFERENCES

1. Gorman B: The scrotum. In Rumack C, Wilson S, Charboneau J, et al: ed 4, *Diagnostic ultrasound*, vol. 1, Philadelphia, 2011, Mosby, pp 840–877.
2. Gilligan TD, Seidenfeld J, Basch EM, et al: American Society of Clinical Oncology Clinical Practice Guideline on uses of serum tumor markers in adult males with germ cell tumors, *J Clin Oncol* 28:3388–3404, 2010.
3. Lin K, Sharangpani R: Screening for testicular cancer: an evidence review for the U.S. Preventive Services Task Force, *Ann Intern Med* 153:396–399, 2010.
4. Sesterhenn IA, Davis CJ: Pathology of germ cell tumors of the testis, *Cancer Control* 11:374–387, 2004.
5. Vijayaraghavan SB: Sonographic differential diagnosis of acute scrotum: real-time whirlpool sign, a key sign of torsion, *J Ultrasound Med* 25:563–574, 2006.
6. Karmazyn B, Steinberg R, Livne P, et al: Duplex sonographic findings in children with torsion of the testicular appendages: overlap with epididymitis and epididymoorchitis, *J Pediatr Surg* 41:500–504, 2006.
7. Dubinski T: ACR appropriateness criteria, acute onset of scrotal pain—without trauma, without antecedent mass, *Ultrasound Q* 28:53–54, 2012.

Neck Mass

Kathryn M. Kuntz

CLINICAL SCENARIO

A 23-year-old man is referred to the sonography department for evaluation of a palpable neck mass. The left-sided mass was incidentally noted by the patient during shaving. The patient is in good general health and has no significant medical history; laboratory blood test evaluation results are normal. The mass is not tender and does not appear to have grown over the last year. A high-resolution neck sonogram reveals not only the palpable left-sided thyroid nodule but also three right-sided thyroid nodules. The predominant nodule is 1.5 cm and solid, and the sonographer notes tiny flecks of nonshadowing calcifications. The other three nodules all are less than 0.5 cm, are also solid, and lack the calcifications detected in the large predominant nodule. Numerous visible lymph nodes also are noted bilaterally along the carotid-jugular chain. The patient is concerned about thyroid cancer. Because the mass was already known, how is the diagnosis of carcinoma confirmed or discounted? What significance do the incidental nodules and the presence of enlarged lymph nodes have?

OBJECTIVES

- Name the most common neck masses encountered on sonographic examinations.
- List risk factors associated with the development of neck masses.
- Describe the sonographic appearances of the most commonly seen neck masses.
- Identify sonographic features that suggest a thyroid nodule is benign or malignant.
- List the risk factors, laboratory values, and sonographic features of parathyroid adenoma.
- Describe less common cystic neck pathologies that can be diagnosed with sonography.

High-frequency sonography has been acknowledged as an important screening and diagnostic imaging method for evaluation of the thyroid and parathyroid glands of the neck. The advantages of sonography over other imaging methods include high degree of accuracy, ready availability, fast examination time, and relatively low cost. Sonography requires no patient preparation, and no ionizing radiation is used. The performance of interventional procedures with sonographic guidance, including fine-needle aspiration (FNA) of thyroid nodules, is an important application of sonography. In addition to thyroid and parathyroid disease, other, less common congenital, cystic, and solid neck masses and lymph node diseases should be considered by any practitioner of sonography.

THYROID GLAND

Normal Sonographic Anatomy

The thyroid gland is part of the endocrine system, which helps the body to maintain a normal metabolism.

The thyroid consists of paired right and left lobes in the lower anterior neck. The lobes are joined at the midline by a thin bridge of thyroid tissue called the isthmus, which is draped over the anterior aspect of the trachea at the junction of the middle and lower thirds of the gland (Fig. 29-1). A midline pyramidal lobe that arises from the isthmus and tapers superiorly, anterior to the thyroid cartilage, is seen in some patients. Anterior to the thyroid surface are the strap muscles of the neck, the sternohyoid and sternothyroid. The large sternocleidomastoid muscles are located anterolaterally. The carotid sheath, which contains the common carotid artery and the jugular vein, is located laterally. The wedge-shaped longus colli muscles are located posteriorly. In the midline, the shadowing air-filled trachea generally hides the esophagus, but the esophagus may be seen protruding slightly laterally and can be confused with a parathyroid adenoma with imaging in the transverse plane only.

The normal thyroid has a fine homogeneous echotexture that is more echogenic than the adjacent muscles. In its periphery, the gland's echotexture is interrupted by

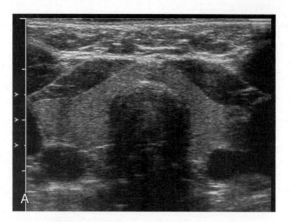

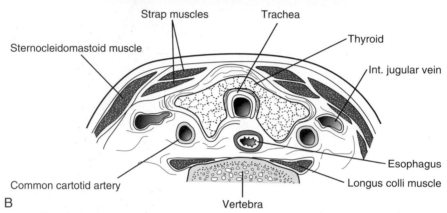

FIGURE 29-1 Transverse image **(A)** and line drawing **(B)** of thyroid anatomy.

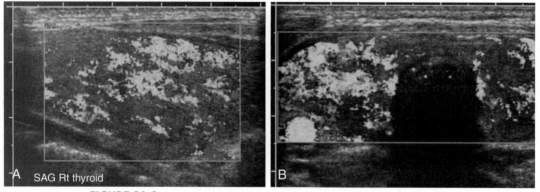

FIGURE 29-2 Color Doppler of thyroid inferno seen with Graves' disease.

vascular structures. Color Doppler imaging of the normal thyroid shows minimal flow signal, which usually is located near the poles of the gland.

Diffuse Disease

Goiter is the most common cause of diffuse thyroid hyperplasia with gland enlargement. Goiter is caused by inadequate iodine ingestion and is not a significant problem in the United States. The most commonly encountered diffuse thyroid diseases in the United States are Hashimoto's disease (chronic thyroiditis) and Graves' disease (diffuse toxic goiter). Although these are distinctly different conditions, the sonographic findings are relatively nonspecific. Visualization of a thyroid isthmus thicker than a few millimeters suggests a diffusely enlarged gland. A sonogram that reveals involvement of the entire gland can alert the physician to consider diffuse rather than focal disease.

Graves' disease is an autoimmune disorder characterized by thyrotoxicosis and is the most frequent cause of hyperthyroidism. Graves' disease usually produces a diffusely hypoechoic thyroid texture, with accompanying contour lobulation but without palpable nodules. A characteristic increase in color flow Doppler in the thyroid is present on examination, both in systole and in diastole, leading to the term "thyroid inferno," coined by Ralls et al.[1] (Fig. 29-2; see Color Plate 48).

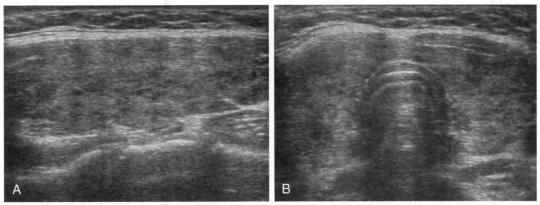

FIGURE 29-3 Transverse **(A)** and longitudinal **(B)** images of Hashimoto's disease.

Hashimoto's disease is the most common form of thyroiditis. The typical clinical presentation is a painless, diffusely enlarged gland in a young or middle-aged woman. The sonographic appearance of Hashimoto's thyroiditis is well recognized. The gland is often diffusely enlarged, and the parenchyma is coarsened, hypoechoic, and often hypervascular. Also seen are multiple ill-defined hypoechoic areas separated by thickened fibrous strands (Fig. 29-3). A micronodular pattern on sonography is highly diagnostic of Hashimoto's thyroiditis. Color Doppler imaging usually demonstrates increased vascularity. In the final stages of the disease, a fibrotic gland may be seen that is small, ill-defined, and heterogeneous. Because of the increased risk for malignant disease associated with Hashimoto's disease, follow-up examinations are recommended.

Discrete thyroid nodules with Hashimoto's thyroiditis are less common. However, discrete nodules may also occur within diffusely altered parenchyma or within sonographically normal parenchyma.[2] The sonographic features and vascularity of nodular Hashimoto's thyroiditis are variable and overlap with the findings typically associated with other benign nodules as well as malignant nodules. A "typical" sonographic appearance for nodular Hashimoto's thyroiditis has not been reported.[2]

Thyroid Mass

Thyroid nodules are very common. In the United States, 4% to 8% of adults are estimated to have thyroid nodules, which can be detected with palpation. Of thyroid nodules, 10% to 41% are visible with ultrasound, and 50% are discovered at autopsy.[3] The prevalence of thyroid cancer increases with age. The likelihood that a nodule is malignant is affected by several risk factors. Thyroid cancer is more common in patients younger than 20 years or older than 60 years.[4] History of neck radiation or a family history of thyroid cancer also increases the risk that a thyroid nodule is malignant. However, thyroid cancer is rare. Most nodules that the sonographer encounters are benign and not clinically significant. In a patient who is referred or has a palpable thyroid

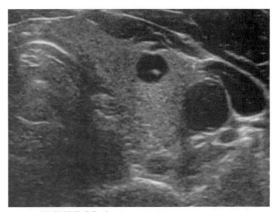

FIGURE 29-4 Cystic follicular adenoma.

nodule, the challenge is to distinguish significant malignant nodules from the many benign ones and to identify patients for whom FNA or surgery is indicated.[3]

Benign Nodules

Sonographic Findings. Benign nodules either are hyperplastic (involution of underlying thyroid tissue) or are adenomas, also called follicular adenomas. Adenomas are true thyroid nodules but are less common than hyperplastic nodules, and follicular adenomas are much more common than follicular carcinomas. In contrast to carcinomas, adenomas have no vascular or capsular invasion but otherwise have similar cytologic features. However, in most clinical cases of suspected follicular neoplasm encountered in day-to-day practice, the sonographic features cannot confidently, prospectively distinguish follicular carcinoma from follicular adenoma.[5]

Sonographically, palpable thyroid nodules can be seen with a high degree of accuracy. However, the differentiation of benign from malignant nodules on the basis of sonographic appearance is challenging. Features that suggest a benign nodule include nodules that are mostly cystic. These cystic nodules almost always contain debris (Fig. 29-4). A nodule with multiple microcystic spaces separated by thin septa or intervening isoechoic parenchyma (a "spongiform" appearance) is also predictive

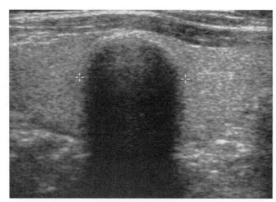

FIGURE 29-5 Longitudinal image of eggshell calcification in benign nodule.

of benignity.[6] Less common types of benign nodules are nodules that are hyperechoic relative to the adjacent thyroid parenchyma and nodules that have peripheral eggshell-type calcification (Fig. 29-5).

Color Doppler, spectral Doppler, and power Doppler all have been applied to the evaluation of thyroid nodules. The presence of increased flow in the periphery of the nodule, or rim vascularity, may help in initial decision making regarding a subtle thyroid mass. However, the characterization of thyroid nodules based on Doppler findings is not definitive. For example, benign hyperplastic nodules show minimal or no flow within the nodule itself and low-velocity flow around the periphery of the nodule. Adenomas show more intralesional and perilesional flow than hyperplastic nodules. However, this is true for some carcinomas as well. In addition, some investigators report no correlation between pathologic findings and the presence or amount of blood flow detected with Doppler.

Malignant Nodules

The sonographic features predictive of malignant nodules have been well reported and include the presence of microcalcifications, hypoechogenicity, irregular (spiculated) margins, the absence of a halo, a predominantly solid composition, a shape taller than wide, and intranodular vascularity. The diagnostic accuracy of the sonographic criteria for malignancy depends on tumor size. Specifically, a lower frequency of microcalcifications in microcarcinomas suggests that microcalcification is not a major predictor of malignancy in nodules 1 cm or smaller.[7]

Sonographic Findings. Most thyroid cancers appear solid and hypoechoic. The significance of peripheral, eggshell or rim calcification for differentiating a benign from a malignant thyroid nodule is debated. Studies have shown that a hypoechoic halo and disruption of peripheral, eggshell calcification are findings that suggest malignancy.[6] A wide, irregular halo surrounding the nodule and fine punctate internal calcifications known as psammoma bodies are features commonly seen with papillary

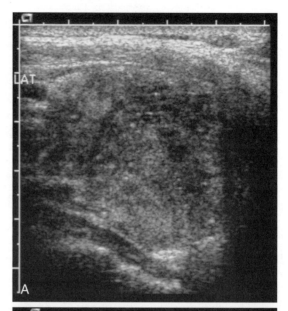

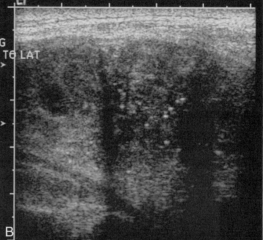

FIGURE 29-6 Transverse **(A)** and longitudinal **(B)** images of psammoma bodies in papillary thyroid cancer.

thyroid cancer (Fig. 29-6). Hypervascularity in the central portion of the nodule has not proven to be useful to predict malignancy with a high degree of confidence.[3] Most follicular tumors are solid and have homogeneous echogenicity. They can be hyperechoic, isoechoic, hypoechoic, or mixed with well-defined areas of different echogenicity within the tumor. Focal cystic components may be present. They usually have a "spoke-and-wheel"–like vascularity with marked circulation in the peripheral halo with vessels converging toward the tumor center.[8] The sonographic features of follicular adenoma and follicular carcinoma are very similar making a sonographic distinction challenging, but larger lesion size, lack of a sonographic halo, hypoechoic appearance, and absence of cystic change favor a diagnosis of follicular carcinoma.[5]

Other types of cancers include anaplastic and medullary cancers. Sonographic findings of these other malignancies are different from the findings of a typical papillary carcinoma (see Table 29-1).[6]

Fine-Needle Aspiration

Because a precise definition of the nature of a thyroid nodule on the basis of its sonographic features is difficult, FNA with cytologic evaluation has become the accepted method for screening a nodule for thyroid cancer. This procedure obtains thyroid follicular epithelial cells and minute tissue fragments for cytologic evaluation. FNA is minimally invasive and provides more direct information than other diagnostic techniques. In most cases, FNA of a thyroid nodule is performed by the clinician as an office-based outpatient procedure. FNA is safe, accurate, and inexpensive. Complications of the procedure, such as hematoma or pain, are rare and usually minor.[3]

Parathyroid Glands

Primary hyperparathyroidism was previously considered to be a rare endocrine disorder but is now recognized as a common disease. The prevalence of primary hyperparathyroidism in the United States is estimated to be 1:1000 with a peak during the fifth and sixth decades. Primary hyperparathyroidism is most frequently identified incidentally on blood screening panels and is very often asymptomatic at the time of diagnosis. Parathyroidectomy remains the definitive cure for the disease. Women have this disease two to three times more frequently than men, and the condition is particularly common in postmenopausal women.

Primary hyperparathyroidism results from inappropriate overproduction of parathyroid hormone from one or many parathyroid glands and manifests with hypercalcemia. Primary hyperparathyroidism usually occurs as the result of sporadic parathyroid adenomas or carcinomas but can also be seen in association with multiple endocrine neoplasias and in rare genetic syndromes and metabolic diseases.

The parathyroid glands are the calcium-sensing organs in the body. They produce parathyroid hormone and monitor the serum calcium. Laboratory values that can raise suspicion for hyperparathyroidism include increased serum levels of calcium and parathyroid hormone, hypophosphatasia, and increased renal excretion of calcium. Nephrocalcinosis or recurrent renal stones may hint at the underlying disorder. Sonography can be used for the preoperative localization of enlarged parathyroid glands in patients with suspected primary hyperparathyroidism from laboratory values. Of the available imaging techniques, the most successful modality is technetium 99m–labeled sestamibi single photon emission computed tomography (SPECT), which identifies 89% of single parathyroid adenomas. Sonography is the second most useful modality; when used with technetium 99m–labeled sestamibi SPECT preoperatively, it can enhance adenoma detection rates.[8]

Primary hyperparathyroidism is caused by a single parathyroid adenoma in 80% to 87% of cases, by multiple gland enlargement in 10% to 20% of cases, and by parathyroid carcinoma in less than 1% of cases. Parathyroid carcinoma is rare. It is seen in less than 1% of patients with hyperparathyroidism.[9] Malignant tumors tend to be more inhomogeneous in echotexture than typical parathyroid adenomas, but no sonographic means of differentiating benign from malignant parathyroid disease exists.

It is important to differentiate primary from secondary and tertiary hyperparathyroidism. Secondary hyperparathyroidism occurs as a normal response to hypocalcemia secondary to diseases affecting the kidney (e.g., renal tubular acidosis), liver, or intestines or vitamin D deficiency. The term "secondary hyperparathyroidism" is used to describe parathyroid glands that show compensatory enlargement and hypersecretion in patients with renal failure or vitamin D deficiency. In secondary hyperparathyroidism, usually all parathyroid glands are affected. Tertiary hyperparathyroidism occurs in patients with long-standing secondary hyperparathyroidism who develop autonomous parathyroid hormone production with hypercalcemia.[10]

Normal Sonographic Anatomy

There are four paired parathyroid glands, two superior and two inferior, located in close proximity to the thyroid gland. Normal parathyroid glands, which typically measure 5.0 mm × 3.0 mm × 1.0 mm in size, are similar in echogenicity to the adjacent thyroid and surrounding tissues and are difficult to visualize sonographically.

Sonographic Findings. Occasionally, normal glands are visualized in young adults. The typical parathyroid adenoma is sonographically seen as a solid oval mass of homogeneous, low-level echogenicity that usually measures slightly more than 1 cm in length (Fig. 29-7). However, the shape, echogenicity, internal architecture, and size can vary.

Parathyroid Adenoma

Color Doppler and power Doppler imaging of a parathyroid adenoma may show a hypervascular pattern or a peripheral vascular arc that can aid in differentiation from hyperplastic regional lymph nodes, which have hilar flow. Superior parathyroid adenomas are located adjacent to the posterior aspect of the midportion of the thyroid. The location of inferior parathyroid adenomas is more variable, but they usually lie in close proximity to the caudal tip of the lower pole of the thyroid. Most of these inferior adenomas are adjacent to the posterior thyroid aspect or in the soft tissues 1 to 2 cm inferior to the thyroid. Most superior and inferior adenomas are found in these typical locations, adjacent to the thyroid. Of adenomas, 1% to 3% are ectopic. Ectopic glands can be a cause of failure to locate adenomas sonographically, which may lead to failed operations. The four most common locations for

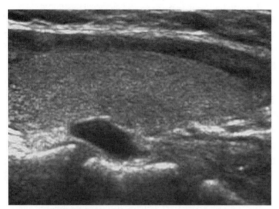

FIGURE 29-7 Parathyroid adenoma.

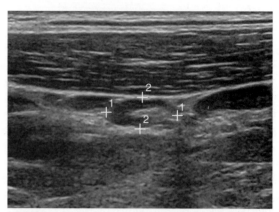

FIGURE 29-8 Longitudinal image of normal cervical lymph node.

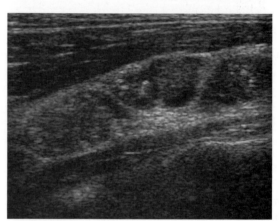

FIGURE 29-9 Abnormal cervical lymph node (malignant).

ectopic parathyroid glands are mediastinal, retrotracheal, intrathyroid, and carotid sheath/undescended.

Hyperparathyroidism and Hyperplasia

Of patients with hyperparathyroidism, approximately 10% have hyperplasia—the enlargement of multiple glands. The cause of parathyroid hyperplasia is not well understood. Although the hyperplasia involves all four glands, the glands are not involved equally, and the enlargement is always asymmetric.

Potential pitfalls in interpretation of parathyroid examinations include normal cervical structures, such as veins adjacent to the thyroid, the esophagus, and the longus colli muscles of the neck, which can simulate parathyroid adenomas and produce false-positive results during neck sonography. Besides these normal structures, pathologies such as thyroid nodules and cervical lymph nodes can also cause false-positive results.

LYMPH NODES

During the course of a neck ultrasound examination, normal, inflammatory, and malignant lymph nodes are readily identified. Adenopathy describes enlarged nodes, and documentation of the size, shape, and internal architecture can be used to help differentiate benign from malignant lymph nodes. Thyroid cancer often metastasizes to cervical lymph nodes, and early detection of metastasis is important for planning surgery and management of patients. Sonography is the imaging method of choice for detecting and characterizing cervical lymph nodes in thyroid cancer. Additionally, sonographically guided FNA of suspicious nodes is safe, accurate, and inexpensive. Complications of the procedure, such as hematoma or pain, are rare and usually minor.[11]

Normal Sonographic Anatomy

Enlarged benign inflammatory nodes occur commonly in the neck. Differentiation of these nodes from malignant nodes in patients with a known cervical malignant disease, such as thyroid cancer, can be difficult. Most normal and inflammatory cervical lymph nodes have a flattened oblong oval shape, with their greatest dimension in the longitudinal axis (Fig. 29-8). This is presumably from compression by the adjacent longitudinally oriented tissue planes in the neck. Most normal nodes measure only a few millimeters in size.

Sonographic Findings. The sonographic characteristics of metastatic lymph nodes of papillary cancer have been widely reported and include the presence of calcification, cystic changes, loss of echogenic fatty hilum, hyperechogenicity, round shape, and abnormal vascularity on color Doppler. Of these, calcification and cystic changes have 100% specificity and positive predictive value, and they are not observed in normal or reactive lymph nodes. In the neck, lymph node shape is probably the best method for this differentiation. It has been suggested that cervical lymph nodes with a short-to-long ratio of greater than 0.5 cm show a much higher prevalence of malignant disease than cervical lymph nodes with a ratio of less than 0.5 cm.[10] The more rounded the shape of the lymph node, the more likely it is to be malignant (Fig. 29-9). Care must be taken not to transfer these principles to other regions of the body; for example, the breast and axilla have normal rounded lymph node appearances because surrounding tissue planes do not constrict the nodes. Malignant nodes often have an abnormal heterogeneous internal architecture. Microcalcifications are often seen in malignant nodes, similar to microcalcifications seen in primary malignant papillary thyroid nodules.

Color Doppler sonography may also demonstrate abnormal flow patterns in malignant cervical lymph nodes compared with benign nodes. However, these differences can be subtle and are unlikely to be definitive. Because of the considerable overlap in the size and appearance of benign and malignant lymph nodes, FNA and biopsy of nodes suspicious for malignant disease can be performed.

OTHER NECK MASSES

Other cystic neck masses may develop from malformations in the cervical thoracic lymphatic system because of the complex embryology of the neck region. Some of these masses are cystic hygroma, cavernous lymphangioma, and simple capillary lymphangioma. Thyroglossal duct cysts are congenital anomalies that form anterior in the midline of the neck (Fig. 29-10). They are the most common, clinically significant congenital anomalies. The cyst can occur anywhere along the course of the duct from the base of the tongue to the pyramidal lobe of the thyroid gland. Branchial cleft cysts are usually located lateral to the thyroid gland along the anterior border of the sternocleidomastoid muscle. Most cysts are located near the angle of the mandible, but they can occur at almost any level in the neck.

Sonographic Findings

Cystic hygromas are most often seen as large cystic masses on the lateral aspect of the neck. They can be multiseptated and multiloculated. Cystic hygroma is differentiated from cavernous lymphangioma, capillary lymphangioma, and other lymphatic malformations based only on the size of its lymphatic spaces.

Thyroglossal duct cysts are oval or spherical masses, located in the midline of the neck, and rarely larger than 2 to 3 cm. These masses, along with cavernous lymphangioma and simple capillary lymphangioma, usually have echolucent cystic internal components and a thin rim; however, they can become infected, significantly changing their sonographic characteristics.

SUMMARY

The ability of high-resolution sonography to detect small, nonpalpable thyroid nodules is unsurpassed by any other imaging method. Thyroid nodules are very common being found in 50% of the population at autopsy. However, only 4% to 8% of the adult population in the United States is estimated to have thyroid nodules that can be detected with palpation.[3] Thyroid cancer is rare. Only 2% to 4% of the nodules that can be detected with palpation represent thyroid malignant disease. Of this small number of thyroid cancers, most have been proven to be tiny, incidentally discovered, occult papillary cancers. Because most papillary carcinomas are slow-growing and remain curable if and when they become clinically apparent at approximately 1.0 to 1.5 cm in size, aggressive pursuit of all small nodules that are detected with high-frequency ultrasound is considered impractical and imprudent. The pathologic conditions discussed in this chapter are summarized in Table 29-1.

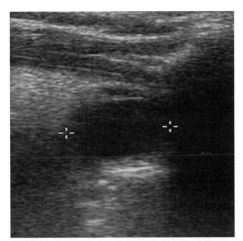

FIGURE 29-10 Transverse image of neck shows thyroglossal duct cyst.

TABLE 29-1	Pathology of Thyroid, Parathyroid, and Neck	
Pathology	**Symptoms**	**Sonographic Findings**
Adenoma	Usually asymptomatic; possibly palpable	Well-marginated, mostly cystic with internal debris
Adenopathy (cervical)	Variable depending on cause; possibly palpable	Loss of normal flattened, elongated oval lymph node shape with increase in anteroposterior dimension; loss of fatty hilum
Anaplastic thyroid cancer	Painful rapid enlargement of nodule; may mimic thyroiditis	Inhomogeneous hypoechoic invasive solid mass
Branchial cleft cyst	Painless mass on lateral neck; if infected, may be tender and painful	Noninfected—thin uniform wall surrounding homogeneous mass; usually fluid-filled; infected—low-level echoes, layering effect, or complex appearance
Thyroglossal duct cyst	Usually asymptomatic; may cause pain if infected	Well-defined, thin-walled, anechoic mass with through enhancement; mass with mixed echogenicity suggests infection of the cyst; midline or just off midline in position; can be found at any level from the base of the tongue to the isthmus of the thyroid gland

Continued

TABLE 29-1	Pathology of Thyroid, Parathyroid, and Neck—cont'd	
Pathology	**Symptoms**	**Sonographic Findings**
Cystic hygroma	Painless, soft, semifirm mass in posterior neck	Usually multiloculated homogeneous cystic masses
Follicular tumors	Usually asymptomatic; possibly palpable	May be hyperechoic, isoechoic, hypoechoic, or mixed with well-defined areas of different echogenicity within; focal cystic components may be present; usually have a "spoke-and-wheel"–like vascularity with marked circulation in peripheral halo*
Goiter	Enlargement of thyroid	Nonspecific
Graves' disease	Symptoms associated with hyperthyroidism	Diffuse hypoechoic thyroid texture; hypervascular
Hashimoto's disease (chronic lymphocytic thyroiditis)	Painless, diffusely enlarging gland	Ill-defined hypoechoic areas separated by thickened fibrous strands; coarse but overall homogeneous thyroid echotexture; frequently hypervascular
Parathyroid adenoma/ parathyroid hyperplasia	Increased levels of serum calcium and parathyroid hormone; hypophosphatasia; increased renal excretion of calcium; nephrocalcinosis and renal stones	Single or multiple oval homogeneous low-echogenicity solid masses; if minimally enlarged, may not be detected with sonography
Medullary thyroid cancer	Possible palpable nodule; increased calcitonin level	Discrete tumor in one lobe or numerous nodules involving both lobes; possible focal hemorrhage, necrosis, coarse calcification, and reactive fibrosis in tumor
Papillary thyroid cancer	Possible palpable mass	Variable, but almost always mass of low echogenicity; wide, irregular halo surrounding nodule often multicentric; internal microcalcifications (psammoma bodies) are a common and specific finding

*Features of follicular adenoma and carcinoma are very similar (adenoma is more common); extensive cytologic and histologic sampling may be necessary for diagnosis, but larger lesion size, lack of a sonographic halo, hypoechoic appearance, and absence of cystic change favor a diagnosis of follicular carcinoma.[5]

CLINICAL SCENARIO—DIAGNOSIS

The patient is a young man, and thyroid nodules are more likely to be malignant in young men. The mass is slow-growing and painless, both also indicative of a malignant nodule. The sonographic appearance of the palpable nodule is solid and hypoechoic with microcalcification versus uninterrupted rim or wall calcification, also pointing toward a papillary thyroid cancer. The patient also has several other nonpalpable masses and cervical lymph nodes visible with high-frequency sonographic techniques, which is not unique. This patient would likely undergo FNA to confirm the diagnosis of papillary thyroid cancer with subsequent thyroidectomy and cervical exploration.

CASE STUDIES FOR DISCUSSION

1. A 40-year-old woman is referred for a sonogram of a palpable neck nodule that is nontender. High-resolution sonography reveals a rounded hypoechoic lymph node that contains microcalcifications and measures 1.0 cm in length and 1.0 cm in anteroposterior dimension that correlates with the palpable lesion. A solid hypoechoic thyroid nodule on the same side of the neck also is noted. What is the most likely diagnosis?

2. A 21-year-old woman is referred for nonspecific neck discomfort. No neck masses are palpable. A mostly cystic thyroid nodule with a "spongiform" appearance is noted on the sonogram. What is the most likely diagnosis?

3. A slender, postmenopausal woman is referred for neck sonogram for evaluation of a palpable, tender right neck nodule. She reports slight pain with palpation; no pain had been noted before the physical examination. Sonographic examination reveals a 1.5 cm, mostly cystic nodule with some solid debris. Uninterrupted, peripheral rim calcification is also noted. What is the most likely diagnosis?

4. A 75-year-old woman is referred to the ultrasound department with elevated serum calcium level. The neck sonogram reveals an oblong hypoechoic mass adjacent to the posterior aspect of the lower third of the left thyroid lobe. What is the most likely diagnosis?

5. A 61-year-old man with a biopsy-proven papillary thyroid cancer is also noted to have several oval, flat, elongated masses in the area between the jugular vein and carotid artery. Hyperechogenicity is noted in the hilar regions of these "masses." What is the most likely diagnosis?

STUDY QUESTIONS

1. A postmenopausal patient with hypercalcemia and hypophosphatasia is referred for sonography of the neck. An oval-shaped, hypoechoic mass is seen posterior to the mid-lower right lobe of the thyroid. The clinical findings of hypercalcemia and hypophosphatasia along with the shape and location of this mass are most suggestive of:
   a. Parathyroid adenoma
   b. Thyroid adenoma
   c. Malignant lymph node
   d. Benign lymph node
   e. Obstructed salivary duct

2. A 31-year-old woman is referred for a sonogram after bilateral neck fullness is noted during a routine physical examination. The sonographic appearance of the thyroid gland is diffuse, hypoechoic enlargement of both lobes and the isthmus and "coarse" parenchyma. The sonographic features of the mass along with the patient's gender and age are suspicious for:
   a. Multiple endocrine neoplasia
   b. Hashimoto's thyroiditis
   c. Graves' disease
   d. Metastatic thyroid cancer
   e. Papillary thyroid cancer

3. A 19-year-old man with no significant medical history is seen with a palpable nodule in the region of the right inferior lobe of the thyroid. On sonographic examination, the corresponding nodule is found to be slightly less echogenic than the surrounding thyroid parenchyma. There is a wide, irregular halo surrounding the nodule and fine punctate internal calcifications throughout the nodule. What is the most likely diagnosis for this nodule?
   a. Parathyroid adenoma
   b. Papillary thyroid cancer
   c. Benign thyroid nodule
   d. Inflammatory lymph node
   e. Malignant lymph node

4. A 63-year-old man in apparent good health is seeking a second opinion for a thyroid nodule that was diagnosed elsewhere. He was told that the nodule contained "psammoma bodies." This finding refers to:
   a. A nodule causing elevated serum calcium
   b. A state of hypothyroidism
   c. Microcystic spaces
   d. Microcalcifications in a nodule
   e. Peripheral rim calcification in a nodule

5. A 10-year-old girl presents with a very tender, high-midline neck mass. Her parents report feeling a "small lump" in this location since she was a baby, but it has enlarged and is now painful. The sonogram reveals an oval, 1.0 cm × 1.5 cm cystic mass with a thin wall and some internal debris. It is located approximately 3 cm superior to the thyroid isthmus. What is the most likely cause of this cystic mass?
   a. Ectopic parathyroid adenoma
   b. Obstructed salivary duct
   c. Branchial cleft cyst
   d. Inflammatory lymph node
   e. Infected thyroglossal duct cyst

6. A 35-year-old man presents with symptoms consistent with hyperthyroidism. He is referred for a neck sonogram. The thyroid appears diffusely hypoechoic with a lobulated contour. No discrete nodules are seen. Color Doppler shows a dramatic increase in flow throughout the gland. What is the most likely cause for these findings?
   a. Secondary hyperparathyroidism
   b. Parathyroid hyperplasia
   c. Goiter
   d. Graves' disease
   e. Cystic hygroma

7. Incidental bilateral thyroid nodules are noted on a 75-year-old man who is undergoing carotid artery evaluation. Because the patient's wife recently died of breast cancer, the patient is concerned about cancer and has asked that these nodules be investigated. The nodule in the right lobe is noted to be mostly cystic but contains debris. The nodule in the left lobe contains multiple microcystic spaces separated by thin septa. These findings almost certainly suggest:
   a. Bilateral papillary cancers
   b. Bilateral benign thyroid nodules
   c. Graves' disease
   d. Bilateral inflammatory lymph nodes
   e. Parathyroid hyperplasia involving more than one gland

8. An elderly man with a painless, palpable thyroid nodule is referred for thyroid sonography. Previous imaging studies have reported "a thyroid nodule with calcification." The images are not available for review. A second sonogram is performed and reveals a 2 cm × 3 cm solid, hypoechoic nodule with a hypoechoic halo and disruption of peripheral, eggshell calcification. These findings make this nodule suspicious for:
   a. Thyroiditis
   b. Inflammatory lymph node
   c. Nodular goiter
   d. Malignant nodule
   e. Benign nodule

9. A young man is referred to the ultrasound department for evaluation of a lateral neck mass that is nontender. The sonogram reveals a solitary thyroid nodule and multiple rounded masses that follow the carotid-jugular areas. Both the intrathyroidal and extrathyroidal masses contain microcalcifications. This should represent:
   a. Metastatic thyroid cancer
   b. Inflammatory reactive lymph nodes
   c. Thyroiditis with reactive lymph nodes
   d. Sternocleidomastoid muscle cysts
   e. Tertiary hyperparathyroidism

10. A young woman presents with a painless, diffusely enlarged thyroid gland on physical examination. The sonographic appearance confirms diffuse enlargement with a micronodular pattern and increased vascularity. Which of the following conditions should the sonographer suggest to the interpreting physician?
    a. Chronic thyroiditis
    b. Tertiary hyperparathyroidism
    c. Toxic goiter
    d. Diffuse hyperparathyroidism
    e. Diffuse parathyroid adenomas

REFERENCES

1. Ralls PW, Mayekawa DS, Lee KP, et al: Color-flow Doppler sonography in Graves' disease: "thyroid inferno." *AJR Am J Roentgenol* 150:781, 1988.
2. Anderson L, Middleton D, Teefey C, et al: Hashimoto thyroiditis: part 1, sonographic analysis of the nodular form of Hashimoto thyroiditis, *AJR Am J Roentgenol* 195:216–222, 2010.
3. Frates MC, Benson CB, Charboneau JW, et al: Management of thyroid nodules detected at US: Society of Radiologists in Ultrasound consensus conference statement, *Radiology* 237:794–800, 2005.
4. Hegedus L, Bonnema SJ, Bennedbaek FN: Management of simple nodular goiter: current status and future perspectives, *Endocr Rev* 24:102–132, 2003.
5. Silleryl JC, Reading CC, Charboneau JW, et al: Thyroid follicular carcinoma: sonographic feature of 50 cases, *AJR Am J Roentgenol* 194:44–54, 2010.
6. Moon W, Jung H, Jung S, et al: Ultrasonography and the ultrasound-based management of thyroid nodules: consensus statement and recommendations, *Korean J Radiol* 12:1–14, 2011.
7. Moon W, Jung S, Lee J, et al: Benign and malignant thyroid nodules: US differentiation—multicenter retrospective study for the thyroid study group, Korean Society of Neuro- and Head and Neck Radiology, *Radiology* 247:762–770, 2008.
8. Pallan S, Khan A: Primary hyperparathyroidism: update on presentation, diagnosis, and management in primary care, *Can Fam Physician* 57:184–189, 2011.
9. Kebebew E, Hwang J, Reiff E, et al: *Thyroid* 18:817–818, 2008.
10. MacKenzie-Feder J, Sirrs S, Anderson D, et al: Primary hyperparathyroidism: an overview, *Int J Endocrinol* 251410:2011, 2011.
11. Sohn Y, Kwak J, Kim E, et al: Diagnostic approach for evaluation of lymph nodes metastasis from thyroid cancer using ultrasound and fine-needle aspiration biopsy, *AJR Am J Roentgenol* 194:38–43, 2010.

Elevated Prostate Specific Antigen

Dan J. Donovan, Diane J. Youngs

CLINICAL SCENARIO

A 56-year-old man presents to the ultrasound department for an examination of his prostate. The patient is apprehensive because his uncle and father both have a history of prostate cancer. Within the past 2 months, he has had lethargy and lower back pain, which precipitated a visit to his physician. His physician performed a physical examination including a digital rectal examination (DRE). DRE revealed a nodule posteriorly on the prostate. Laboratory analysis revealed a free prostate specific antigen (PSA) value of 12 ng/mL. Transrectal ultrasound (TRUS) examination of the prostate is performed to evaluate the nodule, and imaging shows a small hypoechoic mass with slight bulging of the posterior aspect of the capsule. The margins of the mass are poorly defined. What is the possible diagnosis for this lesion?

OBJECTIVES

- Describe the normal sonographic appearance of the prostate.
- Describe the sonographic appearance of benign prostatic hypertrophy.
- Describe the sonographic findings associated with prostatic inflammation.
- Discuss the significance of sonographic evidence of calcifications and cystic areas within the prostate gland.
- List clinical symptoms and sonographic findings associated with prostate cancer.
- Discuss the role prostate specific antigen plays in the detection of prostate cancer and its limitations.

Prostate carcinoma has become the most common cancer affecting North American men and is second only to lung cancer as a cause of cancer-related death. Age, race, ethnicity, and family history affect the risk for prostate cancer. Age is the main risk factor, and most men with clinically diagnosed prostate cancer are older than age 65 years.[1] Because prostate cancer usually occurs at an age when conditions such as heart disease and stroke cause death, many men die with prostate cancer rather than because of it. Mortality rates from prostate cancer have decreased because of the use of new and combined treatments, improved imaging, and advances in biopsy techniques.[2]

In most cases, a patient with prostate cancer is asymptomatic and may undergo further testing after a routine DRE reveals a nodule or if PSA serum levels are elevated. Biopsy is the only means of making a definitive diagnosis of prostate cancer. TRUS examination may be performed to identify prostate abnormalities, measure prostate volume, guide a biopsy procedure, or guide instrumentation for therapy.

PROSTATE ANATOMY

The prostate is located posterior to the inferior arch of the pubic symphysis and anterior to the rectal ampulla. The apex of the prostate is the inferior portion, and the base of the prostate is continuous with the bladder neck. The gland is almost spherical in shape and varies in size depending on whether a disease process is involved. A normal gland is about the size of a walnut.

The anatomic divisions of the prostate are referred to as zones, which have differing embryologic origins and susceptibilities to disease. There are four zones: the peripheral zone, transition zone, central zone, and anterior fibromuscular zone or stroma (Fig. 30-1). The outermost peripheral zone is the largest of the zones, it surrounds the distal urethral segment, and it is the site for most prostate cancers. The transition zone surrounds the proximal prostatic urethra and is most susceptible to

D.J.D. wishes to dedicate this chapter: To my mother Della Donovan who always sought to educate her children. To Betsy, Bridgett, and Collin Donovan for their humor, support, and love.

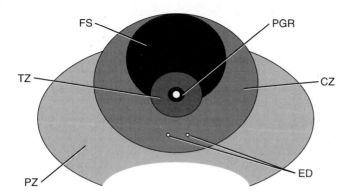

FIGURE 30-1 Prostate zonal anatomy. *CZ,* Central zone; *ED,* ejaculatory ducts; *FS,* fibromuscular stroma; *PGR,* periurethral glandular region; *PZ,* peripheral zone; *TZ,* transition zone.

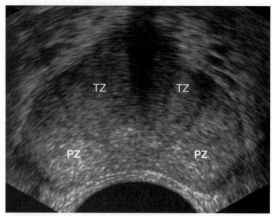

FIGURE 30-2 Normal prostate, transverse plane. *TZ,* Transitional zone; *PZ,* peripheral zone.

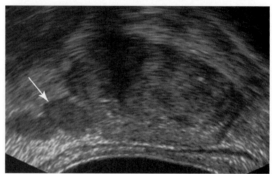

FIGURE 30-3 Normal prostate and seminal vesicle *(arrow),* sagittal plane.

benign prostatic hypertrophy (BPH). When hypertrophy is present, the transition zone may be the largest of the zones. The division between the peripheral and transition zones is called the surgical capsule. The central zone is a cone-shaped region that surrounds the ejaculatory ducts. This zone is rarely the site of prostate cancers and is thought to be relatively resistant to disease.[3] Fibromuscular stroma is located anterior to the transition zone and prostatic urethra.

Sonographic Appearance

The zonal anatomy can be difficult to differentiate sonographically. The peripheral and central zone make up the outer portion of the gland, and the inner gland consists of the transition zone, anterior fibromuscular stroma, and internal urethral sphincter. In young men, the predominant peripheral zone is poorly demarcated because it is isoechoic to the central and transitional zones. When the changes of BPH cause the transitional zone to become enlarged and hypoechoic, the peripheral zone appears relatively hyperechoic and is more easily recognized (Fig. 30-2). The peripheral and transition zones have a homogeneous echotexture; however, the transition zone may become heterogeneous when BPH is present. The surgical capsule is usually hypoechoic, unless corpora amylacea or calcifications have accumulated in this area. The vas deferens and seminal vesicles are visible superior to the base. The seminal vesicles are apparent as hypoechoic, oval, or tubular structures above the prostatic base (Figs. 30-3 and 30-4).

Normal Variants. Normal sonographic findings of the prostate in older men include dilated prostatic ducts (benign ductal ectasia); bright, echogenic foci or clumps representing calcifications; or proteinaceous debris (a precursor of calcific formation) called corpora amylacea. If no acoustic attenuation is present, these bright, echogenic areas may represent corpora amylacea. Calcifications and corpora amylacea are usually found in the periurethral glands and along the surgical capsule, although they can be found anywhere in the prostate (Figs. 30-5

and 30-6). Ductal ectasia may be evident in the peripheral zone. These findings are indicative of a benign process.

The decision to perform TRUS is typically based on the result of a PSA test and a DRE. Table 30-1 lists the components of a typical sonographic evaluation of the prostate.

PROSTATE SPECIFIC ANTIGEN

PSA is a protein produced by the cells of the prostate gland. The PSA test measures the level of PSA in the blood and is considered a valuable screening tool for early, curable, organ-confined prostate cancer. On a volume-per-volume basis, prostate cancer contributes 10 times the amount of PSA to the serum as benign prostate tissue, which is why serum PSA levels are often elevated in patients with prostate cancer.[3] PSA levels also increase with tumor volume and stage. This increase is not the result of increased production of PSA; rather, it is the result of increased diffusion (leaking) of PSA into the serum. The more aggressive the tumor, the more disruption of prostatic architecture and the higher the PSA level.

PSA levels can be elevated for many reasons, including inflammatory changes such as acute bacterial prostatitis, urinary tract infection, chronic prostatitis, and acute urinary retention. BPH (i.e., prostate enlargement) is the most common reason for increased PSA levels. The

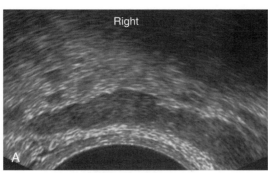
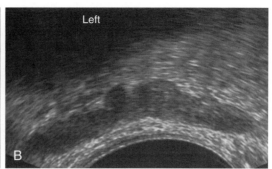

FIGURE 30-4 Normal right and left seminal vesicles, transverse plane.

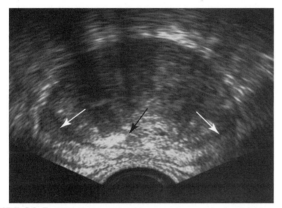

FIGURE 30-5 BPH (100 mL) with corpora amylasia *(black arrow).* Compressed peripheral zone *(white arrows).*

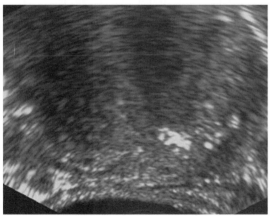

FIGURE 30-6 Prostatic calcifications.

TABLE 30-1	Sonographic Evaluation of Prostate
Imaging of prostate in two planes (sagittal and transverse)
Evaluation of gland for size, echogenicity, and symmetry
Evaluation of periprostatic fat and vessels for asymmetry
Examination of seminal vesicles in two planes for size, shape, position, symmetry, and echogenicity
Evaluation of vas deferens
Survey of perirectal space with attention to rectal wall and lumen

increase in serum PSA levels with gland volume explains most age-related increases in PSA. The net effect is that the bigger the prostate, the higher the PSA level.

Earlier accepted standards placed the normal range for total PSA at 0.0 to 4.0 ng/mL, and it was believed if the PSA level was less than 4.0 ng/mL, a biopsy was not needed. This threshold was adjusted to 0.0 to 2.5 ng/mL; however, a more recent study suggested that both white and African American men with baseline PSA values between 1.5 ng/mL and 4.0 ng/mL are at increased risk for future prostate cancer.[4,5] Because using a specific PSA cut-point can lead to an overestimation of risk in some patients and underestimation in others, the American Urological Association published recommendations that biopsy decisions not only should be based on the results of PSA testing and DRE but also take into account free and total PSA, patient age, PSA velocity, PSA density, family history, ethnicity, prior biopsy history, and comorbidities.[6]

Since PSA testing has become available, it has been shown to be more accurate than DRE and superior to TRUS examination in cancer detection. However, various factors can affect PSA levels, and several methods of evaluation of PSA are being researched to improve sensitivity of this test, including PSA density, PSA velocity, age-adjusted PSA, and free/total PSA ratio.

Prostate Specific Antigen Density

PSA density considers the relationship of the PSA level to the size of the prostate. PSA density is calculated by dividing the PSA level by the volume of the prostate gland determined during TRUS examination (PSA density = serum PSA/prostate volume). In other words, an elevated PSA level in a small gland may be suspicious, whereas an elevated PSA in a larger gland would be considered less suspicious. A PSA density of 0.1 or less is considered normal, a PSA density of 0.10 to 0.15 is intermediate, and a PSA density greater than 0.15 is considered elevated.[3]

Prostate Specific Antigen Velocity

PSA velocity is based on changes of PSA levels over time. A sharp increase in PSA level (>20% per year) is worrisome for malignant disease. Three PSA values over a period of at least 18 months is recommended to establish PSA velocity.[6]

Age-Adjusted Prostate Specific Antigen

Age is an important factor in determination of the meaning of increasing PSA levels. Some experts use age-adjusted PSA levels, which define a different PSA level for each 10-year age group, suggesting that men younger than 50 years old should have a PSA of less than 2.5 ng/mL and that PSA levels up to 6.5 ng/mL would be considered normal for men 70 years old. Opinions on the accuracy of age-adjusted PSA levels vary because increased PSA levels with advancing age are commonly associated with increased volume of the prostate.[3]

Free/Total Prostate Specific Antigen Ratio

PSA circulates in the blood in two forms: free or attached to a protein molecule. Patients with prostate cancer tend to have lower free/total ratios than patients with benign prostate conditions. Using the ratio of free to total PSA may reduce the number of biopsies in men with serum PSA levels between 2.5 ng/mL and 4.0 ng/mL.[6]

PSA is an excellent screening tool; however, it lacks sufficient sensitivity and specificity to consider it the "perfect" tumor marker. Although mortality rates have declined since the introduction of PSA testing, 20% to 40% of men with clinically significant cancer have a normal PSA level.[3] Nonetheless, screening with PSA is the best single test for early detection of prostate cancer.[6]

PROSTATE PATHOLOGY

Benign Prostatic Hypertrophy

BPH is a benign growth of prostate cells that causes the gland to enlarge; it is not considered a precancerous state. BPH is common in men older than age 50 years and rarely causes symptoms in men younger than 40 years. BPH develops almost exclusively in the transitional zone. As the prostate enlarges, the surrounding capsule prevents it from expanding, causing the gland to press internally against the urethra like a clamp on a garden hose. The urinary bladder wall subsequently becomes thicker and more irritable, contracting even when it contains small amounts of urine—leading to frequent urination. As the bladder wall weakens, it loses the ability to empty completely. Narrowing of the urethra and partial emptying of the bladder (bladder outlet obstruction) cause many of the clinical signs and symptoms associated with BPH. Symptoms of urinary obstruction include a hesitant or weak stream of urine, leaking, dribbling, and increased urinary frequency, particularly at night (nocturia).

A patient's symptoms from urinary obstruction caused by BPH may be relieved by undergoing transurethral resection of the prostate (TURP). Other treatments include medical therapy, open surgery, or laser therapy.

Sonographic Findings. The sonographic appearance of BPH varies; however, the most common appearance for BPH is enlargement of the inner gland (transition zone), with hyperechoic or hypoechoic areas or cystic regions. The enlarged transition zone may appear diffusely enlarged, or there may be distinct nodules. BPH may cause compression of the peripheral zone (see Fig. 30-5). Benign nodules may compress both the central zone and the peripheral zone but do not infiltrate beyond the confines of the gland.

Patients who have recently undergone a TURP procedure may have a large surgical defect; however, it rapidly decreases in size. The surgical defect appears as an anechoic region into the base of the gland.

Prostatitis

Inflammation from infection of the prostate can be the result of a bladder or urethral infection. Symptoms of prostatitis include chills, fever, urinary urgency, and frequency. The patient may also have a urethral discharge and pain in the perineal region. During an acute phase of prostatitis, the gland remains normal in size. In severe forms, the gland becomes enlarged with extensive areas of hypoechoic tissue. In patients who are elderly or immunosuppressed, abscess formation may occur.

Sonographic Findings. Prostatitis may be visualized as hypoechoic areas within the prostate, and reactive dilation of the periprostatic vessels may also be identified. An abscess may appear as a cystic region with irregular margins (Fig. 30-7). Color or power Doppler imaging of an inflamed prostate gland may demonstrate increased flow owing to hyperemic changes (Fig. 30-8; see Color Plate 49).

Cysts

The most common prostate cysts are parenchymal degenerative cysts within necrotic, hyperplastic nodules in the transition zone. Other cysts include retention cysts, congenital cysts, and ejaculatory duct cysts. Ejaculatory duct dilation should not be confused with cystic changes.

Sonographic Findings. Cystic changes visualized in the prostate gland usually appear as simple cysts (Fig. 30-9). Cysts that are caused by degeneration usually appear round or ovoid in shape. Ejaculatory duct cysts, which may be teardrop-shaped (in the sagittal plane), are located near the midline (Fig. 30-10). Ejaculatory ductal dilation,

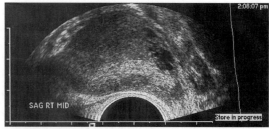

FIGURE 30-7 Irregular hypoechoic lesion, which was confirmed to be an abscess.

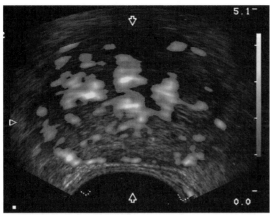

FIGURE 30-8 Prostatitis. Hyperemia evident with power Doppler imaging (see Color Plate 49).

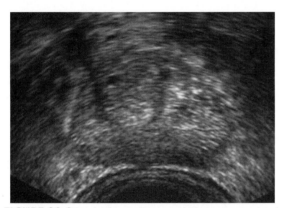

FIGURE 30-9 Multiple small cysts within prostate gland.

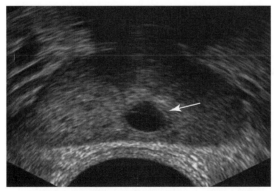

FIGURE 30-10 Ejaculatory duct cyst *(arrow)*.

although rounded when viewed on axial or sagittal images, should appear tubular with rotation of the transducer.

Prostate Cancer

Prostate cancer is particularly prevalent in Western countries such as the United States, and it has become the most frequently diagnosed cancer in men older than 50 years. Prostate cancer is asymptomatic in its early stages, and on average it takes about 10 years to cause death. Microfocal or microscopic prostate cancer is a clinically unimportant form and has been identified in 30% of men older than age 50 who have died of other causes.[7] The American Urological Association recommends a baseline PSA level be obtained at age 40, with subsequent rescreening annually or at intervals based on the initial PSA value.[6] There is great disparity between prostate cancer incidence and mortality, which has created controversy regarding prostate cancer screening and treatment.[2]

Prostate cancers that involve only a small portion of the gland are more successfully treated than cancers that extend throughout the gland. Tumor aggressiveness is determined by the pathologist's examination of the microscopic pattern of the cancer cells obtained during a biopsy. The most common tumor grading system is Gleason grading.[7] Treatment options include watchful waiting, interstitial prostate brachytherapy, external beam radiotherapy, radical prostatectomy, primary hormonal therapy, and other techniques such as cryosurgery.[2]

Sonographic Findings. The classic sonographic appearance of prostate cancer is a hypoechoic nodule in the peripheral zone (Fig. 30-11).[3] Cancerous nodules may also be hyperechoic or isoechoic. Isoechoic prostatic cancers tend to be infiltrative and may be suggested when glandular asymmetry is present, if the tumor is bulging into the capsule, or there is distortion of the contour (Fig. 30-12). Color Doppler imaging may assist in defining these lesions as an area of increased vascularity. However, inflammation can also increase vascularity. Some lesions are subtle in appearance, and comparison of adjacent echogenicity of prostate tissues is imperative. Early cancers may be only a few millimeters in size, and as the tumors increase in size, the echogenicity may change.

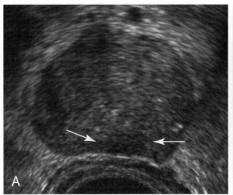
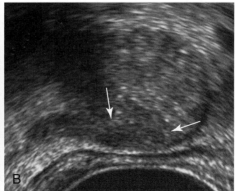

FIGURE 30-11 Prostate cancer. Transverse **(A)** and sagittal **(B)** images demonstrating focal, hypoechoic, solid mass *(arrows)* in the peripheral zone.

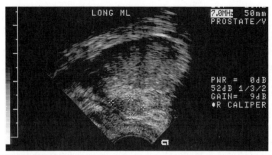

FIGURE 30-12 Prostate cancer causing contour abnormality.

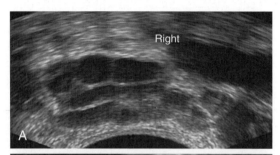

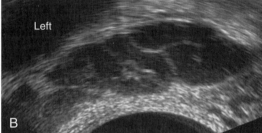

FIGURE 30-13 Cystic changes of seminal vesicles.

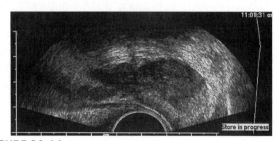

FIGURE 30-14 Seminal vesicle with invasion of prostate cancer.

Tumor extension into the capsule, periprostatic lymph nodes, seminal vesicles, or surrounding tissues may be identified sonographically. If lymph nodes are detected, tumor extension should be suspected.

Cancers occurring in the transition zone are difficult to define against the heterogeneous background of a prostate with hyperplasia. Clues to transition zone cancer include a poorly marginated, hypoechoic area that is different from other BPH nodules and focal loss of the surgical capsule.[3]

Seminal Vesicles

Normal seminal vesicles tend to have moderate echogenicity (see Figs. 30-3 and Fig. 30-4). The seminal vesicles may have increased cystic changes of uncertain clinical significance (Fig. 30-13) or abscess changes visualized as a focal cystic mass with irregular margins, no through-transmission, and possibly gas. Involvement of cancer can be suspected when there is asymmetry between the two seminal vesicles. With tumor infiltration, solid echotexture changes or irregular margins or both may be visualized (Fig. 30-14).

SUMMARY

When combined with DRE and PSA testing, sonography is a valuable tool in evaluation of the prostate. Early treatment of prostate diseases may prevent debilitation to the patient. Sonography may effectively evaluate the prostate for benign and malignant neoplasms, cysts, inflammatory processes, and benign enlargement of the gland, allowing an informed decision on whether to proceed with a prostate biopsy. An understanding of the anatomy, physiology, symptoms, and sonographic characteristics of diseases of the prostate is important for optimal patient care. Table 30-2 summarizes the pathology of the prostate.

CLINICAL SCENARIO—DIAGNOSIS

Clinically, the patient presents with lethargy and lower back pain, which do not fit the clinical picture of BPH. The sonographic examination shows a hypoechoic mass with subtle bulging of the capsule. This finding, coupled with the PSA value of 12 ng/mL, points to a malignant process. A biopsy of the prostate confirms the diagnosis of prostate cancer.

TABLE 30-2	Pathology of the Prostate	
Pathology	**Symptoms**	**Sonographic Findings**
Prostate cancer	Usually asymptomatic; may have various urinary symptoms	Hypoechoic nodule in peripheral zone
Benign prostatic hypertrophy	Hesitant or weak stream of urine, leaking or dribbling, and increased urinary frequency, particularly at night	Enlargement of inner gland with hyperechoic, hypoechoic, or cystic areas
Cysts	Usually asymptomatic	Anechoic, well-defined borders; increased through-transmission
Prostatitis	Chills, fever, urinary urgency and frequency	Enlargement of gland with hypoechoic areas and dilation of periprostatic vessels

CASE STUDIES FOR DISCUSSION

1. A 73-year-old man in otherwise good health has experienced increasing episodes of the need to urinate during the night over the last year. This situation has led to much interruption in his sleep, and finally he saw his internal medicine physician. DRE, urinalysis, and PSA blood test were completed. DRE findings were described as "a generous gland with no palpable nodules," and blood work revealed a high free/total PSA ratio. Given this information, what is likely causing this patient's symptoms?

2. A 32-year-old man woke up with intense pain, which he described as "a constant, deep, throbbing pain behind his scrotum." The patient's temperature had been elevated for a few days, and he had felt intermittent fever and chills for about the same length of time. The primary care physician ordered routine laboratory tests and TRUS examination of the prostate. His laboratory test results showed an elevated PSA and white blood cell count. The sonogram showed a diffuse increase in color flow Doppler in the prostate gland and an irregular, cystic structure at the junction of a seminal vesicle and prostate. What is the most likely diagnosis?

3. An 83-year-old man saw his rural family medicine physician with complaints of overall weakness, joint pain, and generally "not feeling well" for the last 9 months. The patient had been quite active for his age before 1 year ago. After taking a careful history and completing a thorough physical examination, the clinician ordered laboratory tests including PSA. On receiving the PSA results of 23 ng/mL, the physician also requested a prostate sonogram (Fig. 30-15) and a nuclear medicine bone scan. The patient was scheduled for a consultation visit with his physician, who gave the patient what news regarding his current state of health?

4. A 45-year-old patient with a PSA value of 1.5 ng/mL underwent TRUS examination. The patient had been unaware of any prostate or urinary symptoms, and the transrectal sonogram went well for the patient. Sonographic findings are shown in Figure 30-16. What is the most likely diagnosis?

5. A 67-year-old patient had been coping with increasing urinary frequency, increased leaking, and hesitation of the urine stream for more than 3.5 years; he finally scheduled an appointment with his primary care physician. The patient was reluctant to see the physician because a few close friends had received a diagnosis of prostate cancer, and he feared the worst. History, PSA, DRE, and TRUS examination (Fig. 30-17) were completed on this patient. DRE and TRUS examination revealed an enlarged prostate. With this patient's clinical history, elevated PSA results, DRE, and sonographic findings, what is the most likely diagnosis?

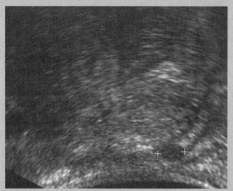

FIGURE 30-15 Prostate findings in an 83-year-old patient with a PSA level of 23 ng/mL.

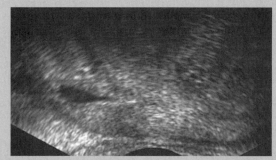

FIGURE 30-16 Prostate findings in a 45-year-old patient with a PSA level of 1.5 ng/mL.

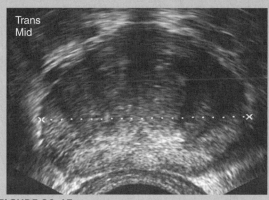

FIGURE 30-17 Prostate findings in a 67-year-old patient.

STUDY QUESTIONS

1. Anatomically, the prostate can be divided into four zones. These include each of the following except:
   a. Transition zone
   b. Medial zone
   c. Central zone
   d. Peripheral zone
   e. Anterior fibromuscular zone

2. The most common reason for elevated PSA is:
   a. Bacterial prostatitis
   b. Urinary tract infections
   c. Chronic prostatitis
   d. Enlarged prostate gland (BPH)
   e. Acute urinary retention

3. The goal of PSA testing is to:
   a. Identify late stage prostate cancers
   b. Identify early stage prostate cancers
   c. Identify prostatitis
   d. Identify bacterial infections of the prostate
   e. Rule out prostate cancer definitively

4. Benign enlargement of the prostate gland occurs almost exclusively:
   a. Throughout the prostate
   b. In the central zone
   c. In the transition zone
   d. In the peripheral zone
   e. In the fibromuscular stroma

5. Symptoms of prostatitis include all of the following except:
   a. Fever and chills
   b. Perineal region pain
   c. Microhematuria
   d. Urethral discharge
   e. Urinary urgency or frequency

6. Transverse imaging of the prostate gland in a 70-year-old man with a history of urinary obstruction demonstrates an anechoic defect into the base of the prostate. This finding most likely represents which of the following?
   a. Prostate cancer
   b. Prostatitis
   c. Cystic degeneration
   d. Urethral cancer
   e. Surgical defect from TURP

7. The PSA density result in an asymptomatic 65-year-old African American man is 0.2, and DRE reveals a nodule. What is the most likely diagnosis?
   a. Enlarged periprostatic lymph node
   b. Prostate abscess
   c. Prostate cancer
   d. Prostatitis
   e. BPH

8. Sonographically, prostate cancers are often visualized as focal, hypoechoic nodules most often found:
   a. In the peripheral zone
   b. In the transitional zone
   c. Anywhere in the prostate
   d. In the central zone
   e. Along the ejaculatory duct

9. Which of the following is a sonographic feature of advanced prostate cancer?
   a. Tumor extension to the periprostatic lymph nodes
   b. Seminal vesicle cysts
   c. Small tumor load confined to the prostate capsule
   d. Tumor involvement to the surrounding tissues
   e. Prostatic calcifications

10. Commonly seen in men older than 50 years of age, symptoms of BPH include:
    a. Leaking or dribbling of urine
    b. Weak or hesitant urine stream
    f Increased urinary frequency
    d. Nocturia
    e. All of the above

REFERENCES

1. American Cancer Society: Learn about cancer, 2011, http://www.cancer.org/Cancer/ProstateCancer/DetailedGuide/prostate-cancer-key-statistics. Date retrieved 12/30/2012.
2. Thompson I, Thrasher J, Aus G, et al: Guideline for the management of clinically localized prostate cancer: 2007 update, *J Urol* 177:2106–2131, 2007.
3. Toi A: The prostate. In Rumack C, Wilson S, Charboneau J, et al: ed 4, *Diagnostic ultrasound*, vol. 1, Philadelphia, 2011, Mosby, pp 547–612.
4. Crawford E, Moul JW, Rove KO, et al: Prostate-specific antigen 1.5–4.0 ng/mL: a diagnostic challenge and danger zone, *BJU Int* 108:1743–1749, 2011.
5. Schroeder F, Roobol M, Andriole G, et al: Defining increased future risk for prostate cancer: evidence from a population based screening cohort, *J Urol* 181:69–74, 2009.
6. Greene K, Albertsen P, Babaian R, et al: Prostate specific antigen best practice statement: 2009 update, *J Urol* 182:2232–2241, 2009.
7. Rietbergen J, Schroder F: Screening for prostate cancer: more questions than answers, *Acta Oncol* 37:515–532, 1998.

PART V

Miscellaneous

Hip Dysplasia

Charlotte Henningsen

CLINICAL SCENARIO

An 8-week-old boy with a grossly abnormal physical examination is seen for a hip sonogram to rule out hip dysplasia. The parents report that their older daughter was also treated for hip dysplasia as an infant. The images of the right hip demonstrated the finding in Figure 31-1, *A-C*, and did not change much with the Ortolani maneuver. Computed tomography (CT) (Fig. 31-1, *D*) is consistent with the sonographic findings. The left hip appeared similar. What is the diagnosis, and what is the possible treatment for this infant?

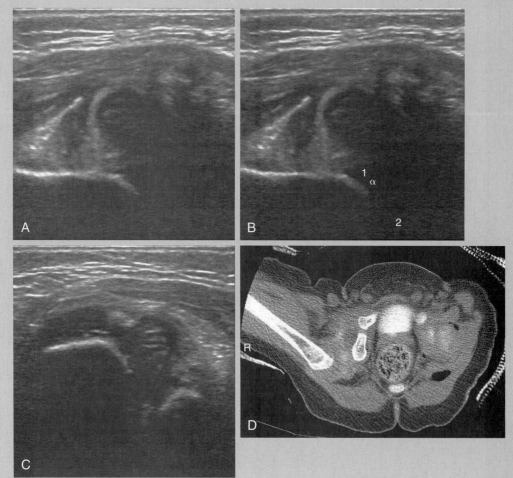

FIGURE 31-1 **(A)**, Coronal view of hip shows relationship of femoral head to acetabulum. **(B)**, The alpha angle was 44 degrees. Transverse/flexion view **(C)** and CT scan **(D)** shows posterior displacement of the femoral head in relation to the acetabulum. *(Courtesy Judith Williams, BS, RDMS.)*

OBJECTIVES

- Identify the normal anatomy of infant hips.
- List the risk factors associated with infant hip dysplasia.
- Describe the clinical maneuvers used in evaluation for hip dysplasia.
- Describe the sonographic protocol for imaging of infant hips.
- Differentiate hip laxity, subluxation, and dislocation.

Every newborn examination includes an evaluation of the infant's hips for assessment for developmental dysplasia of the hip (DDH). This chapter presents the risk factors for DDH and the clinical examination that may be used to identify DDH. The various modes of testing, including ultrasonography, are examined, in addition to the types of treatment available on the basis of the severity of the disease. The sonographic evaluation of infant hips includes a review of normal hip anatomy and imaging protocol for evaluation of DDH.

ANATOMY OF THE HIP

The hip comprises the femoral head and the acetabulum. The femoral head is cartilaginous at birth and begins to ossify between 2 and 8 months, with ossification occurring earlier in girls. The acetabulum comprises cartilage and bone. The bony acetabulum (Fig. 31-2) consists of the ilium, the ischium, and the pubis, which is joined by a growth plate known as the triradiate cartilage. The cartilaginous labrum is located at the acetabular rim and extends over the superolateral aspect of the femoral head.

At birth, the hip has a large cartilaginous component, and the femoral head is more shallow in its relationship to the acetabulum. The hip is subject to molding, especially in the first 6 weeks of life. The normal development of the hip is contingent on the femur having adequate contact with the acetabulum without an abnormal amount of stress. When the femoral head is subluxed or dislocated for a significant amount of time, the acetabulum becomes increasingly dysplastic, the femoral head becomes deformed, and the supporting ligaments deform.

The purpose of early treatment of abnormal hips is to position the hip so that the femoral head and acetabulum can develop normally, avoiding possible surgery and disability. Clinical evaluation and identification of risk factors can be used to identify infants at risk for development of hip dysplasia. Sonographic evaluation can be used to define further infants who would benefit from treatment and to follow their progress. Screening for hip dysplasia is usually reserved for infants with an abnormal clinical examination or for infants with identified risk factors to avoid overtreatment of infants with physiologic laxity.

DEVELOPMENTAL DYSPLASIA OF THE HIP

DDH describes a spectrum of abnormalities that involve an abnormal relationship of the femoral head to the acetabulum, which includes mild instability, subluxation, and frank dislocation. DDH also has been referred to as congenital hip dysplasia, although this is a misnomer because hip dysplasia may develop after birth. The incidence varies depending on whether or not the neonatal population is routinely screened, with a higher incidence in the screened population. In the United States, the incidence is 1.5:1000 to 15:1000 live births.[1] There is also geographic and ethnic variability that may be secondary to environmental or genetic factors or both. An example of this variability is the lower incidence in native Africans versus African Americans; however, the incidence is lower in African Americans compared with the overall prevalence of DDH in the United States.[1]

Hip instability is associated with joint laxity and may be identified in newborns affected by maternal hormones. This laxity often resolves within the first few weeks of birth and necessitates no treatment. Unless there is a significant instability or dislocation, sonographic evaluation

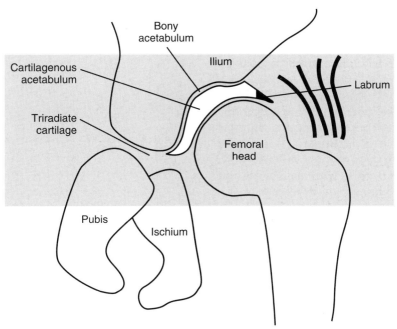

FIGURE 31-2 Normal hip anatomy.

of the infant hip is not recommended before 3 to 4 weeks of age to avoid overtreatment in populations in whom the instability would spontaneously resolve.[2] Subluxation of the hip refers to a femoral head that is shallow in location, allowing it to glide within the confines of the acetabulum. Hip dislocation is defined as a femoral head that is located outside of the acetabulum and may be reducible or irreducible. Hip dislocation can also be associated with congenital neurologic or musculoskeletal anomalies, including spina bifida, scoliosis, arthrogryposis, talipes, and numerous syndromes, and is referred to as teratologic hips.[1,2]

Risk Factors

Many risk factors associated with DDH are related to the inability of the fetus or newborn to move freely. These conditions include pregnancies affected by oligohydramnios (including serious renal anomalies), breech presentation, first pregnancy (primigravida), high birth weight, and postmaturity. Other infants at risk include infants born in the cold seasons of the year, female infants, and infants with torticollis. There is an increase in infants born where swaddling is prevalent, including in Saudi Arabia, Turkey, and Japan as well as Navajo Indians.[1] The left hip is affected more commonly than the right, and DDH is bilateral in 20% of cases.[1] Family history is also an important factor in identification of infants at risk for development of DDH, especially when parents or siblings are affected.

Clinical Evaluation

Evaluation for hip dysplasia is part of every newborn examination. The accuracy of the evaluation is affected by the experience of the physician. Infants in whom hip dysplasia does not develop until after birth may initially have a normal examination. Clinical findings associated with DDH include asymmetric skin folds of the thighs and one knee appearing lower than the other when the hips and knees are flexed. The subluxed or dislocated hip appears shorter (known as the Galeazzi or Allis sign). Also, limited abduction of the hip may be observed.[3]

Clinical maneuvers also can be used to detect hip instability and dislocation, but performance of these maneuvers may be difficult if the infant is not relaxed and are best performed in a warm room after feeding. The two maneuvers are performed with the infant's hips and knees flexed, and one hip should be examined at a time. The Ortolani maneuver (Fig. 31-3) involves abduction of the thigh while the hip is gently pulled anteriorly. If the hip is dislocated, the hip may relocate into the acetabulum with a palpable (and possibly audible) "click." The Barlow maneuver (Fig. 31-4) is performed with adduction of the hip with a gentle posterior push in an effort to solicit subluxation or dislocation in an abnormal hip.[3] These maneuvers are similar to maneuvers performed in a dynamic sonographic evaluation.

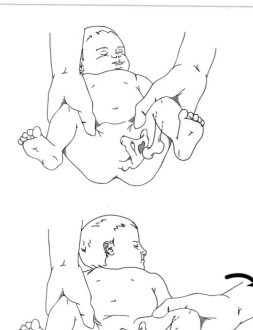

FIGURE 31-3 Ortolani maneuver.

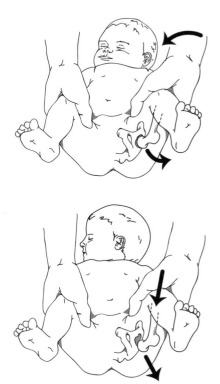

FIGURE 31-4 Barlow maneuver.

SONOGRAPHIC EVALUATION OF INFANT HIPS

The technique for imaging the infant hip was initially described by Graf, who used a static approach. Harcke developed a dynamic approach to sonographic imaging. The two approaches were combined to develop a minimum standard examination.[4] The imaging protocol should incorporate two orthogonal views with one view that includes stress views; this typically includes the coronal/neutral or coronal/flexion view and the transverse/flexion view. Additional views, including anterior views, and measurements are considered optional, although they may be dictated by institutional protocol.[4] Particular care should be taken to image each view in the correct plane and with the appropriate anatomy identified because a minimal shift in the image may lead to an inaccurate diagnosis. This chapter defines the images for the minimum standard examination and describes normal and abnormal findings.

Infant hips may be examined sonographically during the first year of life or until the ossification of the femoral head prevents adequate visualization. A linear transducer is preferred to avoid distortion and to cover a broader field of view. The highest frequency transducer should be used to penetrate the soft tissues of the hip, and this depends on the age of the infant.

A successful examination requires that the infant be relaxed for accurate stress maneuvers. Infants should be imaged in a warm environment with distracters such as toys, pacifiers, or bottles. A parent should be available and visible to the infant to assist in maintaining a relaxed environment. The infant should be placed in a supine or lateral decubitus position to accommodate the lateral and posterolateral position of the transducer. Bolsters should be used as needed to stabilize the infant's position. For easier access, the left hip may be scanned with the right hand while maneuvering the hip with the left hand, and the right hip may be scanned with the left hand while performing stress maneuvers with the right hand. Because two hands are needed to image and maneuver the hip adequately, sonographic evaluation is often a joint effort between the sonographer and radiologist. The second person may assist in maneuvering the hip or producing the images, depending on institutional protocol.

Coronal/Neutral View

The coronal/neutral view of the hip is obtained with placement of the transducer in a coronal plane at the lateral aspect of the hip. The hip is maintained in a physiologic neutral position with approximately 15 to 20 degrees of flexion. By slightly rotating the superior aspect of the transducer posteriorly, the image should demonstrate the midportion of the acetabulum, with the ilium appearing as a straight line parallel to the transducer. The junction of the ilium and triradiate cartilage should be clearly identified, and the cartilaginous tip of the labrum should be visualized.[2] The femoral metaphysis is also seen in this plane, which differentiates this view from the coronal/flexion view. A normal hip (Fig. 31-5, A) shows the hypoechoic femoral head resting against the acetabulum. An abnormal hip (Fig. 31-5, B) migrates laterally and superiorly.

In this view, the alpha angle may be obtained with measurement of a line along the lateral aspect of the ilium with respect to the slope of the acetabulum. According to the Graf classification, a normal hip would have an alpha angle of 60 degrees or more (type I). A type II hip (50 to 60 degrees) would reflect a physiologic immaturity in infants less than 3 months of age and would require follow-up but no treatment. If a type II hip is identified in an infant older than 3 months, treatment would be necessary. A type III hip describes subluxation with a shallow acetabulum and an alpha angle of less than 50 degrees. A type IV hip is a dislocated hip that lacks contact between the acetabulum and the femoral head.[4] With the minimum standard examination, measurements are optional; however, they do provide a quantitative baseline for follow-up purposes.

A more subjective assessment method may be used in this view by noting how deep the femoral head is located within the acetabulum. A normal hip shows at least 50% of femoral head coverage by the acetabulum. This can be assessed by drawing a line across the ilium through the femoral head and identifying whether 50% of the femoral head is below the line. On the basis of the amount of femoral head coverage, the hip can be classified as sitting deep, intermediate, or shallow. A visual assessment of the acetabulum and any irregularities should also be described. The acetabulum becomes progressively deformed (Fig. 31-5, C) when hip dysplasia is present, and fibrofatty tissue develops (appearing as soft tissue echoes) between the femoral head, preventing reduction of the hip.

Coronal/Flexion View

The coronal/flexion view is also imaged from the coronal plane, although the hip is flexed at a 90-degree angle. The sonographic appearance is similar to the coronal/neutral view, with the exception of visualization of the bony metaphysis. The lateral margin of the ilium should appear as a straight line, and the femoral head should be identified resting within the acetabulum (Fig. 31-6, A). As in the coronal/neutral view, the cartilaginous tip of the labrum is visualized. In this view, stress maneuvers can be performed for assessment of instability of the hip, and measurements can be taken (Fig. 31-6, B). The stress maneuvers performed are similar to the Ortolani and Barlow maneuvers to test for the reduction of a dislocated hip or to identify whether or not the hip can be dislocated. The infant must be relaxed for accurate assessment of instability. Gentle guiding of the hip, moving of the hip from a neutral to flexed position, and abducting and adducting while administering a gentle push/pull are also important. The sonographer should observe and document the absence or presence of any instability identified in real time. Notation of whether or not a dislocated hip will reduce is also important. The acetabulum should be evaluated for any evidence of dysplasia.

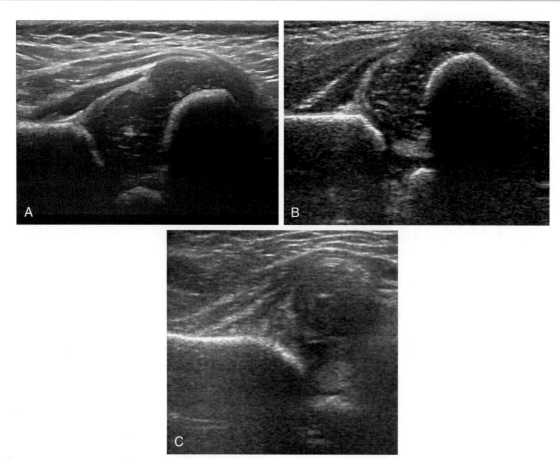

FIGURE 31-5 (A), Normal coronal/flexion view is identified with femoral head resting deep in acetabulum. Calcification of the femoral head is identified in this mature hip. **(B)**, Immature head demonstrates femoral head positioned laterally and superiorly. **(C)**, Displaced hip shows soft tissue echoes in acetabulum that may prevent the hip from being reduced without surgical intervention. *(Courtesy Lorraine Chisari, RDMS, RVT.)*

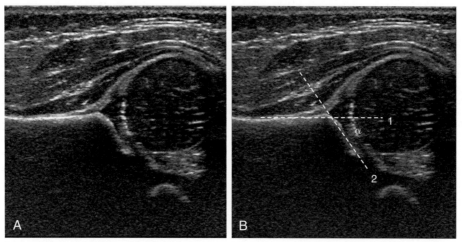

FIGURE 31-6 (A), Graf type II hip is shown in coronal/neutral view. **(B)**, Immature hip with an alpha angle of 55% requires no treatment in this 7-week-old infant. *(Courtesy Judith Williams, BS, RDMS.)*

Transverse/Flexion View

The transverse/flexion view is obtained with the infant's hip flexed at a 90-degree angle. The transducer is rotated 90 degrees from a coronal to a transverse plane and should be positioned slightly posterolaterally over the hip. The infant may need to be moved to a slightly oblique position to accommodate the transducer position. The image shows the femoral head and metaphysis, which is identified anterior to the femoral head; the ischium is identified posterior to the femoral head. The normal hip appears to have a U-shaped configuration (Fig. 31-7, *A*) as the metaphysis and ischium surround the femoral head. An abnormal hip (Fig. 31-7, *B*) lacks

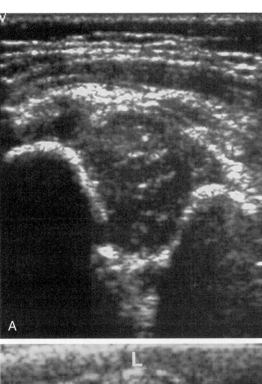

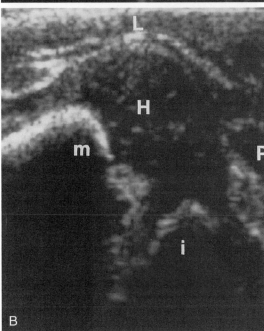

FIGURE 31-7 Normal transverse/flexion view **(A)** shows U-shaped configuration that is not present in dislocated hip **(B)**. *H,* Femoral head; *i,* ischium; *L,* lateral; *m,* femoral metaphysic; *P,* posterior.

this appearance because the femoral head shifts laterally with subluxation and posterolaterally with dislocation. Stress maneuvers should be used as described in the coronal/flexion view to assess for instability and the ability to reduce a dislocated hip.[2,4]

TREATMENT

Treatment of abnormal hips may vary depending on the age at diagnosis and the severity of hip dysplasia. Some degree of laxity may be identified in the newborn period and resolve without intervention, although follow-up

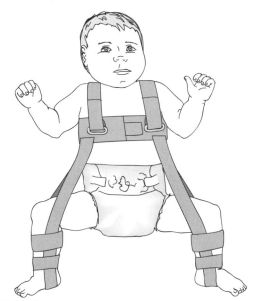

FIGURE 31-8 Pavlik harness is often used in treatment of hip dysplasia.

is necessary to ensure resolution of a subluxation. The double-diaper technique has also been used to prevent adduction but without evidence of improvement and should not be used as a replacement for an abduction brace.[3] Treatment for hip dysplasia is indicated for infants with a persistent subluxation and for infants with hip dislocation.

The Pavlik harness (Fig. 31-8) is the most common device used in the treatment of hip dysplasia; it prevents adduction of the hips and is used for infants with hip subluxations and reducible dislocations. The goal is to maintain a flexed, abducted position of the hip, allowing the stable placement of the femoral head in the acetabulum and encouraging normal modeling of the acetabulum.[1] It is important for trained personnel to adjust the harness, and the harness should not be removed; the success of the harness may depend in part on parental compliance. The treatment period varies; during that time, the infant may be monitored regularly with radiography or sonography, and adjustments to the harness may be made as necessary. When treatment is followed with sonography, the Pavlik harness should initially be left in place. As the infant is weaned from the harness, the sonographer may be directed to perform the examination without the harness. Infants who are not successfully treated with the Pavlik harness and infants with irreducible dislocations may require alternative treatments, including bracing, casting, or operative reduction.

SUMMARY

Early diagnosis and treatment of hip dysplasia can reduce infant morbidity. Risk factors or abnormal clinical examination results can be used to identify infants who would achieve the greatest benefit from sonographic screening. Sonography is an important tool in the diagnosis, especially in infants at risk with normal clinical examination results. A thorough knowledge of imaging technique is necessary to ensure reliability and reproducibility. This is of particular importance when sonography is used to follow the effectiveness of treatment.

CLINICAL SCENARIO—DIAGNOSIS

The femoral head is completely dislocated and did not reduce with stress maneuvers. The CT scan also demonstrates the dislocation, which was also seen on the left side. The Pavlik harness is contraindicated for nonreducible dislocations; alternative treatments including surgery must be considered.

CASE STUDIES FOR DISCUSSION

1. A family practice resident examines a newborn in the first week of life. The left hip feels unstable, and a sonogram is ordered. The evaluation reveals a Graf type II hip with an alpha angle of 56 degrees. What is the appropriate treatment for this infant?
2. An infant is seen with a positive Allis sign on the right side. Clinical examination is limited because the infant is fussy at the time of the appointment. A sonogram is ordered to rule out hip dysplasia.

The sonographer identifies a left hip sitting deep in the acetabulum, and the right hip appears dislocated; however, it reduces with stress maneuvers. What are the treatment options for this infant?

3. A 1-week-old girl is referred for a sonogram to rule out hip dysplasia because of a "click" felt on clinical examination. There is no other pertinent clinical history. Sonographic evaluation reveals the finding in Figure 31-9. What is the diagnosis and treatment plan?

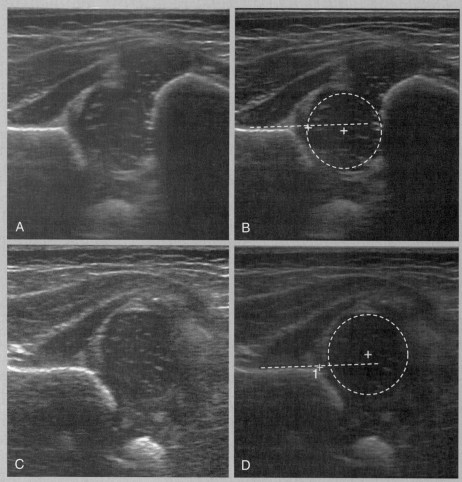

FIGURE 31-9 (A), Coronal/neutral view of right hip. **(B),** Percentage of femoral head contained within acetabulum is 59%. **(C),** Coronal/neutral view of the left hip. **(D),** Percentage of femoral head contained within acetabulum is 38%. *(Courtesy Judith Williams, BS, RDMS.)*

CASE STUDIES FOR DISCUSSION—cont'd

4. A 6-week-old girl is seen for a sonogram to rule out hip dysplasia. The alpha angle for the left hip is 64%, and the alpha angle for the right hip (Fig. 31-10) is 58%. What are the Graf classifications for these hips?

5. A 10-day-old boy is seen for a hip sonogram because of a breech delivery. The mother states that the initial clinical evaluation was normal. Figure 31-11 demonstrates the sonographic findings. What is the appropriate treatment for this infant?

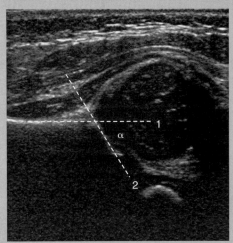

FIGURE 31-10 Coronal view of right hip. *(Courtesy Judith Williams, BS, RDMS.)*

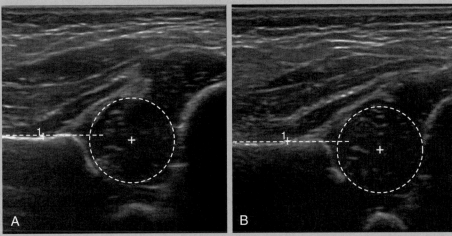

FIGURE 31-11 (A), Coronal view of left hip demonstrates 56% coverage. **(B),** Coronal view of right hip demonstrates 60% coverage. *(Courtesy Judith Williams, BS, RDMS.)*

STUDY QUESTIONS

1. Which term describes the type of hip abnormality in which the femoral head sits outside the confines of the acetabulum?
   a. Dislocation
   b. Dysplasia
   c. Laxity
   d. Subluxation

2. Which of the following views is taken at the lateral aspect of the infant with the transducer oriented parallel to the long axis of the body with the hip at a 90-degree angle?
   a. Coronal/flexion view
   b. Coronal/neutral view
   c. Transverse/flexion view
   d. Transverse/neutral view

3. The risk factors for DDH include which of the following?
   a. Breech position, multigravida, congenital torticollis
   b. American Indian, family history, male gender
   c. Native African, female gender, primigravida
   d. High birth weight, spina bifida, cold season

4. The bony acetabulum consists of which of the following?
   a. Femoral head, ilium, metaphysis
   b. Ilium, ischium, pubis
   c. Ischium, metaphysis, pubis
   d. Pubis, labrum, triradiate cartilage

5. Which maneuver is performed to solicit subluxation?
   a. Allis maneuver
   b. Barlow maneuver
   c. Graf maneuver
   d. Ortolani maneuver

6. Which of the following views are combined with stress maneuvers for evaluation of hip stability?
   a. Anterior/neutral, coronal/neutral
   b. Coronal/flexion, transverse/flexion
   c. Coronal/flexion, anterior/flexion
   d. Transverse/flexion, transverse/neutral

7. Which Graf classification describes an immature hip with an alpha angle of 50 to 60 degrees?
   a. Type I
   b. Type II
   c. Type III
   d. Type IV

8. A 6-week-old infant with a history of a "click" on clinical examination is seen for a hip sonogram. The alpha angle measures 60 degrees on the right and 55 degrees on the left. This would be consistent with which of the following?
   a. Right hip, type II; left hip, type III
   b. Right hip, type I; left hip, type II
   c. Right hip, type III; left hip, type III
   d. Right hip, type III; left hip, type II

9. In which of the following views does the normal hip display a "U" shape?
   a. Anterior/neutral
   b. Coronal/neutral
   c. Coronal/flexion
   d. Transverse/flexion

10. Which of the following would meet the criteria of the minimum standard examination?
   a. Coronal/neutral view with stress maneuvers; coronal/flexion view
   b. Transverse/flexion view with stress maneuvers; coronal/neutral view
   c. Coronal/neutral view with alpha angle; transverse/flexion view
   d. Transverse/flexion view with stress maneuvers; transverse neutral view

REFERENCES

1. Bracken J, Tran T, Ditchfield M: Developmental dysplasia of the hip: controversies and current concepts, *J Paediatr Child Health* 48:963–973, 2012.
2. American Institute of Ultrasound in Medicine: *AIUM practice guideline for the performance of an ultrasound examination for detection and assessment of developmental dysplasia of the hip*, Laurel, MD, 2008, American Institute of Ultrasound in Medicine.
3. Fabry G: Clinical practice: the hip from birth to adolescence, *Eur J Pediatr* 169:143–148, 2010.
4. Casteneda P: Pediatric hip dysplasia and evaluation with ultrasound, *Pediatr Health* 3:465–472, 2009.

Premature Birth: Rule Out Germinal Matrix Hemorrhage

Kimberly Michael

CLINICAL SCENARIO

A woman delivers twins at 27 weeks' gestation. Twin A dies at the time of birth. Twin B is admitted to the neonatal intensive care unit for prematurity and respiratory distress. Cranial sonography is performed at 2 days (Fig. 32-1, *A*). Sonograms performed at 1 and 4 weeks demonstrate the changes noted in Figure 32-1, *B* (1 week) and *C* (4 weeks). What is the diagnosis, and what is the prognosis for this infant?

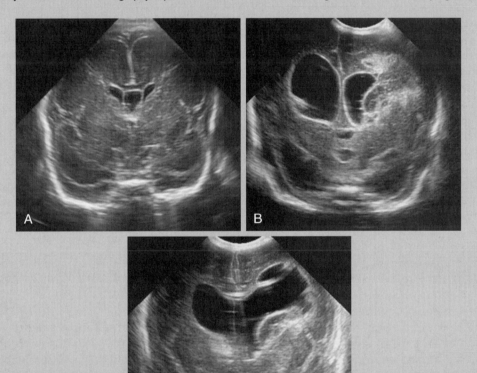

FIGURE 32-1 Girl born at 27 weeks' gestational age. **(A),** Coronal image taken at 2 days. **(B),** Coronal image at taken at 1 week. **(C),** Coronal image taken at 4 weeks.

OBJECTIVES

- List images that should routinely be obtained in the evaluation of a neonatal brain.
- Discuss additional scanning windows for imaging posterior fossa structures.
- Differentiate the sonographic findings of intraventricular hemorrhage and periventricular leukomalacia.
- Identify congenital anomalies seen in the neonatal brain.

Cranial sonography is an effective and reliable imaging tool for assessing the neonatal brain. It is safe, portable, economical, and noninvasive, making it suitable for serial imaging of the brain. Indications for neurosonography of the neonate include follow-up to prenatal abnormalities, prematurity, and abnormal physical examination. Imaging of the neonatal head may also be used to confirm a congenital anomaly or evaluate for changes associated with hypoxic-ischemic encephalopathy. This chapter discusses the most common neonatal brain abnormalities encountered by sonographers. In addition, limited congenital abnormalities of the central nervous system are explored.

NEONATAL HEAD

Imaging Technique and Normal Sonographic Anatomy

Neonatal imaging of the brain is often performed on infants who are premature or critically ill. The infant is examined in the incubator, and care should be taken to maintain body temperature with warm gel, avoidance of unnecessary exposure, and minimization of scanning time. To reduce stress on the infant, a quiet, dark atmosphere is maintained; care should be taken to avoid disruption of that environment. Many infants are immunosuppressed, so proper transducer disinfection and hand washing between infants is imperative for preventing the spread of infection.

Imaging technique should include the selection of the highest frequency transducer possible without sacrifice of adequate penetration. Transducers of 7.5 to 10 MHz are typically selected for premature infants, and 5-MHz transducers are usually adequate for infants with larger heads. A small footprint transducer is needed for imaging through the small fontanelles. Linear array transducers are useful in evaluating superficial structures. Routine neonatal brain imaging is performed through the anterior fontanelle in the coronal, sagittal, and parasagittal planes. Parasagittal views are lateral to the midline (true sagittal) plane but are referred to as sagittal images in this chapter. The posterior and mastoid fontanelles provide additional acoustic windows for further evaluation of the posterior fossa (Fig. 32-2).[1]

For coronal imaging, the transducer is placed transversely in the anterior fontanelle with the right side of the brain displayed on the left side of the image. Sweeping anterior to posterior, six standard coronal views are recorded, as follows:

C1: Frontal lobes of the brain, anterior to the frontal horns of the lateral ventricle (Fig. 32-3, *A*).
C2: Frontal horns of lateral ventricles. Anatomy visualized includes falx, corpus callosum, cavum septi pellucidi (CSP), lateral ventricles, caudate nucleus, putamen, and temporal lobe (Fig. 32-3, *B*).
C3: Lateral ventricles at the level of the third ventricle and foramen of Monro. Structures visualized include

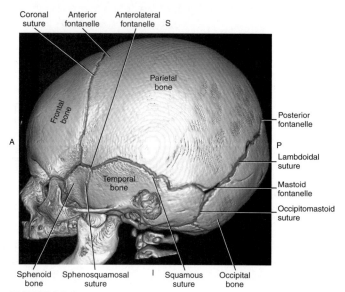

FIGURE 32-2 Diagram demonstrating acoustic scanning windows.

corpus callosum, CSP, frontal horns, foramen of Monro, third ventricle, thalami, sylvian fissure, and brainstem (Fig. 32-3, *C*).
C4: Bodies of the lateral ventricles. Anatomy includes corpus callosum, CSP, choroid plexus in the body of the lateral ventricle, thalami, choroidal fissure, temporal horn, tentorium, cerebellum, and cisterna magna (Fig. 32-3, *D*).
C5: Atria of the lateral ventricles. Anatomic structures include the parietal lobe, glomus of the choroid plexus, and cerebellum (Fig. 32-3, *E*).
C6: Occipital lobe of the brain (Fig. 32-3, *F*).

For sagittal imaging, the transducer is placed longitudinally in the anterior fontanelle so that the anterior aspect of the brain is displayed on the left side of the image. Images are recorded midline and with transducer angulation to the right and left hemispheres, as follows:

Sag ML: Midline image of the brain visualizing the cingulate sulcus, corpus callosum, CSP, third and fourth ventricles, cerebellar vermis, and cisterna magna (Fig. 32-4, *A*).
Sag Left or Right 1: Lateral ventricle demonstrating the caudothalamic notch. Anatomy visualized includes the caudate nucleus, thalamus, and caudothalamic notch (Fig. 32-4, *B*).
Sag Left or Right 2: Entire lateral ventricle showing the frontal, temporal, and occipital horns; glomus of the choroid plexus; caudate nucleus; and thalami (Fig. 32-4, *C*).
Sag Left or Right 3: Periventricular white matter (Fig. 32-4, *D*).
Sag Left or Right 4: Sylvian fissure containing the middle cerebral artery (Fig. 32-4, *E*).

In addition, longitudinal placement of the transducer in the posterior fontanelle, with left and right angulation,

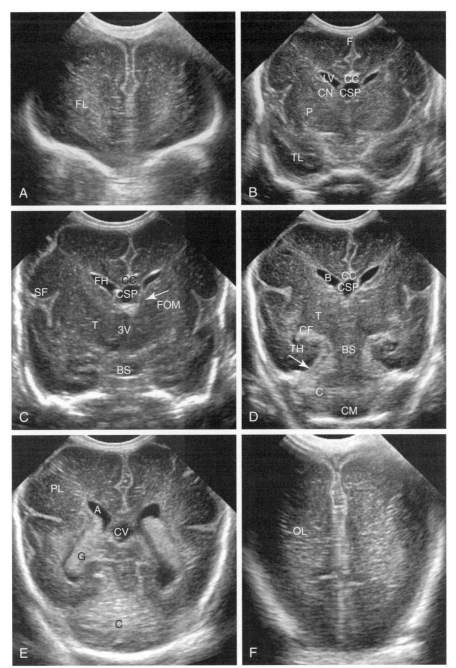

FIGURE 32-3 Coronal views of neonatal head demonstrating standard imaging views. **(A)**, C1. **(B)**, C2. **(C)**, C3. **(D)**, C4. **(E)**, C5. **(F)**, C6, posterior coronal. *A,* Atrium of lateral ventricle; *B,* body of lateral ventricle; *BS,* brainstem; *C,* cerebellum; *CC,* corpus callosum; *CF,* choroidal fissure; *CM,* cisterna magna; *CN,* caudate nucleus; *CSP,* cavum septi pellucidi; *CV,* cavum vergae; *F,* falx; *FH,* frontal horn; *FL,* frontal lobe; *FOM,* foramen of Monro; *G,* glomus of choroid plexus; *LV,* lateral ventricle; *OL,* occipital lobe; *P,* putamen; *PL,* parietal lobe; *SF,* sylvian fissure; *T,* thalami; *TH,* temporal horn of lateral ventricle; *TL,* temporal lobe; *3V,* third ventricle.

allows assessment of the occipital horn for intraventricular hemorrhage. Placement of the transducer in the mastoid fontanelle, with superior to inferior angulation, aids in evaluating the cerebellum and cisterna magna (Fig. 32-5).

INTRACRANIAL HEMORRHAGE

Intracranial hemorrhage may be seen in premature and full-term infants and may be the sequela of an ischemic or hypoxic event, trauma, infarction, vascular malformation, or bleeding disorder. Germinal matrix–intraventricular hemorrhage is the most commonly diagnosed brain lesion in premature newborns.[2] Complications of posthemorrhagic ventricular dilation and parenchymal injury may result in devastating neurologic effects. Cranial sonography is a reliable method for the screening of low-birth-weight (<1500g) or premature (<30 weeks' gestational age) infants at increased risk for development of an intracranial hemorrhage. Approximately 80% of hemorrhages occur within the first 3 days of life, and screening for hemorrhage is usually performed at 1 week of age.[3]

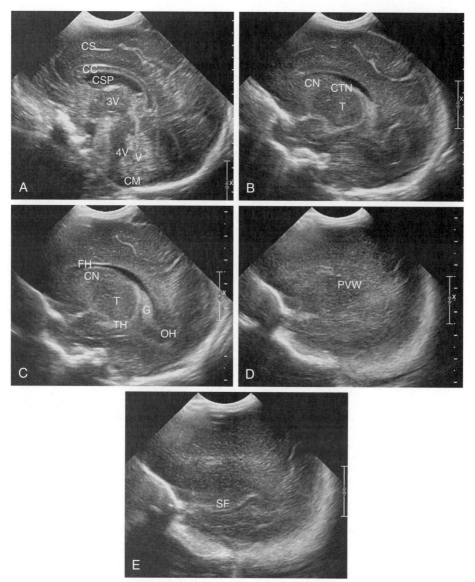

FIGURE 32-4 Sagittal views of neonatal head demonstrating standard imaging views. **(A),** Sag ML. **(B),** Sag Right 1. **(C),** Sag Right 2. **(D),** Sag Right 3. **(E),** Sag Right 4. *CC,* Corpus callosum; *CM,* cisterna magna; *CN,* caudate nucleus; *CS,* cingulate sulcus; *CSP,* cavum septi pellucidi; *CTN,* caudothalamic notch; *FH,* frontal horn of lateral ventricle; *G,* glomus of choroid plexus; *OH,* occipital horn of lateral ventricle; *PVW,* periventricular white matter; *SF,* sylvian fissure; *T,* thalami; *TH,* temporal horn of lateral ventricle; *V,* vermis; *3V,* third ventricle; *4V,* fourth ventricle.

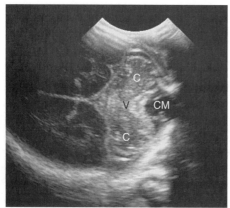

FIGURE 32-5 Mastoid view of neonatal head. *C,* Cerebellum; *CM,* cisterna magna; *V,* vermis.

The most common location for the origin of intracranial hemorrhage in a premature infant is in the germinal matrix, located between head of the caudate nucleus and the thalamus. This embryonic structure contains a fragile network of vessels that are prone to rupture with changes in blood pressure. The germinal matrix is greatest in size between 24 and 32 weeks' gestation and progressively decreases in size with only a small amount present at term, which explains why the risk for hemorrhage is greatest in preterm infants.

The severity of intracranial hemorrhage may be classified by the extent and location of the hemorrhage and the presence of ventricular enlargement. A grade I hemorrhage, also known as a germinal matrix or subependymal hemorrhage, is confined to the subependymal region at the caudothalamic notch. A grade II hemorrhage is

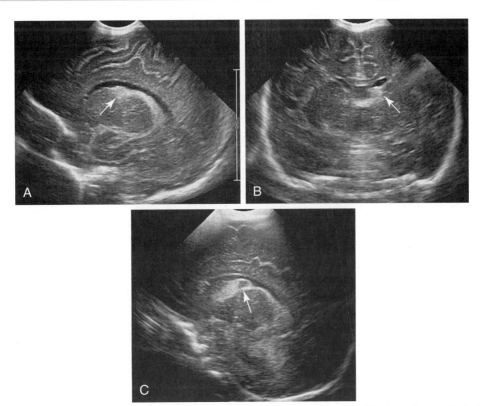

FIGURE 32-6 Sagittal plane **(A)** and coronal plane **(B)** demonstrating echogenic, grade I bleed at the caudothalamic notch *(arrows).* **(C),** Resolving grade I bleed.

defined by extension of the hemorrhage into the ventricle, without ventriculomegaly. A grade III hemorrhage is an intraventricular hemorrhage with ventriculomegaly. A grade IV hemorrhage is defined as parenchymal involvement with or without associated ventriculomegaly.

The prognosis of intracranial hemorrhage is variable depending on the extent of the bleed and includes an increase in morbidity and mortality. Grade I and grade II hemorrhages may spontaneously regress without evidence of long-term effects. Infants with grade III and IV hemorrhages are more likely to have neurologic effects, which range from developmental delays and behavioral problems to spastic motor deficits that may be accompanied by intellectual deficits.

Treatment for intracranial hemorrhage primarily focuses on controlling hydrocephalus to decrease neurologic deficits. Medical management may be used to decrease production of cerebrospinal fluid (CSF). Lumbar and percutaneous ventricular puncture can be used to drain excess CSF. Long-term treatment usually involves the placement of a ventricular shunt for drainage of CSF into the peritoneal cavity. Although this treatment is considered effective, it is not without complications, such as increased infections and shunt blockage.

Sonographic Findings

Sonographic imaging for hemorrhage should identify the absence or presence of hemorrhage, ventricular enlargement, and parenchymal extension. Acute grade I

hemorrhage is identified as a homogeneous, echogenic mass at the caudothalamic groove (Fig. 32-6, *A* and *B*). Subependymal hemorrhages are similar in echogenicity to the choroid plexus. Aging of a grade I hemorrhage may result in the formation of a subependymal cyst (Fig. 32-6, *C*). Grade II intraventricular hemorrhage can be diagnosed by evidence of echogenic material that partially or completely fills the ventricular cavity (Fig. 32-7). Development of ventriculomegaly related to the hemorrhage is classified as a grade III hemorrhage (Fig. 32-8). Grade IV or parenchymal hemorrhage is initially identified as an echogenic, homogeneous mass extending from the ventricle into the adjacent white matter (Fig. 32-9). Over time, the echogenicity of blood decreases, resulting in a cystic cavity extending from the ventricle to the parenchyma. This is known as a porencephalic cyst.

PERIVENTRICULAR LEUKOMALACIA

Periventricular leukomalacia (PVL) is defined as infarction and necrosis of the periventricular white matter. In a premature infant, the periventricular white matter, or watershed area, is poorly supplied because it lies between the distribution of arterial border zones. The lack of vascular maturation in this area makes it especially susceptible to changes in blood pressure. The white matter most affected is adjacent to the trigone of the lateral ventricle and near the foramen of Monro. In addition to prematurity, maternal chorioamnionitis has been identified as a risk factor contributing to the development of PVL. The

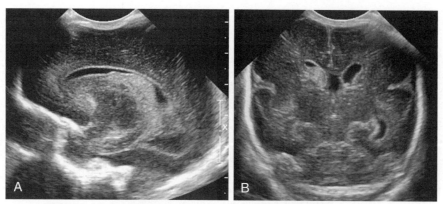

FIGURE 32-7 Sagittal **(A)** and coronal **(B)** views of grade II hemorrhage.

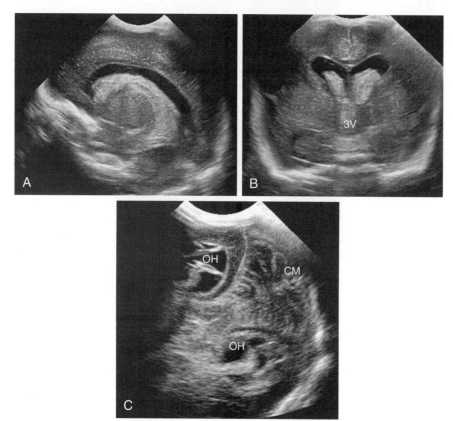

FIGURE 32-8 Grade III hemorrhage with significant ventricular enlargement identified in sagittal **(A)** and coronal **(B)** planes. Image in **(B)** shows hemorrhage extending through the foramen of Monro and into the third ventricle *(3V)*. **(C)**, Mastoid view demonstrates clot in the occipital horns *(OH)* of the lateral ventricles and in the cisterna magna *(CM)*.

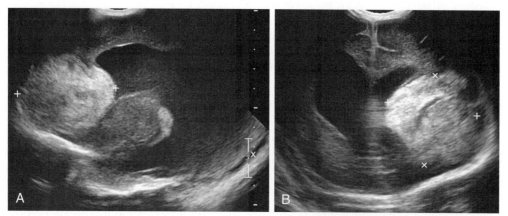

FIGURE 32-9 Sagittal **(A)** and coronal **(B)** images of a large grade IV hemorrhage extending into the left frontal lobe of the brain in an infant born at 30 weeks' gestational age.

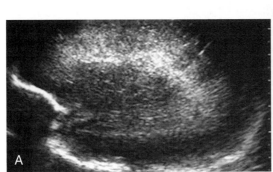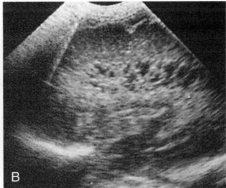

FIGURE 32-10 (A), Sagittal image of PVL in the acute phase. **(B),** Progression to cystic PVL with cavitation of brain parenchyma in a premature infant.

outcome for infants with PVL is variable, depending on the severity and extent of white matter necrosis. Cerebral palsy is a prevalent sequela in infants with PVL. Infants usually have major long-term neurologic deficits, including spastic diplegia, quadriplegia, seizure disorder, visual impairment, and mental retardation.

Sonographic Findings

Sonographic findings of PVL in the acute stage show bilateral areas of increased echogenicity in the white matter superior and lateral to the ventricular margins of the brain (Fig. 32-10, *A*). This finding may resolve or progress to cystic PVL. Cystic PVL typically develops 2 to 3 weeks after the insult and manifests as numerous, small cystic lesions paralleling the lateral ventricle of the brain (Fig. 32-10, *B*). These findings resolve within a few months, with resultant brain atrophy and subsequent ventriculomegaly.

HYPOXIC-ISCHEMIC ENCEPHALOPATHY

Hypoxic-ischemic encephalopathy is a brain injury that is due to birth asphyxia that results in significant mortality and long-term morbidity in neonates.[4] Injury to the brain initially occurs during the hypoxic-ischemic event secondary to decreased blood flow. Additional "reperfusion" injuries also result once the blood flow has been restored. Patterns of brain injury include injuries affecting the deep gray matter, injuries affecting the cortex and subcorticol area, and global brain injury. Diffuse cerebral edema is a common sequela of a hypoxic-ischemic event in a full-term infant. If the hypoxic-ischemic event is severe enough, diffuse brain volume loss occurs within 2 weeks, resulting in ventricular enlargement secondary to brain atrophy.

Sonographic Findings

Sonographic findings associated with hypoxic-ischemic encephalopathy depend on the area of insult. Diffuse cerebral edema is one of the earliest detected changes,

manifesting as a diffusely echogenic brain with slitlike ventricles. The sulci are difficult to differentiate, owing to the overall increased echogenicity of the brain (Fig. 32-11, *A* and *B*). Within a couple of weeks, ventricular enlargement occurs from atrophy of the brain parenchyma, and cystic changes may or may not be demonstrated. Injury to the deep gray matter is characterized by increased echogenicity in the basal ganglion or thalami (Fig. 32-11, *C*).

HYDROCEPHALUS

Hydrocephalus is defined as enlargement of the ventricles with enlargement of the infant's head secondary to increased intracranial pressure. Hydrocephalus may occur from obstruction of CSF, an overproduction of CSF, or abnormal absorption of CSF. Numerous congenital anomalies can contribute to the development of hydrocephalus, including, but not limited to, spina bifida, aqueductal stenosis, Dandy-Walker malformation (DWM), Arnold-Chiari malformation, congenital infections, and hemorrhage.

Sonographic Findings

Sonographic evaluation should include identification of the lateral, third, and fourth ventricles to show the level of obstruction and the identification of associated central nervous system anomalies, if present. Serial sonographic examinations may be used to follow progression or response to shunt placement (Fig. 32-12).

CONGENITAL MALFORMATIONS

Chiari II Malformation

Chiari II malformation, also known as Arnold-Chiari malformation, represents the downward displacement of the cerebellum and brainstem in association with a myelomeningocele, resulting in a small posterior fossa. The intracranial findings related to this anomaly include elongation and caudal displacement of the brainstem

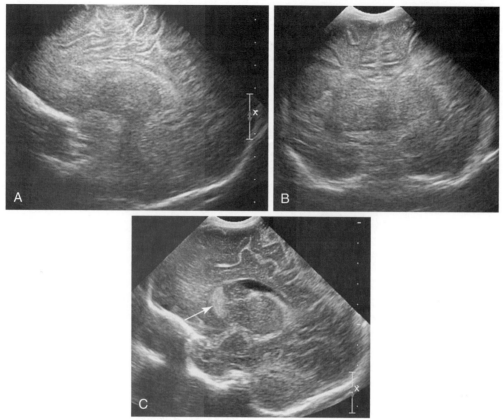

FIGURE 32-11 Hypoxic-ischemic encephalopathy. **(A)** and **(B)**, Findings of diffuse cerebral edema in a term infant with severe birth hypoxia: increased brain echogenicity, silhouetting of the sulci, and compression of the ventricles. **(C)**, Hypoxic injury to the basal ganglion in another term infant.

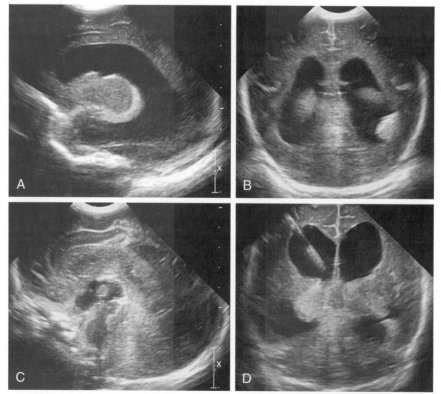

FIGURE 32-12 (A-C), Sagittal and coronal images demonstrate posthemorrhagic hydrocephalus with enlargement of the lateral and third ventricles in a preterm infant. **(D)**, Coronal image shows a shunt in the body of the right lateral ventricle.

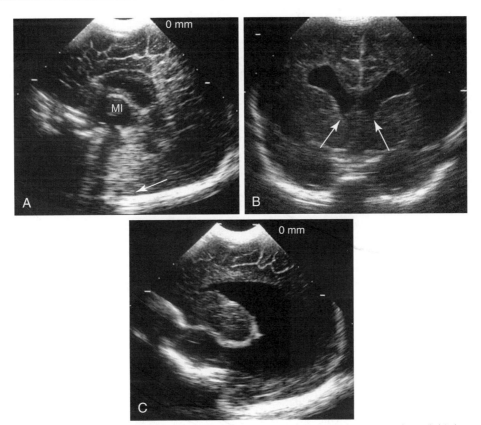

FIGURE 32-13 Findings associated with Chiari II malformation. **(A)**, Midline sagittal image shows an enlarged third ventricle and massa intermedia *(MI)*. The cerebellar tonsils are obliterating the cisterna magna *(arrow)*. **(B)**, The frontal horns of the lateral ventricles are pointed, giving them a "bat wing" appearance in the coronal plane *(arrows)*. **(C)**, Colpocephaly is present in the sagittal plane.

and cerebellum through the foramen magnum and into the cervical canal, with obliteration of the cisterna magna. Hydrocephalus is commonly associated with this anomaly.

Sonographic Findings. Midline sagittal views of the neonatal head may show partial or complete absence of the CSP; large massa intermedia; caudal displacement of the brainstem, fourth ventricle, and vermis; and absent cisterna magna (Fig. 32-13, *A*). Lateral ventricles demonstrate a "bat wing" configuration, with anterior and inferior pointing of the frontal horns (Fig. 32-13, *B*). Colpocephaly may also be present (Fig. 32-13, *C*).

Agenesis of the Corpus Callosum

The corpus callosum is a tract of fibers that connects the cerebral hemispheres and allows the transfer of sensory, motor, and cognitive information between them. Development occurs between 8 and 20 weeks' gestational age, with formation occurring anterior to posterior. An insult during this time period may result in complete or partial agenesis of the corpus callosum (ACC). ACC is present in 2% to 3% of neuropediatric patients.[5] ACC may be found in isolation but is often associated with other anomalies of the central nervous system, including Chiari II malformation, holoprosencephaly, encephalocele, and DWM. It is also associated with more than 80

chromosomal, genetic, and sporadic syndromes.[6] The outcome is variable, ranging from normal to severely impaired, depending on the severity of other anomalies.

Sonographic Findings. Midline sagittal images demonstrate absence of the corpus callosum and CSP, resulting in radial arrangement of the medial sulci above the third ventricle (Fig. 32-14, *A*). The lateral ventricles have a teardrop appearance, with slitlike frontal horns and colpocephaly (Fig. 32-14, *B*). Coronally, ACC results in widely spaced, parallel lateral ventricles (Fig. 32-14, *C*). Superior displacement of the third ventricle with dilation may also be present.

Dandy-Walker Malformation

DWM is characterized by the absence of the cerebellar vermis and dilation of the fourth ventricle, with connection to a posterior fossa cyst. A less severe form, referred to as Dandy-Walker variant, may occur with dysplasia of the cerebellar vermis without enlargement of the posterior fossa. DWM is associated with other central nervous system anomalies in 70% of cases. Chromosomal anomalies occur in 50% of cases.

The prognosis for infants born with DWM is variable, depending on associated abnormalities and the absence or presence of an abnormal karyotype. Overall, the prognosis is considered to be poor, with high morbidity

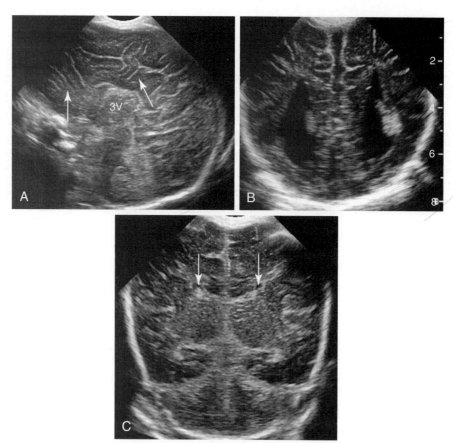

FIGURE 32-14 (A), ACC and CSP are noted in a midline sagittal image of a preterm infant. The cingulate gyri have a radial arrangement above the third ventricle *(3V)*. **(B)** and **(C)**, Coronal images demonstrate teardrop-shaped lateral ventricles that are displaced laterally.

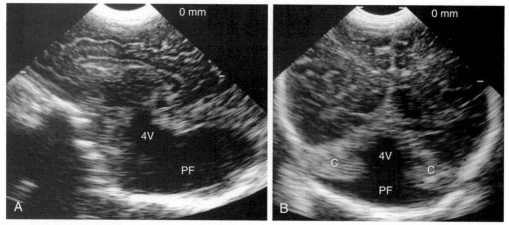

FIGURE 32-15 DWM in a term infant whose mother received no prenatal care. **(A)** and **(B)**, Enlarged fourth ventricle communicating with posterior fossa cyst. Splaying of the cerebellar hemispheres is also visualized in the coronal image.

and mortality rates. Patients may have severe mental and physical disabilities, although infants with Dandy-Walker variant may function normally.

Sonographic Findings. The diagnosis of DWM is made by identification of an enlarged fourth ventricle communicating with a posterior fossa cyst. The cerebellar vermis is hypoplastic or absent, resulting in splaying of the cerebellar hemispheres (Fig. 32-15). Hydrocephalus and ACC frequently accompany this malformation. Sonographic imaging through the mastoid fontanelle is useful in further assessment of the fourth ventricle and cerebellar vermis.

Holoprosencephaly

Holoprosencephaly is a midline malformation that results from failure of the forebrain to separate or cleave into two cerebral hemispheres. It is the most common congenital malformation of the forebrain and midface. The etiology includes genetic and environmental factors.

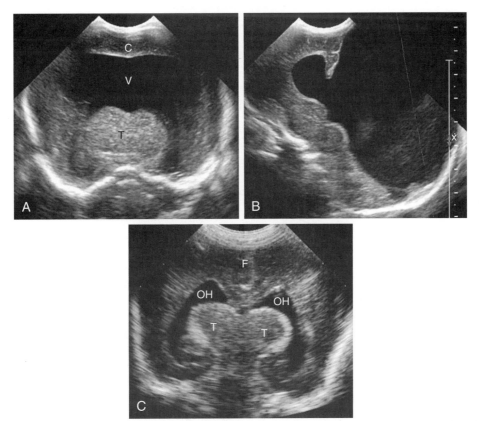

FIGURE 32-16 Holoprosencephaly. **(A)** and **(B)**, Findings associated with alobar holoprosencephaly: horseshoe-shaped ventricle and absent falx, corpus callosum, and CSP. The infant had severe facial anomalies and died shortly after birth. **(C)**, Posterior coronal view in an infant diagnosed with lobar holoprosencephaly. Note the presence of a falx and separation of the occipital horns and thalami.

Approximately 70% of patients with trisomy 13 have holoprosencephaly. Environmental factors linked to the malformation include maternal diabetes, in utero radiation exposure, TORCH (*t*oxoplasmosis, *o*ther [syphilis, varicella-zoster, parvovirus B19], *r*ubella, *c*ytomegalovirus, *h*erpes simplex virus) infection, and retinoic acid.[7] There are three forms of holoprosencephaly, which are categorized according to severity. The most severe form, alobar holoprosencephaly, has complete failure of forebrain separation with a single, midline ventricle, surrounded by a thin rim of cerebral cortex. The falx, corpus callosum, and third ventricle are absent. The thalami are fused. This form is associated with severe facial anomalies, including cyclopia, ethmocephaly, cebocephaly, and facial clefts. Semilobar holoprosencephaly has partial cleavage of the forebrain. The monoventricle is still present but posteriorly; midline structures develop including the falx and portions of the corpus callosum. Separation of the thalami and occipital and temporal horns may be noted. The mildest form, lobar holoprosencephaly, has almost complete separation of the cerebral hemispheres. Box-shaped frontal horns are seen in conjunction with fused frontal lobes. The falx is present, but the genu and rostrum of the corpus callosum, along with the CSP, are absent. Facial anomalies are mild with these forms. The outcome is variable depending on the severity, but infants with alobar holoprosencephaly usually die during the first year of life.[7]

Sonographic Findings. Sonographically, alobar holoprosencephaly appears as a single, horseshoe-shaped ventricle surrounded by brain parenchyma. The falx, corpus callosum, and CSP are absent, and the thalami are fused (Fig. 32-16, *A* and *B*). In semilobar holoprosencephaly and lobar holoprosencephaly, variable degrees of fusion may be identified with absence of the corpus callosum and CSP (Fig. 32-16, *C*).

Hydranencephaly

Hydranencephaly is characterized by in utero destruction of the cerebral hemispheres, most likely related to internal carotid artery occlusion. The cerebral hemispheres are replaced with CSF. Portions of the brain that are not supplied by the internal carotid circulation are present, including the falx, thalami, cerebellum, and brainstem. Hydranencephaly is usually an isolated anomaly, and these infants appear normal at birth. The outcome is poor, with death occurring shortly after birth, although survival for several months has been reported.[8]

Sonographic Findings. The sonographic findings of hydranencephaly include a fluid-filled calvaria with identification of the thalamus, cerebellum, and brainstem. The

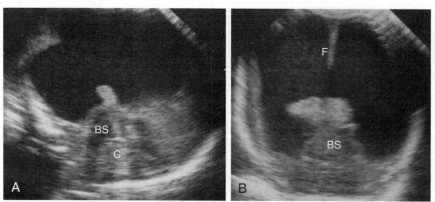

FIGURE 32-17 Hydranencephaly. **(A)** and **(B)**, Cerebral hemispheres are replaced with CSF. Brainstem and structures of posterior fossa appear normal. Identification of the falx aids in the diagnosis.

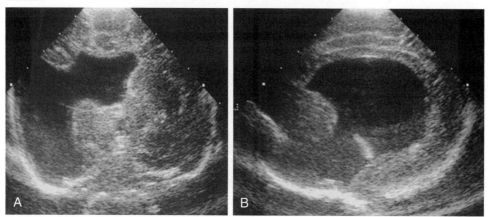

FIGURE 32-18 Schizencephaly. **(A)** and **(B)**, Right-sided cleft in the brain extending from the midline to the calvaria.

falx is usually identified, and documentation is important for differentiation from alobar holoprosencephaly. The absence of the cortical mantle helps differentiate hydranencephaly from severe hydrocephalus, which has a thin rim of cerebral cortex (Fig. 32-17). Color Doppler shows absence of flow in the carotid arteries.

Schizencephaly

Schizencephaly is a rare disorder resulting from a destructive process in utero that leads to clefts in the cerebral cortex extending from the midline to the calvaria. The clefts may be open or closed and unilateral or bilateral. The clefts are lined with abnormal gray matter, although that is not distinguished sonographically. Absence of the corpus callosum and CSP are frequently seen. The outcome for infants born with schizencephaly is variable. Closed-lip clefts carry a better prognosis, as do unilateral clefts. Patients may have seizures, blindness, and motor and mental deficits.

Sonographic Findings. Sonographic evaluation of open schizencephaly reveals a fluid-filled cleft extending from the midline to the calvaria (Fig. 32-18). Ventricular enlargement and absence of the corpus callosum and CSP may be present.

Lissencephaly

Lissencephaly is a disorder of neuronal migration. In the normal brain, the cerebral cortex is composed of six layers. With lissencephaly, there is an abnormal migration of neurons from the germinal matrix to the cortical surface, with formation of only four cortical layers. The result is a lack of sulci and gyri, giving the brain a smooth appearance. Syndromes associated with lissencephaly include Miller-Dieker, Norman-Roberts, and Walker-Warburg syndromes. The prognosis is poor for infants with this anomaly.

Sonographic Findings. Sonographic findings of lissencephaly include a smooth cerebral cortex, with no sulci or gyri. Dilation of the third ventricle and colpocephaly may also be noted (Fig. 32-19). The diagnosis cannot be made in premature infants until after 26 to 28 weeks' gestational age, owing to the normal lack of sulcation at this age.

SUMMARY

Sonography is an effective diagnostic imaging method for evaluation of the neonatal head. An understanding of the normal anatomy and the most common pathologies (Table 32-1) assists the health care team in making an accurate diagnosis so that appropriate treatment can be provided.

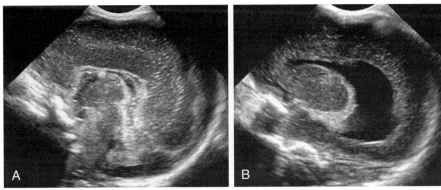

FIGURE 32-19 Lissencephaly. **(A)** and **(B)**, Sagittal images demonstrate sonographic findings associated with lissencephaly in a term infant. Smooth brain with lack of sulci and gyri, ACC, and colpocephaly.

TABLE 32-1	Pathology of Neonatal Head
Diagnosis	**Sonographic Findings**
Hemorrhage	Grade I: Echogenic subependymal bleed
	Grade II: Blood within ventricle
	Grade III: Blood within ventricle with ventricular enlargement
	Grade IV: Intraventricular blood extending to parenchyma
PVL	Increased echogenicity in periventricular parenchyma that becomes cystic over time
Hypoxic-ischemic encephalopathy	Increased echogenicity of cerebral hemispheres, slitlike ventricles; ventricular enlargement as brain atrophies
Hydrocephaly	Enlarged ventricles with enlarged head
Chiari II malformation	Absence of cisterna magna, inferiorly displaced cerebellum, enlarged ventricles, "bat wing" sign
ACC	Absent corpus callosum and CSP, mild ventriculomegaly with dilated occipital horns; lateral displacement of lateral ventricles and superior displacement of third ventricle; dilated third ventricle; cingulate gyri radiate in sunburst pattern
DWM	Posterior fossa cyst communicating with fourth ventricle, enlarged cisterna magna, splaying of cerebellar hemispheres with absent or dysplastic vermis; commonly associated with hydrocephalus
Holoprosencephaly	Single ventricle, fused thalami, absent CSP and corpus callosum, absent falx; variable fusion with less severe forms
Hydranencephaly	Fluid-filled cranium; falx and brainstem may be identified
Schizencephaly	Cleft in brain parenchyma from midline to calvaria
Lissencephaly	Smooth brain

CLINICAL SCENARIO—DIAGNOSIS

The initial sonogram is normal. At 1 week, the echogenic region identified in the anterior coronal view of the head suggests an intraventricular hemorrhage that extends into the parenchyma, which would classify this hemorrhage as a grade IV bleed. The follow-up sonogram demonstrates necrosis of the intraparenchy-mal hemorrhage, with formation of a porencephalic cyst in the left cerebral hemisphere. This finding is consistent with a poor prognosis, which may include death. If this infant survives, she will probably have long-term neurologic deficits and may need shunt placement.

CASE STUDIES FOR DISCUSSION

1. A head sonogram is ordered on a 4-day-old boy for the indication of premature delivery at 25 weeks' gestation. The infant experienced episodes of apnea after delivery and was intubated but is otherwise stable. What sonographic finding is present in Figure 32-20, and what anomaly is associated with it?

2. A boy is born prematurely at 32 weeks' gestational age. Prenatal screening showed an abnormal quad screen, but no amniocentesis was performed. A cranial sonogram is ordered. What is the most likely diagnosis based on Figure 32-21?

3. A sonogram is performed on a premature infant born at 26 weeks' gestational age. Delivery was complicated by severe birth asphyxia. Previous sonograms have documented a grade I hemorrhage. What is the new diagnosis in Figure 32-22?

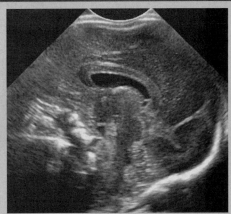

FIGURE 32-20 Sagittal image of the neonatal brain.

CASE STUDIES FOR DISCUSSION—cont'd

4. A sonogram is performed in the neonatal intensive care unit on a premature infant born at 32 weeks' gestational age. The results are shown in Figure 32-23. What is the most likely diagnosis?

5. Figure 32-24 shows a normal head sonogram. Based on these images, is this a premature or term infant? Discuss why or why not.

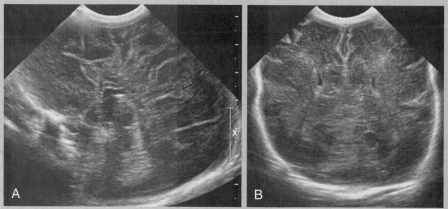

FIGURE 32-21 **(A)** Sagittal image of the neonatal brain and **(B)**, Coronal image of the neonatal brain.

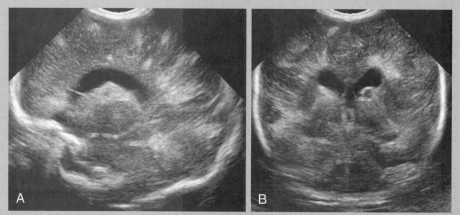

FIGURE 32-22 **(A)** Sagittal image of the neonatal brain and **(B)**, Coronal image of the neonatal brain.

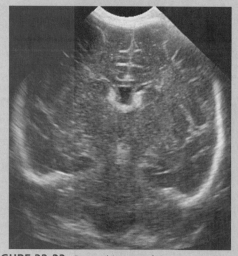

FIGURE 32-23 Coronal image of the neonatal brain.

CASE STUDIES FOR DISCUSSION—cont'd

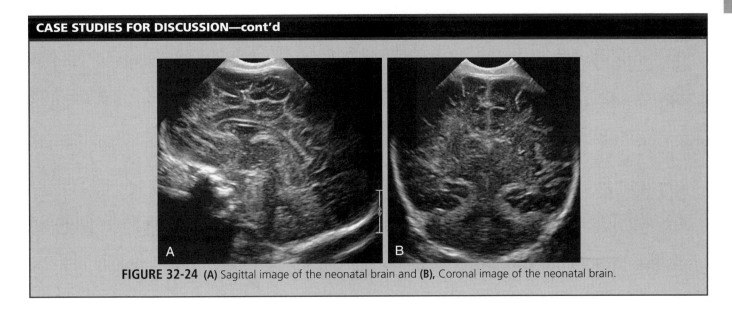

FIGURE 32-24 **(A)** Sagittal image of the neonatal brain and **(B)**, Coronal image of the neonatal brain.

STUDY QUESTIONS

1. The sonographic "bat-wing" sign is associated with which cranial anomaly?
   a. ACC
   b. DWM
   c. Chiari II malformation
   d. Holoprosencephaly
   e. Lissencephaly

2. Which anatomic structure would aid in the differentiation of alobar holoprosencephaly from hydranencephaly?
   a. Falx
   b. Cerebral cortex
   c. Corpus callosum
   d. Vermis
   e. Cisterna magna

3. A coronal image of the neonatal head demonstrates the lateral ventricles at the level of the third ventricle and foramen of Monro. The transducer should be angled in which direction to visualize the glomus of the choroid plexus?
   a. Medial
   b. Lateral
   c. Anterior
   d. Posterior
   e. Superior

4. A premature infant born at 28 weeks' gestational age is scanned to rule out intracranial hemorrhage. The sonogram demonstrates echogenic material within normal-sized ventricles. This finding would be consistent with which pathology?
   a. Grade I hemorrhage
   b. Grade II hemorrhage
   c. Grade III hemorrhage
   d. Grade IV hemorrhage
   e. PVL

5. A cranial sonogram is performed because of an abnormal prenatal scan. Routine coronal and sagittal views are performed through the anterior fontanelle. Additional scanning through the mastoid fontanelle reveals hypoplasia of the cerebellar vermis and communication between the fourth ventricle and posterior fossa. These findings would be consistent with which anomaly?
   a. Holoprosencephaly
   b. ACC
   c. Chiari II malformation
   d. Dandy-Walker variant
   e. Lissencephaly

6. Failure of the sulci and gyri to develop in a term infant is associated with which cranial anomaly?
   a. PVL
   b. Porencephaly
   e. Schizencephaly
   d. Lissencephaly
   e. Holoprosencephaly

7. A premature infant born at 26 weeks' gestational age undergoes scanning at 4 weeks of age for routine follow-up to prematurity. The sonogram reveals symmetric regions of increased echogenicity in the watershed area. This would be consistent with which?
   a. Hypoxic-ischemic encephalopathy
   b. Holoprosencephaly
   c. PVL
   d. Porencephaly
   e. Schizencephaly

8. Radial arrangement of the sulci superior to the third ventricle is a sonographic finding associated with which anomaly?
   a. ACC
   b. Holoprosencephaly
   c. Hydrocephaly
   d. Porencephaly
   e. Schizencephaly

9. Which of the following defines a grade III hemorrhage?
   a. Subependymal hemorrhage without extension into the ventricle with ventriculomegaly
   b. Subependymal hemorrhage without extension into the ventricle without ventriculomegaly
   c. Subependymal hemorrhage with extension into the ventricle with ventriculomegaly
   d. Subependymal hemorrhage with extension into the ventricle without ventriculomegaly
   e. Subependymal hemorrhage with extension into the ventricle and adjacent brain parenchyma

10. A boy born at 32 weeks' gestational age is diagnosed with hydranencephaly. Which cranial structure would be absent?
   a. Cerebrum
   b. Cerebellum
   c. Thalami
   d. Brainstem
   e. Falx

REFERENCES

1. Rumack CM, Wilson S, Charboneau J, et al: *Diagnostic ultrasound*, ed 4, Philadelphia, 2011, Mosby.
2. O'Leary H, Gregas MC, Limperopoulos C, et al: Elevated cerebral pressure passivity is associated with prematurity-related intracranial hemorrhage, *Pediatrics* 124:302–309, 2009.
3. Furlow B: Neonatal imaging, *Radiol Technol* 72:577–597, 2001.
4. Wintermark P: Current controversies in newer therapies to treat birth asphyxia, *Int J Pediatr* 2011:848413, 2011.
5. Mangione R, Fries N, Godard P, et al: Neurodevelopmental outcome following prenatal diagnosis of an isolated anomaly of the corpus callosum, *Ultrasound Obstet Gynecol* 37:290–295, 2011.
6. Winter C, Kennedy A, Byrne J, et al: The cavum septi pellucidi, why is it important? *J Ultrasound Med* 29:427–444, 2010.
7. Lin CH, Tsai JD, Ho YJ, et al: Alobar holoprosencephaly associated with cebocephaly and craniosynostosis, *Acta Neurol Taiwan* 18:123–126, 2009.
8. Tsai JD, Kuo HT, Chou IC: Hydranencephaly in neonates, *Pediatr Neonatol* 49:154–157, 2008.

33

Neonatal Spinal Dimple

Kathryn Kuntz, Emily Smith

CLINICAL SCENARIO

An 8 lb boy is delivered by cesarean section to a young mother. On initial examination, he was found to have an undescended left testicle, bluish colored nevi on the lower back, and a sacral dimple.

A sonogram of the spine was performed 3 days after delivery. The findings are shown in Figure 33-1. What diagnosis is revealed by these sonographic findings?

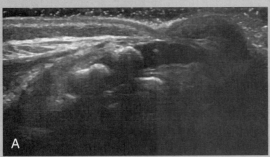 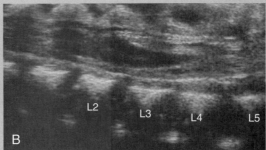

FIGURE 33-1 **(A)** and **(B)**, Longitudinal neonatal spine and level of sacral defect.

OBJECTIVES

- Recognize the normal sonographic anatomy of the neonatal spine.
- Discuss the clinical indications for sonography of the neonatal spine.

- Define the sonographic criteria for occult spinal dysraphism.
- Recognize specific sonographic features of tethered cord, lipoma, hydromyelia, meningocele and myelomeningocele, and diastematomyelia.

Sonography is the preferred imaging modality in cases of suspected abnormal growth or development of the spinal cord and adjacent structures known as occult spinal dysraphism.[1] It is a useful tool for evaluating the neonatal spine because of its portability, low cost, noninvasiveness, and lack of radiation. Common clinical indications for neonatal spinal sonography include atypical sacral dimple, palpable subcutaneous sacral mass, hair tuft, skin tag, hemangioma, sinus tract, and skin pigmentation; spinal sonography is also indicated in neonates with multiple congenital anomalies. Congenital spinal dysraphisms can be classified on the basis of the presence or absence of a soft tissue mass and skin covering. Congenital spinal dysraphisms without a mass include tethered cord, diastematomyelia, anterior sacral meningocele, and spinal lipoma. Dysraphisms with a skin-covered soft tissue mass include lipomyelomeningocele and

myelocystocele. Dysraphisms with a back mass but without skin covering include myelomeningocele and myelocele. The most common request for spinal sonography is to search for occult tethered cord. This chapter discusses the clinical and sonographic findings of tethered cord and other spinal dysraphisms.

NORMAL ANATOMY

On a sonogram, the spinal cord appears hypoechoic with an echogenic central canal. The cord is centrally positioned within the spinal canal. The echogenic nerve roots demonstrate oscillation with respiration or infant movement. The tip of the conus medullaris normally tapers and is positioned at the level of L2 (Fig. 33-2, *A*). The filum terminale is normally echogenic and measures 2 mm or less in thickness (Fig. 33-3). The spinal cord

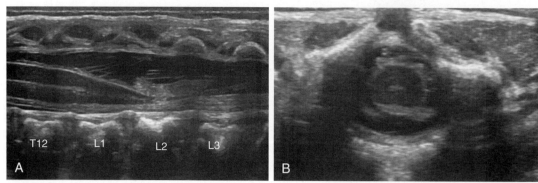

FIGURE 33-2 (A), Normal spinal cord. Sagittal view shows posterior and anterior aspects of thoracic spinal cord. Normal thoracic spinal cord is more anteriorly positioned within the vertebral canal. **(B),** Transverse view shows normal conus medullaris.

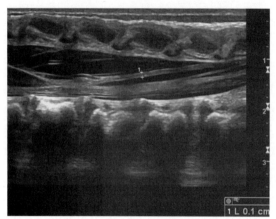

FIGURE 33-3 Normal filum terminale measures less than 2 mm.

should remain round in the axial plane through the thoracolumbar region (Fig. 33-2, *B*).

The main purpose of neonatal spine imaging for tethered cord is the identification of the level of the conus medullaris, which should be located above the interspace of the second and third lumbar vertebrae (see Fig. 33-2). A low conus medullaris, below the level of L2, should lead the clinician to suspect a tethered cord.

To identify the level of the conus medullaris, an understanding of the normal spinal anatomy is essential. The normal spinal cord in the longitudinal plane is visualized between the posterior vertebral processes as an elongated hypoechoic structure surrounded by anechoic cerebrospinal fluid (CSF) (see Fig. 33-2). The cord contains one or two echogenic linear structures, known as the central echo complex. The spinal cord tapers at the caudal end, resembling the end of a carrot. Surrounding and distal to the conus medullaris, the echogenic distal nerve branches, known as the cauda equina ("horse's tail"), are visualized (Fig. 33-4). A normal spine demonstrates pulsations of the cauda equina during real-time sonographic evaluation.

SONOGRAPHIC EVALUATION

The sonographic evaluation is usually performed with the infant in the prone position and the spine flexed; this may

be accomplished by extending the infant over a rolled sheet or pillow. A high-frequency, linear transducer is preferred because a larger transducer footprint is needed to visualize adequately multiple vertebrae along the longitudinal axis. When available, extended field of view, virtual convex, or split-screen imaging (Fig. 33-5, *A-C*) can also be used to maximize the display of the spine.

The neonatal spine should be scanned in both sagittal and axial planes. If a cutaneous dimple is present, a stand-off pad or a thick layer of gel should be used to determine whether the dimple is part of a sinus tract extending from the skin to the spinal cord (Fig. 33-5, *D*).

When scanning the spine, it is recommended to initiate the scan in the sagittal plane, at the level of the sacrococcygeal region. The sacral vertebral bodies, which have begun to ossify, are easily seen. The coccyx appears hypoechoic because it is still cartilage (Fig. 33-6).

The sonographer can identify the relevant anatomy by counting the sacral vertebral bodies. The vertebral level is determined by counting down from the 12th rib and confirmed by counting up from S1, the L5-S1 junction, or the tip of coccyx. The first sacral body can be identified because of its posterior angulation (Fig. 33-7). If the vertebral level is unclear, correlation with radiographs (possibly with a marker) may help.

The tapering tip of the conus medullaris (see Fig. 33-2, *A*) should be identified at the level of L2; a normal conus medullaris tip terminates at the L2 level. After scanning in a sagittal plane, the spinal cord should be imaged in the axial plane and scanned from the level of the coccyx to the level of L1. The transverse cord in the lumbar region appears rounded, and the central echo complex appears as echogenic dots (see Fig. 33-2, *B*). The movement of the filum and cauda equina can be documented with a cine loop or with M mode.

TETHERED CORD

The imaging diagnosis of tethered spinal cord is distinct from the clinical diagnosis of tethered cord syndrome. The clinical signs of tethered cord syndrome include pain (especially with flexion), bowel and bladder dysfunction, weakness, sensory changes, gait abnormalities, and

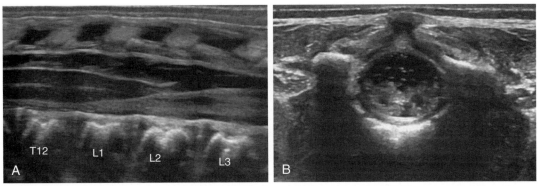

FIGURE 33-4 **(A)**, Longitudinal lower end of spinal cord and cauda equina. **(B)**, Transverse cauda equina.

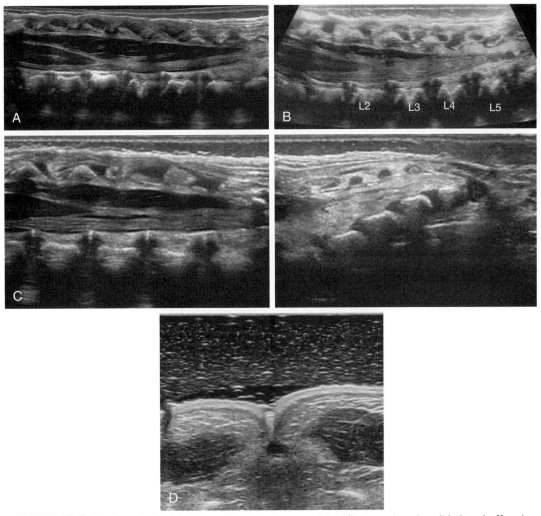

FIGURE 33-5 **(A)**, Extended field of view. **(B)**, Virtual convex. **(C)**, Split screen imaging. **(D)**, Stand-off pad.

musculoskeletal deformities of the feet and spine such as clubfoot and scoliosis. Cutaneous stigmata signifying an underlying congenital defect of the spinal cord also are common.[2]

Over time, the term "tethered cord" has been used interchangeably to include both imaging and clinical findings. Tethered cord is now defined as an abnormal attachment of the spinal cord to the tissues that surround it.[2] A tethered cord may be suspected when cutaneous markers are identified on visual inspection of the infant, including sacral dimple. High-risk, atypical dimples are greater than 5 mm in diameter and greater than 2.5 cm above the anus.[1,4]

Sonographic features of a tethered spinal cord include the low-lying position of the conus medullaris, below the level of L2, and the spinal cord adhered to the posterior wall or dorsal aspect of the spinal canal (Fig. 33-8). Adherence results in reduced or absent nerve root

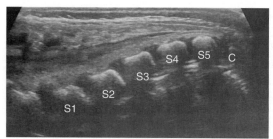

FIGURE 33-6 Calcified sacral vertebral bodies; nonossified coccyx.

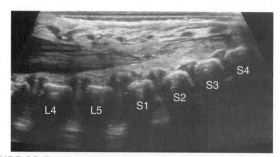

FIGURE 33-7 Comparison of angulation between L5 and S1 vertebral bodies.

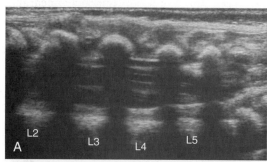

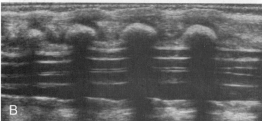

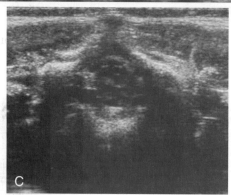

FIGURE 33-8 (A), Longitudinal view of conus medullaris extending to L5. **(B),** Posterior placement of spinal cord. **(C),** Axial view of tethered cord.

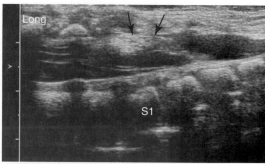

FIGURE 33-9 Longitudinal echogenic lipoma posterior to level of S1 *(arrows).*

oscillation with patient respiration or movement in real-time scanning that is identified in a normal spinal cord. In older patients, clinical correlation is required because the conus medullaris may be normally positioned but still be tethered (tight filum syndrome). In this situation, assessment of normal nerve root motion at real-time imaging is more important than the level of the conus medullaris.[4]

Left untreated, as the infant grows, the increased tension placed on the cord leads to increasing neurologic dysfunction, although the infant may be asymptomatic until he or she begins to ambulate. Symptoms associated with tethering of the cord include bladder and bowel incontinence, leg weakness and atrophy, abnormal gait, abnormal posturing of the lower extremities, and sensory loss. Early treatment can prevent the development of neurologic dysfunction. Nonneurologic anomalies are common as well, including tracheoesophageal fistula, congenital heart disease, and renal anomalies (VATER syndrome [*v*ertebral defects, imperforate *a*nus, *t*racheoesophageal fistula, *r*enal defects]).[3]

OTHER ABNORMALITIES

Lipoma

Spinal lipomas are caused by embryologic errors of development. A spinal lipoma is an encapsulated deposit of fat, neural tissue, meninges, or fibrous tissue. It extends from the posterior subcutaneous tissue through a midline defect of the fascia, muscle, or bone to communicate with the spinal canal or meninges. Lipomas may grow significantly during the first year of life and may change in size as the child's weight increases. They may be intradural, extradural, or a combination of both. Associations include tethered cord, dysraphism, fatty filum or lipoma of filum, and vertebral anomalies. Sonographically, a spinal lipoma appears as an echogenic mass extending from the spinal canal into the subcutaneous tissues (Fig. 33-9).[1,4] If the sonogram reveals a lipoma, magnetic resonance imaging is typically performed to determine attachment to the cord for surgical planning.

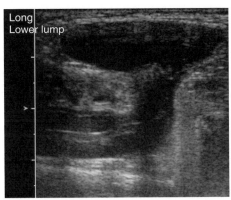

FIGURE 33-10 Longitudinal meningocele with communication to spinal canal.

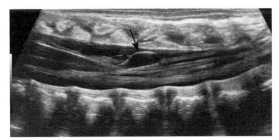

FIGURE 33-11 Filar cyst (arrow).

Hydromyelia

Hydromyelia is the abnormal widening of the central canal by CSF. This condition may be either focal or diffuse, extending through the entire length of the spinal cord. Sonographically, the echogenic lines of the central canal of the spinal cord appear separated, with the central canal appearing widened. It can be associated with several congenital abnormalities, including diastematomyelia, Arnold-Chiari malformation, myelomeningocele, and lipomeningocele.

Myelomeningocele

Meningocele is a condition in which only the meninges herniate through the vertebral column. A myelomeningocele is the herniation of meninges *and* neural tissue through a defect in the vertebral column. Sonography can be useful to differentiate a closed meningocele from a closed myelomeningocele. Sonographically, a meningocele appears as an anechoic sac containing CSF, protruding posteriorly from the spinal canal. It may also contain a few echogenic strands representing the membrane layers of the meninges (Fig. 33-10). A myelomeningocele appears as a sac containing echogenic material representing neural tissue and membranes.

Diastematomyelia

Diastematomyelia is an incomplete or complete longitudinal split or cleft through the spinal cord. The spinal cord divides into two hemicords. Sonographically, there appears to be two separate, smaller spinal cords within the spinal canal. These hemicords are hypoechoic with an echogenic central canal similar to a normal spinal cord but smaller. Diastematomyelia is commonly associated with a vertebral column abnormality and a tethered spinal cord.[3]

Filar Cyst

Filar cyst is an incidental finding that has been studied more recently. The nomenclature for this lesion is confusing in that it has been termed both "ventriculus terminalis" and "filar cyst" by various authors.[4] It is a normal variant that has no known clinical significance when it occurs alone (Fig. 33-11).

Caudal Regression Syndrome

Caudal regression syndrome affects 1 in 7500 children.[4] It occurs most often in children of diabetic mothers and is associated with various other genitourinary, anal, vertebral, and limb anomalies. The imaging appearance varies with the degree of deformity, ranging from minimal to severe regression of the coccyx, sacrum, and lumbar spine. Progressive absence of bone structures occurs in a caudal-to-cranial direction.

SUMMARY

A sonogram of the neonatal spine may be ordered when the clinical examination reveals a complicated sacral dimple, hemangioma, tuft of hair, or other cutaneous lesion on the infant's back because these may be associated with tethering of the spinal cord and other spinal dysraphisms. Sonography is employed in imaging a range of spinal dysraphic disorders, with the most severe anomalies imaged in the perinatal period and less severe anomalies usually evaluated in the neonatal period. The most common request for neonatal spinal sonography is to search for occult tethered cord.

Table 33-1 reviews spinal pathology, symptoms, and clinical and sonographic findings.

CLINICAL SCENARIO—DIAGNOSIS

The area of the conus medullaris in the longitudinal image is extending to the fourth lumbar vertebra. Although impossible to demonstrate without a real-time example or M mode, decreased pulsations were observed in the cauda equina; these met the criteria for diagnosis of tethered cord. At approximately 3 months of age, the infant was taken to surgery, and the cord was untethered. He has no neurologic deficits.

TABLE 33-1	Spinal Pathology, Symptoms, Clinical Findings, and Sonographic Findings	
Spinal Pathology	**Symptoms and Clinical Findings**	**Sonographic Findings**
Tethered cord	Atypical sacral dimple, palpable subcutaneous sacral mass, hair tuft, skin tag, hemangioma, sinus tract, skin pigmentation	Low-lying position of conus medullaris below level of L2; spinal cord adhered to posterior wall or dorsal aspect of spinal canal; absence of pulsation of cauda equina with real-time observation
Lipoma	May be associated with tethered cord, dysraphism, fatty filum or lipoma of filum, vertebral anomalies	Echogenic mass extending from spinal canal into subcutaneous tissues
Diastematomyelia	Commonly associated with vertebral column abnormality and tethered spinal cord	Appearance of two separate smaller spinal cords within spinal canal; hemicords are hypoechoic with echogenic central canal similar to normal spinal cord but smaller
Hydromyelia	Can be associated with several congenital abnormalities including diastematomyelia, Arnold-Chiari malformation, myelomeningocele, lipomeningocele	Echogenic lines of central canal of spinal cord appear separated; central canal appears widened
Myelomeningocele	Cutaneous stigmata, sacral dimple; possible loss of bladder or bowel control; possible partial or complete paralysis of legs; weakness of hips, leg s, or feet; possible clubfoot; possible hydrocephalus	Sac containing echogenic material representing neural tissue and membranes
Filar cyst	Incidental finding	Well-defined, midline, cystic collection
Caudal regression	Occurs most often in children of diabetic mothers and is associated with various other genitourinary, anal, vertebral, and limb anomalies; neurologic impairment; bowel or bladder incontinence may occur in severe cases	Appearance varies with degree of deformity

CASE STUDIES FOR DISCUSSION

1. A 5-day-old boy undergoes a sonogram of the spine. The indication was sacral dimple. The sonogram reveals the findings shown in Figure 33-8. What other physical findings might this infant have displayed?

2. A newborn was noted to have a hemangioma in the area of the sacrum. At 5 days of age, he underwent a sonogram to rule out spinal dysraphism. The sonogram revealed abnormal widening of the central canal by CSF. What is the most likely diagnosis?

3. A 1-year-old girl who was adopted from Haiti was seen by the primary care physician for an abnormal gait and abnormal posturing of the lower extremities. On physical examination, the child was also found to have a skin tuft and nevi in the region of the sacrum. Based on the clinical symptoms and lack of medical attention from

birth to age 1, what spinal dysraphism might the sonographer expect to find? Discuss the clinical implication of delayed medical attention.

4. A 4-day-old infant is referred for sonography of the spine for clinical suspicion of spinal dysraphism. The sonogram shows two separate smaller spinal cords within the spinal canal. What sonographic appearance does this describe?

5. A 1-day-old infant is referred for spinal sonography after physical examination reveals a palpable subcutaneous sacral mass. The sonogram reveals a highly echogenic mass arising from the spinal canal (see Figure 33-9). The conus medullaris is identified at the level of L2. What is the most likely cause of this echogenic mass?

STUDY QUESTIONS

1. All of the following are indications for neonatal spine sonography except:
   a. Lipoma
   b. Osteosarcoma
   c. Sacral dimple
   d. Sacral skin defect

2. Which of the following is an acceptable termination point of the conus medullaris in a normal patient?
   a. L1
   b. L3
   c. L4
   d. S1

3. In a normal patient, the cauda equina nerve branches are the nerve fibers arising from the distal end of the spinal cord and sonographically appear:
   a. Echogenic and oscillate with respiration
   b. Hypoechoic and adherent to the conus medullaris
   c. Complex and adherent to the walls of the canal
   d. Heterogeneous and may move with suspended respiration

4. When scanning to determine the presence of tethered cord, the vertebral level is determined by counting down from the _____ and confirmed by counting up from the _____.
   a. L1; the tip of the coccyx
   b. Xyphoid; umbilicus
   c. Umbilicus; symphysis pubis
   d. Twelfth rib; L5-S1 junction

5. A pathologic fixation of the spinal cord in an abnormal caudal location is the definition of:
   a. Filum terminale
   b. Caudal regression
   c. Tethered cord
   d. Hydromyelia

6. An incomplete or complete longitudinal split or cleft through the spinal cord is the definition of:
   a. Meningocele
   b. Tethered cord
   c. Filum terminale
   d. Diastematomyelia

7. As an infant grows, a tethered cord causes increasing tension leading to:
   a. Ambulation problems
   b. Dysplasia
   c. Shortened limb
   d. Failure to thrive

8. The key to the diagnosis of tethered cord is the sonographic visualization of the level of the:
   a. Central echo complex
   b. Conus medullaris
   c. Sacrum
   d. Cauda equina

9. Suspected abnormal growth or development of the spinal cord and adjacent structures is known as:
   a. Neonatal dysraphism
   b. Occult spinal dysraphism
   c. Dysraphic spinal syndrome
   d. Tethered cord syndrome

10. A normal variant that has no known clinical significance when it occurs alone is a:
    a. Filar cyst
    b. Hydromelia
    c. Lipoma
    d. Diastematomyelia

REFERENCES

1. Fitzgerald K: Ultrasound examination of the neonatal spine, *Austral J Ultrasound Med* 14:9–41, 2011.
2. Agarwalla PK, Dunn FI, Scott RM, et al: Tethered cord syndrome, *Neurosurg Clin N Am* 18:531–547, 2007.
3. Hung P, Wang H, Lui T, Wong AM: Sonographic findings in a neonate with diastematomyelia and a tethered spinal cord, *J Ultrasound Med* 29:1357–1360, 2010.
4. Lowe AJ, Johank AJ, Moore CW: Sonography of the neonatal spine part 2, spinal disorders, *AJR Am J Roentgenol* 188:739–744, 2007.

Carotid Artery Disease

Jenni Taylor, Kelly Mumbert

CLINICAL SCENARIO

A 45-year-old woman is seen in the emergency department with a 1-week history of chest pain, right hand pain, right arm paresthesia, and severe dizziness. She has no prior history of a transient ischemic attack (TIA) or cerebrovascular accident. She has a significant history for tuberculosis, HIV, and tobacco abuse. Blood pressure is 127/80 mmHg in the left arm and 75/43 mmHg in the right arm.

The physician requests a carotid sonogram. Common (Fig. 34-1, *A*; see Color Plate 50, *A*), internal, external, and vertebral arteries are examined bilaterally. All vessels appear patent. Spectral Doppler analysis shows all velocities within normal limits. Color Doppler demonstrates retrograde flow in the right vertebral artery (Fig. 34-1, *B* and *C*; see Color Plate 50, *B* and *C*). A comparison with the left vertebral artery is provided (Fig. 34-1, *D* and *E*, see Color Plate 50, *D* and *E*). What do these findings suggest?

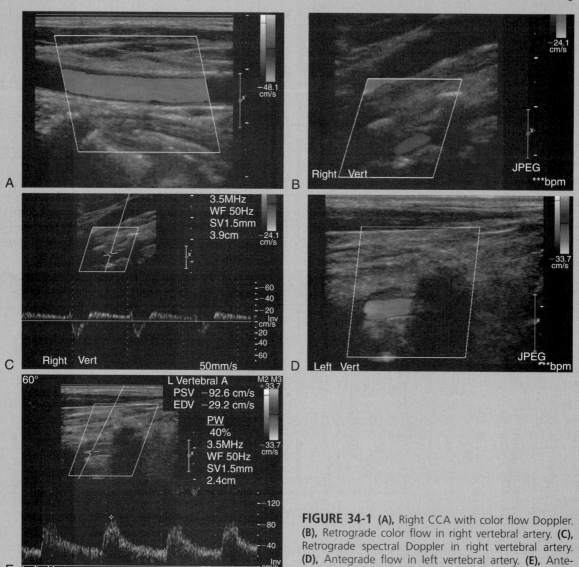

FIGURE 34-1 **(A)**, Right CCA with color flow Doppler. **(B)**, Retrograde color flow in right vertebral artery. **(C)**, Retrograde spectral Doppler in right vertebral artery. **(D)**, Antegrade flow in left vertebral artery. **(E)**, Antegrade flow in left vertebral artery.

Special thanks to Lisa Mullee, Ruben Martinez, James Graven, and Leslie Youngman for their contributions.

OBJECTIVES

- Identify risk factors associated with disease of the carotid or vertebral arteries.
- Identify signs and symptoms associated with abnormalities of the carotid or vertebral arteries.
- Recognize the sonographic appearances of normal and abnormal carotid arteries.

- Differentiate Doppler findings from normal to hemodynamically significant lesions.
- Distinguish rare forms of cerebrovascular disease and cerebrovascular accidents.

Stroke, also known as cerebrovascular accident, is the fourth leading cause of death in the United States, preceded by heart disease, cancer, and chronic lower respiratory diseases. Each year, approximately 795,000 people have a first stroke and an additional 185,000 have a recurrent stroke. On average, someone in the United States has a stroke every 40 seconds, which accounts for approximately 1 of every 18 deaths. Approximately three-fourths of all strokes are the result of ischemia, and one-fourth are hemorrhagic.[1,2]

Carotid sonogram has proved to be a useful and cost-effective method of evaluation of the cervical carotid and vertebral arteries. Knowledge of risk factors, signs, symptoms, and presentation of impending stroke is key in patient outcome. Disease of the carotid arteries affects the ipsilateral side of the head and the contralateral side of body.

Risk factors for stroke include hypertension, cigarette smoking, heart disease, diabetes, and history of TIA or reversible ischemic neurologic deficit. Common warning signs of stroke are unilateral weakness or numbness of the face, arm, or leg; difficulty speaking; loss of vision, particularly in one eye; and a bruit heard by

a physician. Additional generalized symptoms include dizziness, syncope, headache, and confusion.

NORMAL ANATOMY

The aortic root leaves the left ventricle with the left and right coronary arteries immediately branching off near the aortic cusp. The innominate, or brachiocephalic, is the first major branch off the aortic arch. The innominate splits into the right subclavian and right common carotid artery (CCA). The right CCA bifurcates into the right internal carotid artery (ICA) and external carotid artery (ECA). The right vertebral artery branches off the right subclavian and travels cephalad until it joins the left vertebral artery to form the basilar artery. The left CCA is the next branch directly off the aortic arch. It also bifurcates into the ICA and ECA. The third branch off the arch is the left subclavian artery, which supplies blood to the left arm. The left vertebral artery branches off the left subclavian artery and combines with the right vertebral artery to form the basilar artery, which provides blood for the posterior circulation of the brain (Fig. 34-2).

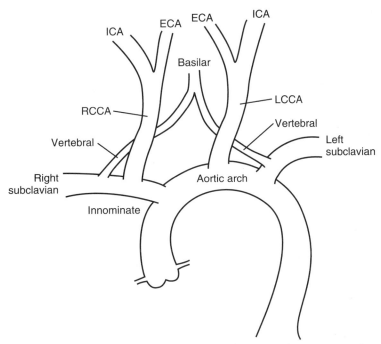

FIGURE 34-2 Schematic drawing of cerebrovascular anatomy as it branches off aortic arch. *ECA*, External carotid artery; *ICA*, internal carotid artery; *LCCA*, left common carotid artery; *RCCA*, right common carotid artery.

SONOGRAPHIC IMAGING TECHNIQUES

A typical carotid sonogram begins with a focused history obtained from the patient or chart. Some laboratory protocols require bilateral arm blood pressures; others may require only blood pressures if retrograde flow is seen in one of the vertebral arteries. The patient is placed in a supine position with the head turned away from the side being scanned. Although consistency is the only necessary factor, most sonographers begin the examination on the

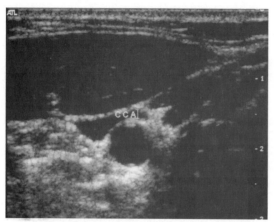

FIGURE 34-3 Transverse view of proximal CCA.

right side. A 7 MHz linear transducer is most frequently used, but a 5 or 10 MHz transducer may be preferred, depending on the size of the patient.

The examination begins with gray-scale interrogation from a transverse plane. The transducer is usually placed in an anterolateral position near the supraclavicular notch and moved cephalad to the angle of the mandible (Fig. 34-3). During scanning in the transverse plane, notation of the orientation of the ICA and ECA as they split just past the bulb (Fig. 34-4) is helpful. The location and amount of plaque also should be noted when present. Area measurements for determination of the percent of stenosis are taken from this plane.

Longitudinal views are obtained, starting again at the proximal CCA near the clavicle (Fig. 34-5). The widening of the artery at the bifurcation is identified as the carotid bulb (Fig. 34-6), seen at the more cephalad portion of the vessel. The artery splits into the ICA and ECA (Fig. 34-7). Plaque characterization should take place. Diameter measurements of a stenotic lesion should also be taken in this view.

The ICA is typically the larger vessel compared with the ECA. In most patients, the ICA is posterior and lateral to the ECA and very rarely has branches off the vessel

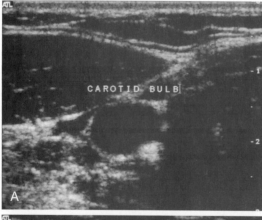

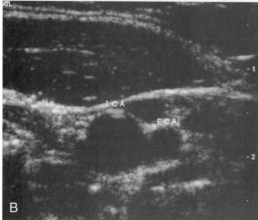

FIGURE 34-4 Transverse views of carotid bulb just before bifurcation of ICA and ECA **(A)** and ICA and ECA just past carotid bulb **(B)**.

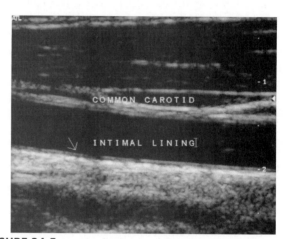

FIGURE 34-5 Longitudinal view of CCA showing intimal lining.

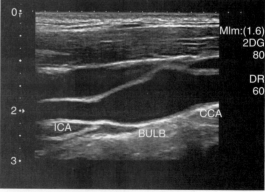

FIGURE 34-6 Longitudinal view of CCA, bulb, and proximal ICA. *(Courtesy Deziree Rada-Brooks, BSHS, RDMS, RVT.)*

seen in the neck. The ECA may be identified by the superior thyroid artery branching off in the cervical area. The vertebral arteries originate from the subclavian artery and are imaged posterolaterally directing the sound beam until the vertebral bodies are identified. The vertebral artery is seen running between the vertebral processes (Fig. 34-8). Color and spectral Doppler are instrumental in visualization of the vertebral artery.

DOPPLER IMAGING: SPECTRAL ANALYSIS

Doppler spectral analysis is valuable in determination of the hemodynamic significance of a stenotic lesion; the signal is both visual and auditory. The CCA, the ICA, and the ECA all have distinct flow characteristics that can be evaluated with peak systolic velocities (PSVs), diastolic velocities, or velocity ratios.

The ICA receives approximately 80% of the blood supplied by the CCA and is needed to supply an adequate amount of blood to the brain. The Doppler spectral waveform has a low-resistance appearance, demonstrating antegrade flow in diastole (Fig. 34-9).

The ECA supplies blood to the facial musculature and demonstrates a high-resistance Doppler waveform. The ECA waveform shows a sharp systolic rise and a sharp diastolic fall with a brief diastolic flow reversal. The ECA can be distinguished from the ICA with a temporal tap, which can be accomplished by locating the superficial temporal artery near the ipsilateral ear and providing quick sequential taps; this can be seen on the ECA spectral waveform during diastole (Fig. 34-10).

The CCA has flow characteristics of both the ICA and the ECA. Similar to the ICA, it has antegrade flow during diastole (Fig. 34-11).

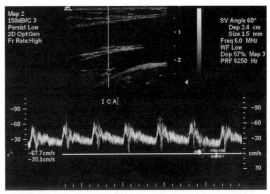

FIGURE 34-9 Doppler flow seen in normal ICA. Note antegrade flow seen in diastole.

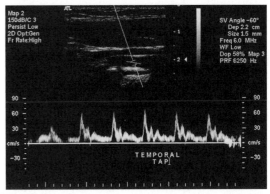

FIGURE 34-10 Doppler flow seen in normal ECA. Diastolic pulsations seen during temporal tap confirm ECA flow.

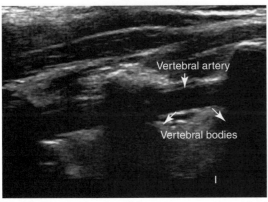

FIGURE 34-7 Longitudinal view of bulb, proximal ICA, and ECA.

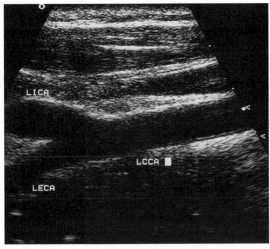

FIGURE 34-8 Vertebral artery identified between shadowing *(arrows)* from vertebral bodies.

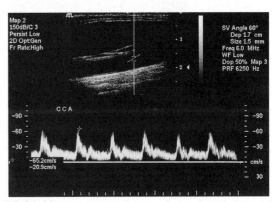

FIGURE 34-11 Normal Doppler waveform of CCA shows characteristics of both ICA and ECA.

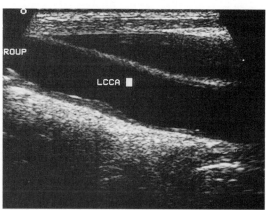

FIGURE 34-12 Minimal homogeneous plaque seen in lining wall of CCA.

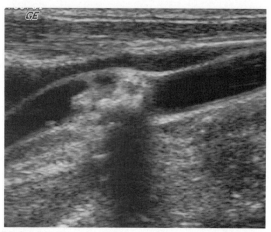

FIGURE 34-13 Significant ICA stenosis shows complex heterogeneous plaque with area of intraplaque hemorrhage. *(Courtesy GE Medical Systems.)*

COLOR DOPPLER

Color Doppler imaging is very helpful in quickly distinguishing between laminar and turbulent flow. The cervical arteries are typically displayed in shades of red that represent antegrade flow. With laminar flow, the lighter color shades are seen in the center of the vessel, showing the highest velocity flows. Turbulent flow is easily identified by the mixture of color shades that represent blood flow traveling at higher speeds and variable directions.

Color Doppler in the CCA and ICA shows a continuous flow pattern that indicates flow throughout the cardiac cycle. The ECA has diminished diastolic flow that can be described with color Doppler as having a "blinking" appearance.

CAROTID ARTERY STENOSIS

A carotid sonogram examination consists of gray-scale imaging, Doppler, and color flow analysis, with each one providing support in determination of the percent of stenosis. Direct imaging of the vessel allows evaluation and characterization of plaque. A homogeneous layer along the intimal lining with smooth borders may indicate a minimal stenosis, sometimes referred to as a "fatty streak" (Fig. 34-12). A more complex plaque may show echogenic areas composed of calcium mixed with soft echoes, reflective of collagen and fibrous tissue. Sonolucent areas seen within a complex plaque would indicate areas of intraplaque hemorrhage (Fig. 34-13). Calcific plaque can be identified easily with distal acoustic shadowing (Fig. 33-14, *A*). Shadowing from a calcific plaque can make determination of vessel patency difficult with sonographic

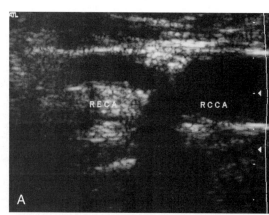

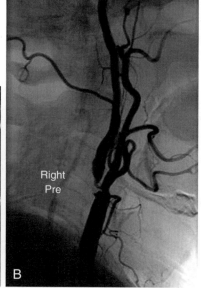

FIGURE 34-14 (A), Critical stenosis in proximal ICA. Note systolic and diastolic velocities at 401 cm/s and 94.2 cm/s, with an ICA/CCA ratio of 8.61. **(B),** Angiogram of critical stenosis in ICA. *(Courtesy Patrick A. Washko, BSRT, RDMS, RVT.)*

imaging techniques. Angiography may be used to define the degree of stenosis further (Fig. 33-14, *B*).

Plaque texture should be described as homogeneous or heterogeneous, and borders should be described as smooth or irregular. Careful attention should be given to irregular borders to evaluate for areas of ulceration (Fig. 34-15). Ulcer craters allow for thrombus formation and embolic possibilities.

Depending on department protocol, area or diameter measurements may be taken for determination of percent stenosis. Area measurements are taken from a transverse plane by tracing the residual and original lumens and calculating the percent stenosis: Area reduction = (1 × residual/original) × 100. Diameter measurements are also taken from a transverse plane, measuring the residual and original lumens: % Diameter reduction = (1 − residual/original) × 100 (Fig. 34-16). Diameter reductions of greater than 50% and area reductions of greater than 70% are considered significant enough to cause an increase in flow velocities.

Color flow Doppler should be used to interrogate the common, internal, and external carotid vessels. Areas of flow disturbance can be identified easily with color Doppler, with aliasing representing the highest velocity shifts, which aids in quick identification of stenosis and determination of placement of the Doppler sample volume.

Doppler spectral analysis helps in quantification of a stenotic lesion. Doppler measurements should be taken in a sagittal view, with the sample volume placed in the area of the greatest color Doppler shift. For accurate spectral information, a Doppler angle between

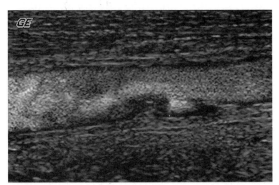

FIGURE 34-15 Area of ulceration seen in CCA. *(Courtesy GE Medical Systems.)*

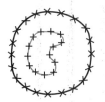
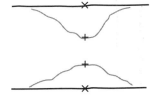

Area measurement   Diameter measurement

FIGURE 34-16 Schematic drawing shows difference between area and diameter measurements.

45 and 60 degrees should be used. Department protocols should be established and followed for consistency and reproducibility.

Spectral waveforms should be obtained in the CCA, bulb, proximal and distal ICA, and ECA. PSVs and end-diastolic velocities (EDVs) of CCA and ICA should be obtained. PSVs should be obtained in the ECA and vertebral vessels (Fig. 34-17, see Color Plate 51). Systolic ratios can also be obtained by dividing the highest PSV of a stenotic ICA by the distal PSV of the ipsilateral CCA. End-diastolic ratios can also be useful in prediction of stenoses greater than 80%. The velocity ranges in Table 34-1 correlate well with quality assurance data. Department-specific protocols and quality assurance data should be established for each laboratory.

When performed correctly, Doppler spectral analysis is an accurate determination of stenosis within the ICA. Soft plaque or thrombus may be difficult to see with imaging techniques alone; Doppler plays a vital role in evaluation for blockage.

In the past, the most common treatment for hemodynamically significant lesions was carotid endarterectomy. However, carotid angioplasty with stenting is a relatively new, increasingly used, less invasive treatment for symptomatic carotid artery stenosis.[3] The randomized Carotid Revascularization Endarterectomy versus Stenting Trial (CREST) compared carotid endarterectomy and stenting for symptomatic and asymptomatic carotid stenosis.[4] There was no overall difference in the primary endpoint of stroke, myocardial infarction, or death. Clinical trials of carotid artery revascularization methods such as carotid endarterectomy and carotid artery stenting provide guidance to clinicians about the choice of therapy based on individual patient need.

CAROTID ARTERY OCCLUSION

Carotid artery occlusion may be suspected when echogenic material appears to fill the vessel lumen totally (Fig. 34-18). Occlusion is also indicated by absence of color and Doppler flow. Doppler within the CCA has a thumping or "drumbeat" sound in systole. The ipsilateral ECA may take on an internal flow pattern as it tries to compensate for the occlusion. The ECA can be identified with a temporal tap. ICAs that are chronically occluded appear reduced in size.

SUBCLAVIAN STEAL

Subclavian steal syndrome is a result of stenosis or occlusion proximal to the vertebral artery. The pressure in the arm decreases from diminished blood flow, resulting in reversal of flow in the ipsilateral vertebral artery. Subclavian steal syndrome is found in men more frequently than in women and usually affects individuals older than 50 years. Subclavian steal syndrome is commonly

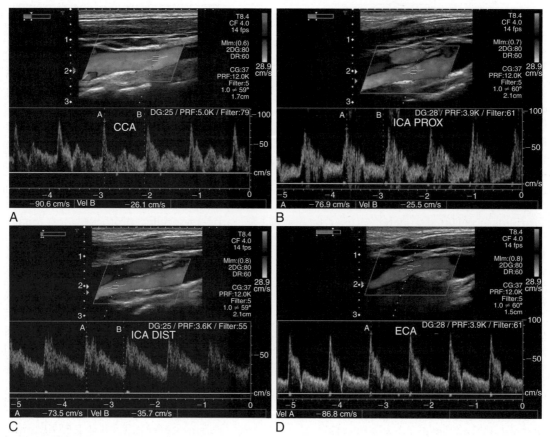

FIGURE 34-17 Spectral Doppler waveforms taken in CCA **(A)**, proximal ICA **(B)**, distal ICA **(C)**, and ECA **(D)**. PSV and EDV measurements are seen in CCA and proximal and distal ICA. *(Courtesy Deziree Rada-Brooks, BSHS, RDMS, RVT.)*

TABLE 34-1	Carotid Artery Stenosis			
Percent Stenosis	PSV (cm/s)	EDV (cm/s)	Systolic Velocity Ratio (ICA/CCA)	Diastolic Velocity Ratio (ICA/CCA)
<49%	<140	<100	<1.8	<2.6
50%-79%	>140	<100	>1.8	>2.6
80%-99%	>140	>100	>3.7	>5.5
100%	Absent	Absent	Absent	Absent

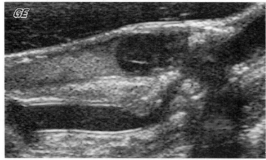

FIGURE 34-18 Completely occluded ICA. *(Courtesy GE Medical Systems.)*

asymptomatic and found incidentally during a carotid sonogram examination. Symptomatic patients may have arm pain with exercise or at rest. Signs of vertebrobasilar ischemia may include ataxia, vertigo, or bilateral visual disturbances.

Subclavian steal syndrome can be diagnosed with reversal of flow in the vertebral artery, which is usually proven with color flow Doppler and confirmed with spectral Doppler. For proven flow reversal in the vertebral artery, antegrade flow should be demonstrated in the CCA. A difference in bilateral blood pressures of greater than 20 mmHg is also an indication of subclavian steal syndrome.

CAROTID DISSECTION

Carotid artery dissection should be considered a possible cause of symptoms associated with a stroke in patients younger than 40 years. Carotid dissection is seen slightly more often in men than in women. Morbidity from a carotid dissection varies in severity from transient ischemic neurologic deficit to death. A 75% mortality rate is associated with dissections that extend intracranially.[5]

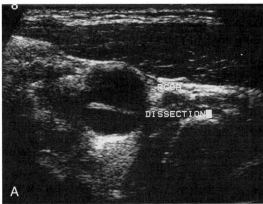

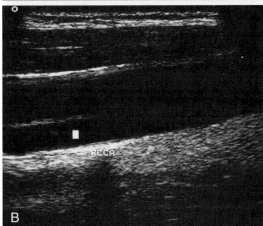

FIGURE 34-19 Carotid artery dissection seen in transverse **(A)** and sagittal **(B)** views. Intimal flap creates double lumen. *(Courtesy Erin Simard, Florida Heart Group, Orlando.)*

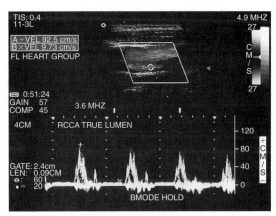

FIGURE 34-20 Doppler waveform seen in the presence of carotid dissection. Although it is an ICA waveform, it has the appearance of high-resistance flow with little to no diastolic flow noted. *(Courtesy Erin Simard, Florida Heart Group, Orlando.)*

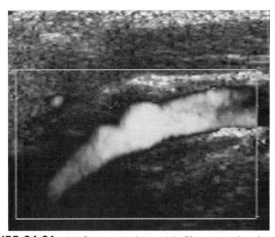

FIGURE 34-21 ICA from a patient with fibromuscular dysplasia. Note "peapod" appearance of artery. *(Courtesy Doug Marcum, Orlando Ultrasound Associates, Inc., Orlando.)*

Predisposing factors associated with carotid artery dissection may include Marfan syndrome, fibromuscular dysplasia, syphilis, or atherosclerosis, or the condition may be familial. Carotid dissection should be considered in patients with a neurologic deficit with sustained injury or trauma. Chiropractic manipulation, blunt trauma, and injury from seat belts in motor vehicle accidents all have been associated with carotid artery dissection.

Dissection of the cervical carotid arteries can be diagnosed when an intimal flap creates a double lumen (Fig. 34-19). The formation of thrombus may be visualized within the false lumen. The vessels should be carefully interrogated in an attempt to determine the extent of the dissection.

Doppler analysis is helpful in identification of a stenosis or occlusion caused by the false lumen. A dissected ICA may have an appearance of a high-resistance waveform with a decreased velocity (Fig. 34-20). With color Doppler, red and blue may be seen within the lumen in a transverse view.

FIBROMUSCULAR DYSPLASIA

Fibromuscular dysplasia is a noninflammatory disease of unknown cause that has been found to affect several members of the same family, implying a hereditary factor. Fibromuscular dysplasia can involve both systemic and cervicocerebral vessels, with the most common being the renal arteries and ICAs. Fibromuscular dysplasia is seen more often in women and is typically diagnosed between the ages of 30 and 50 years. The diagnosis may not be made until the development of hypertension from affected renal arteries or symptoms of TIA or stroke from affected ICAs.

Sonographic evaluation of the ICA reveals expanded and narrowed areas of the arterial lumen often described as having a "string-of-beads" or a "peapod" appearance (Fig. 34-21; see Color Plate 52). The distal portion of the ICA is usually affected. The expanded areas provide an environment for blood to swirl and have a pooling effect that allows for clot formation. Smaller clots may travel, causing TIAs. The narrowed segments of fibromuscular dysplasia may have varying degrees of stenosis and must be interrogated carefully, particularly with Doppler. Because fibromuscular dysplasia commonly involves the distal ICA, a follow-up angiogram is necessary for further evaluation and diagnosis.

Patients with fibromuscular dysplasia affecting the ICAs are typically placed on antiplatelet and anticoagulation therapy to prevent thrombus formation or undergo a carotid endarterectomy to revascularize stenosed segments.[6] Because of the nonatherosclerotic nature of fibromuscular dysplasia, carotid stent grafting has become an additional treatment option for patients with this condition. Carotid artery stenting is a relatively new procedure, and additional clinical trials are needed to determine long-term benefit and complications.

SUMMARY

Carotid sonogram is a safe and cost-effective method for evaluation of vessels that supply blood to the brain. In the hands of a skilled and knowledgeable sonographer, carotid sonogram has been accurate in determination of disease of the carotid or vertebral arteries. Early detection and prevention of impending stroke has the potential for saving millions of dollars in health care and rehabilitation costs.

CLINICAL SCENARIO—DIAGNOSIS

The patient was found to have proximal subclavian arterial stenosis on the right side. In this condition, flow is reversed or retrograde in the right vertebral artery to feed the subclavian artery distal to the stenosis. Normal flow is seen in the right CCA, which suggests the obstruction is restricted to the proximal region of the right subclavian artery causing subclavian steal syndrome.

The patient underwent a thrombectomy along with a carotid subclavian transposition. After rehabilitation, she fully recovered from her paresthesia. After 1 year, the patient has not encountered any dizziness or arm pain associated with her surgical recovery.

CASE STUDIES FOR DISCUSSION

1. During a routine cardiac work-up, a 65-year-old man with a history of smoking and hypertension admits he has experienced some intermittent loss of the use of his left arm. The cardiologist orders a carotid sonogram. Sonographic findings include decreased color flow in the right ICA with a high-pitched Doppler signal measuring a PSV of 600 cm/s and EDV of 140 cm/s. What do these findings suggest? What would be the next step in treatment?

2. A noncompliant 58-year-old woman with depression and hypertension presents to the emergency department with aphasia, left hemiplegia, and possible left hemianopia. The patient communicates that her symptoms started early in the morning. While waiting for further testing that day, the neurologic deficits resolve. What is the most likely diagnosis?

3. A man stumbles into the emergency department showing signs of dysarthria and problems with gait and stance. The front desk personnel assume the man is severely intoxicated and do not assist him right away. Why is this possibly a detrimental mistake?

4. A 67-year-old man developed acute blindness in the left eye while at work. When he arrived at the hospital, he claimed to have gotten lost in the elevator. Staff noticed he appeared uncoordinated and confused and had trouble expressing himself. A carotid sonogram demonstrated the finding in Figure 34-22 (see Color Plate 53) in the left CCA. The left vertebral artery was found to be occluded. After 3 days, the patient's symptoms completely resolved. What do these findings suggest?

5. A 67-year-old man is taken to the hospital via ambulance. His symptoms include confusion, loss of memory, aphasia, and left-sided hemiparesis. His history includes hypertension, hypercholesterolemia, and smoking. A carotid sonogram revealed echogenic material within the right internal carotid lumen. Images are provided in Figure 34-23. No flow was seen with spectral Doppler. What do these findings indicate?

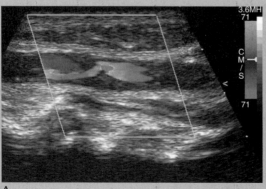
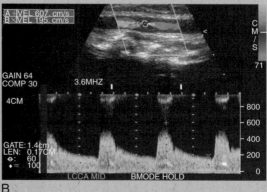

FIGURE 34-22 Images of left CCA with color Doppler **(A)** and spectral analysis **(B)** demonstrating PSV of 607 cm/s and peak diastolic velocity of 195 cm/s.

CASE STUDIES FOR DISCUSSION—cont'd

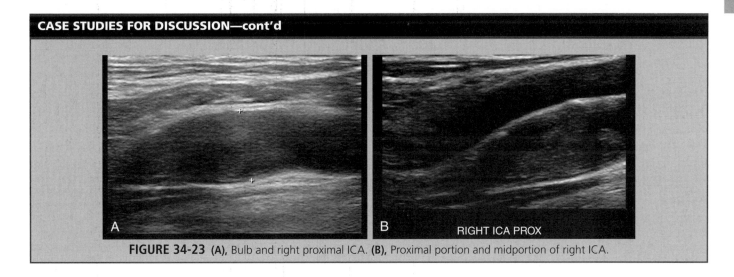

FIGURE 34-23 **(A)**, Bulb and right proximal ICA. **(B)**, Proximal portion and midportion of right ICA.

STUDY QUESTIONS

1. A patient presents with left arm paralysis; which artery is the most likely cause?
a. Right ICA
b. Left ICA
c. Right vertebral artery
d. Left vertebral artery
e. Right ECA

2. A patient describes loss of vision in the left eye as "someone pulling the shade down." What term describes this transient monocular blindness?
a. Aphasia
b. Vertigo
c. Diplopia
d. Amaurosis fugax
e. Syncope

3. Sonographic findings of a carotid sonogram reveal moderate heterogeneous plaque in the left CCA. Spectral Doppler revealed a PSV of 224 cm/s and EDV of 85 cm/s. Which of the following accurately describes the sonographic findings?
a. <49% stenosis
b. 50% to 79% stenosis
c. 80% to 99% stenosis
d. >99% stenosis
e. Total occlusion

4. What is the first sign of subclavian artery stenosis?
a. Change in bilateral brachial pressures
b. Change in vertebral artery waveform
c. Left-sided weakness
d. Increase in carotid velocity
e. Increase in jugular vein compliance

5. A 40-year-old woman presents to the emergency department with uncontrolled hypertension and abnormal laboratory values. Bilateral carotid bruit is noted on cervical auscultation. Renal angiogram results reveal multiple bulbous, luminal irregularities in the renal arteries bilaterally. What is the most likely cause of this patient's carotid bruit?
a. TIA
b. Carotid body tumor
c. Ehlers-Danlos syndrome
d. Fibromuscular dysplasia
e. Cystic medial necrosis

6. When performing a duplex carotid examination, a vessel is encountered demonstrating a continuous low-velocity signal with irregular and varying shape. This most likely represents what vessel?
a. ICA
b. External carotid vein
c. Subclavian artery
d. Subclavian vein
e. Jugular vein

7. A neurologic deficit that lasts longer than 24 hours but completely resolves is a:
a. TIA
b. Reversible ischemic neurologic deficit
c. Cerebrovascular accident
d. Permanent ischemic attack

8. How can the ICA Doppler flow be best described?
a. High flow and low resistance signal
b. High flow and high resistance signal
c. Low flow and low resistance signal
d. Low flow and high resistance signal

9. Which of the following is the percentage of stenosis of the RCCA on a transverse image with a true diameter of 10 mm and a residual diameter of 2 mm?
a. 5%
b. 20%
c. 50%
d. 80%

10. Following are the PSVs for a patient's carotid sonogram. What is the right ICA/CCA ratio?

Right CCA proximal: 98 cm/s
Right ICA proximal: 145 cm/s
Right CCA distal: 88 cm/s
Right ICA distal: 160 cm/s

a. 1.10
b. 1.82
c. 1.63
d. 1.48

REFERENCES

1. Roger VL, Go AS, Lloyd-Jones DM, et al: Heart disease and stroke statistics—2012 update: a report from the American Heart Association, *Circulation* 125:e2–e220, 2012.

2. Kochanek KD, Xu JQ, Murphy SL, et al: Deaths: preliminary data for 2009. *National Vital Statistics Reports*, vol. 59, no 4, Hyattsville, MD, 2011, National Center for Health Statistics.

3. Nederkoorn PJ, Brown MM: Optimal cut-off criteria for duplex ultrasound for the diagnosis of restenosis in stented carotid arteries: review and protocol for a diagnostic study, *BMC Neurol* 9:36, 2009.

4. Brott TG, Hobson RW 2nd, Howard G, et al: CREST investigators: Stenting versus endarterectomy for treatment of carotid-artery stenosis, *N Engl J Med* 363:11–23, 2010.

5. Henderson SO, Kilaghbian T: Dissection, carotid artery, *eMedicine J* 2, 2001.

6. Finster J, Strassegger J, Haymerle A, et al: Bilateral stenting of symptomatic and asymptomatic internal carotid artery stenosis due to fibromuscular dysplasia, *J Neurol Neurosurg Psychiatry* 69:683–686, 2000.

Leg Pain

Jennifer Kurnal-Herring

A 45-year-old man presents to the emergency department with dyspnea that has been getting worse within the last week. He also states his right leg became swollen and painful a little over a week before the emergency department visit. In getting ready for work this morning for his sedentary job, he quickly became short of breath and called an ambulance. En route to the hospital, he began coughing up blood (hemoptysis). History includes hypertension, renal disease, sleep apnea, and back pain.

The emergency department physician ordered a computed tomography (CT) scan of the chest, which showed a large saddle pulmonary embolus. The patient denied any history of thromboembolism, smoking, or drinking. At the time of the initial physical examination, the patient had a pulse of 71 beats per minute and a respiratory rate of 18. Despite a history of hypertension and noncompliance with medication, the patient's blood pressure was 115/72 mmHg. A low blood pressure can indicate a pulmonary embolus. After administering anticoagulation, the physician ordered a lower extremity venous Doppler (LEVD) examination to identify where the pulmonary embolus may have arisen. LEVD demonstrated echogenic matter in the lumen of the right popliteal vein, along with a lack of compression (Fig. 35-1). In the longitudinal plane, color Doppler revealed no internal blood flow (Fig. 35-2, see Color Plate 54).

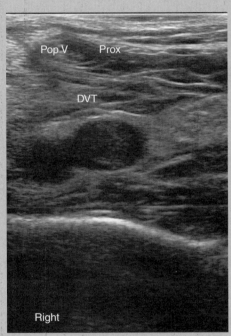

FIGURE 35-1 Transverse right popliteal vein with compression. Note the lack of wall coaptation during the compression and internal echogenic matter. *(Courtesy Maureen O'Neil DiGiorgio, RDCS, RVT.)*

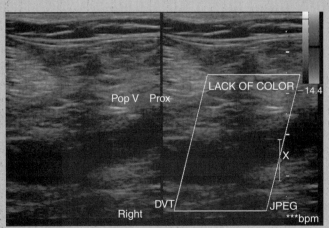

FIGURE 35-2 Longitudinal image of right popliteal vein with lack of color Doppler flow. *(Courtesy Maureen O'Neil DiGiorgio, RDCS, RVT.)*

OBJECTIVES

- Differentiate between the various causes of leg pain.
- Describe the sonographic appearance of thrombosis of the deep venous system.
- Discern the various sonographic appearances of acute and chronic thromboses.
- Explain the differential diagnoses of deep vein thrombosis (DVT).
- Describe the physiologic changes to the venous system that help in the diagnosis of DVT.
- Explain the treatment options for DVT.
- Differentiate between acute and chronic venous thrombosis.

This chapter describes a variety of causes of leg pain, especially causes secondary to venous disease, and the role of sonography in diagnosis of these diseases. Protocols may vary depending on whether these examinations are performed in a radiology-based sonography department versus a dedicated vascular laboratory. This chapter focuses more on the protocols followed in a radiology department. A brief explanation of normal anatomy is included (Fig. 35-3 and Box 35-1), but the focus is on the pathology and diseases that lead to leg pain. The radiology-based sonography department concentrates

primarily on the diagnosis of deep vein thrombosis (DVT) and posterior knee masses.

B-mode and Doppler evaluation in the vascular laboratory can be quite useful in diagnosis of venous causes of leg pain. Bony fractures; tendinous sprains; ligamental ruptures and tears; muscle strains, tears, and ruptures; nerve impingement; and trauma are the most common sources of lower extremity pain. However, these diagnoses are left to plain film radiography, CT, and magnetic resonance imaging (MRI). Figure 35-4 shows how a physician would decide which imaging

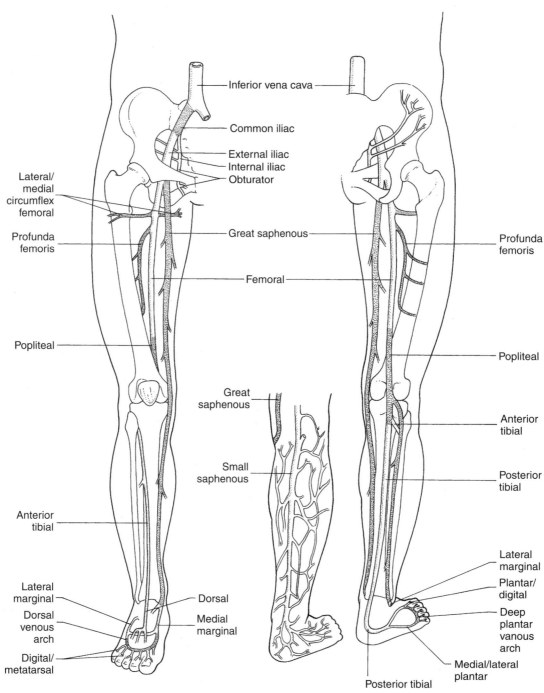

FIGURE 35-3 Normal deep and superficial venous anatomy of the legs.

BOX 35-1 | Normal Lower Extremity Venous Anatomy

Deep Veins
Inferior vena cava
Common iliac vein
External iliac vein
Common femoral vein
Femoral vein
Deep femoral vein (profunda)
Popliteal vein
Posterior tibial veins
Anterior tibial veins
Peroneal (fibular) vein

Superficial Veins
Lesser saphenous vein
Great saphenous vein

Laboratory Value
D dimer

examination would best assess the patient's condition based on history, symptoms, and physical examination.

NORMAL VASCULAR ANATOMY

Veins and arteries contain three layers. The innermost layer is the intima, which comprises endothelial tissue lining the inside of the vein, and extends inward to form the venous valves. The valves in the veins are bicuspid but can have one to three leaflets. These valves keep blood flowing in one direction, upward toward the heart. The muscular layer is the tunica media. The reason that veins are much more compressible than arteries is that the tunica media is much thinner in veins because they do not vasodilate or vasoconstrict. The lower venous pressure also does not need to support the amount of pressure that the arteries need to endure. The outer, protective layer is the tunica adventitia.

In most instances with a single vein, an artery is found with the same name. Two exceptions to this rule are that the veins of the calf distal to the popliteal vein are normally paired, and an artery does not accompany the superficial

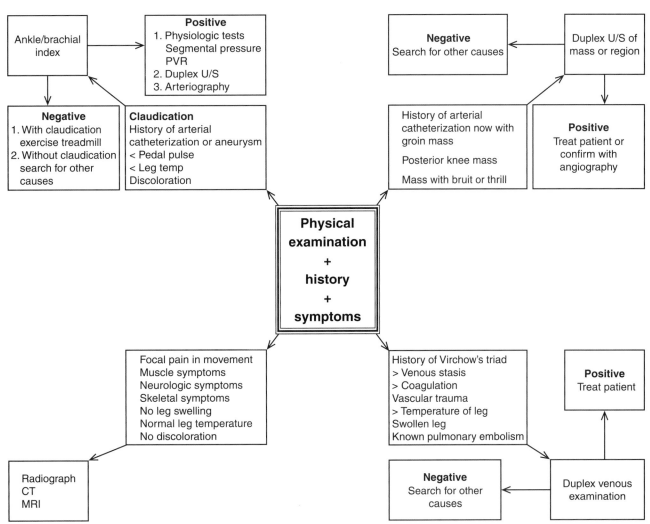

FIGURE 35-4 Leg pain examination selection protocol. *Hx,* History; *PVR,* peripheral vascular resistance; *U/S,* ultrasound.

saphenous vessels. The veins of the leg can be divided into superficial and deep veins. Although they are called deep veins, they are actually superficial enough to be well visualized on most patients with 5- to 7-MHz linear transducers.

Starting at the iliac bifurcation, the veins are listed in a retrograde order (see Fig. 35-3). The two common iliac vessels branch into the inferior vena cava (IVC) and from the aorta at the level of the umbilicus. They continue to the level of the sacroiliac joints before the internal iliac (hypogastric) veins angle steeply into the pelvis draining the rectum, sigmoid, and genitals. After the internal iliacs have departed, the external iliac vein proceeds along the lateral wall of the pelvis before leaving the pelvis at the inguinal canal. After passing the inguinal ligament, the vein is called the common femoral vein (CFV). After about 4 cm, the CFV is joined by the greater saphenous vein (GSV) from an anterior medial direction. The area where the GSV becomes confluent with the CFV is known as the saphofemoral junction (SFJ). Within a few centimeters of the SFJ, the CFV branches into the femoral vein and the deep femoral vein. The deep femoral vein is also called the profunda femoris, or simply the profunda. The profunda serves the upper lateral thigh. The femoral vein continues along the anterior medial leg until it dives deep through the ligaments of the adductor muscles, known as the adductor hiatus or Hunter's canal.

The popliteal vessels are located in the popliteal fossa and can quickly start branching into other veins of various sizes, known as the trifurcation area. From the popliteal vein, moving inferiorly, the sonographer should be able to visualize the tibioperoneal trunk, from which the anterior tibial vein and peroneal (fibular) vein arise. The trifurcation is found a little more inferior after those two vessels separate. The trifurcation consists of the anterior and posterior tibial veins and the peroneal veins. Located posterior to the trifurcation are the gastrocnemius vessels. These are not usually evaluated unless they appear dilated and prominent, or the patient has pain in that area. The trifurcation should be identified by following it from the popliteal, so as to avoid mistaking it for the more posterior gastrocnemius vessels (Fig. 35-5). The anterior tibial vessels branch off anteriorly and laterally, passing through the space formed between the tibia and fibula then laterally to the tibial shaft with a single artery and paired veins. The popliteal continues for a few centimeters before the peroneal (fibular vessels) and posterior tibial veins branch off. The peroneal vessels run deeper and more laterally with a single artery and paired veins, and the posterior tibials (one artery and two paired veins) continue more medially and superficially, down to the area just posterior to the medial malleolus.

A superficial vein that is routinely visualized is the GSV, which travels, without an accompanying artery, along the superficial medial aspect of the leg, starting near the ankle and continuing up to its insertion into the CFV just inferior to the groin crease at the SFJ. Connecting the

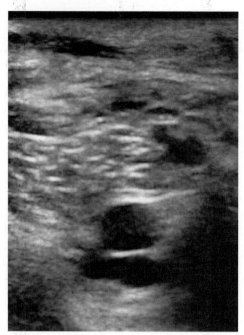

FIGURE 35-5 Trifurcation is anterior to gastrocnemius vessels, and these vessels can be easily mistaken for the trifurcation.

superficial veins to the deep veins are the small perforators, which contain only one venous valve.

Artery or Vein?

Numerous assessments are useful in determining whether an extremity vessel is an artery or a vein.

- The arteries maintain a round shape when viewed in cross section.
- The veins change shape with patient respirations.
- The veins compress much more easily than arteries.
- The veins are ovoid unless distended.
- The arteries pulsate with each heartbeat.
- The veins dilate during a Valsalva maneuver or when the patient's trunk is elevated in relation to the extremity.
- The vein has the potential of being larger than the accompanying artery. In a thrombus-filled state, it is larger; but in a healthy patient, it may appear slightly smaller.

Anatomic Variance

Venous anatomy can demonstrate a variance from normal textbook anatomy. It is fairly common to see a bifid system, in which there are two veins, where traditionally there would be only one. A Giacomini vein is an anatomic variant seen running posteriorly down the leg and is an extension of the small saphenous vein, which normally becomes confluent with the popliteal vein. In either case, the sonographer must evaluate all veins because anatomic variants are also prone to DVT and other venous pathology.

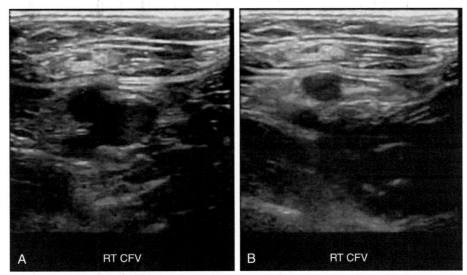

FIGURE 35-6 **(A)**, CFV without compression. **(B)**, CFV is completely compressed. *(Courtesy Patrick A. Washko, BSRT, RDMS, RVT.)*

Normal Sonographic Appearance

Normal veins should appear anechoic on gray-scale imaging, be easily compressed (Fig. 35-6), show intraluminal color Doppler, and be able to demonstrate a distal augmentation on pulsed wave Doppler. On pulsed wave Doppler, the sonographer should be able to appreciate the spontaneous flow and the respiratory phasicity. Normally, when a patient inspires, that pushes the diaphragm inferiorly, increasing intraabdominal pressure on the IVC. Given that the IVC collapses during inspiration, the same occurs distally within the veins of the lower extremity. When the patient expires, that pressure is relieved, and venous flow can resume. If the venous valves are competent, that can also be demonstrated by pulsed wave Doppler by having the patient perform the Valsalva maneuver, or the sonographer can perform a proximal compression. If either technique works to cut off the Doppler signal, the valves are considered competent.

Clinical Evaluation

Before beginning a LEVD, the sonographer should visually examine the limb and make note of any edema, varicose veins, palpable cordlike areas, and skin pigmentation changes, such as stasis dermatitis. Edema is very general symptom, not specific to DVT. Varicose veins, also known as spider veins, indicate venous valve insufficiency in the superficial veins, which can cause pain in addition to the cosmetic issue. A palpable cordlike area can be indicative of superficial thrombophlebitis. Stasis dermatitis lends a brownish appearance to the gaiter zone of the leg as a result of a pooling of blood and a breakdown of hemosiderin. The clinician may also note if the patient has a positive Homan's sign, which is when the patient performs a dorsiflexion of the ipsilateral foot that elicits a pain response.

VENOUS DISEASE

Deep Vein Thrombosis

Pulmonary embolism has a high rate of morbidity and mortality (600,000 hospitalizations and 200,000 deaths each year).[1] The primary source of pulmonary embolism is thrombosis of the deep venous system in the lower extremities. The primary symptom of DVT of the lower extremity is a painful, swollen leg. Duplex sonography is accurate in determination of the presence or absence of venous clot. The advantages of sonography over venography in diagnosing a DVT include better patient tolerance, similar accuracy, lower risk, and lower cost. The current "gold standard" to diagnose a pulmonary embolus is pulmonary angiography. Because it is associated with a high risk of morbidity and mortality, other, less invasive and lower risk modalities usually are used for diagnosis. A nuclear medicine ventilation-perfusion scan can be performed to detect circulation of air and blood within a patient's lung, and CT angiography of the chest can detect a pulmonary embolus. Although sometimes large emboli can be seen in the heart during an echocardiogram, sonography does not usually evaluate the presence of pulmonary emboli directly. Sonography is useful to help identify the location of the origin of the embolus and to help determine the effectiveness of thrombolytic therapy. When DVT in the lower extremity is the culprit, the origin often can be identified; however, any vein can have a DVT and embolization of the thrombus can occur, such as a central vein that is not easily seen on sonography, so not every patient with a pulmonary embolus has a positive DVT in the lower extremity.[1]

Certain patient populations are at increased risk for development of thrombosis in the legs. Blood that is not moving tends to clot. The combined factors of muscle contraction and venous valve action and the effects of respiration propel venous blood in the extremities. Any event that immobilizes the leg (trauma, surgery, advanced age, obesity, prolonged sitting), damages the deep venous valves (varicose veins, venous insufficiency, progression of superficial vein thrombosis [SVT]), increases a patient's coagulability (oral contraceptive use, coagulation disorders, recent surgery, cancer), or decreases natural flow pressures (congestive heart failure [CHF]) increases the possibility of venous thrombosis. The three primary factors that lead to venous thrombosis—vessel damage, flow stasis, and hypercoagulability—are known as Virchow's triad. The most prominent part of Virchow's triad is venous stasis. If the erythrocytes stagnate for too long, natural clotting factors take effect and begin to clot, or stick together. This sticky lump of erythrocytes can be seen on sonographic evaluation. They appear as a swirling mobile hypoechoic mass, termed "rouleau formation." Rouleau, a French term, means "coil" or "roll," which is how the cells begin to appear as they all clump together—a roll. Rouleau formation is a precursor to a thrombosis. The vein fully compresses, and Doppler signals appear normal, but note should be made that slow-moving blood flow was seen.[2,3]

Leg pain can arise from numerous areas other than the venous system—arterial, muscle, connective tissue, nerve, trauma, infection, or skeletal. The role of the sonographer is as much to rule out different possible causes as to determine what exactly may be the etiology of pain. Clinical history is as critical to successful diagnosis as the sonographic study itself. Nevertheless, adherence to strict criteria enables the sonographer to help diagnose venous occlusion.

Patients with DVT may have symptoms directly related to the leg (acutely swollen, painful leg) or symptoms of pulmonary embolism (shortness of breath). The examination consists of viewing the deep veins of the leg with B-mode, compressing the vessels to assess for coaptation, and documenting the changes in the spectral Doppler waveform during Valsalva maneuver or distal augmentation.

The patient should be positioned with the trunk slightly elevated, as in a reverse Trendelenburg position, with the lower extremity slightly rotated outward. Some experts suggest having the patient dangle the affected leg during examination of the calf vessels. The sonographer should start high in the groin crease, documenting the common femoral artery and CFV. The sonographer can use the SFJ or the origin of the GSV and move superiorly to begin scanning correctly in the CFV. If imaging inferior to the SFJ, the femoral vein is seen. Spectral Doppler of the veins should demonstrate phasic flow that varies with respiration, augmentation, and Valsalva maneuver. If the patient's trunk is elevated, the vein appears distended, but there should be no evidence of thrombus within the vein. When moderate probe pressure is increased, the walls of the vein should fully coapt. Probe pressure is adequate if the accompanying artery begins

to deform. (This maneuver must be done in a transverse plane and should not be done with the transducer in a longitudinal plane because it is too easy to slide off the side of the vessel in the longitudinal plane).[4]

The sonographer should begin moving inferiorly on the leg at close intervals to confirm the absence of intraluminal echogenic material, the continuation of phasic flow that varies with respiration, and coaptation of the vein walls. Doppler analysis can be helpful in documenting thrombus that has progressed to a size that can interrupt flow. Doppler signals that show a continuous flow pattern or lack of increased flow during distal augmentation suggest flow-restricting thrombus. If the pulsed wave Doppler demonstrates a dampened, monophasic waveform, that suggests a proximal stenosis. The most common reason for a monophasic waveform seen in an entire unilateral lower extremity is venous thrombosis in the ipsilateral iliac veins. Other causes for a monophasic waveform down an entire lower extremity include a partial thrombus in a more proximal vein; extrinsic compression, such as a fluid collection, mass, pregnancy, or ascites; intrinsic luminal narrowing owing to a hypoplastic vein; or prior thrombus. However, bilateral dampened waveforms mean that there is an issue of obstruction at the level of the IVC.[4]

The vessels that should be interrogated include the CFV, SFJ, GSV, profunda, femoral vein, and popliteal veins to the popliteal trifurcation. Controversy exists regarding the value of continuing through the calf vessels. Most dedicated vascular laboratories also interrogate the anterior tibials, posterior tibials, and peroneals, but many radiology-based sonography department protocols do not include these venous trees. In addition, when DVT is identified, the sonographer should interrogate cephalad to document the extent of the thrombus, which may include imaging of the iliac vessels.

Imaging hints include the following:

- Keeping the focal zone at the level of the vessel being viewed
- Imaging the vessel from an approach that is closest to the skin for that vessel at that level
- Keeping the vessel in the middle of the transducer face
- Carefully adjusting the gain so that soft internal plaque is visualized and not "blacked out" by incorrect gain settings
- Changing the sonographic window if a compression cannot be completed because a ligament may make compression difficult

The study is considered positive for DVT if the walls of the vein do not coapt when the artery has begun to deform or if thrombus can be documented as echogenic matter within the vein (Fig. 35-7). A DVT exhibits a lack of color Doppler flow. The spectral Doppler proximal to the thrombus is continuous with distal augmentation, having little or no effect on the proximal waveform.[5]

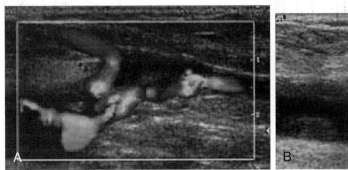
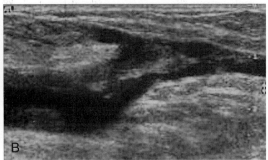

FIGURE 35-7 (A), Color flow is used to show flow in saphenofemoral junction. **(B),** Low-level echoes are identified within vessel walls.

Beyond the discovery of venous thrombosis, the clinical course can be significantly altered by the determination of the age of a clot. Chronic clot is not treated aggressively, and acute clot may respond favorably to aggressive use of antiembolytic/antithrombolytic therapy. Sonographic findings can strongly suggest whether a clot is acute or chronic, insuring that the patient receives appropriate treatment (Fig. 35-8).

The sonographic findings for acute and chronic thrombus are listed subsequently.

- Acute thrombus:
  - Is uniform in texture, with low-level echoes that may be difficult to visualize
  - Is soft, or slightly compressible
  - Is poorly attached; may sometimes "flap about" within the vessel
  - Distends the vessel
- Chronic thrombus:
  - Is heterogeneous, with bright echoes
  - Does not compress
  - Is rigidly attached
  - Tends to contract the vessel and may show a partial recanalization of the vein with a tortuous flow channel with well-developed collateral circulation[1]

Risk factors include the following:

Trauma
Immobility or paralysis
Prior DVT
Recent major surgery
Cancer or chemotherapy
Family history
CHF
Pregnancy
Oral contraceptives
Hypercoagulability
Prolonged bed rest

Superficial Vein Thrombosis

SVT is usually diagnosed clinically with a painful superficial cord with surrounding erythema. This condition

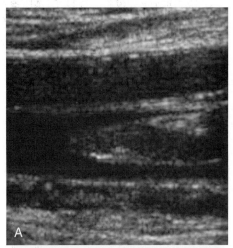
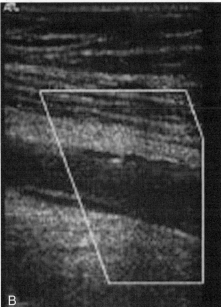

FIGURE 35-8 (A), DVT of femoral vein may show tongue of intraluminal material that may move within vessel. **(B),** Acute DVT shows homogeneous, low-level echoes.

is treated with anticoagulation therapy or ligation of the offending vessel at its proximal attachment to the deep system. Sonography can be useful to ensure that the swelling, pain, and redness are not caused by other underlying causes, such as soft tissue infection or

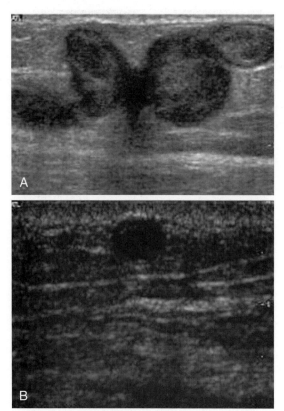

FIGURE 35-9 Superficial venous thrombosis is seen as a palpable, tender cord. **(A)** and **(B)**, Low-level echoes are shown within affected vessels.

hematoma. Sonography is also valuable in determining the extent of the thrombosis and monitoring of progression or regression with therapy.[6]

There is a higher prevalence in women of increasing age that also have concomitant varicose veins. Of SVT, 60% to 80% is seen in the GSV.[6] If the vessel becomes inflamed as a result, it is termed phlebitis, or in this case superficial thrombophlebitis. Although embolization is less likely to occur, SVT may be treated similar to a DVT, especially if it extends into the SFJ or popliteal vein. SVT has a recurrence rate of 15% to 20%.[6] The hallmark of SVT is a very painful but palpable cordlike structure. The sonographic appearance of SVT is similar to findings seen in DVT but is located within a superficial vessel (Fig. 35-9).

Venous Insufficiency

Venous insufficiency, or reflux, occurs when the valves are incompetent. This incompetence allows blood to flow backward toward the ankles, which increases distal venous pressure. The superficial venous system is a common site of valvular insufficiency that leads to varicose veins. Superficial veins that have increased pressure from failure of downstream valves tend to enlarge and shift to a superficial location. They can become infected and are unsightly. If the venous insufficiency occurs because of DVT, it is termed secondary, whereas

if venous insufficiency exists without DVT, it is termed primary.[7] Secondary venous insufficiency can also be termed postphlebitic syndrome, meaning that the DVT damaged the valves beyond their functional capacity. Of patients with a DVT, including patients treated with anticoagulants, 25% to 50% eventually have postphlebitic syndrome. Postphlebitic syndrome is also known as postthrombotic syndrome. High-frequency linear transducers can be used to document the valves in motion on B-mode. Spectral Doppler shows reversed flow during Valsalva maneuver and after augmentation. A proximal compression or Valsalva should halt all venous return.[8]

Sonographers can evaluate for venous insufficiency, or venous reflux, by performing a proximal compression with pulsed wave Doppler to note a complete lack of flow during the proximal compression or having the patient perform the Valsalva maneuver to terminate venous flow. If the valves are competent, there is no Doppler signal until pressure is relieved. A sonographic finding of venous insufficiency is the leakage, as demonstrated by a Doppler signal during the proximal compression or Valsalva. The hallmark of venous insufficiency is when the aforementioned provocative maneuvers cannot halt blood flow.[7]

Varicose Veins

Varicose veins are veins in which the valves become damaged and are leaking to the point of venous wall distention and includes spider veins. The veins appear very superficial and dilated and can be seen bulging out from under the skin. The two types of varicose veins include primary and secondary. Primary varicose veins occur as a congenital absence or malformation of the valves that have no other underlying etiology. Secondary varicose veins are veins that sustained acquired damage from an underlying disease, such as damage from a DVT, as in postphlebitic syndrome. Overweight women of increasing age with a family history of varicose veins are the most susceptible. Other contributing factors are professions that include standing and walking most of the day.[9]

Historically, the treatment for varicose veins was vein stripping, which involved making an incision to remove the vein. Current treatment involves less invasive procedures, including injections, lasers, and radiofrequency energy. Sclerotherapy is used for treating spider veins and small varicose veins; this involves the injection of a type of chemical or irritant foam into the vein to make it stick together, essentially ligating it to become a thread of connective tissue eventually. Foam sclerotherapy can be guided using sonography and has been shown to interact with the vein wall for a greater length of time, eliciting a vasospastic response to ligate the vein faster than liquid sclerotherapy. The foam creates tiny air bubbles, which increase the impedance mismatch, showing up better in a sonographic image. Laser therapy emits a specific wavelength of light to heat up the vein to the point of destruction. Radiofrequency involves emitting an energy to ligate the vein by shrinking it closed.[9]

Phlegmasia Cerulea Dolens

"Cerulea" means blue, which in this case refers to the color of the affected limb. Phlegmasia cerulea dolens (PCD) results from an uncommon but severe form of acute DVT, which is usually proximal, in the outflow area of the limb. Because the blood cannot leave the leg owing to a DVT, it pools and accumulates, causing the bluish tone of the limb. Other signs include a painful limb that is edematous. If left untreated, it can lead to venous gangrene, phlegmasia alba dolens, limb amputation, and death. There is a high risk of amputation and mortality with PCD. Because the lower extremity veins are capacitance vessels that hold a large portion of a person's blood supply, a large amount of blood is being taken out of circulation, which can cause circulatory failure and lead to shock and eventually death.[10]

PCD is more common in men and has a strong correlation in patients with a history of malignancy. Other risk factors include a hypercoagulable state, venous stasis, and contraceptive use. PCD can occur in conjunction with a pulmonary embolism. The left limb is usually affected. The fastest and most reliable modality to evaluate and diagnose PCD is duplex imaging. Sonographic findings would be very similar to DVT, but the patient's clinical history would have to be taken into consideration to help diagnose this rare condition.[10]

Phlegmasia Alba Dolens

"Alba" means white, which is the color of the affected limb. Phlegmasia alba dolens results from an untreated PCD, where the DVT is so massive that it compresses the adjacent artery. It causes the affected artery to vasospasm, or constrict. Because the artery is constricting, not enough blood can reach the limb, so it appears white. This condition is also rare, but it has a high amputation and mortality rate, as does PCD. In addition to a DVT, sonographic findings include the adjacent artery seen as deformed in shape, with a low color Doppler signal and an abnormal arterial waveform to demonstrate the arterial compromise.

May-Thurner syndrome

May-Thurner syndrome accounts for 2% to 23% of cases of lower extremity DVT cases. May-Thurner syndrome is also known as iliocaval compression syndrome. The syndrome comprises compression of the venous outflow that can cause a range of symptoms from mild to severe and has an increased risk of vascular complications. Most commonly, it manifests as compression of the left iliac vein between the right iliac artery and the spine or pelvic brim. This syndrome occurs more often in

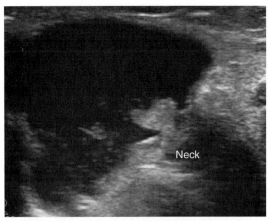

FIGURE 35-10 Image of hemorrhagic Baker's cyst demonstrating the neck that communicates with popliteal space. *(Courtesy Margaret D. Couture, RDCS, RVT.)*

young women, likely secondary to the wider pelvic brim and greater lumbosacral lordosis in that body region. It occurs more frequently on the left because of how the iliac arteries anatomically normally lie anterior and left of the veins. This is a fairly common condition, noted in about 33% of cadavers. The pressure on the iliac vein irritates the vein, causing intimal changes including fibrosis, stenosis, venous occlusion from weblike adhesions, and thrombosis. The weblike adhesions can act as a filter to help prevent pulmonary embolus. Intervention is currently recommended when femoral venous pressure increases 5 mmHg with exercise. Treatment includes anticoagulation, therapy, stents, and bypass grafts.[11]

DIFFERENTIAL DIAGNOSES

Alternative diagnoses are presented here with a brief explanation because these are often the most common causes of leg pain. The other reason is derived from Virchow's triad: venous stasis, trauma, and hypercoagulability. These conditions can make a patient less active, leading to venous stasis, the most significant portion of Virchow's triad. These differential diagnoses can be seen concomitantly with a DVT because they increase risk factors.

Baker's Cyst

For a patient with pain in the area of the popliteal fossa, the culprit may be a Baker's cyst, which is also known as a synovial cyst. This cyst has a high association in patients with concomitant rheumatoid arthritis, which is an autoimmune disease that attacks joints. Small Baker's cysts can be an incidental finding. They are not true cysts but a dilation of the bursa between the gastrocnemius and semimembranous tendon that are in communication with the knee joint. Acquiring the image of the communication validates this diagnosis (Fig. 35-10). These may hemorrhage or rupture, appearing complex on sonography.[12]

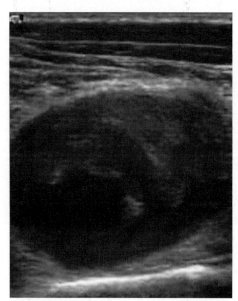

FIGURE 35-11 Large popliteal aneurysm.

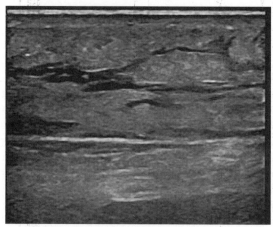

FIGURE 35-12 Cobblestone appearance of cellulitis. *(Courtesy Patrick A. Washko, BSRT, RDMS, RVT.)*

Aneurysm

A weakening in a vessel wall can cause an aneurysm. True aneurysms are classified as fusiform, saccular, and ruptured. A fusiform aneurysm is an overall dilation (Fig. 35-11), whereas a saccular aneurysm is a protruding sac. A ruptured aneurysm is an emergency and occurs when the wall is so weak and thin that it bursts open. These patients can become hypotensive quickly. A pseudoaneurysm, or false aneurysm, is usually iatrogenic in nature and is termed false because there is no vessel wall surrounding it; it is a break in the vessel wall.

Trauma and Hematoma

Sonographically, hematomas appear complex in nature. Because they are a collection of dried blood, they have no internal color Doppler and can be found in an area of trauma. Because trauma is a precursor to DVT, according to Virchow's triad, the patient may be monitored diligently to prevent a DVT. Compression stockings may be worn and the feet elevated to encourage blood flow to the heart.

Neuropathy

Neuropathy is found in many patients with diabetes mellitus. It is a condition of pain from damaged nerves. The nerve damage is chronic in nature caused by metabolic damage to the afferent neurons of the nerves. Symptoms include pain, numbness, and burning of the limbs.[13]

Sciatica

The largest nerve in the body is the sciatic nerve that runs posteriorly down the buttock into the back of the legs. Sciatica is pain radiating from the sciatic nerve. This pain can be caused by neuropathy of the nerve, a herniated disk in the lumbar spine, a trapped piriformis muscle, compression of the inferior gluteal artery, and trauma.

Congestive Heart Failure

A patient with CHF is in a state of volume overload. The heart cannot keep up with the demands of the body, and a backup in the IVC can occur. The IVC becomes dilated and loses respiratory variance; this also causes the veins of the lower extremity to lose respiratory phasicity. If the IVC continues to be dilated, it can transmit the cardiac pulsations down the IVC into the veins of the lower extremity. Sonographic findings of CHF include bilateral pulsatile veins in the lower extremity with a loss of respiratory variance.[14]

Cellulitis

Cellulitis is a bacterial infection of the skin and is common. Symptoms include pain and redness. It can be differentiated from DVT because redness secondary to a DVT is usually localized. Redness from cellulitis usually affects a significant portion of the leg. Significant edema can be visualized sonographically, and cellulitis has been described as having a cobblestone appearance (Fig. 35-12). Sonography can also identify abscess formation and guide needle aspiration, if needed.

Psoriasis

Psoriasis can range from mild to severe. It manifests as a generalized erythema, or redness, with shiny, silvery, thickened skin that flakes and peels easily. People with this condition have an increased growth of skin cells, leading to a buildup of drying and dead skin. It is usually seen in patients with a weakened immune system and can lead to a skin infection.

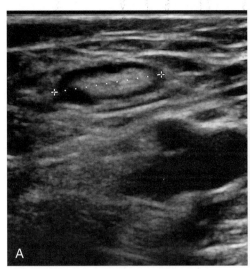
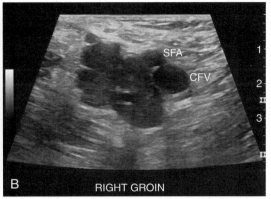

FIGURE 35-13 (A), Image of a normal-appearing lymph node showing the reniform shape with classic fatty hilum. This patient underwent knee surgery 4 days prior. **(B),** Multiple enlarged lymph nodes in the groin adjacent to the CFV. *((B), Courtesy Patrick A. Washko, BSRT, RDMS, RVT.)*

Lymphadenopathy

Lymphadenopathy is inflammation of the lymph nodes. Lymph nodes help to filter the body and are located in multiple areas throughout the body, including axilla, neck, abdomen, and groin. Lymph nodes in the groin may be identified when performing LEVD. Normal lymph nodes appear reniform in shape with an echogenic fatty hilum in the center (Fig. 35-13, *A*) and normally measure less than 1 cm. Some amount of internal flow may be seen that is increased with inflammation. Inflammation can be due to multiple etiologies that may include an infection or, less likely, cancer. An inflamed lymph node increases in size and appears round in shape with a loss of the fatty hilum (Fig. 35-13, *B*).

SYMPTOMS AND SEQUELAE

Symptoms and sequelae include the following:

Shortness of breath
Chest pain
Pulmonary embolism
Limb swelling or pain
Palpable "cord"
Edema
Venous hypertension
Stasis dermatitis
Venous ulcer
PCD
Phlegmasia alba dolens
Postthrombotic syndrome

TREATMENTS

Prevention

The best way to treat a DVT is with prevention. Because the part of Virchow's triad with the greatest impact is

venous stasis, it is best to use the calf venomotor pump fully to keep blood flowing. Elevating the lower extremities to aid gravity in getting venous blood back to the heart helps, as does compression stockings. Compression stockings keep the vein at a smaller diameter, pushing blood upward and not allowing it to pool into stasis dermatitis, which is a precursor to venous ulcers.[14]

Anticoagulation

Medications such as heparin are considered anticoagulants, or blood thinners. Although anticoagulants are a standard of care for acute DVT and are very effective in preventing a thrombus, these medications are not effective in dissolving an already formed thrombus. Bleeding becomes a major risk in patients taking anticoagulants.[14]

Thrombolytics

"Clot-busters," also known as thrombolytics or fibrinolytics, are medicines that effectively break up and dissolve thrombi to restore vessel patency. These medications work by activating fibrin to bind to plasminogen to create the active enzyme plasmin, which can dissolve blood clots. Thrombolytics leave less residual thrombus and aid in the prevention of postphlebitic syndromes. The first "clot-buster" was streptokinase. The next generation was urokinase. Newer thrombolytics or fibrinolytics include tissue plasminogen activator. These agents can be administered systemically or locally with catheter-directed administration. Although fibrinolytics are a treatment for DVT to achieve patency, they have not been proven to reduce risk of venous thromboembolism or pulmonary embolism. Bleeding becomes a major risk in patients receiving thrombolytics.[15]

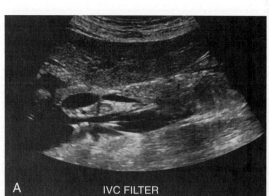
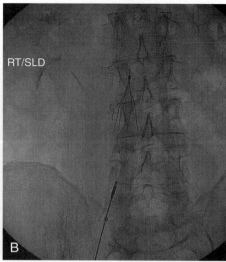

FIGURE 35-14 (A), Image of a filter in the IVC. **(B),** Radiograph confirms the placement of IVC filter. *(Courtesy Patrick A. Washko, BSRT, RDMS, RVT.)*

Thrombectomy

Removal of a clot is termed a thrombectomy. Ways to remove a thrombus include percutaneous mechanical thrombectomy and pharmacomechanical thrombolysis. Historically, a patient had to undergo a surgical thrombectomy. With newer advances in technology, less invasive methods exist. With percutaneous mechanical thrombectomy, the thrombus can be mechanically removed via a catheter inserted into the CFV. This procedure macerates the thrombus and suctions it away and can be used along with medicines to prevent clot formation, as in pharmacomechanical thrombolyis.[15]

Inferior Vena Cava Filter

For patients with venous thromboembolism, a filter can be placed in the IVC to filter clots and allow the body time to break them up before blocking the arteries of the lungs. IVC filters are also indicated in patients in whom anticoagulants are contraindicated and patients with recurrent venous thromboembolism. These filters are typically placed with imaging guidance and percutaneously placed in the IVC infrarenally. IVC filters can be either temporary or permanent.[16]

Intravascular ultrasound (IVUS) is an emerging technology that can aid in the placement of IVC filters. IVUS uses a catheter with an ultrasound transducer on the tip and can image a vessel from the inside. IVUS has been found to correlate with the current "gold standard" of angiography. IVUS can evaluate the severity of vessel disease without prolonged radiation exposure, nephrotoxic contrast agents, and potential allergic reactions, which are advantages of IVUS over angiography. This technology can be used to place the IVC filter, which appears echogenic on sonographic evaluation (Fig. 35-14, *A*).

The patient undergoes LEVD to confirm vein patency before the procedure, which requires puncture of the CFV and the filter to be fed up to the IVC, which can also be visualized on a radiograph (Fig. 35-14, *B*). IVUS was found to be effective in identifying vein confluences with the IVC, accurately measuring lumen diameter of the IVC, and identifying any thrombus in the IVC. Identification of the renal veins is important because proper placement of the filter should be infrarenal.[16]

Surgery, Balloon Dilation, and Stents

If a DVT persisted despite medical treatment, historically the patient had to undergo surgical bypass reconstruction. Now, with the advent of balloon dilations and stents, treatment is much less invasive. A venous balloon dilation involves introducing a catheter into a vein near the groin and feeding it through the venous system to the obstruction. The deflated balloon on the end is pushed through, and the balloon is quickly inflated, manually relieving the obstruction. A stent can also be placed via catheter to keep the vessel patent. Some stents release anticoagulants to prevent further obstruction.[17]

SUMMARY

Vascular leg pain is a serious symptom. Venous vascular disease has a high mortality rate because of pulmonary embolism. A complete and thorough patient history is crucial in effective sequencing of examinations. When sequenced properly, sonography is a quick and effective method of determining vascular causes of leg pain. Sonographic evaluation of the lower extremity veins has proven to be an effective method of determining not only the presence but also the age of thrombus within the deep venous system.

CLINICAL SCENARIO—DIAGNOSIS

This 45-year-old man with a sedentary lifestyle is already at an increased risk because of lack of the calf venomotor compressions during the day to push blood back up to the heart. The leg pain 1 week ago was most likely due to a DVT that was ignored. As the patient continued his activities of daily life, movement dislodged the clot, either fully or partially, and it traveled up into the IVC and into the right side of the heart, lodging in between the right and left pulmonary arteries. Emboli that are seen at the end of the main pulmonary artery at the bifurcation of the right and left pulmonary arteries are termed "saddle" emboli because they appear to be sitting, or saddling that

area. Patients with a pulmonary embolus often experience chest pain, shortness of breath, and hemoptysis. The patient's blood pressure of 115/72 mmHg, although normal, is not normal for a noncompliant patient with a history of hypertension, so the embolus was causing this patient to head toward hypotensiveness. After the patient was treated for the pulmonary embolus, the clinician ordered LEVD to identify if possible the origin of the pulmonary embolus, which was located in the right popliteal vein. Various treatment options for this patient include anticoagulants, thrombolytics, IVC filter, and serial LEVD to monitor therapy effectiveness.

CASE STUDIES FOR DISCUSSION

1. A 52-year-old woman with a painful left leg is seen by her physician. Physical examination reveals a red swollen leg with "tough cords" running just below the skin surface. B-mode examination shows dilated, superficial vessels filled with low-level echoes. These vessels are identified as superficial because their course lies within the first fascial plane. The deep veins of the upper and lower leg are compressible and show normal flow without evidence of internal thrombus. What is the most likely diagnosis?

2. A 32-year-old woman presents to the emergency department with excruciating right lower extremity pain for the past 3 hours. Patient history includes a morbid increase in body habitus, sedentary lifestyle, and mild to moderate right lower extremity pain for the past week that has gotten much worse within the past 3 hours. The clinician notes a bluish tinge to the massively enlarged leg. Her toes and foot are becoming increasingly white. What is the most likely diagnosis?

3. A 39-year-old man presents for a bilateral LEVD for leg pain that has persisted for the past month. Patient history includes diabetes mellitus, hypertension, and hyperlipidemia. This patient is noncompliant and does not take medications, including insulin, as directed. Sonographic findings included fully compressible veins bilaterally with adequate color Doppler. Pulsed wave Doppler revealed

halting proximal compressions with an augmented distal compression bilaterally. What is the most likely diagnosis?

4. A 63-year-old man presents to the emergency department with bilateral lower extremity edema and shortness of breath. Patient history is limited because of lack of medical records, and he appears very confused. Sonographic findings for bilateral LEVD revealed fully compressible veins bilaterally, with adequate color Doppler. Pulsed wave Doppler revealed halting proximal compressions with an augmented distal compression bilaterally. Pulsed wave imaging also noted a lack of respiratory phasicity with very pulsatile veins bilaterally. What is the most likely diagnosis?

5. A 42-year-old man presents to the emergency department for right lower extremity pain and edema. Patient history includes smoking 3 packs of cigarettes per day, alcohol abuse, and diabetes. He is noncompliant in his diabetes monitoring and treatment, partly because he is homeless. Right LEVD revealed intraluminal echoes in the proximal femoral vein with lack of color flow, which were difficult to identify, and a noncompressible trifurcation that is small and hyperechoic. Proximal compressions revealed that blood flow could not be halted. On locating difficult-to-identify intraluminal echoes in the proximal femur, distal compressions were ceased. What is this patient's most likely diagnosis?

STUDY QUESTIONS

1. A 62-year-old man presents to the emergency department with chest pain and sudden onset of shortness of breath. Findings of a bilateral lower extremity Doppler reveal noncompressible veins from the CFV to popliteal vein. Intraluminal echogenic matter is very difficult to visualize. Doppler signals are lacking as well. What is the most likely diagnosis?
   a. Acute DVT
   b. Chronic DVT
   c. Baker's cyst
   d. Venous reflux

2. An 84-year-old woman presents for a bilateral LEVD for pain posterior to the right knee for 6 months. The patient has bilateral ankle edema; she denies any chest pain or shortness of breath. Each vein appears

compressible, with no intraluminal echogenic matter seen. Color Doppler appears adequate. Pulsed wave Doppler reveals pulsatile veins bilaterally. A complex area was noted in the popliteal fossa that measured 5.4 cm × 3.7 cm × 4.0 cm. What is the most likely diagnosis?
   a. Chronic DVT with CHF
   b. Baker's cyst
   c. Baker's cyst with CHF
   d. Chronic DVT

3. An 18-year-old pregnant woman presents to the emergency department with bilateral lower extremity pain for the past 2 days. Sonographic findings include fully compressible veins with adequate color Doppler signals. Proximal compression halts blood flow, whereas the distal compression demonstrates adequate augmentation. Pulsed wave

Doppler reveals monophasic waveforms down the entire lower extremities bilaterally. What is the most likely diagnosis?
a. Acute DVT
b. Iliac vein thrombosis
c. IVC obstruction
d. Chronic SVT

4. A 54-year-old man presents to the emergency department with a large, weepy ulcer on his right lower extremity. The clinician notices stasis dermatitis with pitting edema in the right gaiter zone. The patient denies any chest pain or shortness of breath. Sonographic findings include fully compressible veins, demonstrating adequate color Doppler flow. Proximal compression cannot halt blood flow, but distal compression yields augmentation. What is the most likely diagnosis?
a. Acute DVT
b. Chronic DVT
c. May-Thurner syndrome
d. Venous insufficiency

5. A 51-year-old man with ankle pain for the last 4 years presents for an outpatient left LEVD. The patient does not appear to have any edema, stasis dermatitis, or varicose veins. He states that his ankle has been hurting since a fall from a ladder 4 years ago. The patient is still very active despite the pain. Sonographic findings include a fully compressible CFV, proximal GSV, and femoral vein. Color Doppler reveals adequate blood flow with normal pulsed wave Doppler signals. The sonographer is trying to compress the popliteal vein but cannot. No intraluminal echogenic matter can be seen within the popliteal vein, and Doppler reveals normal signals. What should the sonographer do next?
a. Change sonographic window
b. Note acute DVT
c. Note chronic DVT
d. Have the patient perform a Valsalva maneuver

6. A 23-year-old woman with a morbid increase in body habitus complains of left lower extremity pain with swelling and edema. During the examination, she becomes short of breath with hemoptysis. Sonographic findings include a dilated femoral vein with walls that do not coapt on extrinsic transducer pressure. The lumen of the vessel demonstrates echogenic matter that is difficult to visualize. Doppler signals are absent. What is the most likely diagnosis?
a. May-Thurner syndrome
b. PCD
c. Phlegmasia alba dolens
d. Pulmonary embolus

7. A 34-year-old woman who is 4 hours postpartum complains of sudden onset of left lower extremity pain. Clinical history reveals she has experienced left lower extremity pain for the past 7 years. Left LEVD reveals fully compressible veins and no intraluminal echogenic matter with an adequate color Doppler signal. On pulsed wave Doppler, proximal compressions fully halt blood flow, and distal compression demonstrates a good augment. However, Doppler reveals a dampened waveform down the entire left lower extremity. What is the most likely diagnosis?
a. May-Thurner syndrome
b. PCD
c. Phlegmasia alba dolens
d. Superficial thrombophlebitis

8. A 61-year-old man presents to the emergency department for severe leg pain and generalized erythema, or redness. Silvery, scaly skin that is severely flaking is noted bilaterally from the lower abdomen to the toes. Patient history revealed that he is currently undergoing chemotherapy treatments. LEVD appeared negative for any echogenic matter. What is the most likely diagnosis?
a. Cellulitis
b. CHF
c. Phlegmasia alba dolens
d. Psoriasis

9. A 23-year-old man arrived by ambulance to the emergency department from a motorcycle accident 4 days ago. Portable left LEVD revealed dilated proximal femoral vein with slow-moving flow seen. Intraluminal hypoechoic matter was located in the left popliteal vein, extending down to the distal posterior tibial vein. What is the most likely treatment?
a. Anticoagulants
b. Fibrinolytics
c. Foam sclerotherapy
d. Vein stripping

10. A 22-year-old man with an extensive history of DVT with pulmonary emboli presents to his primary care physician to follow up a hospital stay because of DVT. What is the most likely treatment the physician will prescribe in an attempt to prevent future DVT?
a. Anticoagulants
b. Fibrinolytics
c. Vein stripping
d. Venous bypass

REFERENCES

1. Rubin JM, Xie H, Kim K, et al: Sonographic elasticity imaging of acute and chronic deep venous thrombosis in humans, *J Ultrasound Med* 25:1179, 2006.

2. Kumar DR, Hanlin ER, Glurich I, et al: Virchow's contribution to the understanding of thrombosis and cellular biology, *Clin Med Res* 8:168, 2010.

3. Faitelson IA, Jakobsons EE: Aggregation of erythrocytes into columnar structures ("rouleaux") and the rheology of blood, *J Eng Physics Thermophys* 76:214, 2003.

4. Lin EP, Bhatt S, Rubens D, et al: The importance of monophasic Doppler waveforms in the common femoral vein, *J Ultrasound Med* 26:885, 2007.

5. Society for Vascular Ultrasound: *Vascular Technology Professional Performance Guidelines: Lower Extremity Venous Duplex Evaluation*, Lanham, MD, 2011, Society for Vascular Ultrasound.

6. Litzendorf ME, Satiani B: Superficial venous thrombosis: disease progression and evolving treatment approaches, *Vasc Health Risk Manage* 7:569, 2011.

7. Garrison KL: Sonographic evaluation of venous insufficiency and sonography-guided radiofrequency ablation of the great saphenous vein, *J Diagn Med Sonogr* 23:272, 2007.

8. Corrao D, Schultz SM: Lower extremity sonography detects complex mass, *J Diagn Med Sonogr* 19:114, 2003.

9. Kompally GR, Bharadwaj S, Singh G: Varicose veins: clinical presentation and surgical management, *Ind J Surg* 71:117, 2009.

10. Chinsakchai K, ten Duis K, Moll FL, et al: Trends in management of phlegmasia cerulea dolens, *Vasc Endovasc Surg* 45:5, 2011.

11. Sulzdorf L: May-Thurner syndrome presenting with venous claudication, *J Diagn Med Sonogr* 22:243, 2006.

12. Boodt CL: Infected popliteal (Baker's) cyst, *J Diagn Med Sonogr* 24:233, 2008.

13. Koroschetz J, Rehm S, Gockel U, et al: Fibromyalgia and neuropathic pain—differences and similarities: a comparison of 3057 patients with diabetic painful neuropathy and fibromyalgia, *BMC Neurol* 11:55, 2011.

14. Abbas M, Yahya MM, Hamilton M, et al: Sonographic evaluation of chronic venous insufficiency in right heart failure, *J Diagn Med Sonogr* 21:238, 2005.

15. Lensing WA, Prandoni P, Prins MH, et al: Deep vein thrombosis, *Lancet* 353:479, 1999.

16. Davenport DL, Xenos ES: Early outcomes and risk factors in venous thrombectomy: an analysis of the American College of Surgeons NSQIP dataset, *Vasc Endovasc Surg* 45:325, 2011.

17. Kassavin DS, Constantinopoulos G: The transition to IVUS-guided IVC filter deployment in the nontrauma patient, *Vasc Endovasc Surg* 45:142, 2011.

Claudication: Peripheral Arterial Disease

Rebecca Madery, Nicole Strissel

CLINICAL SCENARIO

A 35-year-old man presents to the emergency department in mid-January in the upper Midwest. The patient complains of severe left foot pain, which is intermittently accompanied by numbness and tingling. The patient states he has experienced some leg pain during exercise over the past year but notes the pain is especially intense while he is resting, and the pain has progressed as the weather has grown colder. His pain is not relieved by over-the-counter pain medication. On physical examination, both feet display pallor, are cool to the touch, and have diminished pulses. The left fifth digit is also noted to have a small, painful sore, which he attributes to "breaking in new shoes." The patient leads an active lifestyle and, aside from his feet, appears in overall good health. He admits to occasional alcohol use and smokes about one pack of cigarettes per day over the past 10 years.

A physiologic, noninvasive lower extremity arterial study is ordered. During the continuous wave Doppler examination, the vascular technologist notes biphasic signals in the common femoral artery, superficial femoral artery, and popliteal artery. Slightly reduced but patent flow is also detected in the posterior tibial artery at the medial malleolus. Distal phalanx flow studies do not demonstrate detectable arterial Doppler tracings in the left second, fourth, and fifth digits. The first and third distal phalanges demonstrate reduced, monophasic flow. Temperatures are 21° C in the second, fourth, and fifth digits with no postwarming increase. What is the most likely diagnosis?

OBJECTIVES

- Identify anatomic landmarks for proper vessel identification in the calf.
- Differentiate between various causes of arterial disease in the leg.
- State symptoms associated with arterial disease.
- Describe the duplex Doppler and indirect physiologic studies that can be used to detect arterial disease of the lower extremity.

- Describe the sonographic appearance of arterial disease in the lower extremity.
- Characterize Doppler waveforms associated with arterial disease.

This chapter describes various causes of arterial disease in the leg and the role of sonography and other vascular testing in diagnosing these diseases. Specific protocols may vary depending on the vascular laboratory. This chapter focuses on general protocols and expected Doppler waveforms associated with each disease. A brief explanation of normal anatomy is included, but the focus is on the pathology, waveforms, and risk factors that lead to arterial disease.

For the lower extremity, gray-scale, spectral, and color Doppler imaging and indirect physiologic testing are used to diagnose vascular causes of leg pain in the noninvasive vascular laboratory. Some of the arterial pathologies diagnosed sonographically include atherosclerosis obliterans (ASO), pseudoaneurysm, arteriovenous fistula (AVF), and compartment and entrapment syndromes.

NORMAL VASCULAR ANATOMY

Lower extremity arteries are accompanied by a single vein or, distal to the popliteal artery, paired veins with the same name. Most of the anatomy can be well visualized on most patients with a 6 to 9 MHz linear transducer. Imaging of the distal aorta and iliac arteries requires the use of a curvilinear transducer with frequencies ranging from 3 to 6 MHz. Starting at the aortic bifurcation and working distally to the foot, a normal artery gradually tapers as it gives rise to branches until it terminates as an arteriole.

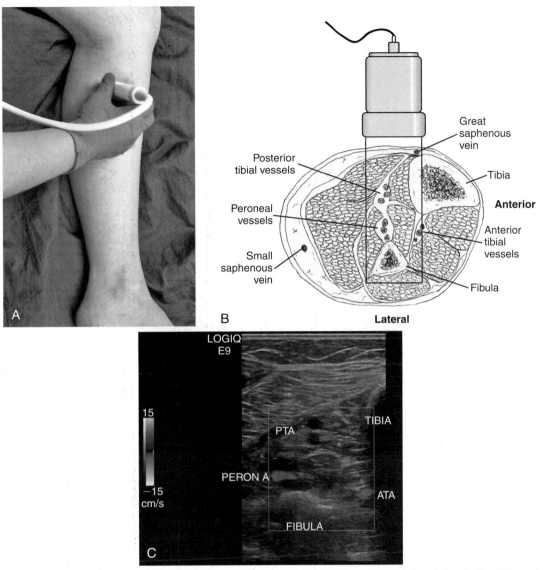

FIGURE 36-1 (A), Approach used to scan the left calf vessels. **(B),** Cross section of the calf vessels in relation to the tibia and fibula. From a medial approach, the posterior tibial artery is the most superficial, and the peroneal artery lies just above the fibula. Occasionally, the anterior tibial artery is visualized between the tibia and the fibula. **(C),** Sonographic cross-sectional (transverse) image of the calf vessels. Note the relationship of the vessels to the tibia and fibula (see Color Plate 55).

The common iliac arteries originate at the level of the umbilicus from the aortic bifurcation and bifurcate into the external and internal (hypogastric) iliac arteries. The hypogastric artery branches deep into the pelvis to perfuse the sigmoid colon, rectum, and reproductive organs. The external iliac artery continues through the pelvis to become the common femoral artery at the inguinal canal, which bifurcates into the deep femoral artery (profunda) and femoral artery. At the level of the adductor canal, the femoral artery becomes the popliteal artery as it courses posterior to the knee and bifurcates into the anterior tibial artery and the tibioperoneal trunk. The anterior tibial artery branches anteriorly and laterally, passing through the space formed between the tibia and fibula then lateral to the tibial shaft where it eventually terminates on the dorsal side of the foot as the dorsalis pedis artery. The tibioperoneal trunk bifurcates into the posterior tibial

artery and peroneal (fibular) artery. From a medial scanning approach, the posterior tibial artery continues more superficially than the peroneal artery, which runs deeper and lies just medial to the fibula. (Fig. 36-1; see Color Plate 55). Arteries of the ankle and foot commonly used for Doppler samples or pulses include the posterior tibial, which can be found about 1 inch posterior to the medial malleolus, and the dorsalis pedis, which is found in the anterior midfoot just over the proximal third metatarsal.

SYMPTOMS AND TESTING

Claudication

Claudication, or intermittent claudication, is defined by repetitive cramping, aching, and pain a patient experiences, especially during exercise, with cessation of

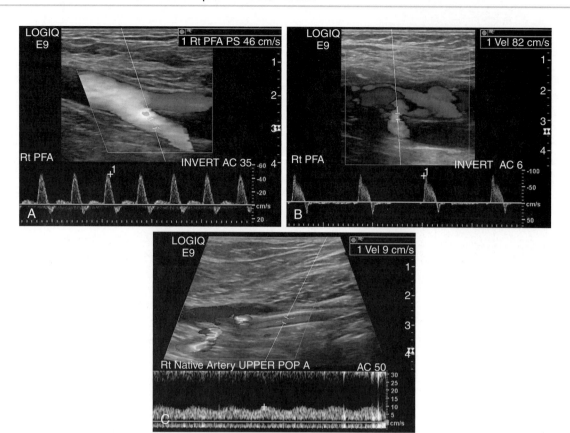

FIGURE 36-2 (A), Normal triphasic signal in the profunda femoris artery *(PFA)* of a healthy individual. **(B),** Biphasic tracing in the profunda femoris artery. The biphasic signal implies a loss of normal elasticity in the vessel wall, which is an early sign of atheromatous disease. **(C),** Monophasic tardus-parvus waveform seen in the popliteal artery *(POP A)* distal to a significant stenosis in the femoral artery.

symptoms on rest. Typically, patients have a set distance they can travel before needing to stop and rest and then can continue with movement. If left untreated, this condition progresses to a severe condition known as rest pain. Symptoms of rest pain are similar to claudication and persist during periods of inactivity. Rest pain can be alleviated by placing the foot in a dependent position, which allows gravity to aid in distal limb perfusion (i.e., tilt the cart in a reverse Trendelenburg position when possible).

Claudication is caused by various factors. Arterial diseases include, but are not limited to, ASO, popliteal entrapment, arterial embolus, and aneurysmal disease. Other nonarterial causes that may mimic arterial disease include vein disease such as deep venous thrombosis, spine-related conditions, pulled muscles, tendinitis, trauma, fibromyalgia, and other musculoskeletal conditions.

Vascular Test Findings. Diagnostic examinations used in assessing lower limb arterial disease include physiologic nonimaging vascular studies (segmental pressures, ankle-brachial index [ABI], pulse volume recording [PVR]), sonography, computed tomography angiography, magnetic resonance angiography, and angiography. To include or rule out vascular claudication as a differential diagnosis, the first examination is typically a physiologic test involving continuous wave Doppler and segmental pressures before and after exercise. Using

continuous wave Doppler, the patient should have a qualitative analysis of the common femoral artery, femoral artery, popliteal artery, posterior tibial artery, and dorsalis pedis artery to determine if the blood flow is triphasic, biphasic, or monophasic in nature (Fig. 36-2). To determine the approximate level of disease, segmental pressures and/or PVR's should be taken. Normally, the pressure gradient between adjacent cuffs, or at the same level on the contralateral extremity, does not exceed 20 mm Hg. A pressure gradient greater than 30 mm Hg is indicative of a significant obstruction between or beneath the cuffs.[1] Segmental pressures are taken by measuring blood pressures from the thigh, calf, and ankle (three-cuff method) and comparing that number with the highest brachial pressure (both arms should be assessed unless contraindicated). A four-cuff method may also be used with two cuffs placed on the thigh with the awareness that the cuff closest to the groin may be artificially elevated because of the discrepancy in cuff size and thigh circumference.

An ABI can be used if a quick study is necessary or for follow-up of a prior physiologic test. A normal ABI ratio generally is 0.90 to 1.40. An ABI ratio less than 0.90 is considered abnormal; however, individuals with values between 0.90 and 1.10 and greater than 1.40 may be at a slightly higher risk for disease.[1] After baseline values have been obtained, the patient should exercise (at the prescribed protocol of that vascular laboratory) and the ABI measurements should be repeated. Patients presenting with a normal ABI may unmask arterial disease after exercise due to the increased demand for blood in the working extremity. The ABI should increase or remain constant in a normal extremity. If pressures decrease significantly but return within 2 to 6 minutes, single-level disease should be considered. However, a significant decrease in pressures after exercise for 10 minutes is highly suggestive of multilevel disease. Symptoms of claudication are not likely to be vascular in origin if they do not correlate with a decrease in pressures.

If sonographic imaging is requested, assessment of the lower extremity arteries from the common femoral artery to the dorsalis pedis artery should be performed. Careful attention should be paid to the vessel walls in gray-scale and the flow patterns and waveforms in color and spectral Doppler imaging. Sonographic findings associated with arterial disease are discussed in further detail throughout the chapter.

Pseudoclaudication

Patients with pseudoclaudication can present with symptoms similar to claudication, but the symptoms are not as reproducible as true vascular claudication; leg pain may occur while the patient is sitting or standing still rather than during exercise. The indirect, nonimaging vascular test with exercise can verify whether or not vascular disease is the source of the symptoms. In the absence of arterial disease, waveforms do not display significant variation in either velocity or shape after exercise.

ARTERIAL DISEASE

Atherosclerosis

Peripheral arterial disease is the process in which arteries become narrowed and impede blood flow to the limbs, generally the lower extremities. Arteriosclerosis is a general term describing the hardening of arterial walls and the associated loss of elasticity. Arteriosclerosis results in a reduced arterial lumen and, ultimately, decreases blood pressure and flow to the distal limb or organ. A stenosis is considered hemodynamically significant if there is a 50% reduction in diameter or a 75% reduction in cross-sectional area.[2] The most common cause of arteriosclerosis is atherosclerosis (ASO). ASO is the result of increased fatty deposits (atheromatous plaque) along the arterial walls. Patients may experience various symptoms depending on the severity of the disease ranging from asymptomatic to debilitating distal ulcerations and eventual limb loss.

Sonographic Findings. The sonographic appearance of ASO in both gray-scale and color Doppler imaging includes thickened arterial walls and a decreased vessel diameter secondary to atheromatous plaque bulging into the lumen. To support color and gray-scale findings, an angle-corrected spectral Doppler cursor should be placed proximal, at, and distal to the area of visual narrowing. It is generally accepted that a stenosis is hemodynamically significant if the peak systolic velocity doubles between a diseased segment and the normal area just proximal to the disease. Waveforms may show signs of spectral broadening and a loss of normal triphasic or biphasic flow patterns. In severe cases of claudication, arteries may be occluded. To demonstrate an occlusion sonographically, gray-scale imaging should show thrombus or calcified plaque within the arterial lumen, while color and spectral Doppler will demonstrate an absence of flow. Because of the confusing nature of collateral arteries that are typical in ASO cases, it is helpful to use the corresponding veins as landmarks when identifying the occluded arteries. It is necessary to document the absence or presence of flow below the occluded segment because it can change the possible treatment for the patient (i.e., a good distal arterial segment is needed for a bypass graft).

Popliteal Aneurysm

An aneurysm is a localized bulging or focal enlargement of a vessel by approximately 50%; the popliteal artery is the most common location for a peripheral aneurysm to occur.[3] The accepted measurement criterion for a popliteal artery aneurysm is 1.5 to 2.0 cm. However, because the normal popliteal artery diameter measures from 0.4 to 0.9 cm, several studies suggest that, in correlation with an increased diameter of 50%, a focal area of 1.0 cm may be considered an aneurysm if the normal arterial diameter is 0.6 cm.[3] Isolated aneurysms are rare in the iliac and femoral arteries. Lower extremity aneurysms increase the patient's risk of having an abdominal aortic aneurysm. Close monitoring is necessary as significant risks are associated with lower extremity aneurysms including: distal embolization, acute occlusion and rupture.

Sonographic Findings. A common indication for sonography is a palpable lump behind the knee on physical examination. Gray-scale imaging should be used to obtain accurate outer wall-to-outer wall longitudinal and transverse measurements. Color Doppler imaging can be used to determine luminal flow and to depict hypoechoic mural thrombus. Spectral Doppler demonstrates blood flow quantity and quality (i.e., triphasic, biphasic, monophasic). It is common to see turbulent flow within the aneurysm. During gray-scale surveillance of the artery, it is important to consider a popliteal cyst (Baker's cyst) as a diagnosis because of its close proximity to the artery. A cyst does not demonstrate any flow by color or spectral Doppler.

Pseudoaneurysm

A pseudoaneurysm is a collection of fluid extending off an artery by a communicating channel or neck. Patients typically present with a pulsatile mass and bruising after an interventional procedure, trauma, surgery, or infection.

Sonographic Findings. Examination requires interrogation of the mass in gray-scale, color, and spectral Doppler. A saccular defect adjacent to the artery is visualized with a swirling flow pattern (often referred to as the "yin-yang" sign) and a neck connecting directly to the artery (Fig. 36-3, *A* and *B*; see Color Plate 56, *A* and *B*). Spectral Doppler of the neck reveals a to-and-fro waveform and elevated velocities (Fig. 36-3, *C*). If a pseudoaneurysm does not spontaneously thrombose, maintaining pressure with the transducer or injecting thrombin near the neck promotes coagulation and eventual resolution.

Arteriovenous Fistula

An AVF is an anomalous communication directly between an artery and a vein. An AVF can be a congenital defect, intentionally created to use for dialysis, or the result of trauma or iatrogenic injuries (i.e., a puncture wound involving an artery and vein).

Sonographic Findings. When imaged with color Doppler, an AVF often displays a ghosting artifact, or tissue thrill, from high-pressure flow coursing throughout the vein (Fig. 36-4, *A*; see Color Plate 57). The waveforms

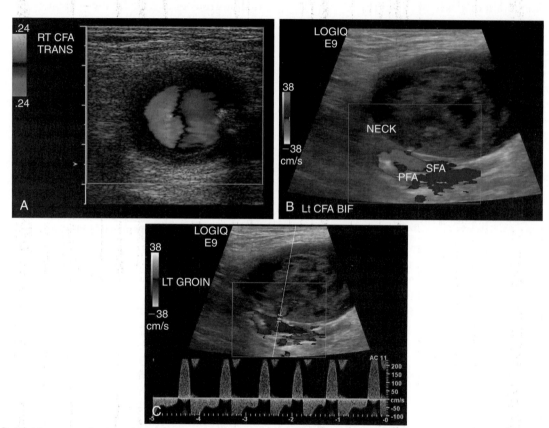

FIGURE 36-3 **(A)**, Yin-yang color Doppler flow pattern seen in aneurysms of the native vessels or within a pseudoaneurysm (see Color Plate 56, A). **(B)**, Pseudoaneurysm with evidence of internal thrombus formation and a visible neck connecting to the superficial femoral artery *(SFA)* (see Color Plate 56, B). **(C)**, To-and-fro spectral waveform is an important sign in diagnosing a pseudoaneurysm.

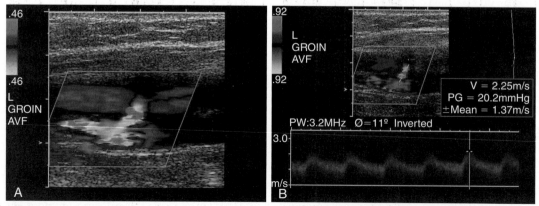

FIGURE 36-4 **(A)**, AVF with clear communication between the artery and vein. Also supporting the diagnosis is the presence of a tissue bruit as is evident by the ghosting, or flash artifact in color Doppler (see Color Plate 57). **(B)**, Low-resistive, high-velocity waveform typically found within an AVF. The waveform continues into the outflow vein above the AVF.

associated with an AVF are low resistance and high velocity in the artery just proximal to the fistula, within the fistula, and in the outflow vein above the fistula (Fig. 36-4, *B*). It is also necessary to document patency and waveforms of the native arteries distal to the AVF to ensure the extremity is adequately perfused. Waveforms in the native artery distal to an AVF demonstrate much slower velocities and may revert back to a normal triphasic signal.

Popliteal Entrapment Syndrome

Popliteal entrapment syndrome is a rare arterial cause of intermittent claudication that generally occurs in young, athletic patients. Typically, it is caused by external compression of the popliteal artery by the medial head of the gastrocnemius muscle. Magnetic resonance imaging is the standard for determining the anatomy causing the compression; however, sonography and indirect testing using a hand-held continuous wave Doppler can be used to verify the severity of the entrapment.

Sonographic Findings. During sonographic examination, the distal portion of the popliteal artery should be located in the longitudinal position. Spectral Doppler should be performed in the neutral, dorsiflexion (toes are pulled back toward the shin), and plantar flexion (toes pointed) positions with angle-corrected, peak systolic velocities recorded. Additional workload can be placed on the muscles by having a second technologist available to pull or push on the foot. With continuous wave Doppler studies, flow should be assessed at both the posterior tibial artery in the ankle and the dorsalis pedis artery in the foot. Diminished or absent waveforms with exercise indicate a positive finding. Care should be taken to ensure the sample volume has not fallen from the artery during manipulation of the foot.

Compartment Syndrome

Compartment syndrome results from nerves, blood vessels, and muscle within a focused area (compartment) of the body being compressed, typically, the forearm or lower leg. Each compartment is separated by thick, rigid fascial tissue. If swelling is present, the inflexibility of the fascia increases pressure, which may impede blood flow and lead to tissue death and possibly require limb amputation. Acute onset of the disease is extremely painful and commonly associated with trauma and swelling of the components within the fascial layers. Chronic disease can be a result of repetitive motions such as running.

Sonographic Findings. Occasionally, sonography is requested to assess blood flow within the diseased area. However, the definitive test for compartment syndrome uses a needle connected to a pressure meter placed into the area of concern. Associated Doppler waveforms would be high resistive proximal to and within the affected area with the potential for diminished flow as well.

Bypass Grafts and Stents

Graft or stent failure is a serious complication that can potentially lead to limb amputation. Assessment of the lower extremity arterial system after the procedure can be performed with both physiologic vascular studies and imaging examinations. Combining the two studies allows for a physiologic examination and the ability to assess accurately the anastomotic sites and surrounding areas for fluid collections, infections, and stenoses developing after the procedure. A major contributing factor to graft and stent failure is a stenosis that develops within the treated area or graft.

When beginning a bypass graft or stent examination, it is important to research the surgical history of the patient. Items to consider include the anastomosis sites, type of anastomosis (end-to-side or side-to-side), and the type of graft material used (vein or synthetic). Vein grafts are autogenous to the patient and can be difficult to distinguish from the native artery if anastomosed in an end-to-end fashion. If a reversed vein graft is used, it is common to note a size discrepancy between the native artery and graft at the distal anastomosis. Synthetic grafts are typically made of polytetrafluoroethylene and are easily differentiated from native vessels. If an adequate segment is available, vein grafts are generally preferred over synthetic because they have a more successful rate of long-term patency.[4]

Sonographic Findings. When surveying a bypass graft or stent, it is necessary to rule out any pathology that may inhibit flow and lead to graft failure. Patency should be documented in the native artery proximal to the anastomosis, in the proximal anastomosis (Fig. 36-5, *A*), throughout the graft or stent, in the distal anastomosis (Fig. 36-5, *B*; see Color Plate 58), and in the native artery beyond the anastomosis. Backflow into the native vessel proximal to the distal anastomosis may also be visualized but is of minimal clinical significance. Graft failure within the first month of surgery often occurs because of surgical defects or in patients with a poor prognosis before intervention. Beyond the first month, vein graft failure can be attributed to intimal hyperplasia caused by the increased arterial pressure on the venous wall. Although a stenosis of the graft or stent may occur at any point, it is most commonly seen at the end points or anastomoses. A stenosis associated with a graft after 12 months is likely due to progression of atheromatous disease in the native vessels above and below the graft. Waveforms within a graft or stent also vary depending on the age of the graft. A recent repair may have monophasic flow as the surrounding, hyperemic tissue heals from the intervention. As time progresses and with the absence of complications, the waveforms should eventually become biphasic or triphasic. Slightly elevated velocities within a stent are expected because of the narrowed lumen compared with the native vessel surrounding it.

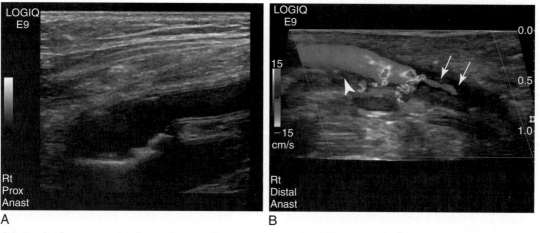

FIGURE 36-5 **(A)**, Proximal anastomosis of a synthetic graft to the native vessel. **(B)**, Distal anastomosis of a vein graft to the smaller caliber native vessel *(arrows)*. Note the normal finding of backflow into the native vessel *(arrowhead)* (see Color Plate 58).

It is also imperative to document and follow any postsurgical fluid collections surrounding a graft. Common fluid collections include seromas, hematomas, and graft infections. The relationship to the graft of a suspected infectious fluid collection should be documented because it may lead to eventual breakdown of the anastomosis and severe bleeding from the site. Graft infections are difficult to treat, and graft removal is the only means to remedy the infection in some cases.

Raynaud's Disease

Raynaud's phenomenon, or disease, consists of two types: primary and secondary. Primary Raynaud's disease implies no underlying condition exists, and secondary Raynaud's disease is a result of an underlying condition such as a connective tissue disorder. Primary Raynaud's disease occurs when the small arteries in the distal extremities go into vasospasm, preventing adequate blood flow. It is the body's extreme reaction to certain conditions, primarily a cold climate or stress, and tends to be more noticeable in the upper extremity but can also occur in the lower extremity. The color changes in the fingers and toes follow the same pattern: white (ischemic), blue (cyanotic), and red (rubor). The patient may also experience pain, tingling, and swelling. In very extreme cases, ulceration and gangrene can result. This condition is more likely to occur in women.

Vascular Test Findings. The upper extremity is easier to test than the lower extremity, so most protocols focus testing on the fingers. Continuous wave Doppler and segmental pressures in the arms should be used to verify adequate flow in the larger arteries and rule out any occlusive disease, followed by a more specific test for Raynaud's disease testing digital pressures and a temperature response test. When performing a temperature response test, baseline photoplethysmography, digital pressure, and temperature of each digit are obtained. Individual laboratory protocols may vary, but generally

when the fingers are warmer than 30° C, they should be immersed to the wrist for 30 seconds in a closely monitored ice bath. The hands should be removed and temperatures repeated immediately at 1 minute, 5 minutes, 10 minutes, 15 minutes, and 20 minutes or until the temperatures have returned to baseline. In a normal response, the fingers should return to baseline temperatures within 5 minutes. Patients with Raynaud's disease tend not to warm up until after the 10-minute post–ice immersion time.[5]

Buerger's Disease

Thromboangiitis obliterans, or Buerger's disease, is a rare disease caused by severe narrowing or obstruction of small and medium-sized blood vessels of the hands and feet owing to inflammation of vessel walls. This disease primarily occurs in men 20 to 40 years old who have a history of heavy smoking or tobacco use. Symptoms include acute, severe pain in the hands and feet, often occurring at rest, and skin changes including ulcerations of the fingers and toes. Prognosis for the patient is improved with smoking cessation. If smoking cessation does not occur, surgical sympathectomy (cutting the nerves) or amputation may be the only course of action for treatment.

Vascular Test Findings. Testing should include duplex sonography of the lower extremity arteries and angiography to view the distal most arteries in their entirety. Photoplethysmography testing should occur only if the digits still have adequate skin coverage. Reduced pressures in the toes and fingers are noted along with abnormal pulse volume recording waveforms with the absence of the dicrotic notch. A temperature response test may also demonstrate minimal change in temperatures after warming the digits. Imaging exhibits normal vessels proximal to the disease and thrombotic occlusions of the arterial walls. Local collateralization with a corkscrew appearance is also a characteristic feature of Buerger's disease.

SUMMARY

Arterial disease of the leg can manifest with a multitude of symptoms and complications. If left untreated, it can lead to painful ulcerations and eventual limb amputation. Obtaining a thorough patient history and having a complete understanding of waveforms and anatomy make recognizing abnormalities instinctive. The ability to anticipate possible findings associated with different disease processes and reacting appropriately to pathology aids in diagnosing and confirming the source of patient complaints.

CLINICAL SCENARIO—DIAGNOSIS

Combined with the significant history of tobacco use and the patient's age, the presenting symptoms of extreme pain (including during periods of inactivity), diminished pulses, and ulcers are the classic signs of thromboangiitis obliterans, or Buerger's disease. The reduced, monophasic arterial signals in the first and third phalanges and absence of flow in the remaining digits support the diagnosis, as do the laser Doppler findings of the lack of a postwarming increase. Definitive diagnosis requires an angiogram showing the distal arteries tapering in a "corkscrew" pattern until eventual occlusion.

CASE STUDIES FOR DISCUSSION

1. A 69-year-old man presents to the emergency department with a 1-day history of a cold, purple left foot. He has a history of a left common femoral artery-popliteal bypass graft. Gray-scale imaging demonstrates low-level echoes within the lumen of the graft. No detectable color or spectral Doppler flow is noted. The native popliteal artery distal to the graft has a monophasic spectral Doppler waveform. What is the most likely diagnosis?

2. A 68-year-old man sees his primary care physician regarding right leg pain during exercise. He mentions he has difficulty walking a single block without the right calf cramping to the point where he has to stop and rest. Gray-scale imaging demonstrates heavily shadowing plaque throughout the right superficial femoral artery. Color Doppler demonstrates flow with luminal irregularities throughout the entire femoral artery except in the midportion where no flow is seen. Spectral Doppler confirms this finding, demonstrating monophasic flow with a good upstroke in the proximal femoral artery, no flow in the mid to distal femoral artery, and tardus parvus flow in the proximal popliteal artery. What is the most likely diagnosis?

3. During his annual physical, a 79-year-old man is noted to have a palpable, nontender, slightly pulsatile mass in the right popliteal fossa. No defect is noted on the left side. He is promptly sent for a sonogram. Gray-scale imaging demonstrates a focal, dilated segment of the right popliteal artery that measures 3.1 cm in all dimensions. Visible echoes can also be seen within a portion of the lumen. Color Doppler shows normal flow in the nondilated segment and a yin-yang appearance in the dilated portion. Spectral Doppler is essentially normal. What is the most likely diagnosis?

4. After a crushing injury to the left calf during a car accident, a 23-year-old woman complains of swelling and severe calf pain, specifically when the area is palpated or she moves her foot. Her pain has not been relieved by medication, and she states she is starting to lose sensation in her foot. Physical examination reveals a swollen calf with shiny skin and an absent pedal pulse. Gray-scale imaging does not reveal any intimal damage; however, spectral Doppler waveforms are high resistive in the popliteal artery and gradually diminish as samples are taken distally in the peroneal and posterior tibial arteries. What is the most likely diagnosis?

5. After a cardiac catheterization, a 72-year-old woman complains of pain in her groin. On physical examination, the physician notes a bruit in the area of arterial access. Spectral Doppler reveals high-velocity, low-resistance waveforms in the common femoral artery proximal to the site of the catheterization and reduced flow distal to the site. The common femoral vein is also noted to have increased pulsatile flow above the puncture site. A thrill can be palpated on the skin, and flash artifact is evident on color Doppler. What is the most likely diagnosis?

STUDY QUESTIONS

1. A man presents to his physician with a large, non-painful mass in the posterior knee fossa. Doppler and gray-scale imaging reveal a patent popliteal artery with a normal biphasic signal. Outer-to-outer wall diameters in the proximal, mid, and distal areas are 0.8 cm, 0.9 cm, and 0.7 cm. There is a 3.0 cm × 4.2 cm × 3.0 cm anechoic mass located medial to the popliteal artery. No color or spectral Doppler is demonstrated in the mass. What is the most likely diagnosis?
   a. Popliteal cyst
   b. Acute deep venous thrombosis of the popliteal artery
   c. Acute thromboembolism of the popliteal artery
   d. Popliteal artery aneurysm

2. An 81-year-old man comes to the emergency department with a blue right toe. His history is positive for long-term tobacco use. On clinical examination, the patient has a right ABI of 0.40 and a left ABI of 0.70. On lower extremity Doppler imaging, the common femoral artery through the popliteal arteries are patent; however, severe, irregular plaque is noted. The peroneal artery is occluded at its origin, but the posterior tibial and anterior tibial arteries are patent; modest plaque buildup is noted. What is the most likely diagnosis?
   a. Peripheral arterial disease
   b. Femoral artery aneurysm
   c. Arterial thromboemboli causing acute ischemia
   d. Both a and c

3. A 66-year-old woman comes for her annual physical and mentions she has been experiencing pain in her legs during exercise. She states it is worse in the left calf but notes mild achiness in the right calf, too. She can walk about 5 minutes then needs to stop for 1 minute before continuing. Her physician orders an ABI. During the test, biphasic waveforms are noted throughout the right leg and the left common and femoral artery, but the left leg demonstrates monophasic signals in the popliteal, posterior tibial, and dorsalis pedis arteries. Before the exercise portion of the test, the ABI values were 1.0 on the right and 0.76 on the left. After exercise, left foot pallor is noted, and the ABI values are 0.80 on the right and 0.35 on the left. What is the most likely cause of her leg pain?
   a. Pseudoclaudication
   b. Mild disease in the right leg and severe arterial occlusive disease in the left leg
   c. Mild disease in both legs
   d. All of the above

4. A young woman in the upper Midwest presents to her physician's office with very painful toes that turn white, blue, and finally red during cold, winter weather; this occurs in a few of her fingers as well. She mentions this happens even in the summer. When quizzed further, she notes this happens in the summer only when she is in an air-conditioned building. An arterial lower vascular laboratory study is performed. Common femoral, profunda, superficial femoral, popliteal, posterior tibial, and dorsalis pedis arteries are triphasic/biphasic with normal blood pressures. Her digital pressure indices all are less than 0.79, her digital temperatures are about 21° C, and her fingers are noticeably discolored. After heating her fingers, her pressures and temperatures improve, and her fingertips are now bright red. What is the most likely diagnosis?
   a. Acute venous thrombosis
   b. Raynaud's disease
   c. Buerger's disease
   d. ASO

5. A 42-year-old man presents to the emergency department with ulcerations on his toes and fingers. He has a known history of extremely heavy tobacco use. A lower extremity Doppler imaging study demonstrates normal Doppler waveforms, and color Doppler demonstrates flow in the common femoral, profunda, superficial femoral, and popliteal arteries. Doppler evaluation also shows a marked velocity decrease in the posterior tibial artery, and flow could not be detected in the dorsalis pedis artery. What is the most likely diagnosis?
   a. Buerger's disease
   b. Chronic deep venous thrombosis
   c. ASO
   d. None of the above

6. A 78-year-old man visits his physician with a chief complaint of an inability to walk long distances anymore. He complains of severe pain in his calves on both sides. This pain also occurs while sitting for long periods. The physician orders a lower extremity venous and arterial sonogram and ABI. The lower extremity venous study demonstrates fully collapsible vessels and wall-to-wall color with color Doppler imaging. The lower extremity arterial sonogram demonstrates minimal plaque formation and no evidence for high-grade stenosis, although the average peak systolic velocity is 70 cm/s. One section in the above-knee popliteal artery demonstrates 112 cm/s. The ABI is 1.1 on the right and 1.2 on the left. What is the most likely cause of the patient's leg pain?
   a. Vascular claudication
   b. Pseudoclaudication
   c. ASO
   d. Popliteal aneurysm

7. A 58-year-old patient is noted to have swelling and discoloration in the groin after balloon angioplasty

of the common iliac artery. Gray-scale imaging demonstrates a cystic mass located adjacent to the common femoral artery. Color and spectral Doppler show turbulent flow within the mass and a to-and-fro waveform in the neck connecting the mass to the artery. What is the most likely diagnosis?

a. AVF
b. Pseudoaneurysm
c. Postoperative seroma
d. Arterial dissection

8. After experiencing a ruptured Achilles' tendon injury, a 34-year-old man complains of severe leg pain and swelling. Spectral Doppler of the veins reveals normal phasicity and complete compressibility from the thigh to just below the knee. Because of the extreme pain, the sonographer is unable to compress the calf or document augmented flow within the veins by color Doppler. The sonographer notes during color Doppler interrogation that arterial signals seem weak. An arterial spectral tracing in the posterior tibial and peroneal arteries confirms the diminished flow and shows that flow disappears entirely in the distal calf. A large hematoma between the gastrocnemius and soleus muscles is incidentally noted. What is the most likely diagnosis?

a. Compartment syndrome
b. Entrapment syndrome
c. Possible deep venous thrombosis of the calf veins
d. Buerger's disease

9. A routine 6-month follow-up examination of a femoropopliteal bypass vein graft reveals a new, moderately echogenic region protruding into the lumen near the proximal anastomosis. Color Doppler shows aliasing and flow disturbance, whereas spectral tracings demonstrate very high velocities and marked spectral broadening. What is the most likely diagnosis?

a. Impending graft failure resulting from infection near the anastomosis
b. Stenosis resulting from technical or surgical error
c. Stenosis secondary to intimal hyperplasia
d. Normal findings in a bypass graft

10. Routine annual follow-up examination of a popliteal artery stent reveals an echo-free lumen by gray-scale. Color Doppler shows aliasing within the stent, and spectral Doppler confirms the mildly elevated velocities. Flow distal to the stent becomes triphasic and demonstrates normal velocities. What is the most likely diagnosis?

a. Impending stent failure resulting from infection near the end points
b. Stenosis resulting from technical or surgical error
c. Stenosis secondary to intimal hyperplasia
d. Normal findings in a stent

REFERENCES

1. Fowkes F, Murray G, Butcher I, et al: Ankle brachial index combined with Framingham Risk Score to predict cardiovascular events and mortality: a meta-analysis, *JAMA* 300:197–208, 2008.
2. McPharlin M, Rumwell C: *Vascular technology: an illustrated review*, ed 4, Pasadena, CA, 2009, Davies Publishing.
3. Wolf Y, Kobzantsev Z, Zelmanovich L: Size of normal and aneurysmal popliteal arteries: a duplex ultrasound study, *J Vasc Surg* 43:488–492, 2006.
4. Klinkert P, Shepers A, Burger D, et al: Vein versus polytetrafluoroethylene in above-knee femoropopliteal bypass grafting: five-year results of a randomized controlled trial, *J Vasc Surg* 27:146–155, 2003.
5. Liedl DM, Liedl DA, Schabauer AM, et al: Effects of ice water immersion on digital temperatures and cutaneous-blood flow, *J Vasc Technol* 20:243–246, 1996.

Abduction act of moving an extremity away from the body

Abscess localized collection of pus surrounded by inflamed tissue that is formed as a result of tissue disintegration from an infection

Acardia rare congenital anomaly in which the heart is absent; this condition is sometimes seen in a conjoined twin whose survival depends on the circulatory system of its twin

Acholic absence of bile

Acini smallest cells of the pancreas that comprise the exocrine portion

Acoustic enhancement image artifact created behind a low-attenuating object such as a cyst

Acute hepatitis hepatitis that resolves within 4 months after the initial infection

Adduction act of moving an extremity toward the body

Adenomas benign neoplasms

Adenomatoid composed of or resembling glandular tissue

Adenomyosis common benign condition in which endometrial tissue invades the uterine muscular layer (myometrium) resulting in abnormal uterine bleeding

Adenopathy enlargement of lymph nodes

Aflatoxin carcinogenic fungus found in grains (corn, wheat) and peanuts

AFP *also* alpha-fetoprotein; plasma protein produced in the fetal liver and by hepatocellular carcinomas. It is measured in th emother's blood to screen for neural tube defects or chromosomal abnormalities. Elevated levels may also be seen in patients with cirrhosis and hepatitis

Albumin by-product of protein metabolism that decreases in cases of parenchymal liver disease

Alcoholic hepatitis *see* cirrhosis

Alfa-fetoprotein plasma protein produced by the yolk sac and liver during fetal development that can be indicative of hepatocellular carcinoma in adults

Alobar holoprosencephaly defect in which interhemispheric fissure and falx cerebri are totally absent, most severe type; monoventricle, fused thalami, microcephaly, may have cyclopia or proboscis or both, absent third ventricle, high association with chromosome abnormalities (trisomy 13)

Alpha fetoprotein glycoprotein synthesized by the embryonic liver that is measured in the mother's blood to screen for neural tube defects or chromosomal abnormalities

ALT alanine aminotransferase; formerly referred to as SGPT (serum glutamate pyruvate transaminase); a liver enzyme

Amaurosis fugax transient blindness described as a shade being pulled over the eye

Amenorrhea lack of menstruation

Amniocentesis procedure of aspiration of an amniotic fluid sample with insertion of a needle through the maternal abdomen into the amniotic sac; the sample may be used to evaluate genetic composition, fetal maturity, or metabolic assays

Amnion thin, smooth innermost membrane of pregnancy enclosing the fetus and the amniotic cavity

Amnionicity refers to the number of amniotic membranes

Amylase pancreas enzyme that converts starches to carbohydrates

Amyloidosis one of the infiltrating testicular cancers

Anaplastic thyroid cancer rare carcinoma of the thyroid

Anastomosis connection between two vessels

Anembryonic pregnancy blighted ovum; occurs when a gestational sac is devoid of an embryo

Anemia condition in which the number of red blood cells is less than normal

Anemia a condition in which the number of red blood cells is decreased. It may be from blood loss, an increase in destruction of red blood cells, or a decrease in production of red blood cells

Aneuploid abnormal chromosome pattern

Aneuploidy abnormal chromosomes

Angiitis inflammation of a vessel

Angiomyolipoma tumor comprising fat, vessels, and muscle tissue that is frequently identified in the kidneys and occurs rarely in the liver

Angiosarcoma most common malignant disease of mesenchymal origin in the liver

Anhydramnios absence of any measureable amniotic fluid

Aniridia absence of the iris

Ankle-brachial index comparison of the blood pressure of the ankle and arms; the ratio of those pressures is called an ankle-brachial index

Anorexia loss of appetite

Anovulation absence of ovulation

Antiradial plane of breast imaging for ultrasound perpendicular to a line radiating from the nipple (the hub) to the periphery of the breast similar to hands of a clock (90 degrees to radial)

Anuria absence of urinary output or production

Aortic aneurysm localized dilation of the aorta

Aphasia inability to communicate, particularly by speaking

Appendicolith fecalith or calcification located in the appendix

Appendix epididymis oval structure located on the head of the epididymis; the remnant mesonephros

Appendix testis small oval structure located on the upper pole of the testis; the remnant müllerian duct

Aqueductal stenosis congenital stenosis of the aqueduct of Sylvius (the part of the ventricular system that connects the third and fourth ventricles) that results in dilation of the lateral and third ventricles

Arachnoid cysts cysts located between the layers of the pia mater and arachnoid

Areola circular area of different pigmentation around the nipple of the breast

Arnold-Chiari malformation constellation of cranial findings associated with spina bifida aperta, with scalloping of the frontal bones, banana-shaped cerebellum, and ventriculomegaly

Ascites accumulation of serous fluid within the potential spaces of the abdomen

Asphyxia severe hypoxia

Asplenia syndrome associated with right atrial isomerism, situs ambiguus, absence of the spleen, and congenital heart disease

AST aspartate aminotransferase; formerly referred to as SGOT (serum glutamate oxaloacetate transaminase); a liver enzyme

Atherosclerosis condition, especially in older persons, in which plaque builds on arterial walls and causes narrowing of the lumen. It can weaken the wall and predispose the artery to aneurysmal dilation

Atrioventricular septal defect (AVSD) failure of the endocardial cushion to fuse; this defect of the central heart provides communication between the ventricles, between the atria, or between the atria and ventricles; subdivided into complete, incomplete, and partial forms

Augmentation external compression of the distal extremity with squeezing of the lower leg or ankle in an attempt to increase proximal venous flow proving no obstruction exists between where the transducer is imaging and the squeeze

Autosomal dominant polycystic kidney disease (ADPKD) hereditary disease characterized by appearance of a large number of cysts in both kidneys and possibly liver, pancreas, and other organs; cysts increase in number and size over time and may leading to renal failure

Autosomal recessive polycystic kidney disease hereditary disease characterized by varying degrees of dilation of the renal tubules and hepatic fibrosis; the most severe manifestations are considered inconsistent with life and are either diagnosed in utero or at birth

Azotemia excess of urea and other nitrogenous waste in the blood

Bacteriuria presence of bacteria in the urine

Baker's cyst communication between the synovial fluid of the knee joint and the tissue spaces of the popliteal fossa

Barium enema radiographic procedure in which barium is introduced into the rectum in a retrograde fashion for visualization of the bowel lining with fluoroscopy

Bear criteria set of criteria for diagnosing autosomal dominant polycystic kidney disease in various age groups

Beat-to-beat variability normal variation of the fetal heart rate seen from the autonomic nervous system control of the fetal heart

Beckwith-Wiedemann syndrome autosomal recessive condition characterized by macroglossia, gigantism, and hemihypertrophy; individuals may also have organomegaly and are at increased risk for development of certain abdominal neoplasms

Benign not malignant; favorable for recovery

Benign prostatic hypertrophy (BPH) enlarged prostate

β-hCG maternal serum test for detection of human chorionic gonadotropin for the diagnosis of pregnancy

β human chorionic gonadotropin laboratory test used for quantification of the amount of circulating human chorionic gonadotropin, which is the "pregnancy hormone" secreted by the placental trophoblastic cells that keeps the corpus luteum producing progesterone after conception occurs

Bicornuate uterus congenital uterine anomaly resulting in varying extents of duplication of the uterine body and cervix

Bilirubin end product of red blood cell metabolism; stored in the liver and used to help metabolize fatty foods

Biometry application of statistics to biologic science, as in assessment of fetal size on the basis of statistics

Blood urea nitrogen (BUN) value used to measure the concentration of nitrogen as urea in the blood

Body cavities pleural, pericardial, and peritoneal; must identify fluid in two body cavities or one cavity and anasarca (tissue edema)

Bosniak classification system set of criteria that aid in patient management by predicting the likelihood of malignancy of renal cysts based on features including septations, wall thickening, and cyst enhancement on computed tomography

Brachial plexus injury damage to the nerves that control arm and hand muscles

Brainstem includes midbrain, pons, and medulla oblongata

Branchial cleft cysts congenital cystic mass in the lateral neck

Budd-Chiari syndrome rare syndrome characterized by the occlusion of the hepatic veins or the inferior vena cava or both

CA 125 cancer antigen 125; the amount of CA 125 in the blood increases with certain types of cancers, including ovarian

Camptomelic dysplasia lethal skeletal dysplasia characterized by bent bones (camptomelia)

Cancer cellular tumor for which the natural course is fatal; has properties of invasion and metastasis and is highly anaplastic

"Candle" sign low continuous ureteral jet flow that is seen with a partial ureteral obstruction or ureterocele

Capillary lymphangioma cystic neck mass caused by malformations of the cervical thoracic lymphatic system

Capsule structure in which something is enclosed; an anatomic structure enclosing an organ or body part

Carcinoembryonic antigen antigen present in trace amounts in adult tissue; when blood test results reveal elevated serum levels, cancer is suspected

Caroli's disease hereditary disease of segmental or diffuse intrahepatic bile duct dilation

Carotid bruit systolic murmur heard in the neck produced by blood flow in the carotid arteries

Catecholamines group of compounds that include epinephrine and norepinephrine

Caudothalamic notch *also* caudothalamic groove; region at which the thalamus and caudate nucleus join; the most common location of germinal matrix hemorrhage

Cavernous lymphangioma cystic neck mass caused by malformations of the cervical thoracic lymphatic system

Cebocephaly hypotelorism with a normally placed nose with a single nostril

Cerebral palsy spectrum of disorders that occurs with brain dysfunction at the time of birth or in the neonatal period; can include spasticity, diplegia, hemiplegia, quadriplegia, seizure disorder, and varying degrees of mental retardation; decreased sight, vision, and impaired speech may also occur

Cerebrovascular accident (CVA) permanent neurologic deficit

"Cervix" sign a term used to describe the appearance of hypertrophic pyloric stenosis which resembles the cervix in pregnancy

Cesarean section   method of fetal delivery with surgical incision of the uterus

Chlamydia   one of the most common sexually transmitted diseases in the United States; it causes discharge, inflammation, and burning during urination

Choledochal cysts   cystic dilations of the biliary tree

Choledocholithiasis   presence of biliary stones in the common bile duct

Cholelithiasis   presence of stones in the gallbladder

Chorioamnionitis   infection that involves the chorion, amnion, and amniotic fluid

Choriocarcinoma   most aggressive germ cell tumor of the testis; very rare

Chorion   outermost extraembryonic membrane composed of trophoblast lined with mesoderm; it gives rise to the placenta and persists until birth as the outer of the two layers of membrane surrounding the amniotic fluid and the fetus

Chorionic villus sampling   procedure of aspiration of a sample of chorionic villi found at the area of implantation and the early placenta

Chorionicity   refers to the number of chorionic membranes, which relates to the number of placentas that develop

Chromosomes   found in the nucleus of a cell; contain DNA and genetic information

Chronic hepatitis   persistence of changes associated with hepatitis for more than 6 months

Chronic hypertension   in a pregnant patient, represents persistent elevated blood pressures identified before pregnancy or before 20 weeks' gestation

Cirrhosis   result of chronic liver disease characterized by the liver tissue becoming fibrotic, nodular, and nonfunctional

Cirrhosis   degenerative disease of the liver in which the hepatocytes are gradually replaced with fibrous and fatty tissues

Cleavage   series of repeated mitotic cell divisions that occurs in an ovum immediately after fertilization

Clinodactyly   permanent curvature or deflection of one or more digits (fingers or toes)

Coapt   when the vessel is subjected to extrinsic pressure, the opposite walls of the vessel touch together completely proving no intraluminal echogenic matter

Collateral circulation   flow of blood through an alternative pathway

Computed tomography (CT)   radiographic technique that allows detailed cross-sectional imaging

Confluence   when a vein joins another vein

Congenital familial anodontia   congenital hereditary anomaly characterized by absence of some or all of the teeth

Conus medullaris   caudal end of the spinal cord

Cooper's ligaments   supporting fibrous structures throughout the breast that partially sheathe the lobes shaping the breast; these ligaments affect the image of the glandular tissue on a mammogram

Corpora amylasia   *also* amyloids; accumulation of dense amounts of calcified materials that are protein-based in nature

Cortex   outer layer of an organ

Couinaud's classification   classification of liver anatomy that divides the liver into eight functionally independent segments

Courvoisier's gallbladder   enlargement of the gallbladder caused by a slow progressive obstruction of the distal common bile duct and is associated with adenocarcinoma of the head of the pancreas

Creatinine   laboratory value and by-product of muscle metabolism

Crenulated   with scalloped projections

Cruveilhier-Baumgarten syndrome   development of para-umbilical collateral flow in cases of portal hypertension

Cryptorchidism   failure of one or both testicles to descend into the scrotal sac

Culdocentesis   transvaginal puncture to remove intraperitoneal fluid, including purulent material

Cutaneous   relating to the skin

Cyanotic heart disease   any heart abnormality or disease that results in cyanosis

Cyclopia   one orbit or fusion of two orbits

Cystadenocarcinoma   predominantly cystic malignant tumor that arises from epithelial cells

Cystadenoma   predominantly cystic tumor composed of epithelial cells

Cystic fibrosis   hereditary disease that causes excessive production of thick mucus by the endocrine glands

Cystic hygroma   cystic or multicystic lesions that occur with lymphatic obstruction and contain loculations and septations of varying sizes and thickness

Cystoscopy   use of a lighted tube to see within the urinary bladder

Cytomegalovirus   group of herpes viruses that infects humans and other animals causing development of characteristic inclusions in the cytoplasm or nucleus; may cause flulike symptoms; congenital infection may cause malformation, fetal growth deficiencies, and death

D-dimer   laboratory value that is increased in blood when there is a degradation of fibrin, which can be a result of thromboembolic disease. A negative value typically excludes thrombosis, while a positive value may be caused by numerous conditions.

Decidua   endometrial lining during pregnancy

Decidua capsularis   portion of the decidua that encloses the chorionic cavity

Decidua parietalis   portion of the remaining decidua other than at the implantation site

Deep vein thrombosis (DVT)   thrombosis located within the deep veins of the extremity; the major, acute concern with DVT is that it can lead to pulmonary embolism, which is a potentially fatal disease; long-term DVT can damage venous valves creating postphlebitic syndrome

Dextrocardia   heart is in the right chest with the apex pointed to the right of the thorax

Dextroposition   condition in which the heart is located in the right side of the chest and the cardiac apex points medially or to the left

Diabetes mellitus   a condition characterized by deficient secretion of insulin that leads to hyperglycemia

Diamniotic   twin pregnancy with two separate amniotic membranes (sacs)

Diaphragmatic hernia (DH)   herniation of abdominal contents through a diaphragm defect; defect is more common on the left side with stomach herniated into the chest or thorax; heart is usually displaced

Diastrophic dysplasia autosomal recessive short-limbed skeletal dysplasia with a characteristic fixed abducted thumb (hitchhiker thumb)

Dichorionic twin pregnancy with two separate chorionic membranes (placentas)

Diplegia paralysis of both sides of the body

Direct bilirubin *also* conjugated bilirubin; bilirubin that has been absorbed by the hepatocytes and is water-soluble

Discordant growth refers to twins with a marked difference in size (>20% difference in weight) at birth; condition is usually caused by an overperfusion of one twin and an underperfusion of the other twin and usually affects monochorionic twins

Dissection (aortic) rupture of the intima of the aorta, which separates from the media, with a column of blood between the two layers

Distal femoral epiphysis small ossification center at the distal end of the femur

Diverticulitis inflammation of pouchlike herniations of the bowel wall

Diverticulum an outpouching of a hollow structure in the body

Ductus deferens *also* vas deferens; transportive duct that propels sperm from the epididymis to the prostatic urethra

Duodenal atresia abnormal development of the proximal duodenum that leads to obstruction; sonographically appears as a double bubble sign

Dysmenorrhea pain that corresponds with menstruation

Dyspareunia painful or difficult sexual intercourse

Dyspnea difficulty in breathing

Dysraphism *also* spina bifida; describes the presence of spine separation

Dystocia difficult birth or labor

Dysuria painful or difficult urination

Eagle-Barrett syndrome (prune-belly) syndrome absence or atrophy of abdominal wall musculature, massive dilation of ureters, normal bladder, thin renal cortex

Ectoderm outer layer of cells in a developing embryo

Ectopia abnormal location of an organ

Ectopic pregnancy pregnancy that occurs outside the uterine cavity

Ehlers-Danlos syndrome hereditary syndrome characterized by hypermotility of the joints and skin laxity and fragility

Eklund maneuver method for imaging augmented breasts that involves pulling the breast tissue away from the implant while displacing the implant posteriorly, excluding it from view and allowing for better visualization of the breast tissue

Elastography diagnostic imaging technique using tissue stiffness to classify masses

Emboli object that breaks off in the vascular system and travels downstream creating a blockage of blood flow; venous emboli that arise from the lower extremity and flow toward and through the heart and then occlude the flow of blood into the lungs are termed pulmonary emboli

Emboli piece of thrombus/emboli, tissue, foreign object or quantity of air (gas) that travels throughout the bloodstream and becomes lodged

Embryonal cell tumor germ cell tumors that can arise in the testis

Endarterectomy surgical removal of plaque or diseased structure to the endothelial or media layer of the vessel wall

Endoderm innermost layer of cells in a developing embryo

Endoleak occurs when blood is allowed to flow into the aneurysm sac after endoluminal graft placement

Endometrial carcinoma uterine malignant disease that originates from endometrial changes related to excessive estrogen stimulation

Endometrial hyperplasia abnormal proliferation (growth) of the endometrium related to estrogen stimulation

Endometrial polyp focal growth of endometrial tissue that projects into the endometrial cavity

Endometritis inflammation of the endometrium

Endometrium the inner lining of the uterus that responds to hormonal stimulation and produces both menstrual and abnormal uterine bleeding

Endoscopic retrograde cholangiopancreatogram (ERCP) imaging procedure used to evaluate bile ducts and pancreatic ducts

Endotoxemia presence of bacterial toxins in the blood that may cause shock

Endovaginal imaging sonographic imaging performed with the introduction of a transducer into the vaginal canal

Epicanthal fold fold of skin at the inner aspect of the eyelid

Epidermoid composed of or resembling epidermal tissue

Epididymal cyst true cyst arising from an epididymal duct

Epididymis convoluted tubular structure that carries sperm cells from the testicle to the ductus deferens

Epididymitis inflammation of the epididymis

Epididymo-orchitis inflammation of the epididymis and testis

Epigastrium area between the right and left hypochondrium that contains part of the liver, duodenum, and pancreas

Epithelioid hemangioendothelioma rare malignant vascular tumor of endothelial origin that sonographically appears as multiple hypoechoic lesions in the periphery of the liver

Epithelium layer of cells that form mucous and serous membranes and the surface of the skin

Erythrocyte sedimentation rate (ESR) nonspecific indicator of inflammation; the rate at which erythrocytes settle in a well-mixed specimen of venous blood

Erythropoietin hormone that promotes the formation of red blood cells

Esophageal veins common collateral pathway for the hepatic circulation in cases of portal hypertension

Esophagitis inflammation of the mucosal lining of the esophagus

Estrogen female sex hormone produced by the ovary

Ethmocephaly cyclopia or hypotelorism with a proboscis or double proboscis

Exsanguination bleeding to death

Extravasation forcing of blood or lymph out of the vessel and into the surrounding tissue

Exudate fluid with a high content of protein and cellular debris that has escaped from blood vessels and has been deposited in tissues; usually as a result of injury or inflammation

Facial palsies   complete or partial loss of voluntary movement of the facial muscles

Familial adenomatous polyposis   hereditary disease characterized by widespread development of polyps in the colon that begin to appear in late adolescence or early childhood and may lead to cancer of the colon

Fasciotomy   surgical procedure in which fascial tissue is cut to relieve pressure within the compartment it surrounds

Fat-sparing   areas of normal liver parenchyma not replaced with fatty tissues occasionally seen in patients with fatty liver disease

Fatty infiltration   accumulation of fat within hepatic parenchyma; often associated with alcoholism, obesity, and diabetes

Fatty liver disease   accumulation of fat within hepatic parenchyma; often associated with alcoholism, obesity, and diabetes

Febrile   having a fever

Fecalith   hard, impacted mass of feces in the colon

Fetal hydrops   refers to fluid accumulation in serous cavities or edema of soft tissue in the fetus

Fibrolamellar carcinoma   rare malignant neoplasm; occurs in younger patients than hepatocellular carcinoma; is of hepatocellular origin, although distinct from hepatocellular carcinoma; serum alpha fetoprotein level is usually normal

Fine-needle aspiration (FNA)   biopsy technique that aspirates cells through a thin, hollow needle

Fitz-Hugh–Curtis syndrome   right upper quadrant pain that occurs with tuboovarian abscess; perihepatitis occurring as a complication of gonorrhea or chlamydial infection, characterized by adhesions between the liver and other sites in the peritoneum

Focal   localized to a point of focus

Follicular cancer   malignant mass in the thyroid

Foramen ovale   *also* fossa ovalis; opening between the free edge of the septum secundum and the dorsal wall of the atrium

Forebrain   *also* prosencephalon; part of the brain that includes the cerebral hemispheres and thalamus

Fundamental frequency   operating or true frequency of a transducer

Gaitor zone   "boot" area of the leg; distal near the ankle

Gallbladder polyp   projection of soft tissue from the wall into the gallbladder lumen

Gastric reflux   abnormal backward flow of gastric fluids into the esophagus

Genotype   genetic composition of an of an individual or group

Germ cell   ovum or sperm cell

Gestational age   age of a fetus, usually expressed in weeks, dating from the first day of the mother's last normal menstrual period; conceptual age plus 2 weeks

Gestational diabetes   temporary type of diabetes that develops in some pregnant women because of an inability to produce enough insulin to keep blood glucose within a safe range

GGT   gamma glutamyl transpeptidase; helps aid in the transport of amino acids across cell membranes; elevates in cases of parenchymal liver disease and is especially sensitive to alcohol-related liver disease; it often parallels alkaline phosphatase

Glycogen storage disease   abnormal storage of fat within hepatocytes

Goiter   enlargement of the thyroid gland that can be focal or diffuse; nodules may be present

Gonorrhea   inflammation of the genital mucous membrane caused by *gonococcus*

Graafian follicle   mature ovum-containing follicle

Granuloma   tumor or growth that results when macrophages are unable to destroy a foreign body; when pertaining to breast implants, a granuloma is a glob of silicone with an associated inflammatory response

Granulosa   layer of cells in the outer wall of a graafian follicle

Graves' disease   autoimmune disorder of diffuse toxic goiter characterized by bulging eyes

Gross hematuria   blood in the urine that can be seen with the unaided eye

Gynecomastia   enlargement of the breast tissue in a male

Haploid   half the normal number of chromosomes found in normal body cells; germ cells are normally haploid

Harmonics   frequencies that are integral multiples of a fundamental or original frequency

Hashimoto's disease   autoimmune disease which is the most common form of thyroiditis

Hemangioma   congenital anomaly in which the proliferation of blood vessels forms a mass that may resemble a neoplasm

Hematocele   hematoma in the peritesticular space

Hematocolpos   menstrual blood within the vagina usually due to obstruction

Hematocrit   measure of the amount of red blood cells

Hematoma   localized walled-off collection of blood that is not in a vessel; the blood is usually clotted

Hematometra   uterine cavity distended with blood from obstruction at the level of the cervix; most commonly from cervical stenosis but may be caused by cervical cancer, cervical fibroids, or endometrial cancer

Hematometracolpos   when the uterine cavity and vagina is distended with blood from obstruction at the level of the vagina, usually from an imperforate hymen

Hematometracolpos   menstrual blood within the vagina and uterus

Hematuria   blood in the urine

Hemianopia   loss of vision in one or both eyes that affects half of the visual field

Hemihypertrophy   an asymmetric overgrowth of the body

Hemiplegia   paralysis of half of the body

Hemoperitoneum   blood in the peritoneal cavity

Hemoptysis   coughing up blood

Heparin   medication administered as an anticoagulant to thin blood

Hepatitis   inflammatory condition of the liver

Hepatitis B and C   viral infections of the liver that cause inflammation, often becoming chronic and resulting in cirrhosis

Hepatoblastoma   malignant solid tumor involving the liver

Hepatocellular disease   dysfunction of the hepatocytes

Hepatofugal   portal vein blood flow away from the liver

Hepatoma   primary liver carcinoma or hepatocellular carcinoma

Hepatopedal   portal vein blood flow toward the liver

Hernia   protrusion of part or all of an organ or structure through the wall that normally contains it

Heterotopic pregnancy   presence of two or more implantation sites that occur simultaneously, with one intrauterine and one extrauterine pregnancy

Heterozygous   inherited from both parents

High-order multiple pregnancy   pregnancy with three or more fetuses

Hirsutism   abnormal excess growth of hair

Hodgkin's disease   malignant disease that involves lymphoid tissue

Holoprosencephaly   absent or incomplete fusion of the forebrain

Homans' sign   when a patient dorsiflexes and complains of leg pain; a clinical method to evaluate a patient for a deep vein thrombosis

Homozygous   inherited from one parent

Hormone replacement therapy   supplemental hormones used with postmenopausal women in preventing osteoporosis and providing cardiovascular benefits

Human chorionic gonadotropin   hormone secreted by the placenta and is commonly used to assess for pregnancy

Hydatid disease   parasitic infestation by the tapeworm *Echinococcus granulosus*; very rarely seen in the United States

Hydatidiform mole   benign form of gestational trophoblastic disease involving the conversion of the chorionic villi

Hydramnios   *also* polyhydramnios; abnormal condition of pregnancy characterized by an excess of amniotic fluid

Hydrocele   accumulation of serous fluid in the peritesticular space

Hydrops   condition of fluid overload that can be diagnosed with the identification of skin edema plus fluid in one body cavity or fluid in two body cavities

Hydrops fetalis   abnormal accumulation of fluid in fetal tissue and organs, leading to anemia and a decreased ability of the blood to carry oxygen

Hydrosalpinx   accumulation of serous fluid in the fallopian tube

Hydrostatic enema   retrograde water enema used as a first attempt at reducing an intussusception

Hydroureter   ureter enlarged with fluid

Hyperemesis gravidarum   abnormal condition of pregnancy characterized by protracted vomiting, weight loss, and fluid and electrolyte imbalance

Hyperemia   excess of blood in part of the body, caused by increased blood flow secondary to an inflammatory response, local relaxation of arterioles, or obstruction of the outflow of blood from an area

Hyperkalemia   greater than normal concentration of potassium ions in the circulating blood

Hyperparathyroidism   disorder associated with elevated serum calcium levels

Hyperplasia   overgrowth or proliferation of cells

Hypertelorism   increased distance between the medial borders of the orbital rims

Hyperthyroidism   oversecretion of thyroid hormones

Hypoglycemia   decreased amount of glucose in the blood

Hypophosphatasia   low phosphatase level that can be seen with hyperparathyroidism

Hypoplastic left heart syndrome   underdevelopment of the left side of the heart

Hypotelorism   decreased distance between the medial borders of the orbital rims

Hypovolemia   decreased amount of blood in the body

Hypoxia   decreased oxygen

Hysterosalpingography   radiologic technique in which dye is infused into the uterus and fallopian tubes for identification of endometrial lesions or tubal blockage

Hysteroscopy   procedure in which a flexible or rigid hysteroscope is inserted into the uterus for direct visualization of the endometrial cavity

Iatrogenic   condition induced by a physician or procedure

Icteric   term used to describe a condition of jaundice

Idiopathic   of unknown cause

Implantation bleeding or spotting   occurs when the blastocyst implants in the endometrium; often mistaken for the normal last menstrual period

In vitro fertilization   infertility treatment involving fertilization of harvested oocytes with sperm in a laboratory setting, followed by transfer of the fertilized embryo back into the uterus

Indirect bilirubin   *also* unconjugated bilirubin, water insoluble; bilirubin present in the bloodstream and not yet absorbed by the hepatocytes

Infarct   area of nonviable tissue

Infarction   interruption in the blood supply to an area that may lead to necrosis of that area

Infundibulum   funnel-shaped portion of a structure

Inguinal canal   canal containing the spermatic cord in males

Inspissated   thickened by evaporation or absorption of fluid; diminished fluidity

Interhemispheric fissure   *also* falx cerebri; separates the cerebral hemispheres

Intraperitoneal   within the peritoneum

Intrauterine device   foreign body placed in the endometrial cavity of the uterus to prevent implantation of pregnancy

Intrauterine growth restriction   abnormal process in which the development and maturation of the fetus are impeded or delayed more than 2 standard deviations below the mean for gestational age, gender, and ethnicity

Intravenous pyelogram   invasive radiographic procedure in which a contrast agent is injected into a peripheral vein and the kidneys, ureters, and bladder are visualized

Ipsilateral   on the same side

Ischemia   local obstruction of the blood supply

Islets of Langerhans   small cells that compose the endocrine portion of the pancreas

Isoechoic   having the same echogenicity when comparing two structures

Isthmus   connection between two larger structures

IVC filter   filter placed in the inferior vena cava to help prevent blood clots from reaching the lungs

Jaundice   yellow discoloration of the skin, mucous membranes, and sclerae of the eyes caused by greater than normal amounts of bilirubin in the blood

Junctional zone   area in the uterus where the endometrium meets the myometrium

Karyotype   the pattern of chromosomes in an individual

Kasai operation *also* portoenterostomy; surgical procedure to correct biliary atresia with establishment of a pathway for bile to flow from the ducts to the intestine

Klinefelter's syndrome congenital endocrine condition of primary testicular failure that usually is not present before puberty; the classic form is associated with the presence of an extra X chromosome; the testes are small and firm; sterility, gynecomastia, abnormally long legs, and subnormal intelligence usually are present

Klippel-Trénaunay-Weber syndrome syndrome characterized by limb hypertrophy with associated large cutaneous hemangiomata

Left atrium filling chamber of the heart

Left ventricle pumping chamber of the heart

Leiomyoma benign smooth muscle tumor that usually occurs in the uterus

Lesions any pathologic or traumatic discontinuities of tissue or loss of function of a part

Lesser sac peritoneal space located posterior to the lesser omentum and stomach

Lethargic sluggish, lazy, or lack of energy

Leukemia cancer of the blood; can metastasize to testes

Leukocytosis increased number of white blood cells that is often associated with infection

Leukoplakia white patch of mucous membrane, commonly considered precancerous

Levocardia normal position of the heart in the left chest with the cardiac apex pointed to the left

Levoposition condition in which the heart is displaced further toward the left chest, usually in association with a space-occupying lesion

Leydig's cell tumor most common non–germ cell tumor of the testis, usually benign

Lipase pancreas enzyme that breaks down fat

Lithotripsy crushing of stones with sound waves or mechanical force that may be used to break down stones in the renal pelvis, ureter, or urinary bladder

Liver function tests group of blood tests that measure enzymes and proteins in the blood; results are used to diagnose and monitor liver disease

Lobar holoprosencephaly defect in interhemispheric fissure, absent septum pellucidum, variable degree of fusion of the lateral ventricles, least severe of three types

Loculation division into small spaces or cavities

Locus relates to the specific location of a gene on a chromosome

Longus colli muscles wedge-shaped muscles posterior to the thyroid lobes

Luteinization development of a corpus luteum within a ruptured graafian follicle

Lymphadenopathy abnormally large lymph nodes

Lymphangioma mass composed of dilated lymph vessels

Lymphoma malignant disease arising from the lymphoid tissues

Lymphosarcoma diffuse lymphoma

Lymphoscintigraphy *also* sentinel node mapping; scintillation scanning of lymph nodes after injection of a radionuclide; the sentinel nodes are the first lymph nodes to absorb the radionuclide, and these lymph nodes are surgically removed to determine whether cancer has metastasized to the lymphatic system

Macroglossia enlarged tongue

Macroscopic hematuria large amount of blood in the urine that can be seen without the aid of a microscope

Magnetic resonance imaging (MRI) type of medical imaging that uses radiofrequencies and allows for excellent resolution and acquisition of data in multiple planes

Malignant tending to become progressively worse and result in death; having the properties of invasion and metastasis

Mammary layer middle layer of the three layers of the breast

Mandibular frenulum normal midline craniofacial structure extending from the vestibular mucosa of the lower lip to the gingival mucosa of the lower jaw

Marfan syndrome autosomal dominant disorder characterized by elongated bones and abnormalities of the eyes and cardiovascular system

Marshall-Smith syndrome disorder characterized by unusually quick physical growth and bone development before birth associated with respiratory difficulties, mental retardation

May-Thurner syndrome iliocaval compression, usually of the left iliac vein by the overlying right common iliac artery

McBurney's sign pain in the right lower quadrant with rebound tenderness, associated with appendicitis

Meckel-Gruber syndrome autosomal recessive disorder involving polycystic kidneys, encephalocele, polydactyly, and cardiac defects

Meckel's diverticulum anomalous sac of embryologic origin that protrudes from the wall of the ileum usually between 30 and 90 cm from the ileocecal sphincter

Meconium initial material passed from the fetal bowels that consists of amniotic fluid debris and cells sloughed from the lining of the gastrointestinal tract during the intrauterine period

Meconium ileus obstruction of the small intestine in the newborn caused by impaction of thick, dry, tenacious meconium, usually at or near the ileocecal valve

Mediastinum testis portion of the tunica albuginea that penetrates the posterior surface of the testis

Medulla central portion of an organ

Medullary cystic disease hereditary condition displaying small medullary cysts resulting from renal tubular atrophy

Medullary sponge kidney condition of multiple ecstatic collecting tubules that may be too small to visualize on sonography; may be associated with nephrocalcinosis

Medullary thyroid cancer uncommon thyroid cancer

Meigs' syndrome ascites and pleural effusion associated with a benign ovarian tumor

Menarchal beginning of the menstrual function

Meningocele defect of the skin, soft tissues, and vertebral arches exposing the neural canal; covered by a thin meningeal membrane (spina bifida aperta)

Menometrorrhagia prolonged or excessive bleeding at irregular intervals

Menopause final menstruation usually occurring around age 52 years; postmenopausal refers to cessation of menstrual periods for 12 months

Menorrhagia   prolonged or excessive uterine bleeding at regular intervals

Mesentery   fold of peritoneum that encircles the small intestines

Mesocardia   atypical location of the heart in the middle of the chest with the cardiac apex pointing toward the midline of the chest

Mesocaval shunt   blood shunted from the superior mesenteric vein directly into the inferior vena cava

Mesoderm   primary embryologic germ layer that lies between the endoderm and ectoderm; from which connective tissue arises

Metabolic alkalosis   abnormal condition characterized by the significant loss of acid in the body or by increased levels of base bicarbonate

Metastasis   spread of cancer from its primary site to another place in the body

Microcalcifications   tiny echogenic foci that may or may not shadow

Micrognathia   small chin

Microlithiasis   tiny nonshadowing calcifications

Microphthalmia   small eyes

Microscopic hematuria   blood in the urine that is seen only with a microscope

Midgut   refers to the primordium of the small intestine, appendix, ascending colon, and most of the duodenum and transverse colon

Mitral valve   atrioventricular valve between the left atrium and left ventricle

Monoamniotic   twin pregnancy with sharing of one amniotic membrane

Monochorionic   twin pregnancy with sharing of one chorionic membrane

Mononucleosis   acute infection caused by Epstein-Barr virus that most commonly affects young persons; symptoms include fever, sore throat, enlarged lymph nodes, abnormal lymphocytes, and hepatosplenomegaly

Monozygotic   derived from one zygote

Morbidity   a state of illness

Morison's pouch   potential space located between the liver and the right kidney

Mortality   state of having died

Mosaicism   presence of two or more karyotypically distinct cell lines in the same tissue or individual

Mucin   glycoprotein produced by mucous membranes

Multicentric   two or more tumors in more than one area of origin

Multicystic dysplastic kidney   multiple, noncommunicating cysts of variable size in a nonfunctioning kidney; usually a unilateral process; may be a cause of an abdominal mass in a newborn

Multifetal   more than one fetus

Multilocular cystic nephroma   rare benign cystic neoplasm consisting of multiple cysts within a defined capsule

Multiparous   defines a woman who has given birth more than once

Multiples of the median   *also* multiples of the mean; a composite measure of an individual's laboratory results compared with matched norms

Murphy's sign   pain on palpation over the area of the gallbladder

Myelomeningocele   meningocele containing neural tissue within the sac (spina bifida aperta); most common site of defect is in lumbosacral region

Myometritis   inflammation or infection of the myometrium of the uterus

Myometrium   middle, muscular layer of the uterus

Necrosis   localized tissue death that occurs in groups of cells in response to disease or injury

Neonate   infant in the first 28 days of life

Neoplasm   any new growth, either malignant or benign

Nephroblastoma   *also* Wilms' tumor; malignant solid tumor involving the kidney usually occurring in pediatric patients

Nephrocalcinosis   calcification within the renal parenchyma that may include the cortex or medulla

Nephrolithiasis   renal calculi

Neural tube   refers to the spinal cord and intracranial contents (brainstem, cerebellum, and cerebrum)

Neuroblastoma   malignant solid tumor involving the adrenal gland usually occurring in pediatric patients

Neuropathy   condition of damaged nerves that can cause pain

Nevus   well-circumscribed benign lesion of the skin

NIHF   nonimmune hydrops fetalis; condition of fluid overload

Nodular regenerative hyperplasia   rare benign process of diffuse liver involvement by nodules composed of hyperplastic hepatocytes; associated with portal hypertension

Nodule   small group of cells

Non-Hodgkin's lymphoma   malignant disease of lymphoid tissue seen in increased frequency in individuals >50 years old

Nonsteroidal antiinflammatory drugs (NSAIDs)   drugs used for pain, including ibuprofen and indomethacin

Nonstress test (NST)   screening test used to monitor the well-being and fetal heart rate of a fetus

Nuclear medicine   medical discipline in which radioactive isotopes are used in the diagnosis and treatment of disease; major fields of nuclear medicine are physiologic function studies, radionuclide imaging, and therapeutic techniques

Obstetrician   physician who treats women during pregnancy and delivery

Obstruction   condition of being clogged or blocked

Obstructive jaundice   excessive bilirubin in the bloodstream caused by an obstruction of bile flow from the liver; characterized by a yellow discoloration of the sclera of the eye, skin, and mucous membranes

Oligohydramnios   a markedly decreased amount of amniotic fluid surrounding the fetus

Oligomenorrhea   decreased menstrual flow

Oliguria   decreased urine output

Omphalocele   defect in the anterior abdominal wall with extrusion of abdominal contents into the base of the umbilical cord

Oocyte   developing female germ cell

Oral contraceptives   medication containing hormones used to prevent pregnancy

Orchiectomy   surgical excision of the testicle

Orchiopexy   surgical correction of cryptorchidism

Orchitis   inflammation of the testis

Ossification   formation of bone substance

Ovulation induction   stimulation of the development of follicles on the ovary

Palliative   treatment given for the comfort of the patient but not as a cure

Papillary thyroid cancer   most common form of thyroid cancer

Paralytic ileus   nonmechanical obstruction of the bowel from paralysis of the bowel wall, usually as a result of localized or generalized peritonitis or shock

Parametritis   inflammation of the tissue of the structures adjacent to the uterus

Parathyroid hormone   hormone that is secreted by parathyroid glands, which regulate serum calcium levels

Parathyroid hyperplasia   enlargement of multiple parathyroid glands

Parenchyma   functioning tissue of an organ

Pathology   condition produced by disease

Peau d'orange   French term meaning "skin of an orange"; a dimpled skin condition that resembles the surface of an orange seen in lymphatic edemas and sometimes over an area of carcinoma of the breast

Pelvic inflammatory disease   inflammation of the female genital tract, especially of the fallopian tubes, caused by any of several microorganisms, characterized by severe abdominal pain, high fever, foul-smelling vaginal discharge, and in some cases destruction of tissue that can result in sterility

Pentalogy of Cantrell   a fetal anomaly comprised by omphalocele, defective sternum, ventral diaphragmatic defect, anterior pericardial deficiency, and intrinsic cardiac disease

Perforation   hole that develops through the membrane wall

Periportal cuffing   Thickening of the portal vein walls

Peritoneum   extensive serous membrane that covers the entire abdominal wall of the body and is reflected over the contained viscera

Peritonitis   inflammation of the peritoneum

Pharyngitis   inflammation of the mucous membrane and underlying parts of the pharynx

Phlegmasia alba dolens   severe, limb-threatening emergency condition, usually preceded by phlegmasia cerulean dolens

Phlegmasia cerulea dolens   severe form of deep vein thrombosis, usually of a proximal outflow area, that causes leg swelling and a bluish tone

PIH   pregnancy-induced hypertension; high blood pressure associated with pregnancy due to either gestational hypertension (hypertension caused only by pregnancy, no other maternal issues) or preeclampsia

Placental abruption   premature separation of the placenta

Placental insufficiency   decreased function of the placenta sufficient to compromise fetal nutrition and oxygen

Placentation   refers to the formation of the placenta

Polycystic disease   multiple cysts of organs usually originating in the kidneys

Polydactyly   extra digits—hands or feet or both

Polyhydramnios   excessive accumulation of amniotic fluid

Polyp   small tumor-like growth that projects from a mucous membrane surface

Polysplenia syndrome   syndrome associated with left atrial isomerism, multiple small spleens, interruption of the inferior vena cava with azygos vein continuation, and situs anomalies

Polyuria   increased urine output

Porcelain gallbladder   calcification of the gallbladder wall; associated with gallbladder cancer

Portal hypertension   increased size and pressure within the portal venous system often leading to splenomegaly, ascites, collateral vessel, and reversed flow within the portal vein

Portocaval shunt   shunts blood from the main portal vein at the confluence of the superior mesenteric vein and splenic vein directly into the inferior vena cava

Postaxial   extra digit by or near fifth digit of hand or foot

Postphlebitic syndrome   syndrome caused by a deep vein thrombosis that damages the venous valves, rendering them incompetent

Preaxial   extra digit by or near first digit of hand or foot

Precocious puberty   thelarche (breast development) and ovulatory activity in a girl <8 years old

Preeclampsia   abnormal maternal blood pressure elevation during the last half of pregnancy, accompanied by proteinuria and edema

Pregnancy induction   process of causing labor and delivery with the use of medication

Premature rupture of membranes (PROM)   rupture of the amniotic membranes before the onset of labor

Primary hyperparathyroidism   oversecretion of parathyroid hormone, usually from a parathyroid adenoma

Primigravida   first pregnancy

Proboscis   Fleshy, trunklike appendage

Progesterone   hormone produced by the corpus luteum and placenta; facilitates implantation of a fertilized ovum

Proliferative phase   refers to the uterine phase of the menstrual cycle between menses and ovulation, approximately days 5 to 14.

Proteinuria   increased presence of protein in the urine

Prothrombin Time (PT, PTT)   determines the time required for blood clotting to occur; increases in cases of parenchymal liver disease or Vitamin K deficiency

Prune-belly syndrome   a condition associated with bladder outlet obstruction consisting of laxity of the abdominal wall, cryptorchidism, and a urethral obstruction, such as posterior urethral valves

Pruritus   itching

Psammoma bodies   fine, punctate, internal calcifications seen in papillary thyroid cancer nodules

Pseudocyst   space or cavity that contains fluid but has no lining membrane

Pseudomyxoma peritonei   condition in which mucinous ascites and peritoneal implants fills the peritoneal cavity in response to a neoplastic process leading to massive abdominal distention and intestinal distress and obstruction

Pulmonary artery   principal artery that carries blood from the right ventricle to the lungs

Pulmonary stenosis   thickening and narrowing of the pulmonary cusps

Pulmonary veins   four pulmonary veins that bring blood from the lungs back into the posterior wall of the left atrium

Purulent   containing, discharging, or causing the production of pus

Pyelectasis   *also* pelviectasis; dilation of the renal pelvis or pelves

Pyloric canal   *also* pyloric channel; muscle that connects the stomach to the proximal duodenum

Pyloromyotomy   *also* Fredet-Ramstedt operation; surgical procedure that involves the cutting of the muscle fibers of the gastric outlet to widen the opening; used as a treatment for pyloric stenosis

Pyocele   peritesticular abscess

Pyosalpinx   condition in which the fallopian tubes are distended with pus

Pyuria   presence of pus in the urine

Quadriplegia   paralysis that includes the upper and lower extremities and the trunk

Radial   plane of imaging the breast for ultrasound that radiates out from the nipple to the periphery of the breast similar to hands of a clock (90 degrees to antiradial)

Radial ray defect   hypoplasia or aplasia of the radius; present in many syndromes

Rebound tenderness   pain that can be produced or intensified with release of pressure

Recanalization   spontaneous opening of an occluded vessel

Recanalized umbilical vein   opening of the potential space located within the ligament of teres left by the fetal umbilical vein

Regression models   tables used to determine gestational age and weight on the basis of measurements

Renal colic   severe pain caused by a stone obstructing or passing through the renal collecting system or ureter

Renal parenchyma   area from the renal sinus to the outer renal surface where the arcuate and interlobar vessels are found

Renal pyramids   portion of the kidney that is composed of a medullary substance consisting of a series of striated conical masses

Retroareolar   area beneath the nipple

Retromammary layer   deepest of the three layers of the breast and layer of the breast that is superficial to the pectoralis major muscle

Retroperitoneum   space posterior to the peritoneal cavity of the abdomen

Reversible ischemic neurologic deficit (RIND)   temporary neurologic deficit, with symptoms lasting >24 hours but <3 weeks

Rhizomelia   shortening of the proximal segment of the extremity

Right atrium   filling chamber of the heart

Right ventricle   pumping chamber of the heart

Rouleaux formation   roll formation; slow-moving erythrocytes that are a precursor to thrombosis and can be seen on two-dimensional ultrasound

Ruvalcaba-Myhre syndrome   rare inherited disorder characterized by excessive growth before and after birth, an abnormally large and narrow head, and benign subcutaneous growths (hamartomas)

Salpingitis   inflammation of the fallopian tubes

Salpingography   radiographic visualization of the fallopian tubes after injection of a radiopaque substance

Sarcoma   malignant tumor of the connective tissues or lymphoid tissues

Sciatica   pain in the lumbosacral area of the spine that radiates posteriorly down the ipsilateral leg from compression of the sciatic nerve

Scrotal pearl   mobile calcified object in the peritesticular space

Scrotum   double pouch that contains the testicles, epididymides, and part of

Sebum   semifluid fatty secretion of the sebaceous glands

Secondary hyperparathyroidism   enlargement of parathyroid glands in patients with renal failure or vitamin D deficiency

Secretory phase   refers to the uterine phase of the menstrual cycle between ovulation and menses, approximately days 15 to 28

Semilobar   larger segments of forebrain absent, larger defect in falx cerebri; the two cerebral hemispheres remain partially separated posteriorly

Seminoma   most common type of germ cell tumor of the testis

Septum primum   first part of the atrial septum to grow from the dorsal wall of the primitive atrium and fuse with the endocardial cushion in the center of the heart

Septum secundum   second part of the atrial septum to grow to the right of the septum primum

Serosa   *also* perimetrium; thin, outermost layer of the uterus

Sertoli's cell tumor   one of the non–germ cell tumors of the testicle, usually benign

Serum calcium   laboratory value that is elevated with hyperparathyroidism

Sexually transmitted disease   disease acquired as a result of intercourse with an infected individual

Shoulder dystocia   condition in which the fetal shoulders become impacted behind the symphysis pubis

Sickle cell anemia   autosomal recessive disease caused by a mutation in the hemoglobin gene; characterized by red blood cells that have an abnormal (crescent) shape and are rigid and sticky; found primarily in descendants of Africa, India, the Mediterranean, Saudi Arabia, and South and Central America; a decrease of oxygen material, such as hemoglobin, from an autosomal dominant disease characterized by crescent-shaped or sickle-shaped erythrocytes and accelerated breaking of erythrocytes

Signet-ring cell   cell type typically contained in a mucus-secreting adenocarcinoma

Situs   relates to the normal location of the organs in the body

"Snowstorm" sign   sonographic sign of implant rupture that appears as echogenic noise or dirty shadowing with a similar sonographic appearance of bowel gas

Sonohysterography   *also* saline-infusion sonography; technique in which sterile saline solution is infused into the endometrial cavity during transvaginal ultrasound for better visualization of endometrial abnormalities

Sonologist   professional educated to perform ultrasound examinations and interpret the findings

Sotos' syndrome   *also* cerebral gigantism; syndrome that is characterized by an enlarged head circumference accompanied by increased birth weight; mental retardation may also be present

Sperm granuloma   extratubular collection of sperm seen mostly in men after vasectomy

Spermatocele cystic lesion containing spermatozoa that can involve the rete testis or epididymal tubules

Splenorenal shunt blood is shunted from the splenic vein into the left renal vein

Splenosis implantation and growth of heterotopic tissue as a result of splenic rupture

Splenunculus accessory spleen (*pl.* spleniculi)

Spontaneous abortion premature expulsion of a nonviable pregnancy from the uterus

Stasis dermatitis brawny edema; limb pigmentation changes causing a brownish patch of edema, usually in the gaitor zone of the leg

Steatohepatitis accumulation of fatty deposits in the liver, linked to obesity and insulin resistance

"Stepladder" sign sonographic sign of implant rupture that appears as parallel echogenic lines within the interior of the implant

Sternocleidomastoid muscles large muscles anterolateral to the thyroid

Strap muscles sternohyoid and sternothyroid muscles that lie anterior to the thyroid

Stroma supporting tissue or matrix of an organ, as distinguished from its functional element or parenchyma

Stuck twin diamniotic pregnancy in which one fetus remains pressed against the uterine wall in a severely oligohydramniotic sac, whereas the other twin is in a severely hydramniotic sac

Subcutaneous layer most superficial of the three layers of the breast located just below the skin

Subphrenic spaces potential spaces located between the liver and the diaphragm

Subseptate uterus congenital anomaly resulting in a septation dividing the endometrial cavity

Superficial vein thrombosis thrombosis located in the superficial veins of the extremity; the thrombosed vein appears as a cordlike structure just below the surface of the skin and on ultrasound examination has the characteristics of a thrombosed vessel; patients with thrombosis localized to the superficial system undergo conservative management but may be monitored to ensure that the thrombus does not progress to the deep system

Superior vena cava venous return from the head and upper extremity into the posterior medial wall of the right atrium

Syndactyly fusion of the extremities or digits; bony or soft tissue fusion

Systemic lupus erythematosus (SLE) connective tissue autoimmune disorder characterized by skin lesions and disseminated vital organ involvement with antinuclear antibodies present; increases the risk of late pregnancy loss owing to hypertension, renal compromise, and premature rupture of membranes; also associated with heart block and neonatal lupus; patients with SLE are at higher risk for the development of intrauterine growth restriction during pregnancy

Talipes clubfoot; abnormal deviation of the foot relative to the lower leg; abnormal relationship of tarsal bones and the calcaneus; 55% of deformities are bilateral; most common deformity talipes equinovarus

Tamoxifen drug given to women with breast cancer to inhibit estrogen stimulation in the breast, but it acts as an estrogen stimulus to the uterus

Tardus parvus describes a waveform with a delayed upstroke and a reduced velocity; seen distal to a significant stenosis

Teratologic caused by a congenital or developmental anomaly

Teratoma congenital germ cell tumor that can contain embryonic elements of all primary germ cell layers

Terminal ductal-lobular unit each of hundreds of individual milk-producing glands within the breast and the terminal end of a lactiferous duct together form the terminal ductal-lobular unit, which is where almost all breast pathology is located

Tetralogy of Fallot congenital heart defect that is the most common form of cyanotic heart disease, characterized by a high, membranous ventricular septal defect; large, anteriorly displaced aorta; pulmonary stenosis; and right ventricular hypertrophy

Theca sheath of membrane forming the outer wall of a structure (e.g., a graafian follicle)

Thrombocytopenia decreased number of platelets

Thrombocytopenia–absent radius syndrome syndrome characterized by thrombocytopenia and absent radii

Thrombosis clotted blood within a vessel

Thyroid inferno increase in color Doppler vascular flow in the thyroid

TIPSS *also* TIPS; transjugular intrahepatic portosystemic shunt

TORCH infections group of infections that may have adverse affects on the fetus—*t*oxoplasmosis, *o*ther [congenital syphilis, viruses] *r*ubella, *c*ytomegalovirus, *h*erpes simplex virus; others have added syphilis and AIDS making the acronym STARCHES

Torsion twisting, twisted

Torticollis condition in which the head tilts to one side because of abnormal contraction of the muscles

Total parenteral nutrition solution administered intravenously to provide nutritional requirement

Transient ischemic attack (TIA) temporary neurologic deficit, with symptoms having lasting a few minutes to several hours, but never >24 hours

Translocation rearrangement of genetic material in which part of a chromosome is located on another chromosome

Transposition of the great arteries abnormal condition that exists when the aorta is connected to the right ventricle and the pulmonary artery is connected to the left ventricle; the atrioventricular valves are normally attached and related

Tricuspid valve atrioventricular valve found between the right atrium and the right ventricle

Triple screen laboratory test that measures not only alpha fetoprotein but also human chorionic gonadotropin and estriol; this test is more accurate than testing of alpha fetoprotein alone and screens for additional genetic problems

Trophoblast outer cell layer of the blastocyst; creates the chorionic membranes and the fetal contribution to the placenta

Trophoblastic disease tumors that arise from an abnormal proliferation of the chorionic villi

Tuberculosis infiltrative neoplasm that can affect the testes

Tuberous sclerosis autosomal dominant or sporadic syndrome characterized by seizures, mental retardation, and cutaneous lesions; associated renal cysts and neoplasms are commonly identified in these patients, as are lesions in the central nervous system, cardiovascular system, and pulmonary and skeletal systems

Tuboovarian abscess (TOA) abscess formed when purulent material escapes the fallopian tube and forms a pocket of abscess near the ovary

Tunica albuginea white, fibrous capsule that surrounds the testicle

Tunica vaginalis serous membrane that covers the front and sides of the testicle, epididymis, and inner scrotal wall

Twin embolization situation in which fetal death of a twin in the second or third trimester results in hypoperfusion and ischemia of the organs of the surviving fetus

"Twinkle" sign color Doppler artifact in which the color rapidly changes posterior to a urinary tract stone with a comet tail appearance

Ulcer breakdown of the skin; a venous ulcer is usually found in the gaitor zone and is large, weepy, and fairly painless

Ulceration circumscribed inflammatory and often suppurating lesion on the skin or an internal mucous surface resulting in necrosis of tissue

Upper gastrointestinal fluoroscopic radiographic imaging of the upper gastrointestinal tract after ingestion of barium

Urachal cysts persistence and distention of the embryologic allantois; midline in location; abuts the bladder

Uremia excess of urea and other nitrogenous waste in the blood

Ureteropelvic junction point at which the ureter joins the renal pelvis

Urolithiasis stone in the urinary system

Uterus didelphys congenital anomaly resulting in complete duplication of the uterine body, cervix, and vagina

Valsalva maneuver maneuver performed by the patient in an effort to stop venous flow to the heart momentarily; the patient is asked to take a breath and bear down as though trying to have a bowel movement and then hold that pressure; the subsequent increase in abdominal pressure causes a cessation of antegrade venous flow and an increase in distal vein size; when the patient releases the pressure, the backed-up venous blood is able to flow rapidly antegrade again

Varicocele dilated pampiniform veins

Varicose veins dilated and tortuous veins of the superficial venous system, usually a result of valve incompetence

Vas deferens ductus deferens

Venous collateral flow alternative circulatory pathways that develop after pathologic changes prevent normal vascular pathways from serving as an adequate source of blood to an organ

Venous insufficiency venous reflux; refers to a vein in which the valves are no longer functioning correctly, allowing blood to flow in a retrograde fashion; the tissues distal to chronic venous insufficiency may become hyperpigmented, indurated, and ulcerative; can be caused by postphlebitic syndrome

Venous ulcer ulceration of the distal, usually lower, extremity with chronic venous insufficiency secondary to venous hypertension

Ventriculomegaly enlargement of the ventricles in the brain

Virchow's triad set of three causative factors described by Virchow in 1862; damage to the venous wall, decrease in flow (stasis), and increase in coagulability increase the probability of venous thrombosis; damage to the vessel wall may be through surgery, trauma, or indwelling lines; decrease in flow may be through immobility, external pressure, varicose veins, congestive heart failure, or other causes; increased incoagulability may be caused by a release of factor III in surgical patients who are healing, by malignant tissues of cancer patients, or by burned damaged tissue

Visceromegaly enlargement of the viscera of the abdomen, such as liver, spleen, stomach, kidneys, or pancreas

Volvulus twisting of the bowel that results in obstruction

von Gierke's disease autosomal recessive disease marked by excessive storage of glycogen in the liver, kidneys, and other parts of the body

von Hippel-Lindau disease autosomal dominant type of phacomatosis that is primarily associated with hemangiomas or hemangioblastomas of the cerebellar fourth ventricle and that may be associated with cysts or hamartomas of the kidneys, adrenal glands, or other organs

von Hippel-Lindau disease autosomal dominant disease characterized by development of various cysts and neoplasms; renal cysts and renal cell carcinoma are prevalent in individuals with this disorder

WBC white blood cell

Weaver's syndrome disorder of large birth size and accelerated growth and skeletal maturation, associated with limb, craniofacial, neurologic, and other abnormalities

Wharton's jelly gelatinous matrix surrounding the umbilical vessels as they course between the placenta and the fetus

Wolffian embryonic structures that develop into parts of the male genitourinary system

X-linked anomalies that are transmitted from the mother to the male fetus

"Yin yang" sign color Doppler pattern in which a vessel examined in a transverse plane shows the swirling pattern flow; the blood coming toward the transducer is color encoded red, and the flow away from the transducer is color encoded blue

Yolk sac structure that develops in the inner cell mass of the embryo and expands into a vesicle with a thick part that grows into the cavity of the chorion; after it supplies the nourishment of the embryo, the yolk sac usually disappears during the seventh week after conception

Zygosity refers to the number of oocytes released from an ovary and fertilized by spermatozoa

Zygote combined cell produced by the union of a spermatozoa and an oocyte at the completion of fertilization until the first cleavage

CHAPTER 1

1. Cholelithiasis was diagnosed in this patient with the possibility of choledocholithiasis. Choledocholithiasis was subsequently confirmed with endoscopic retrograde cholangiopancreatography. The gallbladder and the stones in the ducts were removed.
2. Polycystic disease of the liver and kidneys
3. Cholelithiasis and sludge
4. Gallbladder carcinoma with metastatic disease to the liver
5. Acute cholecystitis

CHAPTER 2

1. This patient with hemorrhagic hepatocellular adenoma has the classic clinical presentation. The sonogram localized the tumor to Couinaud's segment 7, and the next day the patient underwent surgery for excision of that segment.
2. The biopsy report revealed metastatic gastric cancer. Gastric cancer is one of the most common types to metastasize to the liver.
3. The mass is a simple hepatic cyst; most hepatic cysts are asymptomatic and discovered incidentally. No follow-up is required; the cyst is not a cause of concern for the patient.
4. In the setting of chronic hepatitis C and cirrhosis, hepatocellular carcinoma is the most likely diagnosis. A strong correlation between preexisting cirrhosis and hepatocellular carcinoma exists.
5. In this patient with unexplained weight loss and low-grade fever, coupled with the computed tomography (CT) findings, metastatic lung cancer is the most likely diagnosis. Primary lung cancer with metastasis to the liver was revealed at biopsy.

CHAPTER 3

1. Surface irregularities on the liver can indicate the presence of cirrhosis. These irregularities occur as a result of repeated scarring and regrowth of hepatocytic tissue brought on by long-standing disease. The presence of ascites supports the diagnosis of cirrhosis. A complete liver examination should be performed to demonstrate the echogenicity of the liver, the caudate lobe-to-right lobe ratio, and the presence of masses or nodules. Pulsed wave and color Doppler evaluations of the portal circulation to rule out thrombosis or the presence of portal hypertension should be obtained.
2. This patient has fatty liver disease. The appearance of diffuse fatty infiltration of the liver ranges from mild to severe. In the mildest form, the liver may appear slightly echogenic compared with the adjacent kidneys, or it may appear normal. As the fatty replacement becomes more severe, the liver is difficult to penetrate, and the vascular structures are poorly visualized, especially the hepatic veins. Alcoholism, obesity, and diabetes are the most common causes of fatty liver disease; the likely cause for this case is alcohol abuse. This patient has mildly elevated liver enzymes; in most instances of fatty liver disease, liver function is not permanently impaired. However, sustained excessive alcohol consumption can lead to cirrhosis and permanent, irreversible liver damage.
3. The image represents thrombosis of the main portal vein. Reduced portal blood flow caused by hepatocellular disease is one of the major causes of portal vein thrombosis. Portal vein thrombosis is being recognized with increasing frequency with the use of sonography, and patients with hepatocellular disease should undergo a complete evaluation of the portal circulation. In this case, the sonographer should examine the patient for signs of varices that may have formed to bypass the occluded portal vein (cavernous transformation).
4. Although the most common explanation for a solid mass in the liver is metastatic disease, it is common to see focal fat (more hyperechoic) or areas that are fat spared (more hypoechoic). Common areas of focal sparing are the areas anterior to the gallbladder and the right portal vein or within the left lobe; in this case, the focal normal area of liver creates a "mass effect" anterior to the gallbladder. Fatty changes are usually noted in patients with a history of obesity, alcoholism, or diabetes; this patient was noted to be moderately obese. Important considerations in supporting this diagnosis are the findings of normal liver enzymes, obesity, and lack of patient history for a known primary cancer.
5. These images represent recanalization of the umbilical vein, a remnant of fetal circulation that, after birth, resides in the ligament of teres. Flow noted in the location of ligaments, or other potential spaces, often indicates the presence of collateral pathways that have formed in response to portal hypertension. These pathways develop to help alleviate increased flow pressure caused by damage to hepatocytes that prevents portal veins from delivering blood from the intestines and spleen to the liver. Additional changes can be other collateral pathways within the abdominal cavity, notable changes in liver echotexture, and hepatosplenomegaly. Eventually, the portal vein may develop hepatofugal flow (blood flowing out of the liver).

CHAPTER 4

1. The most likely diagnosis is acute pancreatitis. Acute inflammation of the pancreas is generally caused by one of two factors: biliary disease and alcoholism. Other sources may include trauma, pregnancy, peptic ulcer disease, medications, hereditary factors, systemic infections, posttransplant complications, and iatrogenic causes (e.g., endoscopic retrograde cholangiopancreatogram endoscopy). Patients with acute pancreatitis have a sudden onset of persistent midepigastric pain. Fever and leukocytosis accompany the attack. Classically, serum amylase levels increase within 24 hours of onset, and lipase levels increase within 72 hours. Diffuse pancreatitis causes an increase in size and a decrease in echogenicity from swelling and congestion. The borders of the pancreas may appear irregular.

2. This is a pseudocyst. Pseudocysts most often arise from the tail of the pancreas and are located in the lesser sac, as is seen in this case. This patient's pseudocyst may have resulted from pancreatitis caused by her recent biliary surgery.

3. This is a functioning islet cell tumor, specifically, the most common type—insulinoma. Patients with insulinomas may have obesity and hypoglycemic episodes, as was seen with this case. Islet cell tumors are slow-growing, small tumors and are hypoechoic compared with the surrounding pancreatic tissues.

4. Cystic masses of the pancreas include cystadenoma and cystadenocarcinoma. Microcystic serous-type cystadenoma manifests with cysts measuring less than 2 cm, as seen in this case. Cystadenoma may appear similar to pseudocysts; however, the patient history does not support a history of pancreatitis or pseudocyst formation.

5. This solid, hypoechoic mass represents adenocarcinoma; the most common solid pancreatic neoplasm. The most common sonographic appearance of adenocarcinoma is an irregular, hypoechoic mass in the pancreas. Men are more often affected than women, and the peak incidence is between 60 and 80 years of age. Adenocarcinoma is most commonly found in the head of the pancreas. The type and onset of symptoms are related to the location of the tumor; tumors in the pancreatic head may cause obstructive jaundice.

CHAPTER 5

1. This is renal cell carcinoma (RCC). RCC is more common in male patients of advancing age. Hematuria and hypertension are associated signs, and cigarette smoking is a known risk factor. Small RCCs may have variable echogenicity; larger masses are more often hypoechoic to the surrounding renal cortex.

2. Ureteral calculi causing partial obstruction at the ureterovesical junction (UVJ). Stones can cause obstruction of the renal collecting system, or they may pass into the ureter and obstruct it, causing a hydroureter. The two most common sites of obstruction are the ureteropelvic junction and the UVJ. Sonographic documentation of a ureteral stone may be difficult to obtain because of the small size of the calculi, posterior location of the ureter (where the area of interest may not be in the focal zone), lack of fluid surrounding the stone, and adjacent bowel gas. The use of tissue harmonics, when small calculi are suspected, increases the chance of seeing posterior acoustic shadowing. A color Doppler artifact, the "twinkle" sign (see Fig. 5-6, *B*), may be seen with small stones and may be helpful when shadowing cannot be demonstrated.

3. Patients with transitional cell carcinoma (TCC) typically have painless hematuria, but the patient may have pain and hydronephrosis if the lesion involves the renal collecting system. Bladder lesions may cause hematuria and blood clots. TCC occurs more often in men, and an increased incidence is seen with advancing age. The most common presentation of TCC is a bulky, hypoechoic mass in the bladder. In this case, the TCC lesion is in the kidney within the renal sinus. Renal TCC may cause separation and dilation of the renal collecting system, as seen in this case (see also Fig. 5-11). The prognosis for this case was poor; the tumor has invaded the renal vein and inferior vena cava.

4. This mass was an oncocytoma. An oncocytoma is a benign renal cell neoplasm; it accounts for only a small percentage of adult primary renal masses. The imaging characteristics of oncocytomas and renal cell carcinomas (RCCs) overlap, and differentiating an oncocytoma from a RCC and other solid renal neoplasms is not always possible with sonography. Computed tomography (CT) scan or magnetic resonance imaging (MRI) may show the presence of a central scar. The main clinical importance of oncocytoma is the difficulty in distinguishing it from RCC, and a preoperative diagnosis of RCC must be considered for this patient. Most patients with a renal oncocytoma are asymptomatic; symptoms in this patient were likely due to the presence of gallstones. On a sonogram, oncocytoma appears as well-defined, homogeneous, and hypoechoic to isoechoic masses (see also Fig. 5-14).

5. The most likely differential diagnoses are renal cell carcinoma (RCC), transitional cell carcinoma, or oncocytoma. This mass was a RCC with invasion of the renal vein and inferior vena cava. Of the three neoplasms, RCC is known to invade the renal vein and inferior vena cava; transitional cell carcinoma in the kidney arises from the renal sinus, and oncocytoma is less likely to invade the vessels. This

appearance represents a stage 3 RCC. Stage 3 masses extend into the renal vein or vena cava, involve the ipsilateral adrenal gland or perinephric fat or both, or have spread to one local lymph node.

CHAPTER 6

1. Acute glomerulonephritis is an inflammation of the renal glomeruli that frequently occurs as a late complication of an infection, typically of the throat. This patient was recently treated for strep throat and exhibits classic symptoms of acute glomerulonephritis, including malaise, mild hypertension, and edema. Sonographically, in acute glomerulonephritis, the renal cortex may be increased with visualization of the renal pyramids and enlarged kidneys.

2. Chronic kidney disease may have various causes, including diabetes and hypertension. The symptoms of worsening kidney function are nonspecific and might include feeling generally unwell and having a reduced appetite. Patients who are noncompliant with their medications continue to lose renal function. Sonographically, a kidney that has a thin cortex and is echogenic exhibits classic findings of chronic kidney disease.

3. Pyonephritis is a renal infection with pus in the collecting system. This patient developed pyonephrosis as a complication of renal stones, which was a source of persisting infection that occurred spontaneously. Sonographically, pyonephrosis manifests as hydronephrosis with debris in the collecting system. The debris is seen as low-level echoes, and the most common finding is pyonephrosis.

4. Acute kidney injury is a rapid loss of kidney function. Acute kidney injury is caused by conditions that decrease effective blood flow to the kidney; these include systemic conditions, such as low blood volume, hypotension, and heart failure. When there is a decrease in the blood flow to the kidney, it does not function properly. Reduced function results in a decrease of urine output. Despite being pushed fluids and medication, there was neither improvement in renal function nor increased urine production. Sonographically, acute kidney injury appears as normal to enlarged kidneys that are echogenic compared with the liver.

5. Renal artery stenosis is narrowing of the renal artery that can impede blood flow to the kidney. Hypertension and atrophy of the affected kidney may result from renal artery stenosis, ultimately leading to renal failure. The described buttock pain is claudication caused by a significant atherosclerotic process. Although the renal sonogram was unremarkable, the Doppler interrogation of the renal vessels displayed very high velocities with aliasing consistent with renal artery stenosis. It is important to recognize the tardus parvus spectral tracing distal to the stenosis.

CHAPTER 7

1. This is autosomal dominant polycystic kidney disease (ADPKD). The findings meet the unified criteria for ADPKD because there are two or more cysts in each kidney. Note the varied cyst sizes possible in this disease. Associated cysts can be found in the liver, pancreas, and spleen.

2. This is acute renal failure indicated by the presence of an enlarged echogenic left kidney with trace amounts of perirenal fluid. This is a nonobstructive cause of renal impairment. The fluid-filled structures represent multiple parapelvic cysts. Parapelvic cysts are typically asymptomatic and are noted incidentally in this case.

3. The mass is a 5.5 cm × 5.6 cm × 5.9 cm simple cyst arising from the upper pole of the right kidney. The subtle "claw" sign of the renal parenchyma cupping the cyst indicates a renal origin. Note also the line of echogenic retroperitoneal fat separating the kidney cyst from the liver.

4. *Image 1:* The student scanned from an anterior window, with harmonics activated and focus set too shallow. The initial image of the cyst appears to demonstrate internal echoes as the cyst was placed deeper than the focal zone and harmonics may have limited penetration. *Image 2:* The supervising sonographer is scanning the kidney from a more coronal window. This places the cyst shallower in the image and allows for the improved contrast resolution provided by harmonics. The cyst is actually simple and may require only periodic follow-up, if any.

5. This is a Bosniak II cyst. Note the small, minimally complex or atypical renal cyst arising from the lower pole of the left kidney with a solitary, thin septation. No follow-up is warranted.

CHAPTER 8

1. The lesion is round, thin-walled, and anechoic consistent with a cyst. Considering the lesion has not changed over the years further confirms that this mass is a cyst.

2. The patient is asymptomatic and has normal laboratory values, so the most likely reason for the findings is a benign process. The initial appearance illustrates heterogeneity, and with closer inspection, multiple discrete hyperechoic masses can be seen consistent with hemangiomas.

3. Spleen images reveal an anechoic to hypoechoic striated lesion in the lateral portion of the spleen. Knowledge of the clinical history of a gunshot wound, decreased hematocit, absence of free fluid, and imaging appearances support the diagnosis of a

subcapsular hematoma that is contained within the spleen.

4. The most likely cause for the multiple echogenic foci is siderosis (an accumulation of iron and calcium deposits). The presence of portal hypertension creates increased pressure within the splenic vessels causing disintegration of cellular content and resulting in hemorrhage in the red pulp. The deposition of iron and calcium adjacent to the collagen tissue of the red pulp creates Gamna-Gandy bodies.

5. The sonogram revealed multiple splenules consistent with polysplenia. Polysplenia is most often associated with heterotaxy syndrome, which can include partial situs inversus, bilateral left-sidedness, and an interrupted inferior vena cava with azygous/hemiazygous continuation.

CHAPTER 9

1. These findings are consistent with the juvenile presentation of autosomal recessive polycystic kidney disease (ARPKD), also known as infantile polycystic kidney disease. ARPKD can manifest in various forms that range in severity from perinatal (most severe), to neonatal, to infantile, to juvenile. More than 50% of affected children progress to end-stage renal disease, usually in the first decade of life; the 10-year survival of patients who live beyond the first year of life has improved. A few patients present in older childhood or young adulthood with hepatosplenomegaly and evidence of portal hypertension. In childhood and young adulthood, the kidneys are echogenic and large, but massive enlargement is usually not seen. Macrocysts, more typical of autosomal dominant polycystic kidney disease, are often seen in older children.

2. Most pediatric masses are renal in origin. Hepatic and adrenal masses (as well as masses affecting other organs) must also be considered. Determining the organ of origin and relevant laboratory findings should be considered in this case. If the mass is assumed to be adrenal, owing to its suprarenal location, an increased catecholamine level could help to make the diagnosis of suspected neuroblastoma. The clinical presentation of neuroblastoma is highly variable, ranging from a mass that causes no symptoms to a primary tumor that causes critical illness as a result of local invasion, widely disseminated disease, or both.

3. The renal sonogram revealed pyelonephritis with moderate hydronephrosis, marked enlargement of the kidneys, sediment in the renal pelvis, and loss of the corticomedullary interface.

4. Multicystic dysplastic kidney may manifest as a palpable abdominal mass. The sonographic findings of multicystic dysplastic kidney are multiple noncommunicating cysts in the renal bed. The cause is poorly understood, but it may be the result of an obstructive process in utero or a cessation of the embryologic development into the metanephros. Drugs that may cause kidney dysplasia include prescription medicines, such as antiseizure medication and angiotensin-converting enzyme inhibitors and angiotensin receptor blockers.

5. The sonographic findings are consistent with type I choledochal cyst, the most common type. The clinical presentation of choledochal cyst includes jaundice and pain. A palpable mass also may be present. Because abdominal pain and vomiting are nonspecific for this disease process, the prolonged jaundice during the neonatal period raises the suspicion for choledochal cyst. The condition has a higher frequency in Asians. Sonography is useful to differentiate choledochal cyst from other causes of jaundice in infancy, including biliary atresia and hepatitis. Sonographic investigation of a choledochal cyst most commonly shows fusiform dilation of the common bile duct, with associated intrahepatic ductal dilation.

CHAPTER 10

1. Aortic aneurysm with thrombus. Because the aneurysm measures more than 4.5 cm, the patient is referred for a vascular surgical consultation to discuss elective repair.

2. Abdominal aortic aneurysm. Although most aneurysms are found incidentally, they can manifest as pulsatile "masses."

3. Ruptured (or rupturing) aortic aneurysm. The diagnosis is supported by the clinical symptoms. The classic presentation of a ruptured abdominal aortic aneurysm includes the triad of hypotension, abdominal or back pain, and a pulsatile abdominal mass.

4. Aortic dissection. The clinical presentation of dissection is usually an acute onset of severe chest pain. Patients may also have neck or throat pain, pain in the abdomen or lower back, syncope, paresis, and dyspnea. If the patient history includes hypertension, aortic aneurysm, or Marfan syndrome, dissection should be strongly considered. Clinical examination may also reveal absent pulses in the legs.

5. The recommended sonographic surveillance is no further testing for patients with abdominal aortic aneurysms less than 3 cm and annual sonography for patients with aneurysms measuring 3 to 4 cm. When an aneurysm reaches a diameter of 4 to 4.5 cm, screening should be performed every 6 months. Sonography is used in patient follow-up for assessment of an expanding aneurysm for planning of elective surgery. Patients with aneurysms measuring greater than 4.5 cm should be referred to counseling for elective surgical options.

CHAPTER 11

1. Genetically, a history of appendicitis in a first-degree family member is associated with a 3.5% to 10% relative risk for the disorder. The strongest familial associations have been noted when children develop appendicitis at unusually young ages (birth to 6 years).
2. The patient most likely has a periappendiceal abscess, which may be found in cases of rupture either before or after appendectomy and generally appear as vague hypoechoic or complex masses. Abscesses are usually successfully drained after appendectomy with a transrectal biopsy guide on an endocavitary transducer. Insertion of the transducer into the rectum allows for adequate visualization and drainage of the abscess with sonographic guidance.
3. In a male patient, the differential diagnoses would include gallbladder disease, acute pyelonephritis, urinary tract stone disease, and infectious or inflammatory conditions of the cecum or ascending colon. Given this patient's clinical symptoms, the most likely diagnosis is acute appendicitis. A sonogram or computed tomography (CT) scan (or both) focusing on the appendix area should be ordered by the physician.
4. This patient most likely has acute appendicitis.
5. The debris within the appendiceal lumen most likely represents a mucocele. Other sonographic findings include a distended appendix with a cystic structure and debris ("onion" sign) within the lumen and edema in the surrounding tissues. The most likely diagnosis is a mucocele of the appendix.

CHAPTER 12

1. Hypertrophic pyloric stenosis
2. A normal pylorus is seen. The symptoms most likely can be attributed to ongoing gastric distress and a change in formula.
3. Intussusception
4. Hypertrophic pyloric stenosis
5. Intussusception

CHAPTER 13

1. The differential diagnoses for a thickened endometrium in a postmenopausal woman include endometrial carcinoma, endometrial hyperplasia, or polyps. Sonohysterography can help determine if endometrial thickening is the result of a mass, such as a polyp, or if diffuse thickening is present. An endometrial biopsy is the next diagnostic procedure to differentiate between hyperplasia and carcinoma.
2. The hypoechoic mass within the endometrium most likely represents a submucosal fibroid.

3. The endometrium in a postmenopausal patient with bleeding measures less than 5 mm; the most likely diagnosis is endometrial atrophy.
4. The mass demonstrated on the hysterosonogram most likely represents an endometrial polyp.
5. The myometrial mass shown in the image most likely represents a fibroid.

CHAPTER 14

1. Expulsion of the intrauterine device (IUD). A radiograph of the abdomen and pelvis should be ordered to rule out IUD perforation.
2. Proper intrauterine device (IUD) placement. An IUD is identified in the midline of the superior portion of the endometrium consistent with proper placement.
3. Intrauterine pregnancy with an inferiorly located intrauterine device (IUD). A hyperechoic linear structure in the lower uterine segment is identified by the arrow. This finding is most consistent with an improperly located IUD. A gestational sac is visualized in the uterine fundus without evidence of an embryo.
4. Migration of the intrauterine device into the lower uterine segment.
5. Malpositioned intrauterine device (myometrial penetration).

CHAPTER 15

1. The patient had bilateral tuboovarian abscess with an abscess posterior to the uterus. Using endovaginal sonography guidance, the abscess was drained. Close follow-up of the abscess was performed until total resolution was obtained.
2. The patient had left pyosalpinx and abscess formation, but the left ovary appears to be spared.
3. The patient developed pelvic inflammatory disease and bilateral tuboovarian abscess secondary to intrauterine contraceptive device placement.
4. The patient was diagnosed with a peritoneal inclusion cyst.
5. The patient had acute pelvic inflammatory disease with a right tuboovarian abscess.

CHAPTER 16

1. This is a case of a unicornuate uterus with a rudimentary left uterine horn. The left horn does not communicate with the vagina, and the menstrual blood and tissue cannot drain. The debris distends the rudimentary horn and causes increasing pain. Surgical excision of the horn is usually required.
2. This patient has a septate uterus. The septum appears complete on the ultrasound image. The fundal contour is not notched; this does not represent a bicornuate uterus. Uterine septa are associated with

an increased risk of miscarriage. This increased risk is thought to be due to the poor blood supply to the septum, which can lead to problems with implantation of the pregnancy. Additionally, the physical disruption of the normal uterine cavity contour may be another cause for miscarriages associated with a uterine septum.

3. This patient likely has an endometrioma on her right ovary and other implants of endometriosis causing her symptoms. The pain with intercourse may be from endometriosis implants posterior to the uterus. Endometriomas may also cause pelvic pain and usually require surgical excision for adequate treatment.

4. This patient likely has polycystic ovary syndrome given the ovarian appearance, clinical evidence of hyperandrogenism (hirsutism), and anovulatory pattern of menses. Many women with polycystic ovary syndrome are obese; however, this is not a requirement for the diagnosis. This patient would benefit from use of medications to induce ovulation to improve her chances of conceiving a pregnancy.

5. This patient likely has a bicornuate uterus given the fundal notch. Women with bicornuate uteri are at higher risk of having a fetus in breech presentation, likely because of the physical structural constraints within the cavity.

CHAPTER 17

1. The sonographic findings of a cystic mass with low-level echoes could represent a hemorrhagic cyst, endometrioma, or cystic teratoma. The computed tomography (CT) findings of fat within the mass confirm the diagnosis of cystic teratoma.

2. The stable size, cystic nature, and lack of solid components within the mass are suggestive of serous cystadenoma.

3. The low-level echoes represent the classic findings of an endometrioma. Because a hemorrhagic cyst can also have this appearance, the follow-up examination was helpful to rule out a physiologic cyst. The lack of solid components makes it less likely to be a cystic teratoma.

4. Although a history of breast cancer increases the risk for ovarian cancer, the fact that this mass was not evident on follow-up examination suggests a physiologic ovarian cyst.

5. The size and internal components of this mass suggest an ovarian cystadenocarcinoma.

CHAPTER 18

1. The sonographic finding of a thick echogenic ring around an intradecidual fluid collection is suggestive of an early (4 to 4.5 weeks) intrauterine pregnancy. The lack of adnexal pathology and free fluid makes the diagnosis of an ectopic pregnancy less likely.

Follow-up sonographic evaluation should be recommended to ensure the finding represents an intrauterine pregnancy and not a pseudogestational sac.

2. Because crown-rump length provides greater accuracy in gestational dating than patient account of last menstrual period and gestational sac measurements, the pregnancy should be dated as 6.5 weeks.

3. The prognosis is poor because an embryo should be noted when a gestational sac measures 25 mm. A 30-mm gestational sac with a yolk sac but no embryo is consistent with an anembryonic gestation.

4. A nuchal translucency measurement greater than or equal to 3 mm is considered abnormal. Resolution of a thickened nuchal translucency does not guarantee normalcy, and close clinical correlation and counseling should be offered to this patient.

5. The accuracy of fetal biometry is highest earlier in the pregnancy, so the dates should not be changed. By assigning a later due date based on later examinations, fetal growth problems may be overlooked.

CHAPTER 19

1. Osteogenesis imperfecta type II

2. The abdominal circumference. In this case, the new, unregistered sonographer had measured the abdominal circumference at the edges of the ribs and spine rather than at the skin line of the abdominal circumference, excluding the muscles, baby fat, and skin.

3. Incorrect last menstrual period because of early breakthrough implantation bleeding. Early intrauterine growth restriction is also possible but less likely.

4. The ultrasound scan reveals polyhydramnios explaining the increased fundal height. The polyhydramnios was due to anencephaly.

5. A double bubble sign is identified resulting from duodenal atresia and polyhydramnios. The amniotic fluid index is 30.6 cm.

CHAPTER 20

1. The measurements are evidence of intrauterine growth restriction. The Doppler waveforms demonstrate an ominous sign of significant distress. The MCA waveforms show head sparing has occurred. The MCA has a lower RI and a decreased PI compared with the umbilical artery Doppler. Placental insufficiency is clearly demonstrated. The ductus venosus waveform is abnormal with a deep a wave noted. The umbilical vein is pulsatile showing cardiac distress.

2. With evidence of early intrauterine growth restriction and multiple anomalies, one should suspect a chromosomal abnormality or syndrome with probable renal agenesis or bladder obstruction. The umbilical artery waveform is significantly abnormal

demonstrating placental insufficiency. Genetic counseling and testing should be offered. The fetal prognosis is poor.

3. Anhydramnios is a clear sign of a urinary problem or premature rupture of membranes. Right renal agenesis was evident, and the left kidney was dysplastic as well.

4. The distal ureter has an abnormal connection, and the entire ureter demonstrates dilation. This finding is suggestive of an ectopic ureter insertion, and serial sonograms should be performed to evaluate renal size and damage from the hydronephrosis.

5. With low amniotic fluid and a large hydroureter and multicystic kidneys, one should surmise a significant urinary anomaly. With other anomalies also noted, there is a strong suggestion that there may be a chromosomal abnormality or associated syndrome. The fetus had a significant ureterovesical junction obstruction as well as multicystic kidney dysplasia. The amniotic fluid was still low-normal, which is evidence that there is renal function without a bladder outlet obstruction. Genetic counseling and testing should be offered.

CHAPTER 21

1. Placenta previa is identified. The patient will be put on pelvic rest with follow-up sonography to assess for placental migration. If the previa persists, cesarean section will be necessary.

2. Retained products of conception

3. Ectopic pregnancy, most likely in the fallopian tube. The blood that is apparent in the cul-de-sac suggests rupture.

4. An anechoic area is demarcated by arrows in the image. This most likely is a resolving subchorionic hemorrhage. The pregnancy went to term, and delivery was uncomplicated.

5. The intrauterine device is identified within the endometrium, which is filled with blood. There is a large complex mass in the right adnexa and a significant amount of cul-de-sac fluid consistent with a ruptured ectopic pregnancy. The pregnancy test was positive, and the patient was rushed to surgery.

CHAPTER 22

1. The thin intertwin membrane is consistent with a monochorionic, diamniotic twin gestation. However, the empty sac suggests a vanishing twin, which is a common occurrence during the first trimester. First-trimester cotwin death does not pose a significant threat to the survivor.

2. Twin reversed arterial perfusion (TRAP) syndrome should be suspected in monochorionic gestations when one twin is normal and the other twin demonstrates upper body abnormalities. Reversed flow

within the umbilical artery of the abnormal twin confirms the diagnosis of TRAP.

3. The image demonstrates a monochorionic, diamniotic twin gestation, which places it at risk for complications related to shared vasculature, such as growth discordance, twin-twin transfusion syndrome, or twin reversed arterial perfusion sequence.

4. The image demonstrates twin A surrounded by polyhydramnios and twin B positioned by the anterior uterine wall likely restricted by an oligohydramniotic sac. These findings are suggestive of twin-twin transfusion syndrome.

5. The degree of growth discordance and the reversed diastolic flow evident in twin A's umbilical artery is suggestive of intrauterine growth restriction in twin A, which is most commonly caused by placental insufficiency. Because the twins are dizygotic, they do not share placental vascularity, which eliminates twin-twin transfusion syndrome as the cause for intrauterine growth restriction.

CHAPTER 23

1. Anencephaly

2. A diagnosis of a liver-containing omphalocele is made. Other anomalies of organ systems and extremities should be searched for that would suggest aneuploidy. No other anomalies were seen, and amniocentesis revealed a normal karyotype.

3. May recalculate alpha fetoprotein owing to gestational age being less than 21 weeks.

4. The left foot appears grossly malformed and edematous. This asymmetric anomaly is consistent with amniotic band syndrome.

5. Free-floating bowel is noted with the umbilical cord inserting adjacent to the bowel consistent with gastroschisis.

CHAPTER 24

1. Figure 24-14 shows a fetus with a large cystic hygroma, hydrops, and decreased amniotic fluid. These findings have a high association with Turner syndrome. An isolated cystic hygroma can be seen in fetuses with trisomy 18, trisomy 13, trisomy 21, Noonan syndrome, and Turner syndrome and in normal fetuses. The earlier hydrops or anasarca develops, the greater the risk for aneuploidy, and the worse the prognosis for that pregnancy. Early amniocentesis confirmed Turner syndrome.

2. The images demonstrate a small cystic hygroma and clinodactyly of the fifth digit, which are associated with Down syndrome (trisomy 21). Cystic hygroma is associated with other chromosomal abnormalities, and a detailed search for other markers or structural anomalies should be performed. The amniocentesis remains the "gold standard" for identifying which

chromosome abnormality is present because many of these markers and anomalies may be seen in more than one aneuploidy.

3. Omphalocele (see Fig. 24-16, *A*), EIF (see Fig. 24-16, *B*), holoprosencephaly (see Fig. 24-16, *C*), and facial abnormalities (see Fig. 24-16, *D*) in conjunction with polydactyly and early growth delay all are findings associated with trisomy 13. Fetuses with trisomy 13 have multiple midline defects, so a detailed examination must be performed. Also, note the unfused amnion and chorion shown in Figure 24-16, *E*, which is another marker for aneuploidy if seen beyond 15 weeks' gestational age.

4. The sandal gap toes and the atrioventricular defects are markers for Down syndrome (trisomy 21). Amniocentesis confirmed this diagnosis, and the fetus developed polyhydramnios in the third trimester secondary to duodenal atresia.

5. These images demonstrate micrognathia and rocker-bottom feet. The two chromosome abnormalities that have the highest association with these findings are trisomy 18 and trisomy 13. Both have CHDs, but trisomy 13 has a higher association with renal anomalies, polydactyly, and midline defects, whereas trisomy 18 has a slightly higher association with micrognathia. FISH analysis confirmed trisomy 18.

CHAPTER 25

1. What was not disclosed is that the patient has achondroplasia, which is the diagnosis for the fetus. Early measurements can be within normal limits. Although micromelia was noted, it is not the severe or extreme micromelia identified in lethal dwarfisms.

2. Echogenic fetal lung is identified with a flattened diaphragm consistent with congenital cystic adenomatoid malformation. The heart is malpositioned, and an echogenic intracardiac focus is seen. The patient will be monitored for regression of the lesion or the development of hydrops.

3. Extra digits were identified in the upper extremities consistent with polydactyly. Because of her age, the patient desired amniocentesis, which was within normal limits. This was an isolated case of polydactyly.

4. A monoventricle is identified; with the additional findings of multiple echogenic foci in the heart and bilateral cleft lip, holoprosencephaly can be diagnosed with a high suspicion of associated aneuploidy.

5. An enlarged cisterna magna is seen with splaying of the cerebellar hemispheres consistent with Dandy-Walker malformation. Amniocentesis was offered, but the patient declined.

CHAPTER 26

1. Atrioventricular septal defect (AVSD). An incomplete AVSD may result in a cleft mitral valve (the anterior part of the leaflet is divided into two parts, medial and lateral). When the leaflet closes, blood leaks through this hole into the left atrial cavity. The leaflet is usually malformed, causing further regurgitation into the atrium. A complete AVSD may have several variations in valve abnormalities. One of these variations has a single, undivided, free-floating atrioventricular leaflet stretching across both ventricles. The anterior and posterior leaflets are on both sides of the interventricular septum, causing the valve to override or straddle the septum. This is a more complex abnormality to repair because the defect is larger, and the single atrioventricular valve is more difficult to manage clinically, depending on the amount of regurgitation present.

2. Ebstein's anomaly affects the tricuspid valve. The septal leaflet has apical displacement; as a result, massive tricuspid regurgitation is present, causing the right atrial cavity to enlarge. If the regurgitation is severe in the early gestational period, the prognosis is poor. The sonographer should look for signs of cardiac failure, such as decreased contractility, pericardial effusion, and fetal hydrops.

3. Any break in the atrial septum in this view must be confirmed with the short-axis or perpendicular four-chamber view (subcostal view), in which the septum is more perpendicular to the transducer. The area of the foramen ovale is thinner than the surrounding atrial tissue; it is prone to signal dropout during sonographic evaluation, particularly in the apical four-chamber view when the transducer is parallel to the septum. Because of beam-width artifact, the edges of the defect may be slightly blunted and appear brighter than the remaining septum.

4. Muscular defects are usually very small and may be multiple in number. Often these smaller defects close spontaneously shortly after birth. The prognosis is good for a patient with a single ventricular septal defect. However, the association of other cardiac anomalies, such as tetralogy of Fallot, single ventricle, transposition of the great arteries, and endocardial cushion defect, is increased when a ventricular septal defect is found.

5. The underdeveloped left ventricle and aorta is compatible with hypoplastic left heart syndrome. The amount of hypoplasia would depend on when the left-sided atresia developed in the valvar area. Mitral valve atresia would cause the aortic valve to become atretic as well.

CHAPTER 27

1. Invasive ductal carcinoma without metastatic disease was diagnosed in this patient. She opted for bilateral mastectomies and underwent chemotherapy during pregnancy. She delivered a healthy baby girl and is 2 years cancer-free.

2. A juvenile fibroadenoma was diagnosed. The surgeon advised against surgical removal of the mass preferring the asymmetry to surgical scarring.

3. The radiologist obtained biopsy specimens of the lymph nodes even though they were thought to be enlarged because of the patient's HIV status. Both mass and nodes were positive for cancer cells.

4. Invasive ductal carcinoma was diagnosed, and the patient underwent a unilateral mastectomy. Coincidentally, his wife received a diagnosis of invasive ductal carcinoma after undergoing core biopsy in the same facility 1 month prior.

5. Invasive ductal carcinoma was diagnosed. After adjunct chemotherapy, the patient presented for a breast localization in the sonography department. The follow-up sonogram (see Fig. 27-32, *B*) shows a dramatic reduction in the size of the mass. Because of the reduced sonographic visibility, the localization procedure was moved to the mammography suite.

CHAPTER 28

1. The most likely diagnosis is germ cell tumor (seminoma) because the mass is solitary and hypoechoic, and microlithiasis is present.

2. The irregular contour of the testis capsule, the extratesticular soft tissue, and the history of trauma strongly suggest tunica rupture.

3. Partial torsion can cause venous congestion and edema resulting in the enlarged, hypoechoic sonographic appearance demonstrated in Figure 28-28, *A*. In this case, the action of the transducer during the examination resulted in detorsion of the testis and a return to normal perfusion.

4. Acute epididymo-orchitis, which is consistent with the hypervascularity demonstrated in the color Doppler image.

5. A large right-sided varicocele can be caused by extrinsic compression of the right testicular vein, and examination of the right upper quadrant revealed an occult lower pole renal cell carcinoma.

CHAPTER 29

1. Papillary thyroid cancer. Microcalcifications within a nodule or lymph node are highly specific to this diagnosis. Most papillary thyroid cancers are solid and hypoechoic.

2. Benign hyperplasic thyroid nodule. Thyroid nodules are very common. The mostly cystic and "spongiform" appearance is typical of benign disease.

3. Benign hyperplasic thyroid nodule. Benign nodules are mostly cystic, and uninterrupted rim calcification is also reported as a feature of benignity.

4. Parathyroid adenoma. Elevated serum calcium and parathyroid hormone are predictive of primary hyperparathyroidism. The mass is located in the region of a nonectopic gland.

5. Normal cervical lymph nodes

CHAPTER 30

1. Benign prostatic hyperplasia is likely in this patient given the history and clinical and sonographic findings.

2. Prostatitis can cause the "constant, deep, throbbing pain" as described by this patient. The irregular, cystic structure at the junction of the seminal vesicle and prostate coupled with an elevated white blood cell count would lead one to consider abscess.

3. Extremely elevated prostate-specific antigen in this elderly patient with these foreboding symptoms and the sonographic finding of a mass in the peripheral zone likely mean prostate cancer. The bone scan ordered by the physician was to check for metastasis.

4. A teardrop-shaped, midline, cystic mass represents an ejaculatory duct cyst.

5. These symptoms, laboratory results, and sonographic findings are classic for benign prostatic hyperplasia.

CHAPTER 31

1. This finding is consistent with physiologic laxity identified in the first few weeks of life. No treatment is necessary, but the infant should be followed at 4 to 6 weeks of age to confirm whether or not the laxity has resolved.

2. The left hip is normal, and the right hip is dislocatable. Because the right hip reduces with stress maneuvers, treatment with the Pavlik harness can be attempted. If that treatment fails, alternative methods will be required.

3. The right hip is normal with the hip sitting in the acetabulum with 59% coverage. The right hip is subluxable and appears shallow with 38% coverage of the femoral head. Additionally, the left hip was classified as Graf type II. Because the infant is 1 week old, this may be the result of physiologic laxity, and expectant management is appropriate.

4. The left hip would be classified as Graf type I, and the right hip would be classified as Graf type II.

5. Both of the hips are within normal limits, and no follow-up is necessary.

CHAPTER 32

1. There is herniation of the cerebellar tonsils into the cisterna magna; this would be associated with a possible Chiari II malformation and a meningomyelocele.

2. Partial agenesis of the corpus callosum. Sonographic findings include presence of the genu or anterior portion of the corpus callosum and a portion of the cavum septi pellucidi. The body and splenium of the corpus callosum are absent. There is radial arrangement of the sulci, also known as the "sunburst" sign. The coronal image shows widely spaced lateral ventricles.

3. Echogenic areas scattered throughout the brain parenchyma are consistent with infarction and global hypoxic-ischemic encephalopathy.

4. The finding of echogenic hemorrhage in the bodies of the lateral ventricles is consistent with a bilateral grade II hemorrhage.

5. This is a term infant. Note the presence of well-formed sulci and gyri.

CHAPTER 33

1. Common clinical indications for neonatal spinal sonography include atypical sacral dimple, palpable subcutaneous sacral mass, hair tuft, skin tag, hemangioma, sinus tract, skin pigmentation, and multiple congenital anomalies.

2. Hydromyelia is the abnormal widening of the central canal by cerebrospinal fluid. This condition may be either focal or diffuse, extending through the entire length of the spinal cord.

3. A tethered cord may be suspected when cutaneous markers such as skin tags and raised skin lesions are identified on visual inspection of an infant. As the infant grows, increasing tension is placed on the cord, leading to increasing neurologic dysfunction, although the infant may be asymptomatic until ambulation occurs. Left untreated, symptoms associated with tethering of the cord include leg weakness, abnormal gait, and posturing of the lower extremities.

4. Diastematomyelia is an incomplete or complete longitudinal split or cleft through the spinal cord. Sonographically, there appears to be two separate smaller spinal cords within the spinal canal. These hemicords are hypoechoic with an echogenic central canal similar to a normal spinal cord but smaller.

5. A spinal lipoma is an encapsulated deposit of fat, neural tissue, meninges, or fibrous tissue, which extends from the posterior subcutaneous tissue through a midline defect of the fascia, muscle, or bone to communicate with the spinal canal or meninges. Sonographically, a spinal lipoma appears as an echogenic mass extending from the spinal canal. Extension into the subcutaneous tissues maybe difficult to visualize with a sonogram, and complementary magnetic resonance imaging (MRI) may be beneficial.

CHAPTER 34

1. Based on the peak systolic velocity of 600 cm/s and end-diastolic velocity of 140 cm/s, this patient has 80% to 99% stenosis. The next step in treatment is a carotid endarterectomy or carotid angioplasty with stent placement.

2. The patient's symptoms resolved within 24 hours, which suggests a transient ischemic attack.

3. This patient is presenting with strokelike symptoms. The faster the patient receives stroke treatment, the better his chances for reducing long-term disability.

4. The patient has an 80% to 99% stenosis in the left common carotid artery, which most likely is the cause of his aphasia, confusion, and lack of coordination. The blindness was due to left vertebral artery occlusion. The patient's symptoms resolved after 24 hours, and he was given a diagnosis of reversible ischemic neurologic deficit. Because of the stenosis in the common carotid artery, the patient was taken to surgery for a carotid endarterectomy.

5. Echogenic material completely filling the lumen and lack of color and spectral Doppler suggest right internal carotid occlusion.

CHAPTER 35

1. The patient's complaint of leg pain is very nonspecific, but the red, swollen leg with "tough cords" should tip the sonographer that superficial thrombophlebitis would be most likely to be seen. Superficial vessels are close enough to the skin to be palpated. B-mode examination supports the diagnosis of superficial thrombophlebitis because echogenic matter was seen internally within the superficial vessel.

2. The symptoms of the patient are nonspecific, but she does have risk factors of a morbid increase in body habitus with a sedentary lifestyle. With the bluish cast to the leg, the sonographer is thinking that blood is being backed up into the leg, either by venous insufficiency, which would be more chronic in nature, or by an outflow obstruction that is pooling venous blood in the leg. The symptom that signals an emergency is the white toes. This means that blood flow to the toes is being constricted. Because venous insufficiency could not obstruct flow to the toes, it is more likely an outflow obstruction, such as phlegmasia cerulea dolens. The patient did not seek immediate help, and the deep vein thrombosis in the proximal portion of the leg aggravated the artery, causing it to vasospasm, occluding flow to the toes. This is diagnosed as phlegmasia alba dolens.

3. Because this patient is a noncompliant diabetic, he is at increased risk for a multitude of health problems, so this is nonspecific at this point. Also increasing the risk is hypertension and hyperlipidemia. The sonographic findings reveal that the veins are negative for deep vein thrombosis and superficial thrombophlebitis, so the most likely diagnosis for this patient would be neuropathy from the diabetes.

4. Lower extremity edema and shortness of breath can be caused by multiple medical issues, but the

clinician intends to rule out a pulmonary embolus because that is one of the more life-threatening conditions to cause this compilation of symptoms. Because most pulmonary emboli arise from the lower extremity, lower extremity venous Doppler is often the first examination used to evaluate this diagnosis indirectly. However, the lack of respiratory phasicity coupled with very pulsatile veins indicates this patient most likely has congestive heart failure.

5. This patient has multiple risk factors and is non-compliant with medical treatments because he is homeless. Sonographic findings suggest deep vein thrombosus in the femoral vein, extending down into the trifurcation area, which must be treated immediately to prevent a pulmonary embolus. Proximal compressions that could not halt blood flow indicate venous reflux also.

CHAPTER 36

1. Occlusion of the arterial bypass graft with refilling of the popliteal artery versus a large reversed branch (acting as a collateral)
2. Focal occlusion of the native femoral artery in the setting of ASO
3. Popliteal aneurysm with mural thrombus
4. Compartment syndrome
5. Arteriovenous fistula

CHAPTER 1

1. b
2. e
3. d
4. c
5. e
6. e
7. a
8. e
9. c
10. c

CHAPTER 2

1. a
2. c
3. d
4. b
5. e
6. d
7. d
8. d
9. b
10. c

CHAPTER 3

1. d
2. b
3. b
4. a
5. b
6. c
7. b
8. c
9. d
10. d

CHAPTER 4

1. c
2. d
3. c
4. c
5. d
6. c
7. d
8. c
9. b
10. a

CHAPTER 5

1. b
2. b
3. d
4. b
5. a
6. d
7. a
8. a
9. a
10. a

CHAPTER 6

1. a
2. b
3. c
4. b
5. c
6. b
7. c
8. a
9. d
10. b

CHAPTER 7

1. c
2. b
3. d
4. e
5. a
6. b
7. b
8. e
9. d
10. b

CHAPTER 8

1. d
2. b
3. c
4. b
5. d
6. a
7. c
8. b
9. c
10. c

CHAPTER 9

1. b
2. d
3. a
4. c
5. b
6. c
7. d
8. a
9. b
10. b

CHAPTER 10

1. a
2. d
3. a
4. c
5. b
6. d
7. a
8. a
9. c
10. b

CHAPTER 11

1. b
2. c
3. d
4. d
5. a
6. b
7. b
8. a
9. c
10. d

CHAPTER 12

1. d
2. b
3. c
4. d
5. b
6. a
7. d
8. c
9. c
10. a

CHAPTER 13

1. c
2. a

3. d
4. b
5. c
6. d
7. b
8. a
9. b
10. c

CHAPTER 14

1. b
2. e
3. e
4. b
5. d
6. a
7. b
8. a
9. a
10. d

CHAPTER 15

1. b
2. c
3. b
4. a
5. d
6. d
7. b
8. d
9. b
10. a

CHAPTER 16

1. c
2. a
3. d
4. c
5. b
6. a
7. a
8. b
9. d
10. c

CHAPTER 17

1. d
2. b
3. a
4. d
5. c
6. d

7. b
8. c
9. d
10. a

CHAPTER 18

1. d
2. d
3. a
4. a
5. c
6. b
7. c
8. c
9. d
10. b

CHAPTER 19

1. b
2. b
3. d
4. b
5. e
6. b
7. a
8. c
9. a
10. d

CHAPTER 20

1. d
2. a
3. c
4. a
5. d
6. c
7. a
8. b
9. c
10. b

CHAPTER 21

1. a
2. c
3. b
4. c
5. b
6. d
7. a
8. c
9. b
10. b

CHAPTER 22

1. a
2. d
3. d
4. c
5. b
6. a
7. c
8. d
9. b
10. a

CHAPTER 23

1. b
2. b
3. d
4. c
5. d
6. c
7. b
8. c
9. d
10. b

CHAPTER 24

1. a
2. c
3. d
4. b
5. a
6. c
7. b
8. d
9. a
10. b

CHAPTER 25

1. a
2. d
3. b
4. b
5. b
6. b
7. c
8. a
9. c
10. c

CHAPTER 26

1. b
2. b

3. a
4. c
5. a
6. c
7. a
8. c
9. d
10. d

CHAPTER 27

1. c
2. d
3. a
4. c
5. d
6. b
7. c
8. d
9. e
10. b

CHAPTER 28

1. d
2. c
3. d
4. b
5. a
6. b
7. c
8. c
9. d
10. a

CHAPTER 29

1. a
2. b
3. b
4. d
5. e
6. d
7. b
8. d
9. a
10. a

CHAPTER 30

1. b
2. d
3. b
4. c
5. e
6. e

7. c
8. a
9. a
10. e

CHAPTER 31

1. a
2. a
3. d
4. b
5. b
6. b
7. b
8. a
9. d
10. b

CHAPTER 32

1. c
2. a
3. d
4. b
5. d
6. d
7. c
8. a
9. c
10. a

CHAPTER 33

1. b
2. a
3. a
4. d
5. c
6. d
7. a
8. b
9. b
10. a

CHAPTER 34

1. a
2. d
3. b
4. b
5. d
6. e
7. b
8. a
9. d
10. b

CHAPTER 35

1. a
2. c
3. c
4. d
5. a
6. b
7. a
8. d
9. a
10. a

CHAPTER 36

1. a
2. d
3. b
4. b
5. a
6. c
7. b
8. b
9. c
10. d

ILLUSTRATION CREDITS

Callen P: Ultrasonography in Obstetrics and Gynecology, ed 5, St. Louis, 2008, Saunders.
Figures 14-7; 14-10; 14-13

Curry R: Sonography: Introduction to Normal Structure and Function, ed 3, St. Louis, 2011, Saunders.
Figure 4-3

Eisenberg R, Johnson N: Comprehensive Radiographic Pathology, ed 5, St. Louis, 2012, Mosby.
Figure 5-2

Hagen-Ansert S: Textbook of Diagnostic Sonography, ed 7, St. Louis, 2012, Mosby.
Figures 2-3 A&B; 5-14 A-C; 10-3; 13-2; 23-2 B; 23-3 A-C; 25-3 E&F; 25-21; 25-24 B&C; 25-29; 26-1; 26-2; 26-3; 26-4 A&B; 26-5 A&B; 26-7 A-D; 26-8 A&B; 26-9 A&B; 26-10; 26-11; 26-12; 26-13 A&B; 26-14 A-E; 26-15 A-C; 26-16 A-C; 26-17; 26-18 A-D; 26-19 A&B

Hagen-Ansert S: Textbook of Diagnostic Ultrasonography, ed 6, St. Louis, 2006, Mosby.
Figure 26-6 A&B

Hagen-Ansert S: Textbook of Diagnostic Ultrasonography, ed 5, St. Louis, 2007, Mosby.
Figures 1-25 A&B; 1-26 A-C; 4-4; 7-3 A; 11-22; 16-12; 19-3; 19-4; 19-6 A&B; 19-7 to 19-10; 21-5 C; 21-6; A; 22-8; 22-9; 23-5; 23-9; 23-10; 24-17 A; 25-2 A; 25-9; 25-12; 25-15; 25-23; 28-2

Kelley L, Petersen C: Sectional Anatomy for Imaging Professionals, ed 3, St. Louis, 2013, Mosby.
Figure 32-2

Ovel S: Sonography Exam Review: Physics, Abdomen, Obstetrics and Gynecology, ed 2, St. Louis, 2014, Mosby.
Figure 14-9 A

Rumack C: Diagnostic Ultrasound, ed 2, St. Louis, 1998, Mosby.
Figures 1-18; 1-19 B; 1-24; 7-4; 7-10; 8-6B; 8-10; 8-11; 9-2 A&B; 9-6 A-D; 22-10; 27-8; 31-7 B

Rumack C: Diagnostic Ultrasound, ed 4, St. Louis, 2011, Mosby.
Figure 12-13 A&B

Tempkin B: Ultrasound Scanning: Principles and Protocols, ed 3, St. Louis, 2010, Saunders.
Figure 35-3

A

Page numbers wed by *b*, *t* and *f* indicate boxes, tables and figures respectively.